Fundamentals of Fixed Prosthodontics

Fundamentals of Fixed Prosthodontics

Third Edition

Herbert T. Shillingburg, Jr, DDS

David Ross Boyd Professor and Chair
Department of Fixed Prosthodontics
University of Oklahoma College of Dentistry
Oklahoma City, Oklahoma

Sumiya Hobo, DDS, MSD, PhD

Director, International Dental Academy
Tokyo, Japan

Visiting Professor
Department of Fixed Prosthodontics
University of California, Los Angeles
School of Dentistry
Los Angeles, California

Lowell D. Whitsett, DDS

Professor Emeritus
Department of Occlusion
University of Oklahoma College of Dentistry
Oklahoma City, Oklahoma

Richard Jacobi, DDS

Professor
Department of Fixed Prosthodontics
University of Oklahoma College of Dentistry
Oklahoma City, Oklahoma

Susan E. Brackett, DDS, MS

Associate Professor
Department of Fixed Prosthodontics
University of Oklahoma College of Dentistry
Oklahoma City, Oklahoma

quintessence books

Quintessence Publishing Co, Inc

Chicago, Berlin, London, Tokyo, São Paulo, Moscow, Prague, and Warsaw

Library of Congress Cataloging-in-Publication Data

Fundamentals of fixed prosthodontics / Herbert T. Shillingburg, Jr.
... [et al.]. — 3rd ed.
            p.   cm.
      Rev. ed. of: Fundamentals of fixed prosthodontics / Herbert T.
Shillingburg, Jr., Sumiya Hobo, Lowell D. Whitsett. 2nd ed. 1981.
      Includes bibliographical references and index.
      ISBN 0-86715-201-X
      1. Prosthodontics. I. Shillingburg, Herbert T.
      [DNLM: 1. Denture, Partial, Fixed. 2. Prosthodontics—methods.
3. Dental Prosthesis Design. WU 515 F981 1996]
RK651.F86 1997
617.6'9—dc20
DNLM/DLC
for Library of Congress   96-24703
                                                         CIP

© 1997 by Quintessence Publishing Co, Inc

Quintessence Publishing Co, Inc
551 Kimberly Drive
Carol Stream, IL 60188-1881
www.quintpub.com

Editor: Lori A. Bateman
Production Manager: Timothy M. Robbins
Cover Design: Jennifer A. Sabella

Printed in Canada

Contents

Preface

Fixed prosthodontics is the art and science of restoring damaged teeth with cast metal, metal-ceramic, or all-ceramic restorations, and of replacing missing teeth with fixed prostheses. Successfully treating a patient by means of fixed prosthodontics requires a thoughtful combination of many aspects of dental treatment: patient education and the prevention of further dental disease, sound diagnosis, periodontal therapy, operative skills, occlusal considerations, and sometimes, placement of removable complete or partial prostheses and endodontic treatment.

Restorations in this field of dentistry can be the finest service rendered for dental patients, or the worst disservice perpetrated upon them. The path taken depends upon one's knowledge of sound biological and mechanical principles, the growth of manipulative skills to implement the treatment plan, and the development of a critical eye and judgment for assessing detail.

As in all fields of the healing arts in recent years, there has been tremendous change in this area of dentistry. Improved materials, instruments, and techniques have made it possible for today's operator of average skills to provide a service whose quality is on par with that produced only by the most gifted dentist of years gone by. This is possible, however, only if the dentist has a thorough background in the principles of restorative dentistry and an intimate knowledge of the techniques required.

This book was designed to serve as an introduction to the area of restorative dentistry dealing with fixed partial dentures and cast metal, metal-ceramic, and all-ceramic restorations. It should provide the background knowledge needed by the novice, as well as be a refresher for the practitioner or graduate student.

To provide the needed background for formulating rational judgments in the clinical environment, there are chapters dealing with the fundamentals of treatment planning, occlusion, and tooth preparation. In addition, sections of other chapters are devoted to the fundamentals of the respective subject. Specific techniques and instruments are discussed because dentists and dental students must deal with them in their daily work.

Alternative techniques are given when there are multiple techniques widely used in the profession. Frequently, however, only one technique is presented. Cognizance is given to the fact that there is usually more than one acceptable way of accomplishing a particular operation. However, in the limited time available in undergraduate dental training, there is usually time for the mastery of only one basic technique for accomplishing each of the various types of treatment.

An attempt has been made to provide a sound working background in the various facets of fixed prosthodontic therapy. Current information has been added to cover the increasing use of new cements, new packaging and techniques for the use of impression materials, and changes in the management of soft tissues for impression making. New articulators, facebows, and concepts of occlusion needed attention, along with precise ways of making removable dies. The increased usage of periodontally weakened teeth required some tips on handling teeth with exposed root morphology or molars that have lost a root.

Different ways of handling edentulous ridges with defects have given the dentist better control of the functional and esthetic outcome; no longer must metal or ceramics be relied on to somehow mask the loss of bone and soft tissue. The pages devoted to the technique for fabricating gold pontics with cemented, customized, prefabricated porcelain facings have been deleted.

The increased emphasis on esthetic restorations has necessitated expanding the subject of all-ceramic and metal-ceramic restorations from one chapter to three chapters. A chapter has been added to cover resin-bonded fixed partial dentures, a treatment modality whose strengths and shortcomings we are coming to recognize. Changes are based on recent research and on the experiences of the authors and their associates in the treatment of patients and the teaching of students.

Updated references are used to document the rationale for using materials and techniques and to familiarize the student with the literature in the various aspects of fixed prosthodontics. If more background information on specific topics is desired, several books are recommended:

For a detailed treatment of the subject of dental materials, refer to Dr Kenneth Anusavice's book, *Phillips' Science* of *Dental Materials.* For an in-depth study of occlusion, see Dr Peter Dawson's *Evaluation, Diagnosis, and Treatment of Occlusal Problems* (2nd ed) or Dr Jeffrey P. Okeson's *Management of Temporomandibular Disorders and Occlusion* (3rd ed). The topic of tooth preparations is discussed in greater detail in *Fundamentals of Tooth Preparations* by Shillingburg, Jacobi, and Brackett. For detailed coverage of occlusal morphology used in waxing restorations, consult *Guide to Occlusal Waxing* by Shillingburg, Wilson, and Morrison. A wealth of information concerning both the fabrication of porcelain restorations and the materials aspect of porcelain can be found in Dr John McLean's excellent works, *The Science and Art of Dental Ceramics, Volumes I and II;* in *Metal Ceramics—Principles and Methods of Makoto Yamamoto;* and in *Introduction to Metal Ceramic Technology* by Dr W. Patrick Naylor.

Two fine restorative dentists had an important influence on this book. Dr Robert Dewhirst and Dr Donald Fisher have been teachers, colleagues, and most important, friends. Many of their philosophies have steered us through the past 25 years. *The UCLA Fixed Prosthodontics Syllabus,* authored and edited by Dr Fisher and coauthored by Drs Dewhirst and Shillingburg in 1968, was the foundation upon which the first edition of this book was based in 1976.

Acknowledgments

No book is the work of just its authors. It helps immeasurably to be backed by the encouragement of your superiors. Dr Donald A. Welk, chair of restorative dentistry, has supported this project by his interest and his counsel. Dr Russell J. Stratton, dean of the University of Oklahoma College of Dentistry, and his predecessor, Dr William E. Brown, the founding dean, have always been most supportive of this undertaking.

It is difficult to say which ideas are our own and which are an amalgam of the ideas of those with whom we associate. Dr Manville G. Duncanson, Jr, chair of dental materials; Dr Dean Johnson, retired chair of removable prosthodontics; Dr James Roane, former chair of endodontics; and Dr Clyde Sabala, present chair of endodontics, have been forthcoming through the years with their suggestions, criticism, and shared knowledge.

Dr Arthur Vernino, former director of the graduate periodontics program, has helped to expand our horizons regarding the interactions between periodontics and restorative dentistry. He was especially helpful with the section on periodontal surgery.

Special acknowledgment is made to Ms Julie Hall for her typing. Illustrations were produced by Mr Robert Shackleford, Ms Laurel Kallenberger, Ms Jane Cripps, and Ms Judy Amico of the Graphics and Media Department of the University of Oklahoma Health Sciences Center. Artwork was also contributed by the authors, Drs Richard Jacobi and Herbert Shillingburg.

Dedicated to

Connie
Eleanor
Ann
Gregg Wadley

Chapter 1

An Introduction to Fixed Prosthodontics

The scope of fixed prosthodontic treatment can range from the restoration of a single tooth to the rehabilitation of the entire occlusion. Single teeth can be restored to full function, and improvement in cosmetic effect can be achieved. Missing teeth can be replaced with fixed prostheses that will improve patient comfort and masticatory ability, maintain the health and integrity of the dental arches, and, in many instances, elevate the patient's self-image.

It is also possible, by the use of fixed restorations, to render supportive and long-range corrective measures for the treatment of problems related to the temporomandibular joint and its neuromuscular components. On the other hand, with improper treatment of the occlusion, it is possible to create disharmony and damage to the stomatognathic system.

Terminology

A *crown* is a cemented extracoronal restoration that covers, or veneers, the outer surface of the clinical crown. It should reproduce the morphology and contours of the damaged coronal portions of a tooth while performing its function. It should also protect the remaining tooth structure from further damage.

If it covers all of the clinical crown, the restoration is a *full* or *complete veneer crown* (Fig 1-1). It may be fabricated entirely of a gold alloy or some other untarnishable metal, a ceramic veneer fused to metal, an all-ceramic material, resin and metal, or resin only. If only portions of the clinical crown are veneered, the restoration is called a *partial veneer crown* (Fig 1-2).

Intracoronal cast restorations are those that fit within the anatomic contours of the clinical crown of a tooth. *Inlays* may be used as single-tooth restorations for proximo-occlusal or gingival lesions with minimal to moderate extensions. They may be made of gold alloy (Fig 1-3, A) or a ceramic material (Fig 1-3, B). When modified with an occlusal veneer, the intracoronal restoration is called an *onlay* and is useful for restoring more extensively damaged posterior teeth needing wide mesio-occluso-distal restorations (Fig 1-4).

Another type of cemented restoration has gained considerable popularity in the past 10 years. The all-ceramic *laminate veneer*, or facial veneer (Fig 1-5), is used in situations requiring an improved cosmetic appearance on an anterior tooth that is otherwise sound. It consists of a thin layer of dental porcelain or cast ceramic that is bonded to the facial surface of the tooth with an appropriate resin.

The *fixed partial denture* is a prosthetic appliance, permanently attached to remaining teeth, which replaces one or more missing teeth (Fig 1-6). Although the term is preferred by prosthodontists, this type of restoration has long been called a *bridge*. "Bridge" is still in common enough usage that in the most recent listing of ADA insurance codes and nomenclature (1991), components of this restoration are catalogued under "bridge," and the term "fixed partial denture" does not appear in the list.[1] A tooth serving as an attachment for a fixed partial denture is called an *abutment*. The artificial tooth suspended from the abutment teeth is a *pontic*. The pontic is connected to the fixed partial denture *retainers*, which are extracoronal restorations that are cemented to the prepared abutment teeth. Intracoronal restorations lack the necessary retention and resistance to be utilized as fixed partial denture retainers. The *connectors* between the pontic and the retainer may be rigid (ie, solder joints or cast connectors) or nonrigid (ie, precision attachments or stress breakers).

Diagnosis

A thorough diagnosis must first be made of the patient's dental condition, considering both hard and soft tissues. This must be correlated with the individual's overall physical health and psychological needs. Using the diagnostic information that has been gathered, it is then possible to formulate a treatment plan based upon the patient's dental needs, mitigated to a variable degree by his or

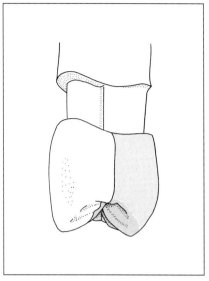

Fig 1-1 A full veneer crown covers all of the clinical crown of a tooth. The example is of a metal-ceramic crown.

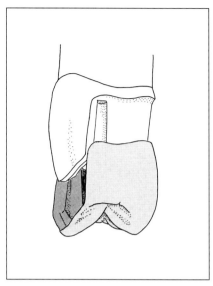

Fig 1-2 A partial veneer crown covers only portions of the clinical crown. The facial surface is usually left unveneered.

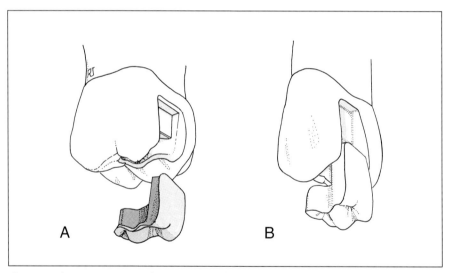

Fig 1-3 Inlays are intracoronal restorations with minimal to moderate extensions made of gold alloy (A) or a ceramic material (B).

her medical, psychological, and personal circumstances.

There are five elements to a good diagnostic workup in preparation for fixed prosthodontic treatment:

1. History
2. TMJ/occlusal evaluation
3. Intraoral examination
4. Diagnostic casts
5. Full mouth radiographs

History

It is important that a good history be taken before the initiation of treatment to determine if any special precautions are necessary. Some elective treatment might be eliminated or postponed because of the patient's physical or emotional health. It may be necessary to premedicate some patients for certain conditions or to avoid medication for others.

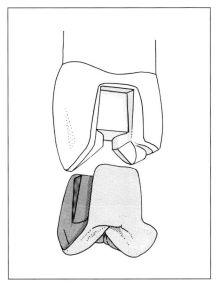

Fig 1-4 An onlay is an intracoronal restoration with an occlusal veneer.

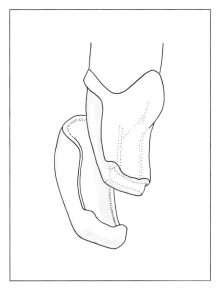

Fig 1-5 A laminate veneer is a thin layer of porcelain or cast ceramic that is bonded to the facial surface of a tooth with resin.

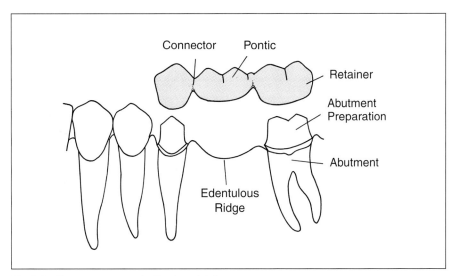

Fig 1-6 The components of a fixed partial denture.

It is not within the scope of this book to describe all the conditions that might influence patient treatment. However, there are some which occur frequently enough or pose a great enough threat to the patient's or dentist's well-being that they merit discussion. A history of infectious diseases such as serum hepatitis and acquired immunodeficiency syndrome must be known so that protection can be provided for other patients as well as office personnel.

There are numerous conditions of a noninfectious nature that also can be important to the patient's well-being. If a patient reports a previous reaction to a drug, it should be determined whether it was an allergic reaction or syncope resulting from anxiety in the dental chair. If there is any possibility of a true allergic reaction, a notation should be made on a sticker prominently displayed on the outside of the patient's record, so that the offending medication will never be administered or prescribed. Local anesthetics and antibiotics are the most common offenders.

The patient might also report a reaction to a dental material. Impression materials and nickel-containing alloys are leading candidates in this area. Do not engage in any "do-it-yourself" allergy testing to corroborate the patient's recollection of previous problems. It is possible to initiate a life-threatening anaphylactic reaction if you challenge the patient's immune system with an allergen to which he or she has been previously sensitized.

The patient should be asked about medication currently being taken. All medications should be identified and their contraindications noted before proceeding with treatment. Question the patient about current medications at each subsequent appointment so that you will have up-to-date information on the medication regimen.

Patients who present with a history of cardiovascular problems may require special treatment. No patient with uncontrolled hypertension should be treated until the blood pressure has been lowered. Generally, a systolic reading above 160 mm of mercury or a diastolic reading above 95 preempts dental treatment and should be cause for referring the patient to his or her physician for evaluation and treatment.[2] Patients with a history of hypertension or coronary artery disease should not receive epinephrine, since this drug has a tendency both to increase heart rate and elevate blood pressure.

An individual with a prosthetic heart valve, a history of previous bacterial endocarditis, rheumatic fever with valvular dysfunction, most congenital heart malformations,[3,4] or mitral valve prolapse with valvular regurgitation[3-5] should be premedicated with amoxicillin or, in the case of allergy, erythromycin or clindamycin following the 1991 guidelines set by the American Heart Association.[3,4] Alternative regimens with other antibiotics administered by injection could be required. Patients with cardiac pacemakers[3,4] or prosthetic joints[6] probably will not require prophylaxis. It is best to check with the patient's physician if there is any question whether prophylactic antibiotics should be employed at all, or if an alternative antibiotic regimen should be utilized.

A patient who is on an antibiotic regimen prescribed to prevent the recurrence of rheumatic fever is *not* adequately premedicated to prevent bacterial endocarditis.[3,4] Tetracyclines and sulfonamides are also *not* recommended.[3,4]

Many patients with prosthetic heart valves are on Coumadin, an anticoagulant. These patients' physicians should be consulted before beginning any procedures that will cause even minor bleeding.

Epilepsy is another condition whose existence should be known. It does not contraindicate dentistry, but the dentist should know of its history in a patient so that appropriate measures can be taken without delay in the event of a seizure while the patient is in the chair. Steps should also be taken to control anxiety in these patients. Long, fatiguing appointments should be avoided to minimize the possibility of precipitating a seizure.

Diabetic patients are predisposed to periodontal breakdown or abscess formation.[7] A well-controlled diabetic may receive routine dental treatment. Those who are poorly controlled, tending toward elevated blood sugar, or hyperglycemia, could be adversely affected by the stress of a dental appointment to the point of falling into a diabetic coma.

Hypoglycemia can also cause problems. A controlled diabetic (on medication) who has missed a meal or has not eaten for several hours may suddenly feel light-headed and appear intoxicated. These patients usually carry some quick source of sucrose, such as candy, which should be administered. For this reason, dental treatment for the diabetic should interfere as little as possible with the patient's dietary routine, and the patient's stress level should be reduced. Any questions about the patient's ability to cope with dental treatment, and whether he or she is properly controlled, should be referred to a physician before proceeding.

The prolonged presence of xerostomia, or dry mouth, is conducive to greater carious activity and is therefore extremely hostile to the margins of cast metal or ceramic restorations. Patients who have had large doses of radiation in the oral region may have drastically diminished salivary flow.[8] It can also occur as a component of Sjogren's syndrome, an autoimmune, collagen disease.[9] It is frequently seen in conjunction with other autoimmune diseases, such as rheumatoid arthritis, lupus erythematosus, and scleroderma.[10]

There are also some 375 drugs capable of producing mild to severe xerostomia.[11] Anticholinergics, anorectics, and antihypertensives may produce this effect. Antihistamines comprise the largest group of such drugs, and chronic allergy sufferers who use them over a prolonged time may suffer from a dry mouth.

The patient should be given an opportunity to describe the exact nature of the complaint that has brought him or her to the dental office for treatment. Attitudes about previous treatment and the dentists who have rendered it offer an insight into the patient's level of dental awareness and the quality of care expected. This will help the dentist to determine how much education the patient will require and how amenable the patient will be to cooperating with a good home-care program.

An effort should be made to get an accurate description of the patient's expectations of the treatment results. Particular attention should be paid to the cosmetic effect anticipated. A judgment must be made as to whether the patient's desires are compatible with sound restorative procedures. Possible conflicts in this area, as well as in the realm of personality, should be noted. The option of not providing care may need to be exercised with some patients.

TMJ/Occlusal Evaluation

Prior to the start of fixed prosthodontic procedures, the patient's occlusion must be evaluated to determine if it is

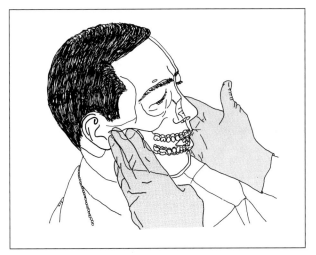

Fig 1-7 The joints are palpated as the patient opens and closes to detect signs of dysfunction.

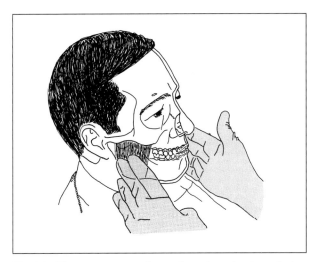

Fig 1-8 The masseter muscle can be palpated extraorally by placing your fingers over the lateral surfaces of the ramus of the mandible.

healthy enough to allow the fabrication of such restorations. If the occlusion is within normal limits, then all treatment should be designed to maintain that occlusal relationship. However, if the occlusion is dysfunctional in some manner, further appraisal is necessary to determine whether the occlusion can be improved prior to the placement of the restorations or whether the restorations can be employed in the correction of the occlusal problem.

Does the patient suffer from frequent occasions of head, neck, or shoulder pain? If so, an attempt must be made to determine the origin of such pain. Many patients suffer from undiagnosed muscle and/or joint dysfunction of the head and neck region, and such a history that has not been adequately diagnosed should be investigated further.

Next is an assessment of the temporomandibular joints themselves. Healthy temporomandibular joints function quietly with no evidence of clicking, crepitation, or limitation of movement on opening, closing, or moving laterally. Palpation of the joints as the patient opens and closes should reveal the existence of any signs of dysfunction (Fig 1-7). Many patients suffer from muscle pain as a result of parafunctional jaw activity related to stress or sensitivity to faults in their occlusion. Habits such as clenching the teeth and "playing with the bite" during the course of the daily routine may result in fatigue and muscle spasm. Observe the physical appearance and activities of this type of patient. Many times they will have a square-jowled appearance, with masseter muscles that are overdeveloped from hyperactivity. They may be clenching their teeth even as they converse with you.

A brief palpation of the masseter (Fig 1-8), temporalis (Fig 1-9), medial pterygoid (Fig 1-10), lateral pterygoid (Fig 1-11), trapezius (Fig 1-12), and sternocleidomastoid

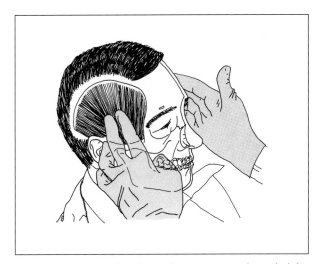

Fig 1-9 Fingers are placed over the patient's temples to feel the temporalis muscle.

(Fig 1-13) muscles may reveal tenderness. The patient may demonstrate limited opening due to spasm of the masseter and/or temporal muscles. This can be noted by asking the patient to open "all the way" (Fig 1-14). If it appears that the opening is limited, ask the patient to use a finger to indicate the area that hurts. If the patient touches a muscle area, as opposed to the temporomandibular joint, there is probably some dysfunction of the neuromuscular system (Fig 1-15).

Evidence of pain or dysfunction in either the temporomandibular joints or the muscles associated with the head and neck region is an indication for further evaluation prior to starting any fixed prosthodontic procedures.

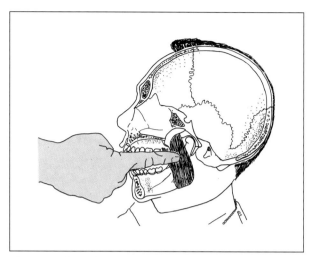

Fig 1-10 The index finger is used to touch the medial pterygoid muscle on the inner surface of the ramus.

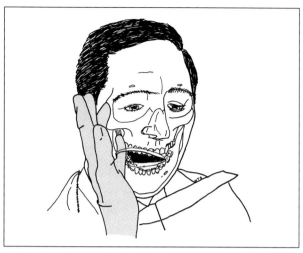

Fig 1-11 The little finger is inserted facial to the maxillary teeth and around distal to the pterygomaxillary, or hamular, notch to palpate the lateral pterygoid muscle.

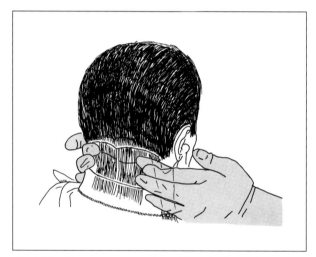

Fig 1-12 The trapezius muscle is felt at the base of the skull, high on the neck.

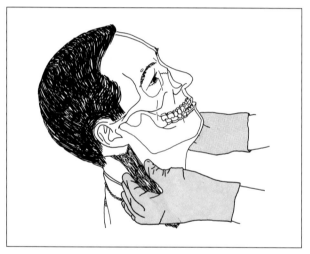

Fig 1-13 The sternocleidomastoid muscle is grasped between the thumb and forefingers on the side of the neck. The muscle can be accentuated by a slight turn of the patient's head.

Intraoral Examination

When the patient's mouth is examined, there are several observations to be made. The first of these is the patient's general oral hygiene. How much plaque can be found on the teeth, and in what areas? What is the general periodontal condition?

Check for a band of attached gingiva around all teeth, particularly around teeth to be restored with crowns. Mandibular third molars frequently do not have attached gingiva around the distal segment (30% to 60%). A prospective abutment that lacks the necessary attached

tissue is a very poor candidate to receive a crown. The prospects of chronic inflammation occurring in response to any minute marginal irregularity in the crown are quite high.

The presence or absence of inflammation should be noted along with gingival architecture and stippling. The existence of pockets should be entered in the record and their location and depth charted. The presence and amount of tooth mobility should also be recorded, with special attention paid to any relationship with occlusal prematurities and to potential abutment teeth.

Examine edentulous ridges and note the relationship

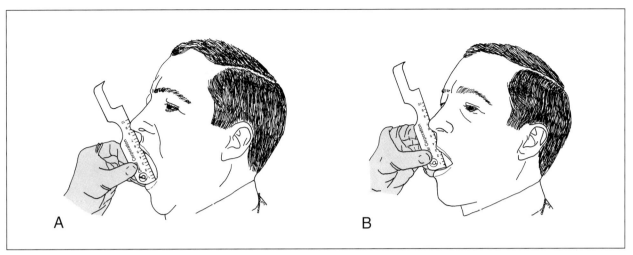

Fig 1-14 The distance between maxillary and mandibular incisors is measured when the patient is instructed to open "all the way" (A). If the patient can only open part way (B), the cause should be determined.

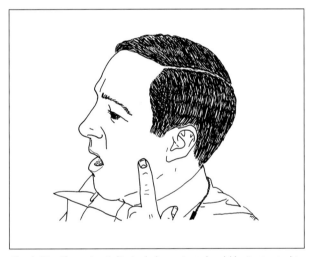

Fig 1-15 If opening is limited, the patient should be instructed to use a finger to indicate the area that hurts.

of spaces if there are more than one. What is the condition of prospective abutment teeth? Note the presence and location of caries. Is it localized or widespread? Are there large numbers of gingival lesions and decalcification areas? The amount and location of caries, coupled with an evaluation of plaque retention, can offer some prognosis for new restorations that will be placed. It will also help to determine the preparation designs to be used.

Previous restorations and prostheses should be examined carefully. This will make it possible to determine their present suitability or their need to be replaced. It will also offer some prognosis for future work to be done.

Finally, an evaluation should be made of the occlusion. Are there large facets of wear? Are they localized or widespread? Are there any nonworking interferences? The amount of slide between the retruded position and the position of maximum intercuspation should be noted. Is the slide a straight one, or does the mandible deviate to one side or the other? The presence or absence of simultaneous contact on both sides of the mouth should be observed. The existence and amount of anterior guidance is also important. Restorations of anterior teeth must duplicate existing guidance or, in some patients, replace that which has been lost through wear or trauma.

Diagnostic Casts

Diagnostic casts are an integral part of the diagnostic procedures necessary to give the dentist as complete a perspective as possible of the patient's dental needs. To accomplish their intended goal, they must be accurate reproductions of the maxillary and mandibular arches, made from distortion-free alginate impressions. The casts should contain no bubbles as a result of faulty pouring, nor positive nodules on the occlusal surfaces ensuing from air entrapment during the making of the impression.

To gain the most from the diagnostic casts, they should be mounted on a semiadjustable articulator. When they have been positioned with a facebow and the articulator adjustments have been set by the use of lateral interocclusal records, or check bites, a reasonably accurate simulation of jaw movements will be possible. The articulator settings should be included in the patient's permanent record to facilitate resetting the instrument when restorations are fabricated for this patient at some future date. Finally, the mandibular cast should be set in a relationship determined by the patient's optimum condylar position (with the disc interposed) to better enable a critical occlusal analysis.

Articulated diagnostic casts can provide a great deal of information for diagnosing problems and arriving at a treatment plan. They allow an unobstructed view of the edentulous spaces and an accurate assessment of the span length, as well as the occlusogingival dimension. The curvature of the arch in the edentulous region can be determined, so that it will be possible to predict whether the pontic(s) will act as a lever arm on the abutment teeth.

The length of abutment teeth can be accurately gauged to determine which preparation designs will provide adequate retention and resistance. The true inclination of the abutment teeth will also become evident, so that problems in a common path of insertion can be anticipated. Mesiodistal drifting, rotation, and faciolingual displacement of prospective abutment teeth can also be clearly seen.

A further analysis of the occlusion can be conducted using the diagnostic casts. A thorough evaluation of wear facets—their numbers, size, and location—is possible when they are viewed on casts. Occlusal discrepancies can be evaluated and the presence of centric prematurities or excursive interferences determined. Discrepancies in the occlusal plane become very apparent on the articulated casts. Teeth that have supererupted into opposing edentulous spaces are easily spotted, and the amount of correction needed can be determined.

Situations calling for the use of pontics which are wider or narrower than the teeth that would normally occupy the edentulous space call for a diagnostic wax-up. Changes in contour plus widening or narrowing of an abutment tooth can also be tried and evaluated on a duplicate of the original cast. This enables the dentist and the patient to see how a difficult treatment will look when finished. The diagnostic wax-up, done in ivory wax, allows the patient to see all of the compromises that will be necessary.

It is far better to discover that the projected result is unsatisfactory to the patient before treatment is begun. If the patient is satisfied and the work proceeds, the wax-up will help the dentist plan and execute the preparations and the provisional, or temporary, restorations.

Full-Mouth Radiographs

Radiographs, the final aspect of the diagnostic procedure, provide the dentist with information to help correlate all of the facts that have been collected in listening to the patient, examining the mouth, and evaluating the diagnostic casts. The radiographs should be examined carefully for signs of caries, both on unrestored proximal surfaces and recurring around previous restorations. The

presence of periapical lesions, as well as the existence and quality of previous endodontic treatments, should be noted.

General alveolar bone levels, with particular emphasis on prospective abutment teeth, should be observed. The crown-root ratio of abutment teeth can be calculated. The length, configuration, and direction of those roots should also be examined. Any widening of the periodontal membrane should be correlated with occlusal prematurities or occlusal trauma. An evaluation can be made of the thickness of the cortical plate of bone around the teeth and of the trabeculation of the bone.

The presence of retained root tips or other pathosis in the edentulous areas should be recorded. On many radiographs it is possible to trace the outline of the soft tissue in edentulous areas so that the thickness of the soft tissue overlying the ridge can be determined.

Protection Against Infectious Diseases

Protecting against cross-contamination of patients and preventing exposure of office staff to infectious diseases have become major concerns in dentistry in recent years. In particular, patients should be queried about a past history of either serum hepatitis (hepatitis B virus, or HBV) or human immunodeficiency virus (HIV). Although AIDS has received the greatest publicity and has generated near hysteria, HBV is the major infectious occupational hazard to health-care professionals.[12]

There is no evidence that either disease is contracted by casual contact with an infected person. However, the nature of dental procedures does produce the risk of contact with blood and tissues. A safe, effective vaccine against hepatitis B is available and is recommended by the Centers for Disease Control[13,14] and the ADA Council on Dental Therapeutics[15] for all dental personnel who have contact with patients.

While special precautions should be observed when treating patients with a history of either disease, *every* patient should be treated as being potentially infectious. Rubber gloves, a surgical mask or full-length plastic face shield, protective eyeglasses (if a shield is not used), and a protective uniform are recommended for the dentist and all other office personnel who will be in contact with the patient during actual treatment (Fig 1-16).

Concern for these matters does not end at the door to the operatory. Any item contaminated with blood or saliva in the operatory, such as an impression, is just as contaminated when it is touched outside the operatory. The days of casually munching on Doritos while waxing and handling a cast recently extracted from a bloody impression are a thing of the past. The specifics of decontaminating impressions will be covered in Chapter 17.

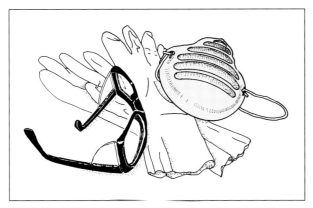

Fig 1-16 Rubber gloves, a surgical mask, and eye protection are important for safeguarding dental office personnel.

Steps must be taken in a receiving area of the laboratory to isolate and decontaminate items coming from the dental operatory.[15] An infection-control program should be established to protect laboratory personnel from infectious diseases, as well as to prevent cross-contamination that could affect a patient when an appliance returns from the laboratory to the operatory for insertion in the patient's mouth.[16] There is more to dental laboratory work than manipulating inert gypsum, wax, resins, metal, and ceramics.

References

1. Council on Dental Care Programs: Code on dental procedures and nomenclature. *J Am Dent Assoc* 1991; 122(3): 91–97.

2. Malamed SF: Blood pressure evaluation and the prevention of medical emergencies in dental practice. *J Prev Dent* 1980; 6:183–198.

3. Dajani AS, Bisno AL, Chung KJ, et al: Prevention of bacterial endocarditis—Recommendations by the American Heart Association. *JAMA* 1990; 264:2919–2922.

4. Council on Dental Therapeutics, American Heart Association: Preventing bacterial endocarditis—A statement for the dental professional. *J Am Dent Assoc* 1991; 122:87–92.

5. Brackett SE: Infective endocarditis and mitral valve prolapse—The unsuspected risk. *Oral Surg Oral Med Oral Pathol* 1982; 54:273–276.

6. Council on Dental Therapeutics: Management of dental patients with prosthetic joints. *J Am Dent Assoc* 1990; 121:537–538.

7. Schlossman M, Knowler WC, Pettit DJ, Genco RJ: Type 2 diabetes mellitus and periodontal disease. *J Am Dent Assoc* 1990; 121:532–536.

8. Frank RM, Herdly J, Phillipe E: Acquired dental defects and salivary gland lesions after irradiation for carcinoma. *J Am Dent Assoc* 1965; 70:868–883.

9. Bertram U: Xerostomia—Clinical aspects, pathology and pathogenesis. *Acta Odontol Scand* 1967; 25 (suppl 49):1–126.

10. Daniels T, Silverman S, Michalski JP, Greenspan JS, Silvester RA, Talal N: The oral components of Sjogren's syndrome. *Oral Surg Oral Med Oral Pathol* 1975; 39:875–885.

11. Sreebny LM, Schwartz SS: A reference guide to drugs and dry mouths. *Gerodontology* 1986; 5:75–98.

12. *Joint Advisory Notice. Protection Against Occupational Exposure to Hepatitis B Virus (HBV) and Human Immunodeficiency Virus (HIV)*. Washington, DC, US Department of Labor, US Department of Health and Human Services, Oct 19, 1987.

13. Centers for Disease Control: Hepatitis B virus vaccine safety—Report of an inter-agency group. *Morbidity and Mortality Weekly Report* 1982; 31:465–467.

14. Centers for Disease Control: The safety of hepatitis B virus vaccine. *Morbidity and Mortality Weekly Report* 1983; 32: 134–136.

15. Council on Dental Materials, Instruments and Equipment; Council on Dental Practice; Council on Dental Therapeutics: Infection control recommendations for the dental office and the dental laboratory. *J Am Dent Assoc* 1988; 116:241–248.

16. National Board for Certification of Dental Laboratories: *Infection Control Requirements for Certified Dental Laboratories*. Alexandria, VA, National Association of Dental Laboratories, 1986.

Chapter 2

Fundamentals of Occlusion

Unfortunately, the occlusion of teeth is frequently overlooked or taken for granted in providing restorative dental treatment for patients. This may be due in part to the fact that the symptoms of occlusal disease are often hidden from the practitioner not trained to recognize them or to appreciate their significance. The long-term successful restoration of a mouth with cast metal or ceramic restorations is dependent upon the maintenance of occlusal harmony.

While it is not possible to present the philosophies and techniques required to render extensive occlusal reconstruction in this limited space, it is essential that the reader develop an appreciation for the importance of occlusion. The perfection of skills required to provide sophisticated treatment of complex occlusal problems may take years to acquire. However, the minimum expectation of the competent practitioner is the ability to diagnose and treat simple occlusal disharmonies. He or she also must be able to produce restorations that will avoid the creation of iatrogenic occlusal disease.

Centric Relation

In restorative treatment, the goal is to create occlusal contacts in posterior teeth that stabilize, instead of creating deflective contacts that may destabilize, the mandibular position. The occlusion in a restoration should be made in harmony with the optimum condylar position, *centric relation*: an anteriorly, superiorly braced position along the articular eminence of the glenoid fossa, with the articular disc interposed between the condyle and eminence.[1]

This position of the condyles in the glenoid fossae has been discussed and debated for years. It is used in dentistry as a repeatable reference position for mounting casts in an articulator.[2,3] The term attempts to define the optimum relative position between all of the anatomic components. Ideally, that condylar position is also coincident with maximum intercuspation of the teeth.[4]

For the concept of centric relation to be meaningful, the basic anatomy of the temporomandibular joint must be understood (Fig 2-1). The bone of the glenoid fossa is

thin in its most superior aspect and is not suited to be a stress-bearing area. However, the slope of the eminence in the anterior aspect of the fossa is composed of thick cortical bone that is capable of bearing stress.

The articular disc is biconcave, is devoid of nerves and blood vessels in the central area, and is tough—much like a piece of shoe leather. It has a few muscle fibers attached in the anterior aspect from the superior head of the lateral pterygoid muscle. The disc is attached to the condyle on its medial and lateral aspects and should be interposed between the condyle and articular eminence as function occurs. The condyle is not spherical, but has an irregular, elliptical shape. This shape helps to distribute stress throughout the temporomandibular joint rather than concentrating it in a small area.

Many methods have been used to guide the mandible into an "ideal" position. Earlier concepts of centric relation involved the most posterior condylar position in the fossa. The condyle was sometimes forcefully manipulated into the rearmost, uppermost, and midmost position within the glenoid fossa, called the *"RUM"* position,[3,5–7] using chinpoint guidance. However, when the condyle is retruded, it may not be seated onto the central area of the articular disc. Instead it may be on the highly vascular and innervated retrodiscal tissues (the *bilaminar zone*) posterior to the disc (Fig 2-2).[8] This can occur if the horizontal fibers of the temporomandibular ligament have been unduly traumatized so that they no longer support the condyle in a more anterior, physiologic position. It is presently thought that rather than being a physiologic position, it is frequently an abnormal, forced position, which could create unnecessary strain in the temporomandibular joint. In this circumstance, the disc is displaced anteriorly, and clicking of the joint is frequently observed as the patient opens and closes.

The more recent concept describes a physiologic position regarding musculoskeletal relationships of the structures[9] (Fig 2-3). It is not a forced position, but is gently guided by the operator using the bilateral method[10] or by allowing natural muscle action to place the condyle in a physiologically unstrained position.[11]

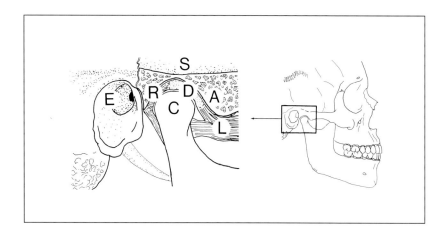

Fig 2-1 Some of the components of the temporomandibular joint are A, articular eminence; C, condyle; D, articular disc; E, external auditory meatus; L, lateral pterygoid muscle; R, retrodiscal tissue (bilaminar zone); S, thin superior wall of the glenoid fossa.

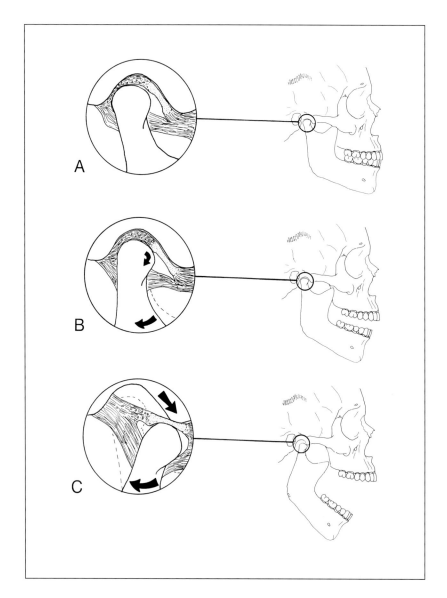

Fig 2-2 In a dysfunctional joint with an internal derangement, the condyle is displaced posterior to the disc at the intercuspal position (A). After initial rotational opening, the condyle is still posterior to the disc (B). In translation of the mandible to maximum opening, the condyle recaptures the disc, clicking into position as it does (C).

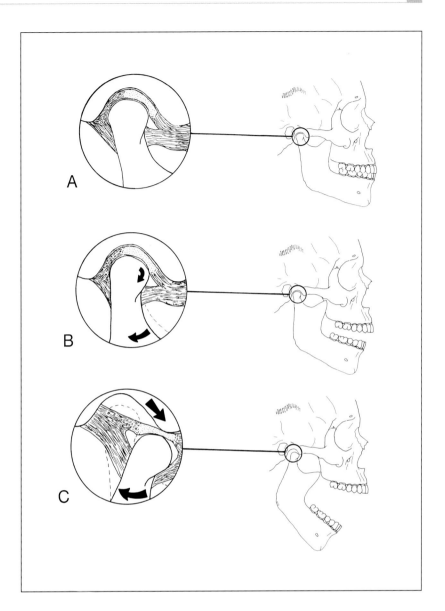

Fig 2-3 In a healthy joint, the condyle is in a superoanterior position in the fossa with the articular disc interposed when the teeth are in maximum intercuspation (A). In the initial stage of opening, the condyle rotates in position, with the disc remaining stationary (B). In maximum opening, the condyle translates forward, with the disc still interposed (C).

Mandibular Movement

Mandibular movement can be broken down into a series of motions that occur around three axes:

1. *Horizontal axis* (Fig 2-4). This movement, in the sagittal plane, happens when the mandible in centric relation makes a purely rotational opening and closing border movement around the *transverse horizontal axis*, which extends through both condyles.
2. *Vertical axis* (Fig 2-5). This movement occurs in the horizontal plane when the mandible moves into a lateral excursion. The center for this rotation is a vertical axis extending through the rotating or working-side condyle.
3. *Sagittal axis* (Fig 2-6). When the mandible moves to one side, the condyle on the side opposite from the direction of movement travels forward. As it does, it encounters the eminentia of the glenoid fossa and moves downward simultaneously. When viewed in the frontal plane, this produces a downward arc on the side opposite the direction of movement, rotating about an anteroposterior (sagittal) axis passing through the other condyle.

Various mandibular movements are composed of motions occurring concurrently about one or more of the axes. The up and down motion of the mandible is a combination of two movements. A purely "hinge" movement occurs as the result of the condyles rotating in the lower compartments of the temporomandibular joints within a 10- to 13-degree arc, which creates a 20- to 25-mm separation of the anterior teeth (Fig 2-3, B). This phenomenon was the basis for the "terminal hinge axis" theory in the early 1920s by McCollum.[2] Kohno verified the pres-

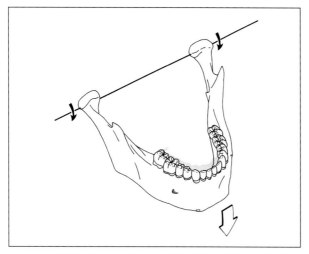

Fig 2-4 The mandible moves about a horizontal axis, as seen in a hinge axis opening.

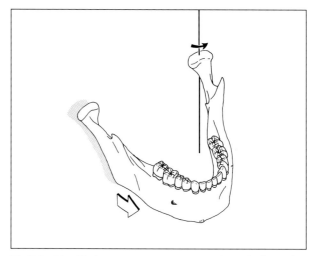

Fig 2-5 Mandibular movement occurs around a vertical axis during a lateral excursion.

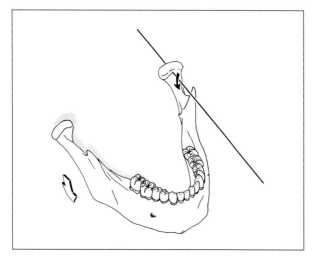

Fig 2-6 The mandible also rotates around a sagittal axis when one side drops down during a lateral excursion.

ence of a transverse horizontal axis, which he termed the "kinematic axis."[12] There is also some gliding movement in the upper compartment of the joint if the mandible drops down farther (Fig 2-3, C). Then the axis of rotation shifts to the area of the mandibular foramen, as the condyles translate forward and downward while continuing to rotate.

When the mandible slides forward so that the maxillary and mandibular anterior teeth are in an end-to-end relationship, it is in a *protrusive* position. Ideally, the anterior segment of the mandible will travel a path guided by contacts between the anterior teeth, with complete disocclusion of the posterior teeth (Fig 2-7).

Mandibular movement to one side will place it in a *working*, or laterotrusive, relationship on that side and a *nonworking*, or mediotrusive, relationship on the opposite side; eg, if the mandible is moved to the left, the left side is the working side, and the right side is the nonworking side (Fig 2-8). In this type of movement, the condyle on the nonworking side will arc forward and medially (Fig 2-8, A). Meanwhile, the condyle on the working side will shift laterally and usually slightly posteriorly (Fig 2-8, B). The bodily shift of the mandible in the direction of the working side was first described by Bennett.[13] The angle formed in the horizontal plane between the pathway of the nonworking condyle, the *mandibular lateral translation*, and the sagittal plane, is called the *Bennett angle* (Fig 2-9). The presence of an immediate or early *lateral translation*, or side shift, has been reported in 86% of the condyles studied.[14] In addition to confirming the predominant presence of the early lateral translation, Lundeen and Wirth, using a mechanical apparatus, showed its median dimension to be approximately 1.0 mm with a maximum of 3.0 mm.[15] Hobo and Mochizuki, using an electronic measuring device, found a lower mean value of 0.4 mm for the immediate lateral translation, with a high of 2.6 mm.[16,17]

Following the immediate lateral translation, there is a further gradual shifting of the mandible, *progressive lateral translation*, which occurs at a rate proportional to the forward movement of the nonworking condyle.[18] At one time this was known as "progressive side shift" or "Bennett side shift." Lundeen and Wirth found slight variation in the direction of the progressive lateral translation or Bennett angle, with a mean value of 7.5 degrees.[15] Hobo and Mochizuki found a much greater variation, ranging from 1.5 to 36 degrees, with a mean value of 12.8 degrees.[16,17]

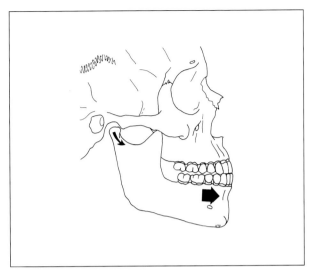

Fig 2-7 A protrusive movement occurs when the mandible moves forward.

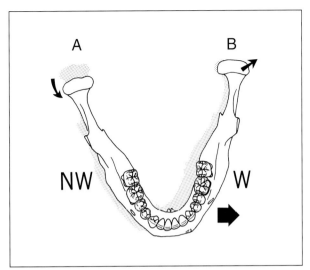

Fig 2-8 When the mandible moves into a left lateral excursion, the right condyle (A) moves forward and inward, while the left condyle (B) will shift slightly in a lateroposterior direction. In this example, the left side is the working side (W), and the right side is the nonworking side (NW).

The Determinants of Mandibular Movement

The two condyles and the contacting teeth are analogous to the three legs of an inverted tripod suspended from the cranium. The determinants of the movements of that tripod are, posteriorly, the right and left temporomandibular joints; anteriorly, the teeth of the maxillary and mandibular arches; and overall, the neuromuscular system.[19]

The dentist has no control over the posterior determinants, the temporomandibular joints; they are unchangeable. However, they influence the movements of the mandible, and of the teeth, by the paths that the condyles must travel when the mandible is moved by the muscles of mastication. The measurement and reproduction of those condylar movements is the basis for the use of articulators.

The anterior determinant, the teeth, provides guidance to the mandible in several ways. The posterior teeth provide the vertical stops for mandibular closure. They also guide the mandible into the position of maximum intercuspation, which may or may not correspond with the optimum position of the condyles in the glenoid fossae. The anterior teeth (canine to canine) help to guide the mandible in right and left lateral excursive movements and in protrusive movements. Anterior teeth are especially suited for guidance by virtue of:

1. Canines having the longest, strongest roots in their respective arches
2. The load being reduced by distance from the fulcrum (Class III lever)
3. The proprioceptive threshold and concomitant reflexes reducing the load [20–22]

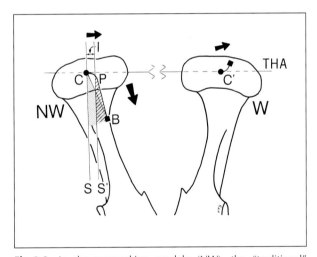

Fig 2-9 In the nonworking condyle (NW), the "traditional" Bennett angle (SCB) measures the angle from the sagittal plane to the endpoint of the movement of the condyle center. The Bennett angle used in articulators with an immediate lateral translation capability (S'PB) is measured from the sagittal plane after the immediate or early lateral translation (I) has occurred. The transverse horizontal axis (THA), or hinge axis of purely rotational movement, extends through both condyles. The working-side condyle (W), slides laterally, or outward, in laterotrusion.

Dentists have direct control over the tooth determinant by orthodontic movement of teeth; restoration of the anterior lingual or posterior occlusal surfaces; and equilibration, or selective grinding, of any teeth that are not in a harmonious relationship. Intercuspal position and anterior guidance can be altered, for better or for worse, by any of these means.

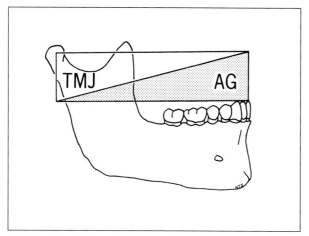

Fig 2-10 The farther anterior a tooth is located, the less the influence of the temporomandibular joint (TMJ) and the greater the influence of the anterior guidance (AG).

The closer a tooth is located to a determinant, the more that it will be influenced by that determinant (Fig 2-10). A tooth placed near the anterior region will be influenced greatly by anterior guidance and less by the temporomandibular joint. A tooth in the posterior region will be influenced partially by the joints and partially by the anterior guidance.

The neuromuscular system, through proprioceptive nerve endings in the periodontium, muscles, and joints, monitors the position of the mandible and its paths of movement. Through reflex action, it will program the most nearly physiologic paths of movement possible under the set of circumstances present. Dentists have indirect control over this determinant. Procedures done to the teeth may be reflected in the response of the neuromuscular system.

One of the objectives of restorative dentistry is to place the teeth in harmony with the temporomandibular joints. This will result in minimum stress on the teeth and joints, with only a minimum effort expended by the neuromuscular system to produce mandibular movements. When the teeth are not in harmony with the joints and with the movements of the mandible, an interference is said to exist.

Occlusal Interferences

Interferences are undesirable occlusal contacts that may produce mandibular deviation during closure to maximum intercuspation or may hinder smooth passage to and from the intercuspal position. There are four types of occlusal interferences:

1. Centric
2. Working
3. Nonworking
4. Protrusive

The *centric interference* is a premature contact that occurs when the mandible closes with the condyles in their optimum position in the glenoid fossae (Fig 2-11). It will cause deflection of the mandible in a posterior, anterior, and/or lateral direction.[23]

A *working interference* may occur when there is contact between the maxillary and mandibular posterior teeth on the same side of the arches as the direction in which the mandible has moved (Fig 2-12). If that contact is heavy enough to disocclude anterior teeth, it is an interference.[24]

A *nonworking interference* is an occlusal contact between maxillary and mandibular teeth on the side of the arches opposite the direction in which the mandible has moved in a lateral excursion (Fig 2-13). The nonworking interference is of a particularly destructive nature.[25–28] The potential for damaging the masticatory apparatus has been attributed to changes in the mandibular leverage, the placement of forces outside the long axes of the teeth, and disruption of normal muscle function.[29]

The *protrusive interference* is a premature contact occurring between the mesial aspects of mandibular posterior teeth and the distal aspects of maxillary posterior teeth (Fig 2-14). The proximity of the teeth to the muscles and the oblique vector of the forces make contacts between opposing posterior teeth during protrusion potentially destructive, as well as interfere with the patient's ability to incise properly.

Normal Versus Pathologic Occlusion

In only slightly more than 10% of the population is there complete harmony between the teeth and the temporomandibular joints.[30] This finding is based on a concept of centric relation in which the mandible is in the most retruded position. With the present concept of the condyles being in the most superoanterior position with the disc interposed, the results could be different. Nonetheless, in a majority of the population, the position of maximum intercuspation causes the mandible to be deflected away from its optimum position.

In the absence of symptoms, this can be considered physiologic, or normal. Therefore, in the normal occlusion there will be a reflex function of the neuromuscular system, producing mandibular movement that avoids premature contacts. This guides the mandible into a position of maximum intercuspation with the condyle in a less than optimal position. The result will be either some hypertonicity of nearby muscles or trauma to the temporomandibular joint, but it is usually well within most people's physiologic capacity to adapt and will not cause discomfort.

However, the patient's ability to adapt may be influenced by the effects of psychic stress and emotional tensions on the central nervous system.[31] By lowering the threshold, frequently parafunctional jaw activity such as

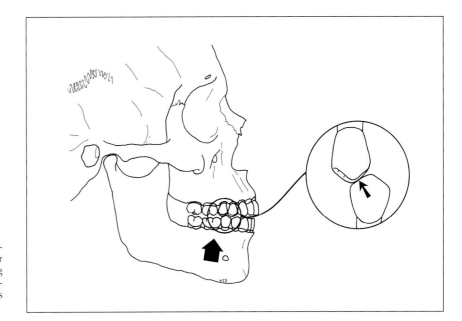

Fig 2-11 A centric occlusal interference often occurs during mandibular closure between maxillary mesial-facing cusp inclines and mandibular distal-facing inclines. As a result, the mandible is deflected anteriorly.

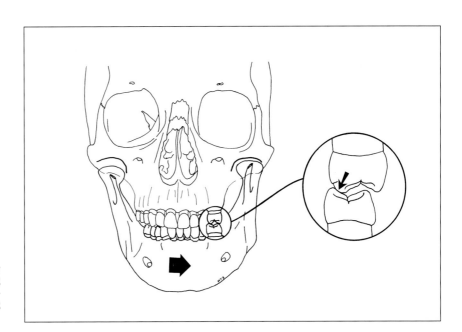

Fig 2-12 A working interference may occur between maxillary lingual-facing cusp inclines and mandibular buccal-facing cusp inclines on the working side.

clenching or bruxing occurs, and a normal occlusion can become a pathologic one (Fig 2-15). Simple muscle hypertonicity may give way to muscle fatigue and spasm, with chronic headaches and localized muscle tenderness, or temporomandibular joint dysfunction may occur. Pathologic occlusion can also manifest itself in the physical signs of trauma and destruction. Heavy facets of wear on occlusal surfaces, fractured cusps, and tooth mobility often are the result of occlusal disharmony. There is no evidence that occlusal trauma will produce a pri-

mary periodontal lesion. However, when occlusal trauma is present, there will be more severe periodontal breakdown in response to local factors than there would be if only the local factors were present.[32]

Habit patterns may develop in response to occlusal disharmony and emotional stress. Bruxism and clenching, the cyclic rubbing together of opposing occlusal surfaces, will produce even greater tooth destruction and muscle dysfunction.

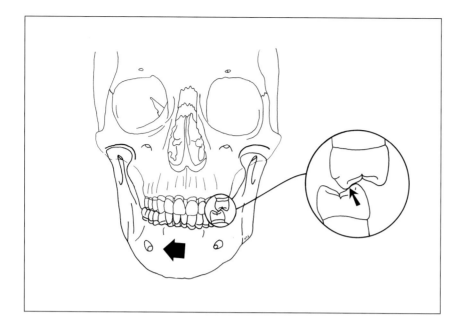

Fig 2-13 A nonworking interference results when there is contact between maxillary buccal-facing cusp inclines and mandibular lingual-facing cusp inclines on the nonworking side.

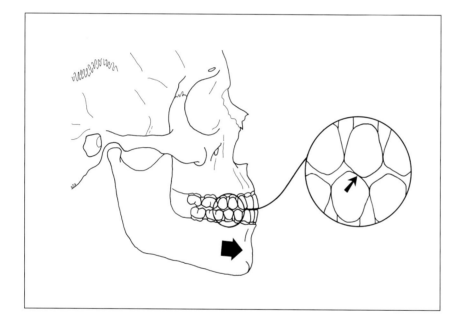

Fig 2-14 A protrusive interference occurs when distal-facing inclines of maxillary posterior teeth contact mesial-facing inclines of mandibular posterior teeth during a protrusive movement.

When the acute discomfort of a patient with a pathologic occlusion has been relieved, changes that will prevent the recurrence of symptoms must be effected in the occlusal scheme. Care must also be taken when providing occlusal restorations for a patient without symptoms. The dentist must not produce an iatrogenic pathologic occlusion.

In the placement of restorations, the dentist must strive to produce for the patient an occlusion that is as nearly optimum as his or her skills and the patient's oral condition will permit. The optimum occlusion is one that requires a minimum of adaptation by the patient. The criteria for such an occlusion have been described by Okeson[33]:

1. In closure, the condyles are in the most superoanterior position against the discs on the posterior slopes of the eminences of the glenoid fossae. The posterior teeth are in solid and even contact, and the anterior teeth are in slightly lighter contact.
2. Occlusal forces are in the long axes of the teeth.
3. In lateral excursions of the mandible, working-side contacts (preferably on the canines) disocclude or separate the nonworking teeth instantly.
4. In protrusive excursions, anterior tooth contacts will disocclude the posterior teeth.
5. In an upright posture, posterior teeth contact more heavily than do anterior teeth.

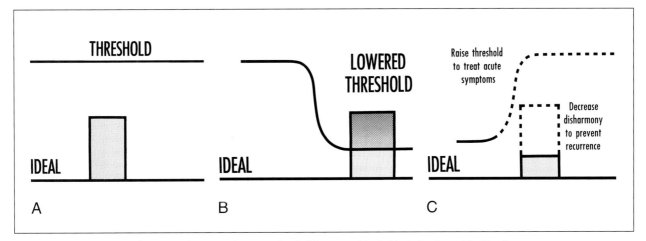

Fig 2-15 There may be an occlusal disharmony (shaded bar) that is not ideal but is tolerated by the patient because it is below his or her threshold of perception and discomfort (A). If the threshold is lowered, the disharmony which had been previously tolerated may produce symptoms in the patient (B). Treatment is then rendered by first raising the patient's threshold and then decreasing or eliminating the disharmony (C).

Organization of the Occlusion

The collective arrangement of the teeth in function is quite important and has been subjected to a great deal of analysis and discussion over the years. There are three recognized concepts that describe the manner in which teeth should and should not contact in the various functional and excursive positions of the mandible. They are bilateral balanced occlusion, unilateral balanced occlusion, and mutually protected occlusion.

Bilateral Balanced Occlusion

Bilateral balanced occlusion is based on the work of von Spee[34] and Monson.[35] It is a concept that is not used as frequently today as it has been in the past. It is largely a prosthodontic concept which dictates that a maximum number of teeth should contact in all excursive positions of the mandible. This is particularly useful in complete denture construction, in which contact on the nonworking side is important to prevent tipping of the denture.[35] Subsequently, the concept was applied to natural teeth in complete occlusal rehabilitation. An attempt was made to reduce the load on individual teeth by sharing the stress among as many teeth as possible.[36] It was soon discovered, however, that this was a very difficult type of arrangement to achieve. As a result of the multiple tooth contacts that occurred as the mandible moved through its various excursions, there was excessive frictional wear on the teeth.[37]

Unilateral Balanced Occlusion

Unilateral balanced occlusion, which is also commonly known as *group function*, is a widely accepted and used method of tooth arrangement in restorative dental procedures today. This concept had its origin in the work of Schuyler[38] and others who began to observe the destructive nature of tooth contact on the nonworking side. They concluded that inasmuch as cross-arch balance was not necessary in natural teeth, it would be best to eliminate all tooth contact on the nonworking side.

Therefore, unilateral balanced occlusion calls for all teeth on the working side to be in contact during a lateral excursion. On the other hand, teeth on the nonworking side are contoured to be free of any contact. The group function of the teeth on the working side distributes the occlusal load. The absence of contact on the nonworking side prevents those teeth from being subjected to the destructive, obliquely directed forces found in nonworking interferences. It also saves the centric holding cusps, ie, the mandibular buccal cusps and the maxillary lingual cusps, from excessive wear. The obvious advantage is the maintenance of the occlusion.

The functionally generated path technique, originally described by Meyer,[39] is used for producing restorations in unilateral balanced occlusion. It has been adapted by Mann and Pankey for use in complete-mouth occlusal reconstruction.[40,41]

Mutually Protected Occlusion

Mutually protected occlusion is also known as canine-protected occlusion or "organic" occlusion. It had its origin in the work of D'Amico,[42] Stuart,[43,44] Stallard and

Stuart,[25] and Lucia[45] and the members of the Gnathological Society. They observed that in many mouths with a healthy periodontium and minimum wear, the teeth were arranged so that the overlap of the anterior teeth prevented the posterior teeth from making any contact on either the working or the nonworking sides during mandibular excursions. This separation from occlusion was termed *disocclusion*. According to this concept of occlusion, the anterior teeth bear all the load and the posterior teeth are disoccluded in any excursive position of the mandible. The desired result is an absence of frictional wear.

The position of maximum intercuspation coincides with the optimal condylar position of the mandible. All posterior teeth are in contact with the forces being directed along their long axes. The anterior teeth either contact lightly or are very slightly out of contact (approximately 25 microns), relieving them of the obliquely directed forces that would be the result of anterior tooth contact. As a result of the anterior teeth protecting the posterior teeth in all mandibular excursions and the posterior teeth protecting the anterior teeth at the intercuspal position, this type of occlusion came to be known as a mutually protected occlusion. This arrangement of the occlusion is probably the most widely accepted because of its ease of fabrication and greater tolerance by patients.

However, to reconstruct a mouth with a mutually protected occlusion, it is necessary to have anterior teeth that are periodontally healthy. In the presence of anterior bone loss or missing canines, the mouth should probably be restored to group function (unilateral balance). The added support of the posterior teeth on the working side will distribute the load that the anterior teeth may not be able to bear. The use of a mutually protected occlusion is also dependent upon the orthodontic relationship of the opposing arches. In either a Class II or a Class III malocclusion (Angle), the mandible cannot be guided by the anterior teeth. A mutually protected occlusion cannot be used in a situation of *reverse occlusion*, or cross bite, in which the maxillary and mandibular buccal cusps interfere with each other in a working-side excursion.

Effects of Anatomic Determinants

The anatomic determinants of mandibular movement, ie, condylar and anterior guidance, have a strong influence on the occlusal surface morphology of the teeth being restored. There is a relationship between the numerous factors, such as immediate lateral translation, condylar inclination, and even disc flexibility, and on the cusp height, cusp location, and groove direction that are acceptable in the restoration. It is beyond the scope of this text to discuss all of the nearly 50 rules that have been written on the subject of determinants.[46] Those which have the greatest effect on morphology should be considered.

Molar Disocclusion

When subjects with normal occlusions perform repeated lateral mandibular movements, they will not trace the same path on electronic recordings, presumably because of the flexible nature of the articular disc. The measured deviation averages 0.2 mm in centric relation, 0.3 mm in working, and 0.8 mm in both protrusive and nonworking movements.[47] To avoid occlusal interferences and nonaxially directed forces on molars during eccentric mandibular movements, molar disocclusion must equal or surpass these observed deviations in mandibular movement.

Healthy natural occlusions exhibit clearances that will accommodate these aberrations. Measurements of disocclusions from the mesiobuccal cusp tips of mandibular first molars in asymptomatic test subjects with good occlusions showed separations averaging 0.5 mm in working, 1.0 mm in nonworking, and 1.1 mm in protrusive movements.[48] Therefore, one of the treatment goals in placing occlusal restorations should be to produce a posterior occlusion with buffer space that equals or surpasses the deviations resulting from natural variations found in the temporomandibular joint.

Condylar Guidance

Chief among those aspects of condylar guidance that will have an impact on the occlusal surface of posterior teeth are the protrusive condylar path inclination and mandibular lateral translation.

The inclination of the condylar path during protrusive movement can vary from steep to shallow in different patients. It forms an average angle of 30.4 degrees with the horizontal reference plane (43 mm above the maxillary central incisor edge).[16,17] If the protrusive inclination is steep, the cusp height *may* be longer. However, if the inclination is shallow, the cusp height *must* be shorter (Fig 2-16).

Immediate mandibular lateral translation is the lateral shift during initial lateral movement. If immediate lateral translation is great, then the cusp height *must* be shorter (Fig 2-17). With minimal immediate translation, the cusp height *may* be made longer.

Ridge and groove directions are affected by the condylar path, particularly the lateral translation. The effects are observed on the occlusal surface of a mandibular molar and premolar with the paths traced by the lingual cusps of the respective opposing maxillary teeth. The working path is traced on the mandibular tooth in a lingual direction, and the nonworking path is in a distobuccal direction. The nearer the tooth is to the working-side condyle anteroposteriorly, the smaller the angle between the working and nonworking paths (Fig 2-18). The farther the tooth is placed from the working-side condyle, the greater the angle between the working and nonworking condyles. When immediate lateral translation is increased, the angle also becomes more oblique.

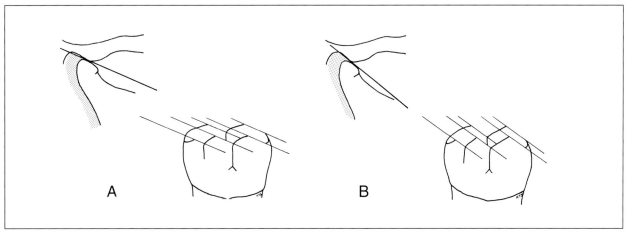

Fig 2-16 A shallow protrusive condylar inclination requires short cusps (A), while a steeper path permits the cusps to be longer (B).

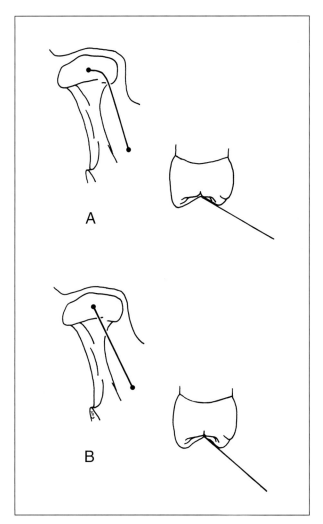

Fig 2-17 A pronounced immediate lateral translation requires that the cusps be short (A), while a gradual lateral translation allows the cusps to be longer (B).

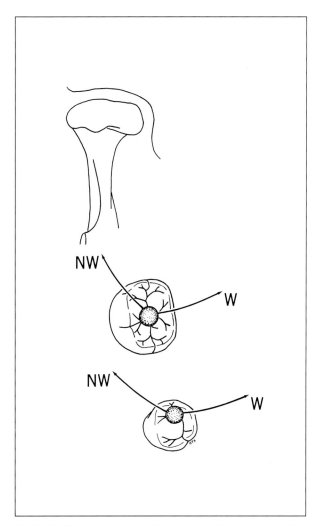

Fig 2-18 The angle between the working (W) and nonworking (NW) paths is greater on teeth located farther from the condyle.

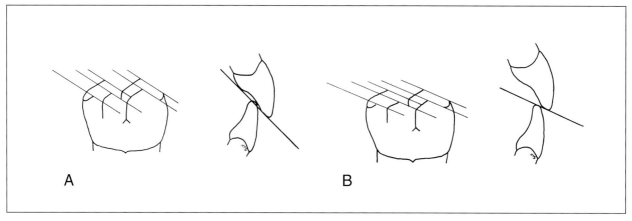

Fig 2-19 A pronounced vertical overlap of the anterior teeth permits posterior teeth to have longer cusps (A). A minimum anterior vertical overlap requires shorter cusps (B).

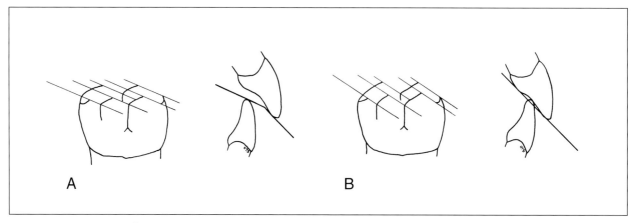

Fig 2-20 A pronounced horizontal overlap of the anterior teeth requires short cusps on the posterior teeth (A). A minimum anterior horizontal overlap permits the posterior cusps to be longer (B).

Anterior Guidance

During protrusive movement of the mandible, the incisal edges of mandibular anterior teeth move forward and downward along the lingual concavities of the maxillary anterior teeth. The track of the incisal edges from maximum intercuspation to edge-to-edge occlusion is termed the *protrusive incisal path*. The angle formed by the protrusive incisal path and the horizontal reference plane is the *protrusive incisal path inclination*, which ranges from 50 to 70 degrees.[49,50] While conventionally regarded as independent factors, there is evidence to suggest that condylar inclination and anterior guidance are linked, or dependent factors.[51–53] In a healthy occlusion, the anterior guidance is approximately 5 to 10 degrees steeper than the condylar path in the sagittal plane. Therefore, when the mandible moves protrusively, the anterior teeth guide the mandible downward to create disocclusion, or separation, between the maxillary and mandibular posterior teeth. The same phenomenon should occur during lateral mandibular excursions.

The lingual surface of a maxillary anterior tooth has both a concave aspect and a convexity, or cingulum. The mandibular incisal edges should contact the maxillary lingual surfaces at the transition from the concavity to the convexity in the centric relation position. The concavity represents a uniform shape in all subjects.[54]

Anterior guidance, which is linked to the combination of vertical and horizontal overlap of the anterior teeth, can affect occlusal surface morphology of the posterior teeth. The greater the vertical overlap of the anterior teeth, the longer the posterior cusp height *may* be. When the vertical overlap is less, the posterior cusp height *must* be shorter (Fig 2-19). The greater the horizontal

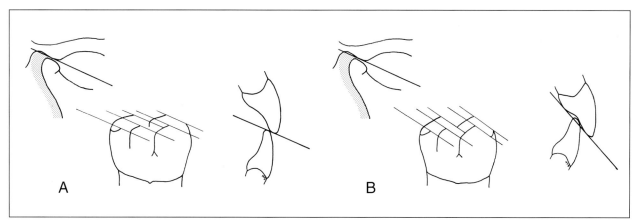

Fig 2-21 While a shallow protrusive path would require short cusps in the presence of minimal anterior guidance (A), the posterior cusps can be lengthened if the anterior guidance is increased (B).

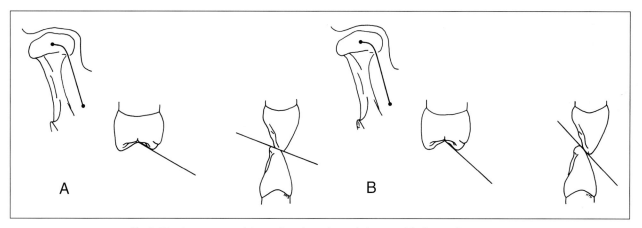

Fig 2-22 A pronounced immediate lateral translation would dictate short cusps where there is little anterior guidance (A). However, the cusps can be lengthened if the anterior guidance is increased (B).

overlap of the anterior teeth, the shorter the cusp height *must* be. With a decreased horizontal overlap, the posterior cusp height *may* be longer (Fig 2-20).

By increasing anterior guidance to compensate for inadequate condylar guidance, it is possible to increase the cusp height. If the protrusive condylar inclination is shallow, *requiring* short posterior cusps, the cusps *may* be lengthened by making the anterior guidance steeper (Fig 2-21). In like manner, increasing anterior guidance will permit the lengthening of cusps that would otherwise have to be shorter in the presence of a pronounced immediate lateral translation (Fig 2-22).

References

1. Nomenclature Committee of the Academy of Denture Prosthetics: *Glossary of Prosthodontic Terms*, ed 5. St Louis, CV Mosby Co, 1987, p 15.

2. McCollum BB, Stuart CE: *Gnathology—A Research Report.* South Pasadena, Calif, Scientific Press, 1955, pp 91–123.

3. Lucia VO: *Modern Gnathological Concepts.* St Louis, CV Mosby Co, 1961, pp 15–22.

4. Dawson PE: *Evaluation, Diagnosis, and Treatment of Occlusal Problems.* St Louis, CV Mosby Co, 1974, p 293.

5. Kornfeld M: *Mouth Rehabilitation.* St Louis, CV Mosby Co, 1967, p 34.

6. Bauer A, Gutowski A: *Gnathology.* Berlin, Quintessence Publ Co, 1975, pp 85–91.

7. Huffman R, Regenos J: *Principles of Occlusion*, ed 8. Columbus, H & R Press, 1980, pp VA1–VB39.

8. Parsons MT, Boucher LJ: The bilaminar zone of the meniscus. *J Dent Res* 1966; 45:59–61.

9. McNeill C: The optimum temporomandibular joint condyle position in clinical practice. *Int J Periodont Rest Dent* 1985; 5(6):53–76.

10. Dawson PE: *Evaluation, Diagnosis, and Treatment of Occlusal Problems*. St Louis, CV Mosby Co, 1961, pp 48–79.

11. Brill N, Lammie GA, Osborne J, Perry HT: Mandibular positions and mandibular movements. *Br Dent J* 1959; 106:391–400.

12. Kohno S: Analyse der kondylenbewegung in der sagittlebene. *Dtsch Zahnärtzl Z* 1974; 27:739–743.

13. Bennett NG: A contribution to the study of the movements of the mandible. *Proc Roy Soc Med, Odont Sec* 1908; 1:79–95 (reprinted in *J Prosthet Dent* 1958; 8:41–54).

14. Aull AE: Condylar determinants of occlusal patterns. Part I. Statistical report on condylar path variations. *J Prosthet Dent* 1965; 15:826–835.

15. Lundeen HC, Wirth CG: Condylar movement patterns engraved in plastic blocks. *J Prosthet Dent* 1973; 30:866–875.

16. Hobo S, Mochizuki S: Study of mandibular movement by means of an electronic measuring system, Part I. *J Jpn Prosth Soc* 1982; 26:619–634.

17. Hobo S, Mochizuki S: Study of mandibular movement by means of an electronic measuring system, Part II. *J Jpn Prosth Soc* 1982; 26:635–653.

18. Nomenclature Committee of the Academy of Denture Prosthetics: *Glossary of Prosthodontic Terms*, ed 5. St Louis, CV Mosby Co, 1987, p 31.

19. Guichet NF: *Occlusion*. Anaheim, CA, The Denar Corporation, 1970, p 13.

20. Manly RS, Pfaffmann C, Lathrop DD, Kayser J: Oral sensory thresholds of persons with natural and artificial dentitions. *J Dent Res* 1952; 31:305.

21. Williamson EH, Lundquist DO: Anterior guidance: Its effect on electromyographic activity of the temporal and masseter muscles. *J Prosthet Dent* 1983; 49:816.

22. Manns A, Chan C, Miralles R: Influence of group function and canine guidance or electromyographic activity of elevator muscles. *J Prosthet Dent* 1987; 57:494–501.

23. Dawson PE: Temporomandibular joint pain-dysfunction problems can be solved. *J Prosthet Dent* 1973; 29:100–112.

24. Dawson PE: *Evaluation, Diagnosis, and Treatment of Occlusal Problems*. St Louis, CV Mosby Co, 1961, p 299.

25. Ramfjord SP: Dysfunctional temporomandibular joint and muscle pain. *J Prosthet Dent* 1961; 11:353–374.

26. Stallard H, Stuart CE: Eliminating tooth guidance in natural dentitions. *J Prosthet Dent* 1961; 11:474–479.

27. Schuyler CH: Factors contributing to traumatic occlusion. *J Prosthet Dent* 1961; 11:708–715.

28. Yuodelis RA, Mann WV: The prevalence and possible role of nonworking contacts in periodontal disease. *Periodontics* 1965; 3:219–223.

29. Whitsett LD, Shillingburg HT, Duncanson MG: The nonworking interference. *J Okla Dent Assoc* 1974; 65:5–8.

30. Posselt U: Studies in the mobility of the human mandible. *Acta Odontol Scand* 1952; 10 (suppl 10): 1–109.

31. Ramfjord SP, Ash MM: *Occlusion*, ed 2. Philadelphia, WB Saunders Co, 1971, p 104.

32. Glickman I, Smulow JB: Alterations in the pathway of gingival inflammation into the underlying tissues induced by excessive occlusal forces. *J Periodontol* 1962; 33:7–13.

33. Okeson JP: *Management of Temporomandibular Disorders and Occlusion*. St Louis, CV Mosby Co, 1989, p 113.

34. von Spee FG: The gliding path of the mandible along the skull. *Archiv f Anat u Phys* 1890; 16:285–294. (Translated by Biedenbach MA, Hotz M, Hitchcock HP: *J Am Dent Assoc* 1980; 100:670–675).

35. Monson GS: Impaired function as a result of a closed bite. *J Am Dent Assoc* 1921; 8:833–839.

36. Schuyler CH: Fundamental principles in the correction of occlusal disharmony, natural and artificial. *J Am Dent Assoc* 1935; 22:1193–1202.

37. Stuart CE, Stallard H: Principles involved in restoring occlusion to natural teeth. *J Prosthet Dent* 1960; 10:304–313.

38. Schuyler CH: Factors of occlusion applicable to restorative dentistry. *J Prosthet Dent* 1953; 3:772–782.

39. Meyer FS: Can the plain line articulator meet all the demands of balanced and functional occlusion in all restorative work? *J Colo Dent Assoc* 1938; 17:6–16.

40. Mann AW, Pankey LD: Oral rehabilitation: Part I. Use of the P-M instrument in treatment planning and in restoring the lower posterior teeth. *J Prosthet Dent* 1960; 10:135–150.

41. Pankey LD, Mann AW: Oral rehabilitation: Part II. Reconstruction of the upper teeth using a functionally generated path technique. *J Prosthet Dent* 1960; 10:151–162.

42. D'Amico A: Functional occlusion of the natural teeth of man. *J Prosthet Dent* 1961; 11:899–915.

43. Stuart CE: Good occlusion for natural teeth. *J Prosthet Dent* 1964; 14:716–724.

44. Stuart CE: Why dental restorations should have cusps. *J South Calif Dent Assoc* 1959; 27:198–200.

45. Lucia VO: The gnathological concept of articulation. *Dent Clin North Am* 1962; 6:183–197.

46. Katz GT: *The Determinants of Human Occlusion*. Los Angeles, Marina Press, 1972, p vi.

47. Oliva RA, Takayama H, Hobo S: Three-dimensional study of mandibular movement using an automatic electronic measuring system. *J Gnathol* 1986; 5:115–182.

48. Hobo S, Takayama H: Pilot study—analysis and measurement of the amount of disclusion during lateral movement. *J Jpn Prosth Soc* 1984; 29:238–239.

49. Gysi A, Kohler L: *Handbuch der Zahnehikunde*. Berlin & Vienna, Scheff, 1929, IV.

50. Gysi A: The problem of articulation. *Dent Cosmos* 1910; 52:1–19, 148–169, 403–418.

51. Takayama H, Hobo S: The derivation of kinematic formulae for mandibular movement. *Int J Prosthodont* 1989; 2:285–295.

52. Takayama H, Hobo S: Experimental verification of the kinematic formulae for mandibular movement (unpublished data).

53. Takayama H, Hobo S: Kinematic and experimental analyses of mandibular movement for clinical application. *Prec Mach Incorp Life Supp Tech* 1989; 2:229–304.

54. Kubein-Meesenburg D, Naegerl H, Meyer G, Buecking W: Individual reconstruction of palatal concavities. *J Prosthet Dent* 1988; 60:662–672.

Chapter 3

Articulators

An articulator is a mechanical device that simulates the movements of the mandible (Fig 3-1). The principle employed in the use of articulators is the mechanical replication of the paths of movement of the posterior determinants, the temporomandibular joints. The instrument is then used in the fabrication of fixed and removable dental restorations that are in harmony with those movements.

The outer limits of all excursive movements made by the mandible are referred to as border movements. All functional movements of the mandible are confined to the three-dimensional envelope of movement contained within these borders.[1] The border movements are of significance in discussing articulation because they are limited by ligaments. As such, they are highly repeatable and useful in setting the various adjustments on the mechanical fossae of an articulator. The more nearly the articulator duplicates the border movements, the more nearly it will simulate the posterior determinants of occlusion. As a result, the harmony between the restoration fabricated and the posterior determinants, ie, the temporomandibular joints, will be improved.

Articulators vary widely in the accuracy with which they reproduce the movements of the mandible. At the lower end of the scale is the nonadjustable articulator. It is usually a small instrument that is capable of only a hinge opening. The distance between the teeth and the axis of rotation on the small instrument is considerably shorter than it is in the skull, with a resultant loss of accuracy.

As the mandible moves up and down in the retruded position, the cusp tip of a mandibular tooth moves along an arc in a sagittal plane, with the center for that rotation located at the transverse horizontal axis, which passes through the condyles (Fig 3-2). If the location of the axis of rotation relative to the cusp tip differs markedly from the patient to the articulator, the radius of the arc of closure of the cusp tip may be different, producing an error. Drastic differences between the radius of closure on the articulator and in the patient's mouth can affect the placement of morphologic features such as cusps, ridges, and grooves on the occlusal surface.

The casts mounted on a smaller articulator will have a much shorter radius of movement, and a tooth will travel a steeper arc during closure of the small articulator (Fig 3-3). If the casts are mounted at an increased dimension of occlusion (ie, a thick interocclusal record), the teeth will occlude in a different intercuspal position on the articulator than in the mouth.[2] A slight positive error resulting in a deflective occlusal contact could develop between the mesial incline of the maxillary teeth and the distal incline of the mandibular teeth.[3]

The mediolateral location of the centers of rotation (ie, the intercondylar distance) will change the radius of tooth movement, which in turn will affect the arc traveled by a tooth cusp in the horizontal plane during a lateral excursion of the mandible. On a small hinge articulator, the discrepancy between the arcs traveled by a cusp on the instrument and in the mouth can be sizable, particularly on the nonworking side (Fig 3-4). The result is an increased possibility of incorporating a nonworking occlusal interference into the restoration.

A semiadjustable articulator is an instrument whose larger size allows a close approximation of the anatomic distance between the axis of rotation and the teeth. If casts are mounted with a facebow using no more than an approximate transverse horizontal axis, the radius of movement produced on the articulator will reproduce the tooth closure arc with relative accuracy, and any resulting error will be slight (Fig 3-5). Placing the casts a small distance closer to or farther from the condyles through the use of an approximate transverse horizontal axis will produce an error of only a small magnitude during lateral excursions (Fig 3-6).

The semiadjustable articulator reproduces the direction and endpoint, but not the intermediate track of some condylar movements. As an example, the inclination of the condylar path is reproduced as a straight line on many articulators, when in fact it usually traverses a curved path. On many instruments, the lateral translation, or Bennett movement, is reproduced as a gradually deviating straight line, although several recently introduced semiadjustable articulators do accommodate the immediate lateral translation.

Intercondylar distances are not totally adjustable on semiadjustable articulators. They can be adjusted to small, medium, and large configurations, if at all. Restorations will require some intraoral adjustment, but it should be inconsequential if the restoration is fabricated carefully on accurately mounted casts. This type of articulator can be used for the fabrication of most single units and fixed partial dentures.

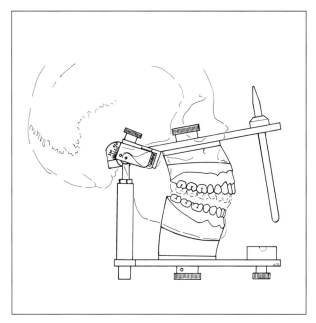

Fig 3-1 The articulator should simulate the movements of the mandible.

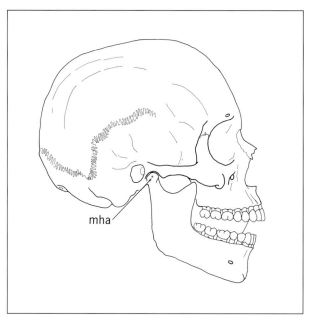

Fig 3-2 As the mandible closes around the hinge axis (mha), the cusp tip of each mandibular tooth moves along an arc. (From Hobo et al.[2])

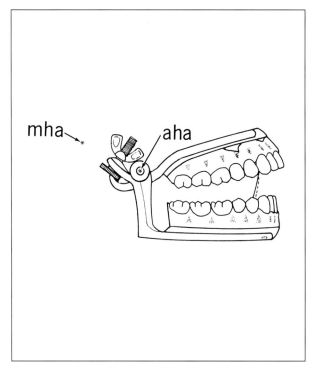

Fig 3-3 The large dissimilarity between the hinge axis of the small articulator (aha) and the hinge axis of the mandible (mha) will produce a large discrepancy between the arcs of closure of the articulator *(broken line)* and of the mandible *(solid line)*. (From Hobo et al.[2])

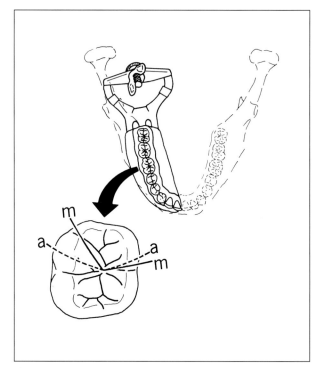

Fig 3-4 A major discrepancy exists between the nonworking cusp path on the small articulator (a) and that in the mouth (m). (From Hobo et al.[2])

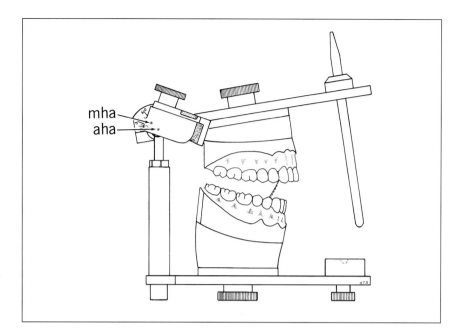

Fig 3-5 The dissimilarity between the hinge axis of the full-size semiadjustable articulator (aha) and the mandibular hinge axis (mha) will cause a slight discrepancy between the arcs of closure of the articulator *(broken line)* and of the mandible *(solid line)*. (From Hobo et al.[2])

The most accurate instrument is the fully adjustable articulator. It is designed to reproduce the entire character of border movements, including immediate and progressive lateral translation, and the curvature and direction of the condylar inclination. Intercondylar distance is completely adjustable. When a kinematically located hinge axis and an accurate recording of mandibular movement are employed, a highly accurate reproduction of the mandibular movement can be achieved.

This type of instrument is expensive. The techniques required for its use demand a high degree of skill and are time consuming to accomplish. For this reason, fully adjustable articulators are used primarily for extensive treatment, requiring the reconstruction of an entire occlusion.

Arcon and Nonarcon Articulators

There are two basic designs used in the fabrication of articulators: arcon and nonarcon. On an arcon articulator, the condylar elements are placed on the lower member of the articulator, just as the condyles are located on the mandible. The mechanical fossae are placed on the upper member of the articulator, simulating the position of the glenoid fossae in the skull. In the case of the nonarcon articulator, the condylar paths simulating the glenoid fossae are attached to the lower member of the instrument, while the condylar elements are placed on the upper portion of the articulator.

To set the condylar inclinations on a semiadjustable instrument, wax wafers called interocclusal records, or check bites, are used (see Chapter 4 for the technique)

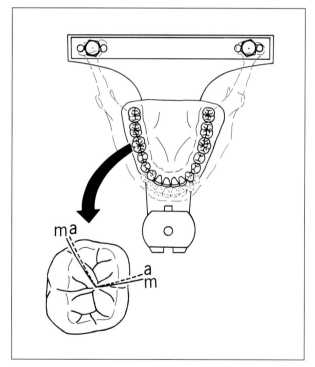

Fig 3-6 There is only a slight difference between cusp paths on a full-size articulator (a) and those in the mouth (m), even though the cast mounting exhibits a slight discrepancy. (From Hobo et al.[2])

to transfer the terminal positions of the condyles from the skull to the instrument. These wafers are 3.0 to 5.0 mm thick, so that the teeth on the maxillary and mandibular casts are separated by that distance when the condylar inclinations are set.

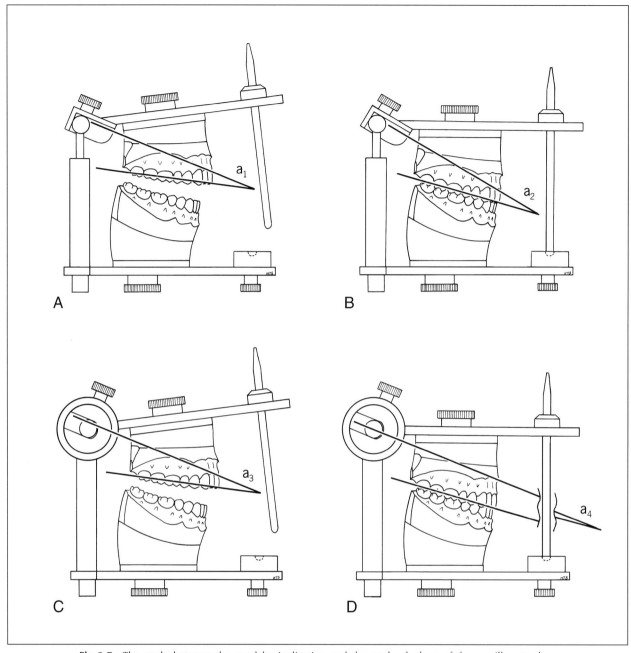

Fig 3-7 The angle between the condylar inclination and the occlusal plane of the maxillary teeth remains constant between an open (A) and a closed (B) arcon articulator $\angle a_1 = \angle a_2$. However, the angle changes between an open (C) and a closed (D) nonarcon instrument $\angle a_3 \neq \angle a_4$. For the amount of opening illustrated, there would be a difference of 8 degrees between the condylar inclination at an open position (where the articulator settings are adjusted) and a closed position at which the articulator is used.

When the wafers are removed from an arcon articulator, and the teeth are closed together, the condylar inclination will remain the same. However, when the teeth are closed on a nonarcon articulator, the inclination changes, becoming less steep (Fig 3-7). Arcon articulators have become more widely used because of their accuracy and the ease with which they disassemble to facilitate the occlusal waxing required for cast gold restorations. This very feature makes them unpopular for arranging denture teeth. The centric position is less easily maintained when the occlusion on all of the posterior teeth is being manipulated. Therefore, the nonarcon instrument has been more popular for the fabrication of dentures. Arcon articulators equipped with firm centric latches that prevent posterior separation will overcome many of these objections.

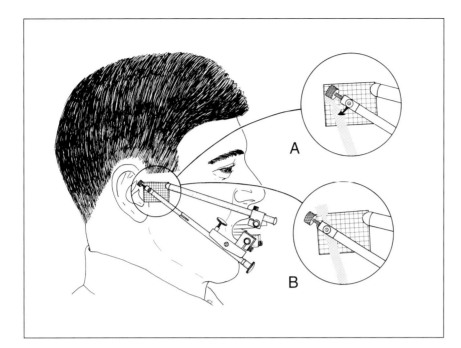

Fig 3-8 After the transverse horizontal axis locator is placed, the patient is assisted in opening and closing on the transverse horizontal axis. An arcing movement of the stylus on the side arm (A) indicates that it is not located over the transverse horizontal axis. The side arm is adjusted so the stylus will rotate without moving during opening and closing (B). This indicates that it has been positioned over the transverse horizontal axis.

The Tooth–Transverse Horizontal Axis Relationship

To achieve the highest possible degree of accuracy from an articulator, the casts mounted on it should be closing around an axis of rotation that is as close as possible to the transverse horizontal (hinge) axis of the patient's mandible. This axis is an important reference because it is repeatable. It is necessary to transfer the relationship of the maxillary teeth, the transverse horizontal axis, and a third reference point from the patient's skull to the articulating device. This is accomplished with a *facebow*, an instrument that records those spatial relationships and is then used for the attachment of the maxillary casts to the articulator.

The more precisely located the transverse horizontal axis, the more accurate will be the transfer and the mounting of the casts. The most accurate way to determine the hinge axis is by the "trial and error" method developed by McCollum and Stuart in 1921.[4] A device with horizontal arms extending to the region of the ears is fixed to the mandibular teeth. A grid is placed under the pin at the end of the arm, just anterior to the tragus of the ear. The mandible is manipulated to a retruded position, from which it is guided to open and close 10 mm. As it does, the pin will trace an arc (Fig 3-8). The arm is adjusted in small increments to move it up, down, forward, or back, until the pin simply rotates without tracing an arc. This is the location of the hinge axis, which may be preserved for future reference by tattooing.

The facebow is attached to the maxillary teeth, and the side arms are adjusted so the pin at the free (posterior)

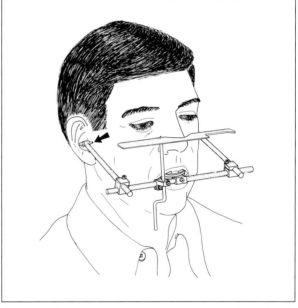

Fig 3-9 When a precision facebow transfer is made, both side arms are adjusted so that the stylus at the end of each arm is located over the transverse horizontal axis *(arrow)*. A third reference point, such as the plane indicator shown here, is used.

end of each side arm will touch the hinge axis mark on its respective side of the face (Fig 3-9). A third reference point is selected on the face and recorded by adjusting a pointer on the facebow. The facebow is removed from the patient and transferred to the articulator. The reference pins on the facebow are placed over the axis of rotation on the articulator condyles. With the anterior ref-

Table 3-1 *Accuracy of Arbitrary Hinge Axis Points*[15]

Measurements and landmarks for arbitrary hinge axis points	Arbitrary points within 6 mm of kinematic hinge axis points (%)	Investigator
13 mm from posterior margin of tragus to canthus	98.0 92.1 58.3	Schallhorn[7] Beyron[8] Beck[9]
13 mm in front of anterior margin of meatus	16.7 40.0	Beck[9] Lauritzen and Bodner[10]
13 mm from foot of tragus to canthus	33.0	Teteruck and Lundeen[12]
10 mm anterior to center of external auditory meatus and 7 mm below Frankfort plane	83.3	Beck[9]
Ear axis	75.5	Teteruck and Lundeen[12]

erence device providing the vertical orientation of the facebow, it can then be used to accurately mount the maxillary cast on the articulator. This technique is most commonly used for facebow transfers to fully adjustable articulators.

A facebow that employs an approximate location of the hinge axis based on an anatomic average can also be used. This technique should provide enough accuracy for the restoration of most mouths, if the occlusal vertical dimension is not to be altered to any significant extent. An error of 5.0 mm in the location of the transverse hinge axis location will produce a negligible anteroposterior mandibular displacement of approximately 0.2 mm when a 3.0-mm centric relation record is removed to close the articulator.[5]

There are numerous techniques used for arbitrarily locating the hinge axis to serve as the set of posterior reference points for a facebow.[6–14] A comparison of the accuracy of arbitrary and kinematically located hinge axis points is shown in Table 3-1.

Facebows must have acceptable accuracy and be simple to apply or they will not be used routinely. Caliper-style ear facebows possess a relatively high degree of accuracy, with 75% of the axes located by it falling within 6 mm of the true hinge axis.[12] There are several caliper-style facebows (Fig 3-10). They are designed to be self-centering, so that little time is wasted in centering the bite fork and adjusting individual side arms. The technique for their use is described in Chapter 4.

Registration of Condylar Movements

To faithfully simulate the condylar movement on an articulator, it is necessary to obtain a precise tracing of the paths followed by the condyle. This can be achieved most accurately by means of a pantographic recording, which will capture all of the characteristics of the mandibular border movement from its retruded position to its most forward and most lateral positions.

The pantograph consists of two facebows. One is affixed to the maxilla and the other to the mandible, using clutches that attach to the teeth in the respective arches. Recording styli are attached to the one member, and small tables upon which the tracings are made are attached to the other member of the instrument, opposite the styli. There are both horizontal and vertical posterior tables attached in the vicinity of the hinge axis on each side of the pantograph. There are also two tables attached to the anterior member of the bow, one on either side of the midline (Fig 3-11).

The mandible goes through a series of right and left lateral, as well as protrusive, excursions. The styli on one facebow scribe on the recording tables the paths followed by the condyles in each movement (Fig 3-12). When the pantograph is attached to the articulator, various adjustments are made until the movements of the articulator will follow the same paths scribed on the tracings during mandibular excursions.

The pantographic tracing can only be utilized to full advantage when used with a fully adjustable articulator. To adjust the settings of a semiadjustable articulator, wax interocclusal records are used. The patient closes into a heat-softened wax wafer in a right lateral protrusive position and maintains that posture until the wax has hardened. The procedure is repeated with another wax wafer for a left lateral protrusive position. The wax wafers are then placed, first one and then the other, on the articulated casts. After the right lateral wafer is used to adjust the condylar inclination for the left condyle, the left lateral wafer is used to adjust the right condylar inclination. Complete details of the technique are described in Chapter 4.

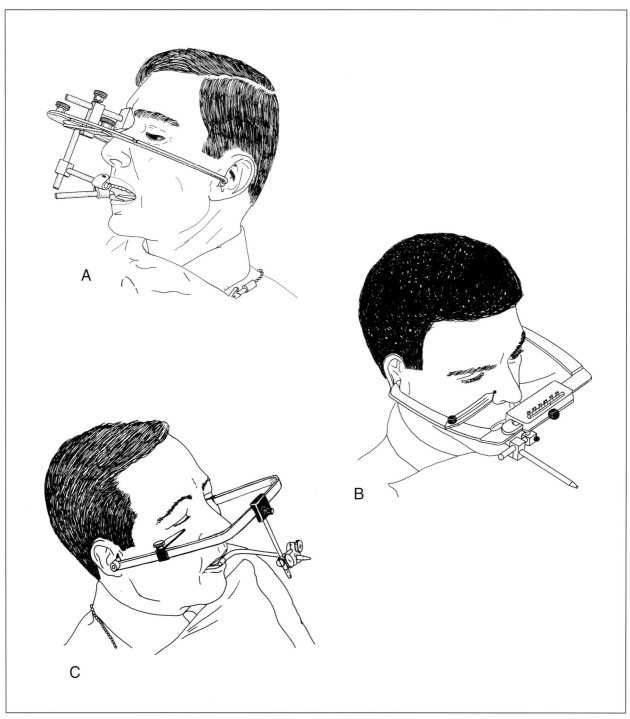

Fig 3-10 These three caliper-style facebows are among those in use at the present time: A, Quick-Mount facebow (Whip Mix Corp, Louisville, KY); B, Denar Slidematic facebow (Teledyne Water Pik, Fort Collins, CO); C, Hanau Springbow facebow (Teledyne Water Pik).

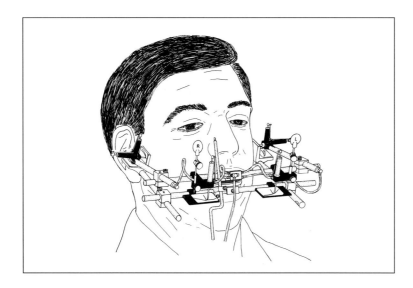

Fig 3-11 An air-activated pantograph for recording mandibular movements.

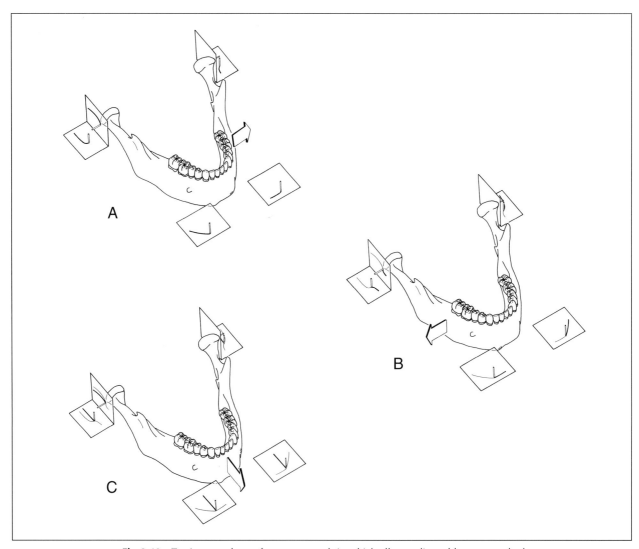

Fig 3-12 Tracings are shown for a pantograph in which all recording tables are attached to the mandible and all styli are attached to the maxilla; A, left lateral excursion; B, right lateral excursion; C, protrusive excursion. Styli are shown in their initial positions.

References

1. Posselt U: *Physiology of Occlusion and Rehabilitation*, ed 2. Philadelphia, FA David Co, 1968, p 55.

2. Hobo S, Shillingburg HT, Whitsett LD: Articulator selection for restorative dentistry. *J Prosthet Dent* 1976; 36:35–43.

3. Hodge LC, Mahan PE: A study of mandibular movement from centric occlusion to maximum intercuspation. *J Prosthet Dent* 1967; 18:19–30.

4. McCollum BB, Stuart CE: *Gnathology—A Research Report.* Ventura, Calif, Scientific Press, 1955, p 39.

5. Weinberg LA: An evaluation of the face-bow mounting. *J Prosthet Dent* 1961; 11:32–42.

6. Kornfeld M: *Mouth Rehabilitation—Clinical and Laboratory Procedures*, ed 2. St Louis, CV Mosby Co, 1974, pp 48, 336.

7. Schallhorn RG: A study of the arbitrary center and the kinematic center of rotation for face-bow mountings. *J Prosthet Dent* 1957; 7:162–169.

8. Beyron H: Orienteringsproblem vid protetiska rekonstruktioner och bettstudier. *Sven Tandlak Tidskr* 1942; 35:1–55.

9. Beck HO: A clinical evaluation of the arcon concept of articulation. *J Prosthet Dent* 1959; 9:409–421.

10. Lauritzen AG, Bodner GH: Variations in location of arbitrary and true hinge axis points. *J Prosthet Dent* 1961; 11:224–229.

11. Gysi A: The problem of articulation. *Dent Cosmos* 1910; 52:1–19.

12. Teteruck WR, Lundeen HC: The accuracy of an ear face-bow. *J Prosthet Dent* 1966; 16:1039–1046.

13. Bergstrom G: On the reproduction of dental articulation by means of articulators—A kinematic investigation. *Acta Odontol Scand* 1950; 9 (suppl 4):1–131.

14. Guichet NF: *Procedures for Occlusal Treatment—A Teaching Atlas.* Anaheim, CA, The Denar Corporation, 1969, p 35.

15. Whitsett LD, Shillingburg HT, Keenan MP: Modifications of a new semi-adjustable articulator for use with a caliper style ear face-bow. *J Calif Dent Assoc* 1977; 5:32–38.

Chapter 4

Interocclusal Records

After the maxillary cast has been accurately affixed to the articulator by using a facebow, the mandibular cast must be oriented to the maxillary cast with equal exactitude to be able to diagnose the patient's occlusion.[1,2] *Centric relation records* are used to replicate, on the articulator, the relationship between the maxillary and mandibular arches that exists when the condyles are in their most anterosuperior position in the glenoid fossae. *Lateral interocclusal records* are used to adjust the condylar guidance of the articulator. Then, it is possible to observe tooth relationships and identify deflective contacts and/or other occlusal discrepancies from the casts on the articulator. When this information has been gathered and assessed, a determination can be made as to what corrective measures, if any, will be performed on the occlusion.

A distinction must be made between mounting for diagnosis and mounting for treatment. The attachment of casts to an articulator for diagnosis will be done with the condyles in a centric relation position. When casts are articulated for restoration of a significant portion of the occlusion, it also may be done with the condyles in the centric relation position. However, the beginning operator usually will be restoring only limited segments of the occlusion at one time. Mounting casts for restoration of only a small part of the occlusion generally will be done with the teeth in a position of maximum intercuspation.

Centric Relation Record

To mount the mandibular cast on the articulator, it is necessary to record the relationship of the dental arches to each other. There are three techniques that are frequently used in locating the centric relation position: chinpoint guidance, bilateral manipulation, and the unguided method. With a computer-assisted three-dimensional mandibular recording device, Hobo and Iwata[3] analyzed condylar position achieved by the three methods. Chinpoint guidance puts the condyles in the most posterior and superior position, while the bilateral and unguided methods allow the muscles to guide the condyles into

a physiologic anterosuperiorly braced position on the articular disc along the articular eminence.

The unguided method produces a physiologic "muscle position," but it can be difficult to achieve consistent results because of the patient's muscle activity. Muscle proprioception is minimized by separating the teeth with a leaf gauge composed of several 0.1-mm-thick plastic strips, which help to eliminate direct proprioceptor responses. While the patient occludes with light pressure, strips are added one at a time in the anterior region until the patient no longer feels any posterior tooth contact. This permits the muscles to act freely and allows the condyles to move into a physiologic position.[4,5] Then the muscles will rotate the mandible anteriorly and superiorly.

Armamentarium

1. Cotton rolls
2. Pink baseplate wax
3. Green stick compound
4. Hollenback carver
5. Scissors
6. Aluwax
7. Bite registration paste
8. Cement spatula
9. Disposable mixing pad
10. Laboratory knife with no. 25 blade
11. 28-gauge green wax
12. No. 10 red-inked silk ribbon

Technique

The most consistent, repeatable results can be accomplished by utilizing the technique of "bimanual manipulation" described by Dawson.[6,7] The neuromuscular system monitors all sensory impulses from the teeth and jaws and programs occlusal contact to occur where the protective stimuli are minimal. This position, through repeated closures, becomes habitual and is maintained at the expense of normal muscle function.[8] To enable the condyles to be placed in an unstrained position, the mus-

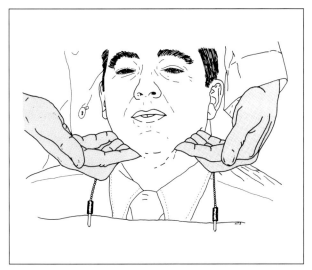

Fig 4-1 The fingers are placed along the inferior border of the mandible.

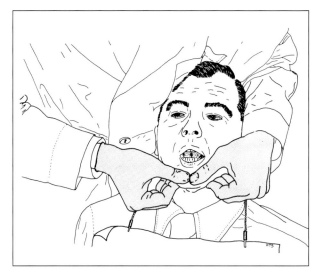

Fig 4-2 With the thumbs in position, the mandible is manipulated into a centric relation position.

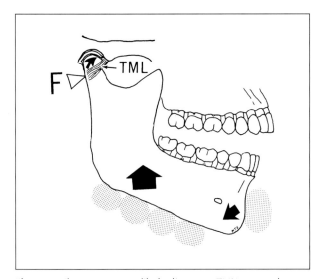

Fig 4-3 The temporomandibular ligament (TML) acts as the posterior limit and fulcrum (F). The downward force of the thumbs and upward force of the fingers help to seat the condyles in the posterosuperior portion of the glenoid fossa (after Dawson[7]).

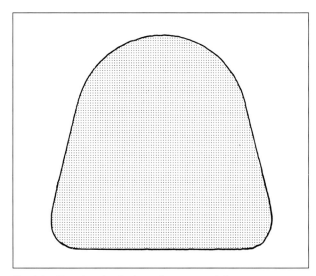

Fig 4-4 Template for the baseplate wax arch form.

culature must first be deprogrammed from its habitual closing pattern.

A simple means of doing this is to place a cotton roll between the anterior teeth and have the patient close with the instructions, "Bite on your back teeth." Check to be sure that there is no contact of the posterior teeth. If the cotton roll is placed as soon as the patient is seated, the operator and assistant can prepare the materials for the subsequent interocclusal record during the 5 minutes that the patient remains closed. After this time, the "memory" of the position in which the teeth intercuspate fully will likely have been lost, and the mandible can be manipulated more easily into its optimum position. As

soon as the cotton roll has been removed, begin the mandibular manipulation. Do not allow the patient to close the teeth together again, as this will allow the musculature to readapt to a tooth-guided closure.

Seat the patient with the chair back approximately 45 degrees from the floor. The head should be tilted back with the chin up so that the face is parallel with the floor. This position tends to keep the patient from protruding the mandible. The dentist should take a position behind the patient that will facilitate stabilization of the patient's head between the dentist's rib cage and forearm. The patient's head must not move while the mandible is being manipulated. Place all four fingers of each hand on the

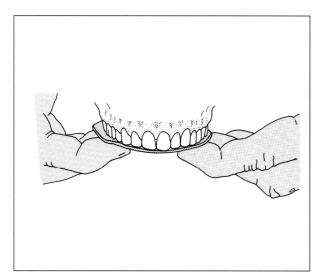

Fig 4-5 Baseplate wax is adapted to the maxillary arch.

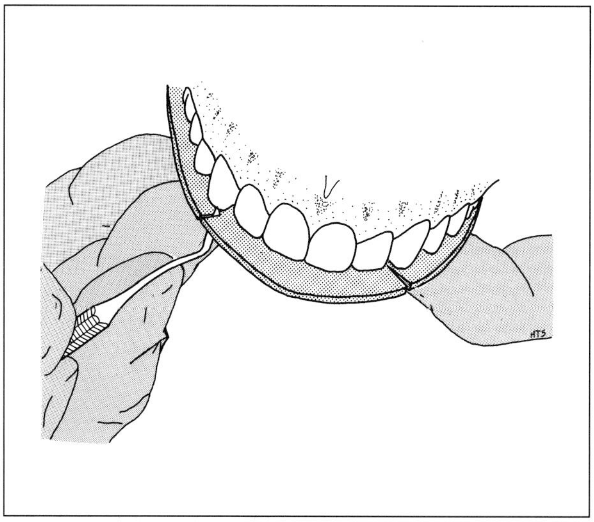

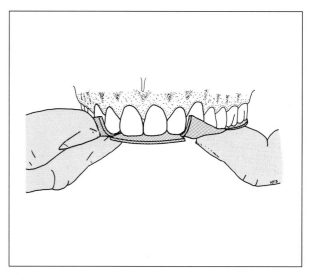

Fig 4-6 Cuts are placed between the lateral incisor and canine on each side.

lower border of the mandible, making sure that the fingertips are in direct contact with bone (Fig 4-1).

Place the thumbs lightly over the mandibular symphysis so that they touch each other at the midline. Instruct the patient to open approximately 35 mm, and then ask him or her to relax the jaw as you close it, guiding the mandible posteriorly into a terminal hinge relationship with a gentle motion (Fig 4-2). Observation of the patient's mandible will demonstrate that it shifts posteriorly with this gentle motion.

When the mandible has "dropped back," firm pressure is applied to seat the condyles anterosuperiorly in the glenoid fossae (centric relation). An upward lifting force is applied on the inferior border of the mandible by the fingers of each hand, while a downward force is applied to the symphysis by the thumbs (Fig 4-3). With firm seating pressure, once again open and close the mandible in small increments of 2.0 to 5.0 mm while gradually closing the mandible to the point of first tooth contact. Do not allow the mandible to deviate from this arc while closing. This position of initial tooth contact with the mandible in the optimum position is the *centric relation contact position* (*CRCP*).

Trim a piece of hard, pink baseplate wax to an arch form, using the template as a guide (Fig 4-4). Minor modifications to make it fit the arch may be necessary after the first try-in. Soften this preformed piece of baseplate wax in hot tap water. Place it against the maxillary arch so that the anterior teeth are approximately 6.0 mm (1/4 inch) inside the periphery of the wax. Carefully but firmly apply finger pressure along the inferior surface of the softened wax so that indentations of all of the maxillary cusp tips will be registered in the wax (Fig 4-5).

Use a Hollenback carver or similar instrument to place a cut in the wax extending from the periphery of the wax sheet to the embrasure between the maxillary lateral

Fig 4-7 Orientation tabs are folded over the labial surfaces of both canines.

incisor and canine on each side (Fig 4-6). Fold the wax distal to the cuts onto the facial surfaces of the canines (Fig 4-7). These tabs will serve as an index to aid in reseating the baseplate wax record later.

Remove the wax record from the mouth while it is still soft. Extend the initial cuts with scissors so that a wedge-shaped piece of wax is removed (Fig 4-8). This will produce space for the compound occlusal programmer later when the wax is reinserted in the mouth. Narrow the wax arch form in its buccolingual dimension by trimming away any wax that lies buccal to the buccal cusp tips from the second molar to the first premolar (Fig 4-9). Take

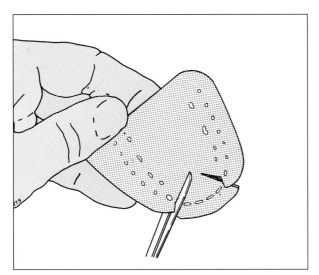

Fig 4-8 The cuts between the lateral incisors and canines are extended to remove an anterior wedge.

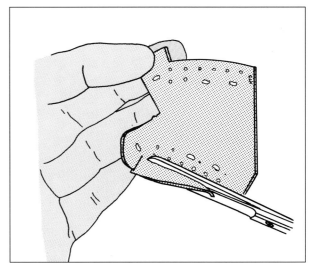

Fig 4-9 Excess wax outside the buccal cusp tips is trimmed.

care to retain the tabs that were folded onto the labial surfaces of the canines. Remove any excess wax distal to the second molars.

Lightly adapt a piece of 28-gauge green wax over both quadrants of the maxillary teeth and again manipulate the mandible to centric relation. At this position, tap the teeth together lightly until perforations are made in the wax at CRCP. Remove and store the wax in a cup of cool water.

An anterior programming device, or jig, is made to establish a predetermined stop to vertical closure with the condyles in optimum position.[2] The absence of deflecting incline tooth contact allows muscle function to be reprogrammed to eliminate the adaptive arc of closure. Soften a 2.5-cm (1.0-inch) length of green stick compound in hot tap water and bend it into a "J." Place the compound over the midline between the two maxillary central incisors with the short leg of the "J" on the facial surface, extending approximately halfway between the incisal edge and the gingiva. While the compound is still quite soft, quickly adapt it to the maxillary teeth in the following three-step procedure:

1. With your thumb, firmly adapt the facial portion of the compound into the labial embrasure, while at the same time thinning out the compound to an approximate thickness of 2.0 mm.
2. Place both thumbs on the facial and both index fingers on the lingual, with approximately 6.0-mm (1/4-inch) space between the tips. Squeeze tightly to mold the compound to the lingual surface (Fig 4-10).
3. While maintaining the finger posture and pressure in Step 2, push the fingertips closer together to form a spine of compound at approximately the midline. (The entire process described should take no more than a few seconds, and the compound should still be soft enough to further mold as the patient's mandible is closed into it.)

While the compound is still soft, repeat the mandibular position previously rehearsed, guiding the patient into a retruded position while arcing the mandible closed until the mandibular incisors have made an indentation in the compound and the posterior teeth are 1.0 mm out of contact. Cool the compound and confirm the accuracy of the programming device. There are two important points to be checked at this time:

1. Be certain that the condyles are in the optimum position in their fossae by lightly tapping the mandibular incisors into the compound. The patient should close precisely into the programming device with no deflection.
2. The patient must not be closed to the point of contact between the maxillary and mandibular teeth. The mandibular teeth should make contact only with the compound programming device and be no closer than 1.0 mm to the maxillary teeth anywhere.

If the patient's posture is maintained with the chair back and the chin up, the face will be parallel with the floor and a well-adapted compound programming device should stay firmly in place. If necessary, it can be held in place by the patient, using his or her index finger (Fig 4-11). It need not be removed until the centric relation registration has been completed.

With the compound anterior programming device still in place, slightly resoften the baseplate wax record and place it in position, using the canine flaps as an index for correct placement. Carefully close the patient's teeth into the programmer, and note that the pink wax has been adequately softened to allow complete closure into the programmer (Fig 4-12). Ideally, the mandibular molars should form slight indentations in the pink wax.

If the increased vertical dimension of occlusion produced by the anterior programming device is great

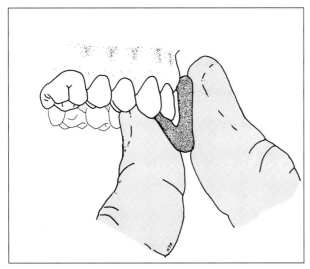

Fig 4-10 Green stick compound is molded to form the anterior programming device.

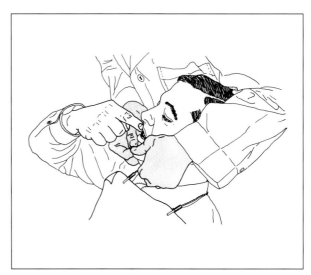

Fig 4-11 The patient holds the programming device in position while the operator manipulates the mandible.

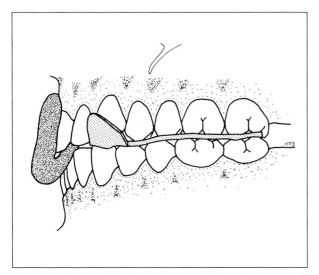

Fig 4-12 The assembled programmer and baseplate wax arch form.

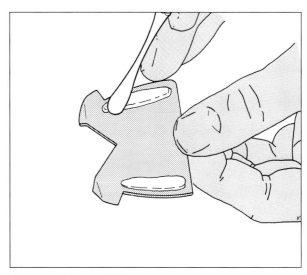

Fig 4-13 If the mandibular cusp tips do not leave indentations, the thickness of the arch form is increased with Aluwax.

enough to prevent contact of the mandibular posterior cusp tips with the pink wax, it will be necessary to flow a layer of Aluwax (Bite and Impression Wax, Aluwax Dental Products Co, Grand Rapids, MI) onto the inferior surface of the wax arch form (Fig 4-13). This will increase the thickness and insure contact of the posterior teeth with the record. Remove the wax arch form from the mouth and cool it by floating it in a cup of water. Replace it in the mouth to confirm that the wax did not distort while being cooled.

Measure out 6.0-mm (1/4-inch) lengths of zinc oxide–eugenol bite registration paste base and accelerator (Bite Registration Paste [Type I, Hard], Kerr

Manufacturing Co, Romulus, MI) on a small mixing pad. Mix thoroughly with a cement spatula (Fig 4-14). Carefully place a small amount of registration paste on the wax arch form over each area where a centric holding cusp has indented the wax (Fig 4-15). Do not place large amounts of paste into the indentations, since it will have to be removed later. The maximum allowable amount over each cusp is approximately the size of a match head.

Replace the wax in the mouth and have the patient close until the mandibular incisors are firmly contacting the programming device. Have the patient hold that position with moderate closing pressure until the registration

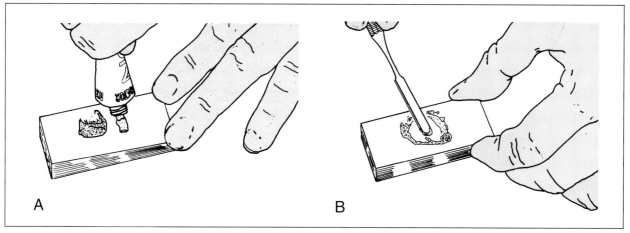

Fig 4-14 One-quarter inch (6.0-mm) lengths of bite registration paste (A) are mixed with a cement spatula (B).

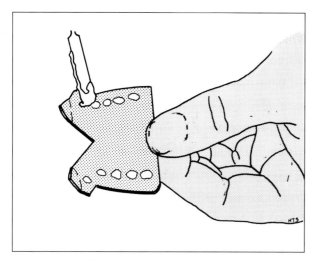

Fig 4-15 A small amount of registration paste is placed in each functional cusp tip imprint.

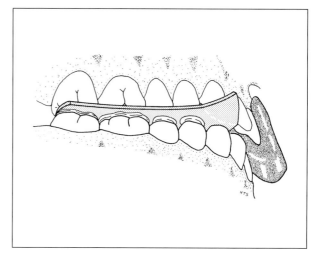

Fig 4-16 Completed interocclusal record consisting of the occlusal programming device and the paste-corrected wax arch form.

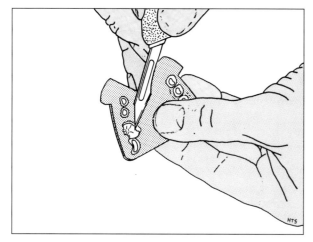

Fig 4-17 Excess registration paste is removed with a sharp knife.

paste is completely set (Fig 4-16). When it has set, remove the complete interocclusal record and compound programmer from the mouth. Use a sharp laboratory knife to remove any excess registration paste that extends more than 1.5 mm from the cusp tip in any direction (Fig 4-17). Excess paste that has spread to occlusal anatomic grooves may prevent the cast from seating completely into the record.

The success of this technique is dependent upon the use of very small quantities of bite registration paste. Because inexperienced operators have a tendency to use too large a quantity, it may be best to eliminate the use of the paste completely when introducing the technique to novices. In that case, the baseplate wax record is well adapted to the maxillary teeth, and Aluwax is placed on the underside of the baseplate wax to accommodate the cusp tips of the mandibular teeth.

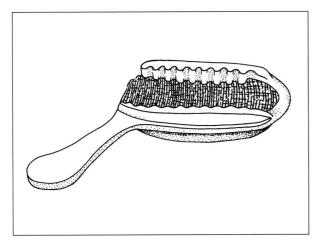

Fig 4-18 The bite registration form.

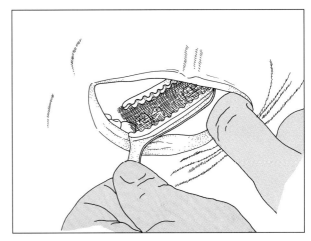

Fig 4-19 The frame is tried in the mouth over the prepared teeth.

Maximum Intercuspation Record

While diagnostic mountings are done with the condyles in a centric relation position, casts that are to be used for the fabrication of restorations for a small portion of the occlusion are attached to the articulator in a position of maximum intercuspation. Mounting them in a retruded position could result in a restoration with a built-in interference.

Armamentarium

1. Plastic registration frame
2. Scissors
3. Polyvinyl siloxane registration material
4. Impression material dispenser
5. Laboratory knife with no. 25 blade
6. Arbor band

Technique

The technique employed to index the intercuspal position for restoration fabrication produces an interocclusal record with the maxillary and mandibular teeth in total contact. Use a plastic registration frame (Triple-Bite Impression Tray, Premier, Inc, Philadelphia, PA) to carry the registration material (Fig 4-18). Try it in the mouth on the side with the prepared teeth (Fig 4-19). This will insure that the patient is able to bring the posterior teeth together completely with the frame in position. The presence of both third molars on one side of the mouth will usually preclude the use of this device. Note any area where the interarch film overlies unprepared teeth. After removing the frame from the mouth, trim away the film that covered the unprepared teeth (Fig 4-20).

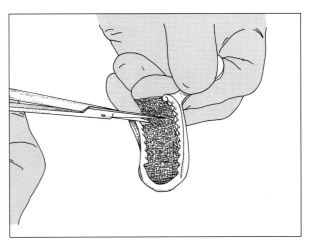

Fig 4-20 Scissors are used to remove any film that overlies unprepared teeth.

Place the twin-barrel cartridge of bite registration material (Stat B-R Registration Paste, Kerr Manufacturing Co) in the gun and lock on a new tip. Then mix the registration material by expressing it from the dispenser with steady pressure on the trigger. Apply the material evenly to both top and bottom of the frame (Fig 4-21). Do not place any in those areas where you have removed the supporting film.

Insert the loaded frame into the mouth, centering the loaded portion over the prepared tooth or teeth (Fig 4-22). Have the patient close firmly until all posterior teeth are contacting normally. Part the lips and verify that the patient has not closed in a protrusive or working relationship. Instruct the patient to keep the teeth together until asked to open. Leave the record in place for 3 minutes. Remove the tray from the mouth, rinse it under running tap water, and then dry it with an air syringe. Inspect it to insure that you have captured all of the necessary teeth (Fig 4-23). Use a laboratory knife with a no. 25 blade to

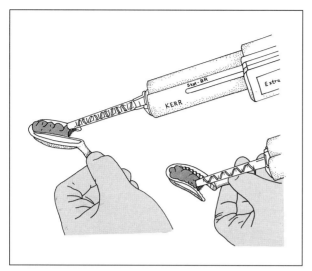

Fig 4-21 Registration paste is injected over the top and bottom of the bite registration frame.

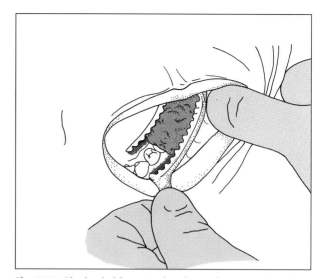

Fig 4-22 The loaded frame is placed over the prepared teeth.

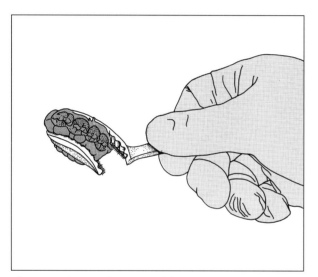

Fig 4-23 The record is inspected for completeness and detail.

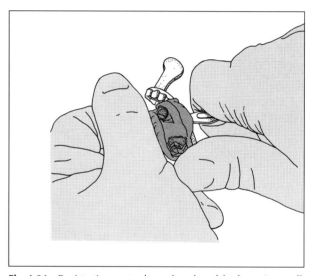

Fig 4-24 Registration paste above the edge of the frame is cut off.

cut off all excess above the edge of the frame (Fig 4-24). Cut off any material that extends over unprepared teeth adjacent to the preparation(s).

Remove excess thickness from the upper and lower surfaces of the record using an arbor band on a lathe (Fig 4-25). On the unprepared teeth opposing the preparation(s), remove enough material so that little more than the cusp tip indentations remain (Fig 4-26). Any material that reproduces edentulous ridges, gingival crevices, or the central fossae of the occlusal surfaces is likely to produce incomplete seating of a cast with imperfections in those areas, so get rid of it. The overall thickness of the record should be approximately 4.0 mm, with an equal amount having been removed from its upper and lower aspects.

So that you will be able to verify seating of the casts

into the record, cut completely through its thickness along the buccal cusps of the mandibular teeth using a laboratory knife with a no. 25 blade (Fig 4-27). Cut all the way through the posterior member of the frame and discard the facial segment of the record.

Set the record on the mandibular cast, making sure that it seats completely (Fig 4-28). Place the teeth of the maxillary cast completely into the index while articulating the teeth on the opposite side of the arch and those near the preparation(s) (Fig 4-29). At this point you will best appreciate why the registration material must be rigid and brittle. If a flexible material were used, it would distort when the casts were compressed and the resultant articulation of casts would be inaccurate. Now use the record to articulate the casts and mount the mandibular cast on the articulator (Fig 4-30).

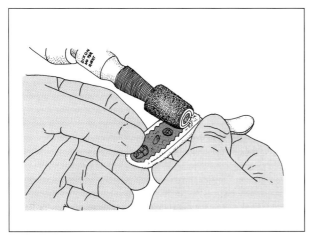

Fig 4-25 Excess thickness of the record is ground off with an arbor band.

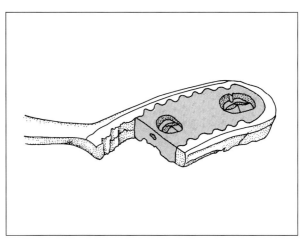

Fig 4-26 Only the imprint of cusp tips should remain on the trimmed record.

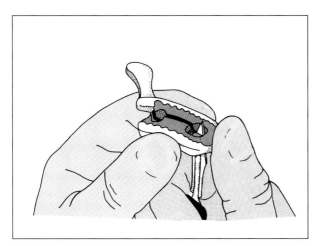

Fig 4-27 The part of the record facial to the mandibular buccal cusp tips is cut off.

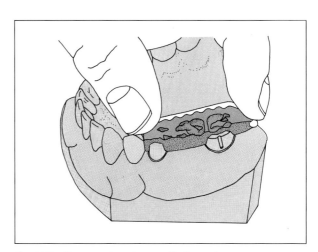

Fig 4-28 The record on the mandibular cast.

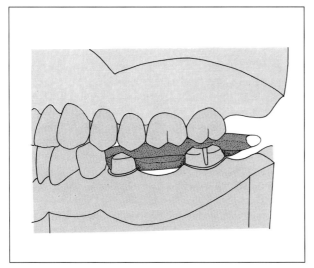

Fig 4-29 The casts are articulated with the aid of the record.

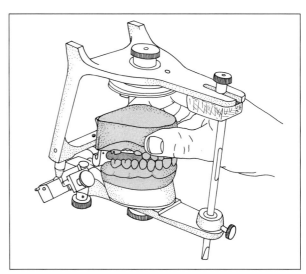

Fig 4-30 The mandibular cast is mounted on the articulator, using the record.

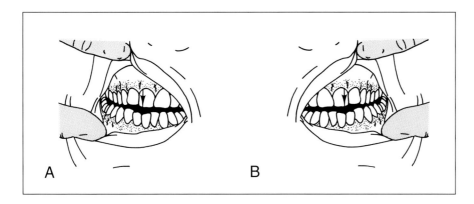

Fig 4-31 The patient is guided into working excursions on the right (A) and left (B) sides.

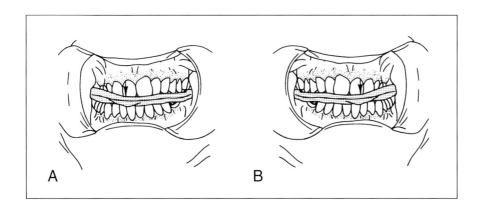

Fig 4-32 Right (A) and left (B) lateral interocclusal records are made in wax wafers.

Lateral Interocclusal Record

Lateral interocclusal records, or check bites, are made in the mouth for the purpose of capturing the position of the condyles in their respective fossae. These records are then used to set the condylar guides to approximate the anatomic limits of the temporomandibular joints. This allows the maximum benefit from using an articulator, facilitating the fabrication of accurate restorations with a minimum of time required for intraoral adjustment when the restoration is cemented.

Because the configuration of the temporomandibular joint has a strong determining influence on the movements of the mandible, the occlusal morphology of any restoration placed in the mouth must be in harmony with the movements of the mandible to prevent the initiation of occlusal disharmony and trauma. Cusp placement, cusp height, groove direction, and groove depth are all features ultimately affected by temporomandibular joint configuration.[9]

Armamentarium

1. Laboratory knife with no. 25 blade
2. Horseshoe wax wafers
3. Plaster bowl

Technique

Guide the patient into a CRCP closure and visually note the position of the lower midline in relation to the maxillary teeth. Measure and mark with a pencil the points on the maxillary teeth that would be opposite the lower midline if the patient moves the mandible 8.0 mm in both a right and left lateral excursion (Fig 4-31). With your hand on the patient's chin, have the patient open slightly. Guide the mandible approximately 8.0 mm to the right and close it until the teeth lightly touch. Explain to the patient that you are going to repeat this procedure with some wax between the teeth and that you want him or her to bite down carefully until told to stop.

Place a slightly warmed wax rim (Surgident Coprwax Bite Wafer, Miles Dental Products, South Bend, IN) against the maxillary teeth approximately 4.0 mm off center to the right. Support the wax with your hand and guide the mandible to the right. Repeat the closure practiced previously until the teeth make indentations in the wax that are approximately 1.0 mm deep (Fig 4-32). Cool the wax rim with compressed air and remove it from the mouth. Place it in a plaster bowl of cold tap water. Repeat the steps with a second wax rim for the left side.

References

1. Lucia VO: Centric relation: theory and practice. *J Prosthet Dent* 1960; 10:849–856.

2. Lucia VO: A technique for recording centric relation. *J Prosthet Dent* 1964; 14:492–505.

3. Hobo S, Iwata T: Reproducibility of mandibular centricity in three dimensions. *J Prosthet Dent* 1985; 53:649–654.

4. Williamson EH, Steimke RM, Morse PK, Swift TR: Centric relation: A comparison of muscle-determined position and operator guidance. *Am J Orthod* 1980; 77:133–145.

5. McHorris WH: Centric relation defined. *J Gnathol* 1986; 5:5–21.

6. Dawson PE: Temporomandibular joint pain dysfunction problems can be solved. *J Prosthet Dent* 1973; 29:100–112.

7. Dawson PE: *Evaluation, Diagnosis, and Treatment of Occlusal Problems.* St Louis, CV Mosby Co, 1974, p 58.

8. Perry HT: Muscular changes associated with temporomandibular joint dysfunction. *J Am Dent Assoc* 1957; 54:644–653.

9. Weinberg LA: Physiologic objective of reconstruction techniques. *J Prosthet Dent* 1960; 10:711–724.

Chapter 5

Articulation of Casts

To properly evaluate a patient's occlusion, it is mandatory that diagnostic casts be placed in an articulator in approximately the same relationship to the temporomandibular joints as exists in the patient.[1] A facebow registration is used to mount the maxillary cast on the articulator so that it is properly located both anteroposteriorly and mediolaterally.[2,3] To be used enough to make a real contribution to the improvement of quality dentistry, a facebow and articulator that possess a modicum of accuracy, are simple to assemble and use, and can be set up relatively quickly should be selected.

In a survey done in 1984, 36% of the responding North American dental schools were using a Whip Mix articulator, 32% were using an arcon Hanau (with another 25% using a nonarcon model employing the same type of condylar track mechanism), and 28% were using a Denar semiadjustable articulator.[4] The percentages add up to more than 100 because some schools use more than one articulator. Two of the three articulators described in this chapter did not exist in 1984, but they do represent the latest advances and the best features for fixed prosthodontics offered by those manufacturers at the present time. Each of the sections on a facebow–articulator combination is meant to stand alone; ie, everything the reader needs to know about the use of a system is contained in that respective section. The one exception lies in the description of a mechanical anterior guide. Although similar devices are available for all three articulators, use of the mechanical anterior guide is described only for the Hanau articulator.

Whip Mix Facebow and Articulator

The technique for the Quick Mount facebow (Whip Mix Corp, Louisville, KY) (Fig 5-1), an ear facebow that possesses the qualities previously described, is presented. Following that is the technique for the use of the Whip Mix 2200 series articulator, a semiadjustable instrument. Casts mounted on one of these articulators can be transferred accurately to another instrument of the same type

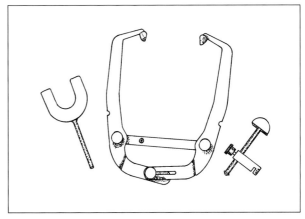

Fig 5-1 The components of a Quick Mount facebow are *(left to right)*: a bitefork, the facebow, and the nasion relator.

that has been set to the same parameters.[5] There are many advantages to this feature, including the ability to send casts to the laboratory without sending the instrument.[6]

Facebow Armamentarium

1. Quick Mount facebow (with bitefork, nasion relator, and hex driver)
2. Whip Mix articulator
3. Plaster bowl
4. Spatula
5. Laboratory knife with no. 25 blade
6. Trimmed maxillary cast
7. Pink baseplate wax
8. Mounting stone

Facebow Record

Heat a sheet of baseplate wax in hot tap water until it becomes soft and flexible. Adapt the wax to the bitefork so that it is uniformly covered. Place the wax-covered bitefork against the maxillary teeth. Center the shaft of the fork with the patient's midline. Support the bitefork

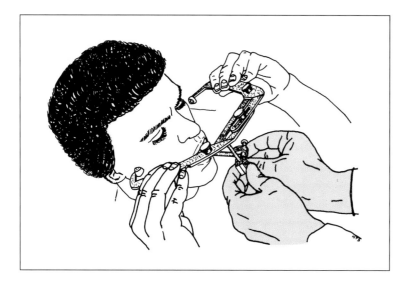

Fig 5-2 The patient guides the earpieces while the dentist inserts the bitefork shaft into the toggle under the facebow.

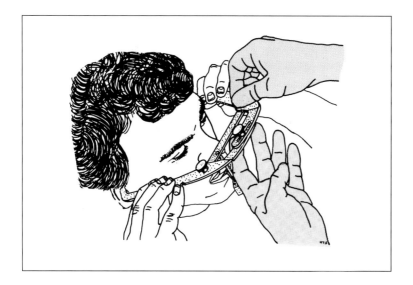

Fig 5-3 The three thumbscrews on the top of the facebow are tightened.

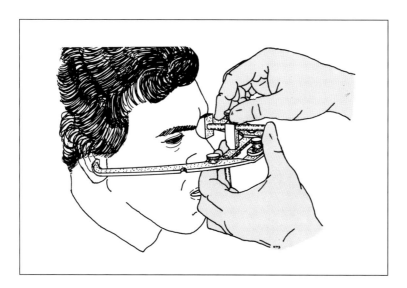

Fig 5-4 Firm pressure is placed on the end of the nasion relator and the thumbscrew is tightened.

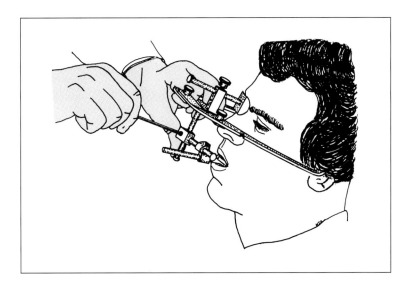

Fig 5-5 The two toggles are tightened with a hex driver or a T-screw.

and have the patient close lightly into the wax to obtain shallow impressions of only the cusp tips. Cool the wax and remove the bitefork from the mouth. Trim away excess wax. Any areas where soft tissue was registered on the wax must be completely removed.

Set the maxillary cast in the bitefork registration to confirm that the cast seats firmly in the index with no rocking or instability. If the cast does not seat, first check the occlusal surfaces of the cast to make sure there are no nodules of stone. If there are none, then either the registration or the cast is distorted and should be remade.

Place the bitefork back in the mouth and have the patient close to hold it securely between the maxillary and mandibular arches. Ask the patient to grasp both arms of the facebow and guide the plastic earpieces into the external auditory meati, much as one would guide the earpieces of a stethoscope (Fig 5-2). At the same time, the operator should slide the toggle onto the shaft of the bitefork, making certain that the toggle is positioned above the shaft. Tighten the three thumbscrews on the top of the facebow (Fig 5-3). Place the nasion relator on the transverse bar of the facebow. Extend the shaft while adjusting the facebow up or down to center the plastic nosepiece on the patient's nasion. Tighten the thumbscrew (Fig 5-4).

Support the facebow with a *firm, forward* pressure and slide the toggle lock on the bitefork shaft until it is near, but not touching, the lips. Tighten it firmly with the hex driver (Model 8600) or T-screw (Model 8645), and then tighten the toggle on the vertical bar in the same manner (Fig 5-5). For extra support and for peace of mind, the patient can hold the side arms of the facebow. Be extremely careful that the facebow does not tilt out of position in any direction during these tightening procedures. Use your free hand to stabilize the assembly against any torquing while tightening.

The patient's approximate intercondylar distance of "small," "medium," or "large" is indicated on the top of

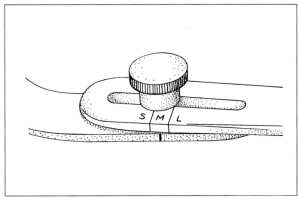

Fig 5-6 The intercondylar distance is indicated on the front of the facebow.

the front edge of the facebow (Fig 5-6). If you are using a Model 8500 articulator, this information should be recorded on the patient's data record to aid in setting the articulator later. It is not necessary for the 2200 series instrument shown here, because it has a permanent non-adjustable intercondylar width of 110 mm. This corresponds to the "M" width shown on the facebow.

Loosen the thumbscrew and remove the plastic nasion relator. Then loosen the three thumbscrews on the top surface of the facebow by one-quarter turn. As the patient slowly opens the mouth, carefully remove the entire assembly from the head. Recheck and securely tighten the toggles. It is sometimes difficult to adequately tighten these toggles while the facebow is on the patient's head.

Mounting the Maxillary Cast

Prepare the articulator to receive the cast. Separate the upper and lower members of the articulator. Set the

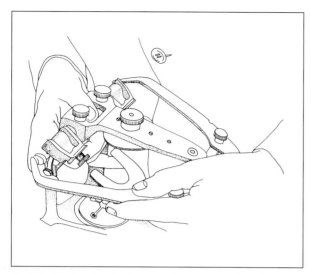

Fig 5-7 The facebow is placed on the upper member of the articulator.

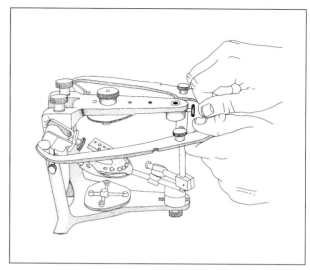

Fig 5-8 The three thumbscrews on the facebow are tightened. The incisal guide pin has been removed.

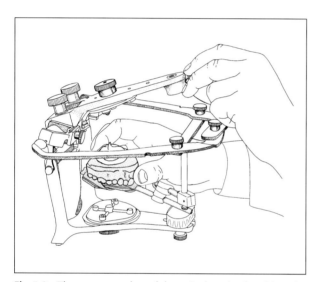

Fig 5-9 The upper member of the articulator is closed into the mounting stone on the maxillary cast.

condylar guides at "FB" in preparation for attachment of the facebow. If your articulator does not have this setting, adjust the guides to an angulation of 30 degrees. Firmly secure clean mounting plates to the upper and lower members of the articulator. Remove the incisal guide pin. The three thumbscrews on the top of the facebow should be slightly loose for the next step. Hold the facebow in one hand and the upper member of the articulator in the other. Guide first one and then the other pin on the outer surfaces of the condylar guides into the holes on the inner surfaces of the plastic earpieces. Hold the facebow against your body while you are doing this (Fig 5-7). Allow the front end of the member of the articulator to rest on the transverse bar of the facebow.

An indirect transfer assembly, which can be removed from the facebow and attached to a transfer base mounted on the articulator base, is available. This permits the facebow to be used on another patient even if the casts for this patient have not yet been mounted.

Hold the facebow firmly against the upper frame and tighten the three thumbscrews on the facebow. Place the upper frame and attached facebow back onto the lower frame of the articulator with the fork toggle of the facebow resting on the plastic incisal guide block (Fig 5-8).

Soak the maxillary cast, tooth side up, in a plaster bowl. There should not be enough water to cover the teeth. Carefully seat the cast into the bitefork registration. Mix mounting stone (Whip Mix Corp) to a thick, creamy consistency. Lift the upper frame of the articulator and apply a golf-ball-sized mound of stone to the base of the cast. Use one hand for support to prevent any movement of the facebow fork or cast, and close the upper frame down until it touches the transverse bar of the facebow (Fig 5-9). This will force the mounting plate into the soft mounting stone.

The mounting stone should engage undercuts on the base of the cast and the mounting plate. If necessary, add more mounting stone into these areas to insure adequate retention for the mounting. When the stone has completely set, remove the facebow from the articulator.

Mounting the Mandibular Cast

Replace the incisal guide pin in the upper frame of the articulator with the rounded end down and set at a 2.0-mm opening. (Align the second mark above the circumferential line of the pin with the top edge of the bushing.) Adjust the plastic incisal guide block slightly so that the pin will rest in the dimple. This compensates for lengthening the straight incisal pin. Snap the centric latch closed at the rear center of the articulator (Fig 5-10).

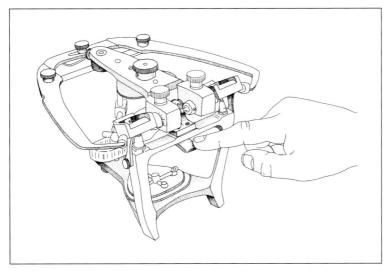

Fig 5-10 To hold the condyles in a retruded position, the centric latch is snapped closed.

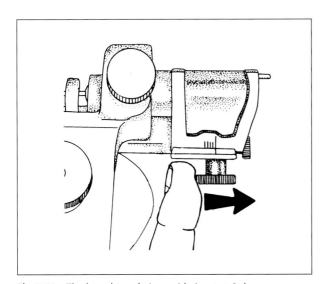

Fig 5-11 The lateral translation guide is set at 0 degrees.

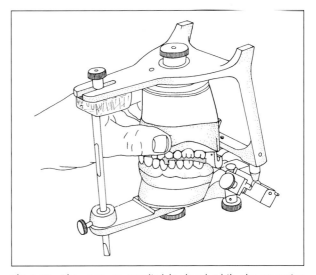

Fig 5-12 The casts are steadied by hand while the mounting stone sets.

Secure the bilateral elastic straps to the lateral, or outer, aspects of the vertical posts of the base frame, using the thumb holding screws attached to the straps.

Place the upper frame of the articulator (with maxillary cast attached) upside down on the laboratory bench with the incisal guide pin extending over the front edge of the bench. Set the centric relation interocclusal record on the maxillary cast. The teeth should seat completely into the depressions in the record.

Now position the mandibular cast in the interocclusal record and confirm that the teeth are fully seated. The maxillary and mandibular casts should not contact anywhere. Remove the mandibular cast and soak it, tooth side up, in a plaster bowl for approximately 2 minutes. There should not be enough water in the bowl to cover the teeth. Move the immediate lateral translation guide on the front of each condylar guide outward to a setting of "0" (Fig 5-11). This will prevent any lateral movement during mounting of the mandibular cast.

After the cast has soaked, reseat it into the record. Mix mounting stone to the consistency of thick cream and place a golf-ball-sized mound of stone on the bottom of the cast. Apply a small portion of stone to the mounting plate on the lower frame, and hinge the lower frame down into the soft stone until contact is made between the incisal guide pin and the incisal guide block. Hold the mandibular cast with your fingers to steady it in the interocclusal record until the mounting stone has set (Fig 5-12).

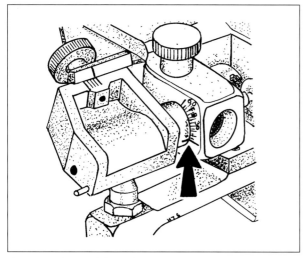

Fig 5-13 The condylar inclination is set at 0 degrees.

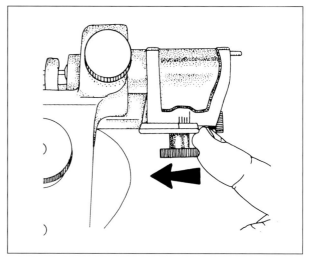

Fig 5-14 The lateral translation controls are set at maximum opening.

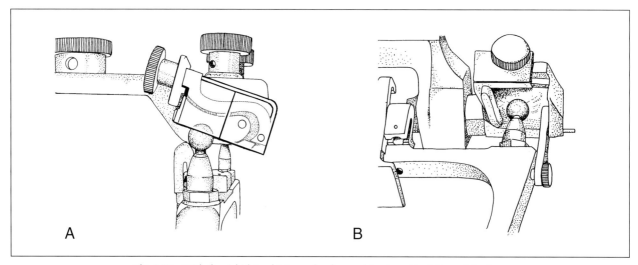

Fig 5-15 With the right lateral interocclusal record in place, the left condyle does not contact the superior wall (A) or the medial wall (B) of the guide.

Check these features:

1. Each condylar element should be against the posterior and superior walls of its condylar guide.
2. The maxillary and mandibular casts should be completely seated in the interocclusal record.
3. The mounting stone should be engaged in the undercuts on both the base of the cast and on the mounting plate.

Allow the mounting stone to set completely. Then confirm the mounting accuracy by opening the articulator, removing the interocclusal record, and raising the incisal guide pin 2.5 cm (1 inch). Place a 5.0-cm (2-inch) strip of no. 10 red-inked silk ribbon between the posterior teeth on both sides and lightly tap the teeth with the condyles retruded. This will leave red dots at CRCP.

Remove the pieces of 28-gauge green wax from the storage cup and carefully place them over the maxillary cast. If the red dots show through the perforations in the wax, the accuracy of the mounting procedure has been confirmed. If they do not show through, recheck the procedure and correct the error.

Remove both casts, with their respective mounting plates, from the articulator. Mix more mounting stone and fill all voids between the casts and mounting plates. Use your finger to smooth over the mounting stone to give it a neat appearance. There must be no stone on the surface of the mounting plate that contacts the articulator frame. The neatness of the casts (or the absence of same) will be interpreted by the technician and the patient as indicators of how much you care about the work that you are doing.

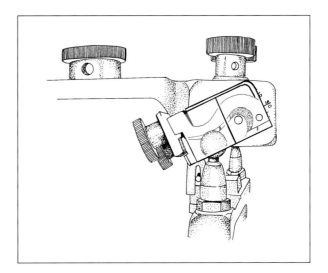

Fig 5-16 The condylar inclination is increased until the condyle contacts the superior wall of the guide.

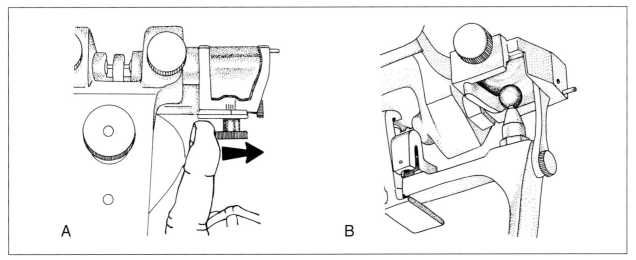

A   B

Fig 5-17 The medial wall of the guide (A) is moved until it contacts the condyle (B).

Setting Condylar Guidance

Loosen slightly the medial pair of thumb clamp screws on the top or back side of the upper frame of the articulator. Set both condylar guides at 0 degrees (Fig 5-13). Now loosen the lateral translation clamp screws on the forward aspect of each condylar guide and set the immediate lateral translation controls at their most open position (Fig 5-14). Raise the incisal guide pin so that it will not touch the plastic incisal stop in any position.

Invert the upper frame, with cast attached, and seat the right lateral interocclusal record on the teeth of the maxillary cast. Be sure that the teeth seat completely in the wax indentations. Hold the upper frame in your left hand and place the right condylar element in the right condylar guide. Gently position the teeth of the mandibu-

lar cast in the indentations of the wax record. Be sure they are seated completely. Support the articulator in this position with one hand on the right side. Notice that the left condylar element has moved downward, forward, and inward. It is not touching the condylar guide at any point (Fig 5-15).

Set the inclination of the left guide by releasing its clamp screw. Rotate the guide inferiorly until the superior wall again touches the condylar element (Fig 5-16). Tighten the holding screw. Accommodate mandibular lateral translation by releasing the lateral translation clamp screw and sliding the lateral translation guide laterally until it touches the medial surface of the condylar element (Fig 5-17). Retighten the clamp screw. Set the right condylar guidance by using the record for the left lateral excursion and repeating these steps.

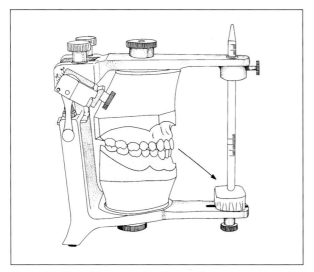

Fig 5-18 The guidance provided by anterior teeth can be recorded in acrylic resin on the incisal guide block.

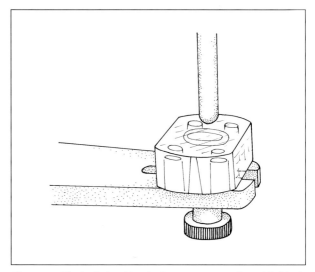

Fig 5-19 The incisal guide pin does not contact the guide block.

Once the lateral interocclusal records have been made for the diagnostic mounting and the articulator has been set, the data are recorded on the patient's information card. On the patient's casts, mark the correct articulator settings for each side. *Example:* A condylar inclination of 40 degrees and a lateral translation of 0.3 mm would be recorded as 40/0.3. When teeth are prepared at some future date and working casts are mounted on the articulator, it will not be necessary to make new lateral interocclusal records. The recorded information from the diagnostic mounting can be used to set the instrument.

Anterior Guidance

The influence of the temporomandibular joint on the occlusal scheme has been noted. The use of lateral interocclusal records in the setting of the condylar guides enables us to transfer some of the influence from the temporomandibular joint to the semiadjustable articulator. The influence of the incisors and canines (ie, anterior guidance) on the occlusion during excursive movements must also be taken into account.[7,8]

The guidance given to mandibular movements by the anterior teeth can be recorded and made part of the setting of the articulator (Fig 5-18). Anterior guidance can, in effect, be transferred from the teeth to the incisal guide block of the articulator. If crowns restoring the lingual contours of the anterior teeth are to be placed, it is extremely important that the anterior guidance be registered on the articulator. If this is not done, restorations may be made whose lingual contours or length will not provide anterior guidance.

The mounted casts should be examined on the articulator to assess the anterior guidance. If there are nonworking interferences on the casts, remove them to enable the articulator to move freely while maintaining contact between the anterior teeth. Examine the anterior guidance to determine its adequacy. If it is not adequate because of wear, fracture, or missing teeth, restore it to an optimum form with inlay wax or denture teeth on the cast.

Raise the incisal guide pin (round end down) so that it will miss contacting the plastic incisal guide by at least 1.0 mm in all excursions (Fig 5-19). Place one or two drops of monomer on the plastic incisal guide. Mix one-half scoop of tray acrylic resin in a paper cup. While it still flows freely, place a small amount on the incisal guide. As the uncured acrylic resin develops more body, add additional material to the block until there is approximately 6.0 mm (1/4 inch) of resin on the plastic incisal guide (Fig 5-20).

Lubricate the round end of the incisal guide pin and the functioning surfaces of the anterior teeth with petrolatum. Close the articulator into full occlusion so that the guide pin penetrates into the soft tray resin (Fig 5-21). Move the articulator repeatedly through all the mandibular movements, making sure that the anterior teeth remain in contact at all times (Fig 5-22). The tip of the incisal guide pin molds the acrylic resin to conform to the various movements. Continue moving the articulator through all the excursions until the tray resin has polymerized.

Trim off excess resin after it has polymerized. The tip of the guide pin has acted as a stylus in forming a registration of the anterior guidance (Fig 5-23). It will now be possible to duplicate the influence of the anterior teeth on the movements of the casts, even if the anterior teeth are prepared and the incisal edges shortened.

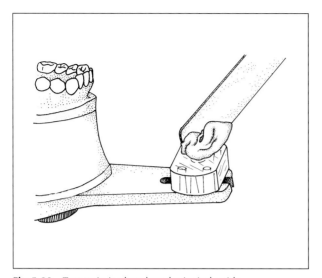

Fig 5-20 Tray resin is placed on the incisal guide.

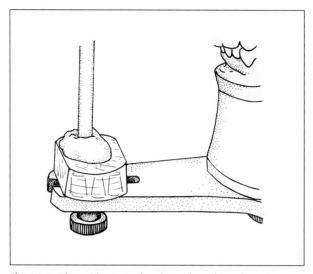

Fig 5-21 The guide pin is closed into the soft acrylic resin.

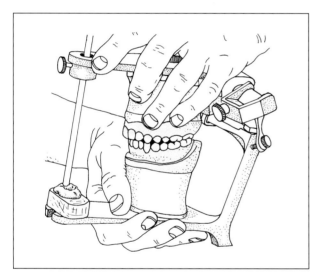

Fig 5-22 The articulator is moved through all excursions.

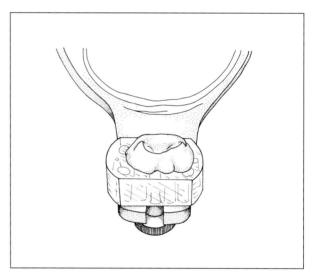

Fig 5-23 An anterior guidance record has been formed on the guide block.

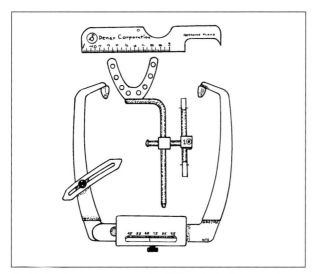

Fig 5-24 The components of a Slidematic facebow are *(top to bottom)*: a reference plane indicator, the bitefork assembly, and the facebow with pointer.

Denar Facebow and Articulator

The Denar Slidematic facebow (Teledyne Water Pik, Fort Collins, CO) is another self-centering ear facebow that is easy to use (Fig 5-24). The technique for its use is described with the Mark II articulator, an arcon semiadjustable articulator. This articulator also allows interchangeability of articulated casts with other Mark II articulators without a loss of accuracy.

Facebow Armamentarium

1. Slidematic facebow (with bitefork, articulator index, reference pin, and reference plane indicator)
2. Felt-tip marker
3. Denar Mark II articulator
4. Plaster bowl
5. Spatula
6. Laboratory knife with no. 25 blade
7. Trimmed maxillary cast
8. Pink baseplate wax
9. Mounting stone

Facebow Record

Use the reference plane indicator to measure a point 43 mm above the incisal edges of the maxillary incisors on the right side. Mark this point with a felt-tip marker (Fig 5-25). This will form the anterior, or third, reference point for the facebow transfer.

Heat a sheet of baseplate wax in a bowl of hot water until it can be easily molded. Adapt the wax to the bitefork to cover all portions of it. Place the wax-covered bitefork between the teeth, with the bitefork shaft to the patient's right. Center the fork by aligning the index ring on the fork with the patient's midline. Instruct the patient to bite lightly into the wax to produce shallow indentations of the cusp tips in the wax. Cool the wax and remove the bitefork from the mouth. Trim any excess wax off the bitefork.

Try the maxillary cast in the wax record to insure that it will seat without rocking. If the cast fails to seat, check the occlusal surfaces of the cast for nodules of stone. If none are evident, there is a distortion in the registration or the cast.

Fasten the reference pin to the underside of the facebow by tightening the set screw with a hex driver (Fig 5-26). Recent models have finger screws rather than set screws. The clamp marked "2" should be on the patient's right (your left as you look at the front of the instrument).

Place the bitefork in the mouth and have the patient hold it securely between the maxillary and mandibular teeth. The patient should grip both arms of the facebow to guide the plastic earpieces into the external auditory meati, in the same manner as one would place a stethoscope into the ears (Fig 5-27). While the patient is inserting the earpieces, the operator should slide the clamp marked "2" onto the shaft of the bitefork. The clamp should be positioned above the shaft. Tighten the single finger screw on the front of the facebow (Fig 5-28).

Extend the anterior reference pointer while moving the facebow up or down. When the pointer is properly aligned with the anterior reference point, tighten the finger screw (Fig 5-29). While continuing to support the facebow, tighten the set screw on clamp "1" on the vertical reference pin with a hex driver (Fig 5-30). Then tighten clamp "2" on the horizontal reference pin. For added stability and peace of mind, the patient can continue to support the facebow by holding the side arms. Do not allow the facebow to torque or tilt during the tightening procedure.

Loosen the finger screw on the front of the facebow by a quarter turn. As the patient opens the mouth, remove the assembly from the head. Recheck and tighten the clamps with a hex driver. Remove the bitefork assembly from the underside of the facebow by loosening the set screw on the clamp by a quarter turn. Only the bitefork assembly need be used for mounting the maxillary cast. The facebow is ready for use on another patient.

Mounting the Maxillary Cast

Remove the incisal guide block from the articulator and replace it with the articulator index (Fig 5-31). Insert the vertical reference pin of the bitefork assembly into the hole on the top of the articulator index. The reference pin has a flat side, which will match a flat side on the hole.

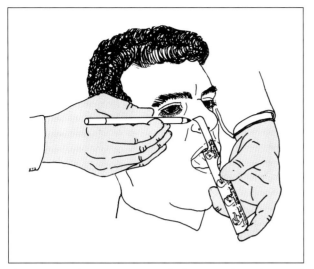

Fig 5-25 A reference point is marked 43 mm above the incisal edges of the maxillary teeth.

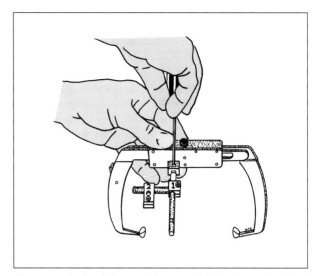

Fig 5-26 The bitefork assembly is attached to the underside of the facebow.

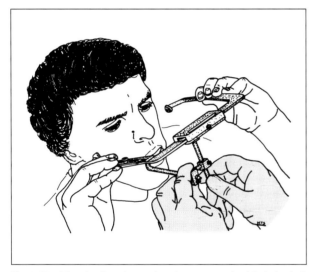

Fig 5-27 The dentist places the clamp over the bitefork shaft while the patient inserts the earpieces.

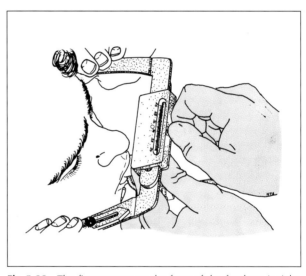

Fig 5-28 The finger screw on the front of the facebow is tightened.

Check to be sure that the numbers "1" and "2" on the clamps of the bitefork assembly are upright. Use a hex driver to tighten the set screw in the front of the index.

Secure clean mounting plates to the upper and lower members of the articulator. Assemble the articulator by placing the fossae over the condyles. Place the incisal pin at the zero position. The long incisal pin for the dimpled guide block will rest in the recessed center of the index. The short pin used for flat guide blocks will contact the sliding metal piece in the middle of the index. The incisal pin with the adjustable foot sits on the posterior section of the index. Remove the upper member of the articulator and set it on the benchtop, with the mounting plate up.

Soak the maxillary cast, tooth side up, in a plaster bowl containing only enough water to wet the sides and bottom of the cast. Seat the cast into the wax registration on the bitefork (Fig 5-32). Mix mounting stone (Whip Mix Corp) to the consistency of thick cream. Apply a golfball-sized mound of stone to the base of the cast and the mounting plate. Assemble the articulator by placing the fossae over the condyles. Close the upper member of the articulator into the soft mounting stone until the incisal guide pin contacts the appropriate spot on the articulator index. Lock the centric latch by pushing it into the down position.

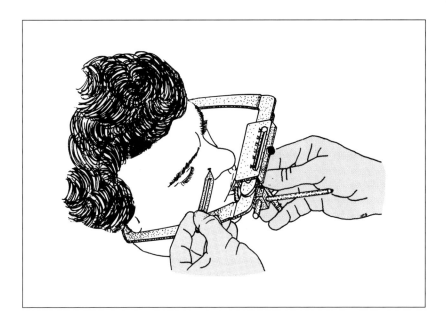

Fig 5-29 The facebow is supported with one hand and extend the reference pointer with the other.

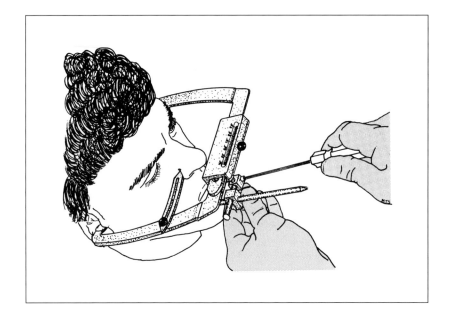

Fig 5-30 The clamps in the facebow assembly are tightened.

The mounting stone will engage undercuts in the mounting plate and cast. Additional stone can be added if needed to secure the mounting. When the stone has set completely, remove the transfer jig from the articulator. Replace the incisal guide block in the articulator.

Mounting the Mandibular Cast

Adjust the incisal pin for a 2.0-mm opening to accommodate the thickness of the interocclusal record. Invert the articulator with the attached maxillary cast, making sure

that the centric latch is engaged. Place the centric relation interocclusal wax record on the maxillary cast. Check to insure that the teeth seat completely into the record.

Place the mandibular cast into the interocclusal record and make sure that the teeth are fully seated. There should be no contact between the maxillary and mandibular casts. Remove the mandibular cast and soak the bottom and sides of it in a partially filled bowl of water for about 2 minutes.

Reseat the soaked mandibular cast into the interocclusal wax record. Mix some mounting stone to a thick, creamy consistency and place a mound of stone on the inverted bottom of the cast. Apply some mounting stone

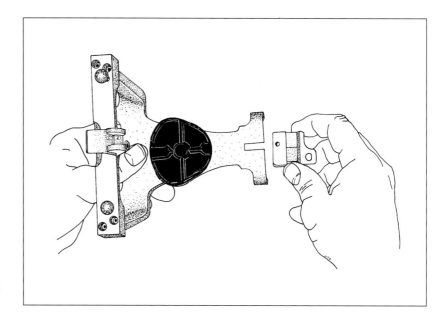

Fig 5-31 The articulator index is placed on the lower member of the articulator.

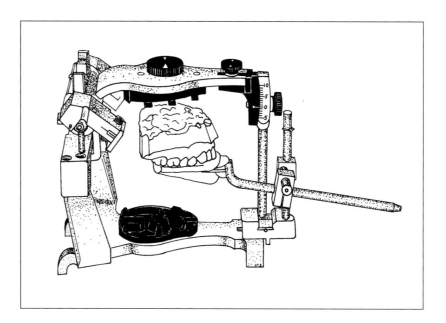

Fig 5-32 The maxillary cast in the bitefork is positioned by the articulator index.

to the mounting plate on the lower member of the articulator and hinge it down into the soft stone on the cast until the incisal guide pin makes firm contact with the incisal guide block. Stabilize the mandibular cast with your fingers to keep it securely in the interocclusal record until the mounting stone sets (Fig 5-33). Rubber bands or sticky wax can also be used, but they are more likely to slip and produce a mounting error.

Examine the casts and articulator for the following:

1. The condyle is located against the posterior and superior walls of the condylar guide.
2. Both casts are completely seated in the interocclusal record.

3. Mounting stone engages undercuts on both the base of the cast and the mounting plate.

When the mounting stone has set completely, confirm the accuracy of the mounting. Open the articulator, remove the interocclusal record, and raise the incisal guide pins 1 inch. Place a 2-inch piece of no. 10 red-inked silk ribbon between the posterior teeth on both sides. Tap the teeth together lightly with the condyles against the posterior wall of the condylar guide, leaving red dots that represent the contacts at centric relation position.

Retrieve the pieces of 28-gauge green wax that have been stored in a cup and lightly place them on the teeth

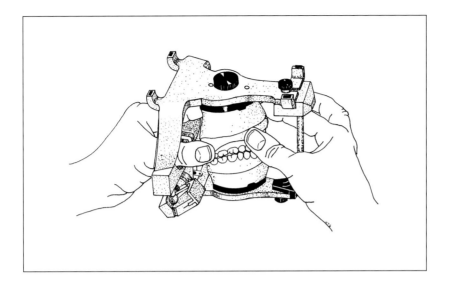

Fig 5-33 The cast is held in the interocclusal wax record until the mounting stone sets.

of the maxillary cast. The accuracy of the mounting will be confirmed if the red dots are visible through the perforations in the wax. If they are not visible, the procedure should be rechecked and the error corrected.

Remove the casts and their mounting plates from the articulator. Mix additional mounting stone to fill any voids between the casts and their mounting plates. Smooth the mounting stone with your finger to give it a neat appearance. No stone should remain on the surface of the mounting plate that will contact the articulator frame. Both the dental technician and the patient will form an impression of you when they see these casts on the articulator. Make sure that it is a positive one.

Setting Condylar Guidance

With a hex driver, loosen the set screw on the underside of each fossa and set the medial side wall to a 6-degree progressive lateral translation. Release the lock screw on each end of the posterior aspect of the upper crossbar of the articulator using a hex driver and set both condylar guides at 0 degrees. Then loosen the set screw on the top of each fossa as far as possible to the medial. Lift the incisal guide pin to prevent it from touching the plastic incisal stop in any position. Release the centric latch.

Seat the right lateral interocclusal record on the maxillary cast attached to the inverted upper member of the articulator. The teeth should seat completely in the wax indentations. Hold the upper member of the articulator in the left hand and place the right condylar element in the right condylar guide. Seat the teeth of the mandibular cast gently but completely into the indentations of the wax record.

Use one hand on the right side of the articulator to support it in this position. The left condylar element will have moved downward, forward, and inward. It should not be touching the condylar guide at any point (Fig 5-34).

Increase the inclination of the right protrusive condylar path by rotating the fossa until the superior wall makes contact with the condylar element (Fig 5-35, A). Tighten the set screw on the back of the upper crossbar with a hex driver. Set the immediate lateral translation by moving the medial wall of the fossa outward or laterally until it contacts the medial surface of the condylar element (Fig 5-35, B). Retighten the set screw. The wax interocclusal record for the left lateral excursion is used to set the right condylar guidance in the same manner.

After setting the articulator, record the data on the patient's information card. Mark the articulator settings for each side on the respective side of the patient's cast. *Example:* A condylar inclination of 35 degrees and an immediate lateral translation of 0.6 mm would be recorded as 35/0.6. When teeth are prepared at some future time, working casts can be mounted on the articulator without making new records. The instrument can be reset using the recorded information from the diagnostic mounting.

Anterior Guidance

Examine the mounted casts on the articulator. Remove any nonworking interferences from the casts so that the articulator can move freely while the anterior teeth remain in contact. If the guidance is inadequate for any reason, restore it to an optimum configuration with a diagnostic wax-up.

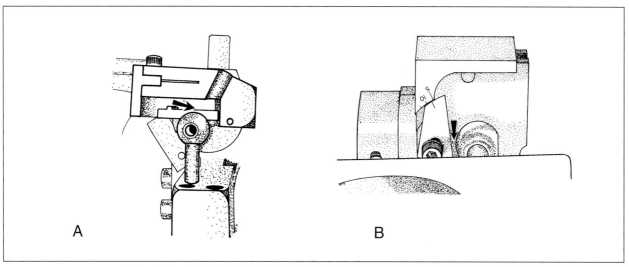

Fig 5-34 The right lateral interocclusal record causes the left condyle to move away from the superior wall (A) and the medial wall (B) of the guide.

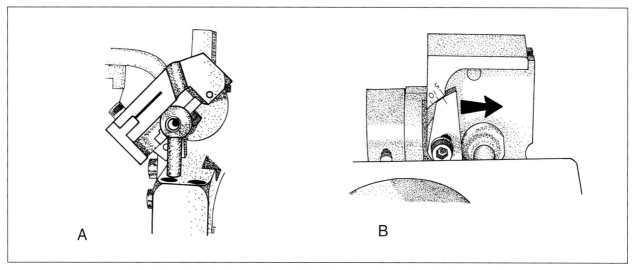

Fig 5-35 To adjust the condylar guide: (A) the condylar inclination is increased until the superior wall contacts the condyle and (B) the medial wall is moved into contact with the condyle.

Raise the incisal guide pin so that it will be at least 1.0 mm off the plastic incisal guide block in all excursions (Fig 5-36). Moisten the surface of the guide block with monomer. Mix one-half scoop of tray resin and, while it is still free-flowing, place a small amount on the incisal guide. As the polymerizing resin becomes stiffer, add more until there is about 1/4 inch of it covering the guide block (Fig 5-37). Lubricate the end of the incisal guide pin and all contacting surfaces of the anterior teeth with petrolatum. Close the articulator so that the teeth occlude completely. The guide pin will penetrate the soft acrylic resin (Fig 5-38). Move the articulator through all excursions repeatedly, keeping the teeth contacting at all times (Fig 5-39). The tip of the guide pin will mold the acrylic resin to record the pathway of the various movements. Continue the movements until the resin is completely polymerized. Trim off the excess. A record of the anterior guidance has now been formed on the incisal table (Fig 5-40).

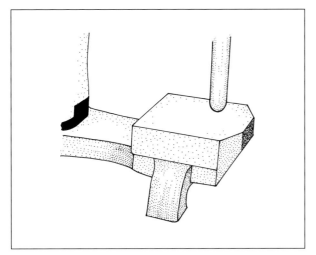

Fig 5-36 The incisal guide pin should not contact the guide block.

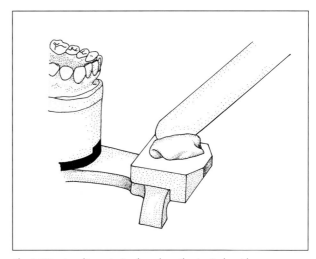

Fig 5-37 Acrylic resin is placed on the incisal guide.

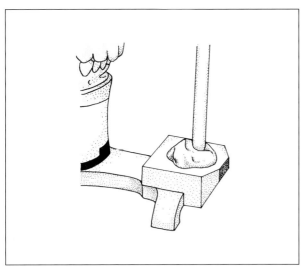

Fig 5-38 The guide pin is allowed to close into the soft resin.

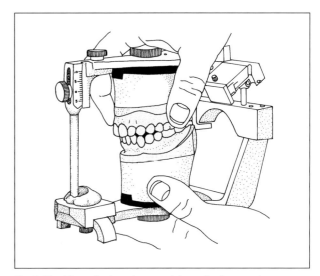

Fig 5-39 The articulator is moved through all excursions.

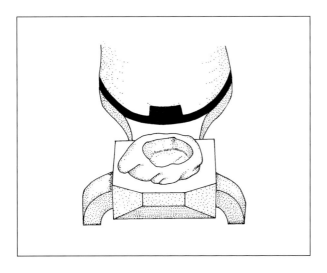

Fig 5-40 An anterior guidance record exists on the guide block.

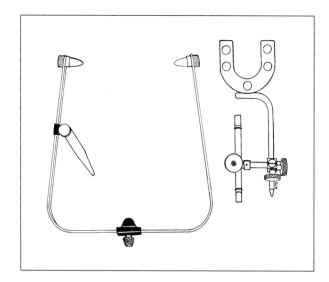

Fig 5-41 The components of a Spring-Bow are *(left to right)*: the facebow with orbital pointer and the bitefork assembly.

Hanau Facebow and Articulator

The Hanau Spring-Bow (Teledyne Water Pik, Fort Collins, CO) is an ear facebow that utilizes a one-piece spring-steel bow (Fig 5-41). It is simple in design and can be used either as a direct-mount or an indirect-mount device with the removable bitefork assembly and mounting platform.[9] The technique for its use is described with the Hanau Series 184 Wide-Vue Articulator, an arcon semi-adjustable instrument.

Facebow Armamentarium

1. Spring-Bow (with bitefork assembly and mounting guide)
2. Hanau Wide-Vue articulator
3. Plaster bowl
4. Spatula
5. Laboratory knife with no. 25 blade
6. Trimmed maxillary cast
7. Pink baseplate wax
8. Mounting stone

Facebow Record

Soften a sheet of baseplate wax in hot water and completely cover the bitefork with it. Position the wax-covered bitefork against the maxillary teeth and have the patient close until the mandibular teeth contact the wax on the underside of the fork. The shaft of the bitefork will be to the left of the patient's midline.

Cool the wax in the mouth with an air syringe. Remove the fork from the mouth and finish cooling it in a bowl of cold tap water. Trim off excess and any areas imprinted by soft tissue. Seat the maxillary cast in the wax record to be sure that it is stable. If there is any rocking of the cast, check the occlusal surfaces of the cast for nodules of stone. If there are none, either the cast or the record is distorted and must be remade.

If the bitefork assembly is separate from the facebow, insert the transfer (vertical) rod of the assembly into the bow socket on the underside of the black centerpiece on the front of the facebow. Make sure the flat surface on the front of the rod faces you as you place it in the socket. The assembly should be to your right, with the knobs facing you (Fig 5-42). Tighten the thumbscrew on the front of the centerpiece.

While the patient grips the bitefork between the maxillary and mandibular teeth, position the loosened bitefork clamp over the bitefork shaft 4.0 cm (1.5 inches). The facebow should be pointed upward during this action (Fig 5-43). Open the bow by pulling outward on the arms and swing it down into position, placing an earpiece gently into each external auditory meatus. Have the patient adjust the earpieces to the most comfortable seated position (Fig 5-44).

Mark the orbitale (infraorbital notch) on the patient's face with a felt-tip marker to provide an anterior reference point (Fig 5-45). Loosen the thumbscrew that holds the orbital pointer and gently swing it in toward the reference mark (Fig 5-46). Elevate the front of the facebow along the transfer (vertical) rod of the bitefork assembly until the pointer is at the plane of the anterior reference point. Grasp the bow to resist torquing (Fig 5-47) and tighten the three thumbscrews in order from left to right (Fig 5-48):

1. Transfer (vertical) rod/transverse (horizontal) rod

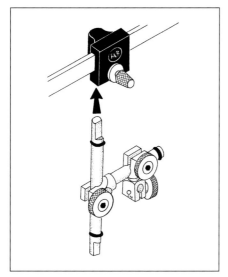

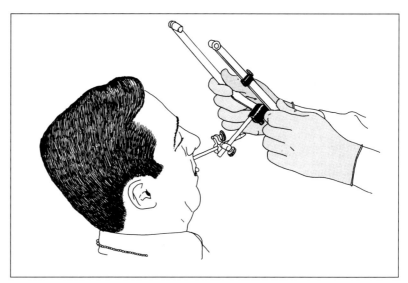

Fig 5-42 The vertical rod of the bitefork assembly is inserted into the bow socket. The flat side should face you, with the empty bitefork clamp to your right.

Fig 5-43 The bitefork clamp is slid onto the shaft.

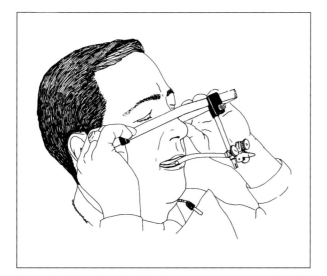

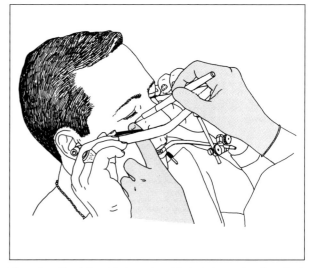

Fig 5-44 The patient should adjust the facebow for comfort. The earpieces should be checked to make sure they are still seated.

Fig 5-45 The infraorbital notch (orbitale) is located and marked.

2. Transverse rod clamp (upper)
3. Bitefork clamp (lower)

Be sure that they are tight. Use an Allen wrench if necessary.

Now rotate the reference pointer back over the right temple of the bow and tighten the thumbscrew enough to hold it there. Have the patient open while you grasp the ends of the bow and remove the earpieces from the auditory meati. Make sure that you have a firm hold, since the bow is made of spring steel and could snap back. Slide the bow away from the patient.

Mounting the Maxillary Cast

Prepare the articulator to accept the casts by setting the inclination of the enclosed condylar track mechanisms at 30 degrees on each side (Fig 5-49). The "Bennett angle" ring for the progressive mandibular lateral translation should be set at 30 degrees (Fig 5-50).

Use petrolatum to lubricate the surfaces of the upper and lower members of the articulator around the threaded mounting studs. Then firmly secure a clean mounting plate to the mounting stud on the upper member of the

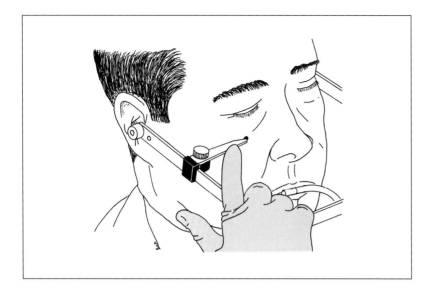

Fig 5-46 The pointer is rotated toward the reference mark.

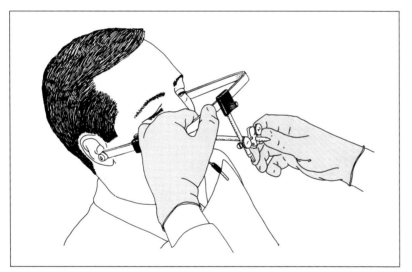

Fig 5-47 The bow is secured with one hand while tightening the thumbscrews on the bitefork assembly with the other.

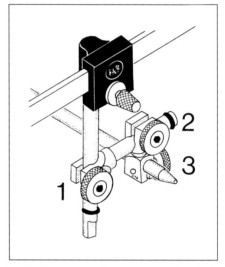

Fig 5-48 The thumbscrews are tightened in order: 1, 2, 3.

articulator. Attach a mounting guide or platform to the lower member of the articulator. Loosen the thumbscrew on the front of the facebow and remove the bitefork assembly. Place the vertical transfer rod of the assembly into the hole at the front of the mounting guide and secure it by tightening the screw. Adjust the cast support to touch the underside of the wax on the bitefork (Fig 5-51).

Soak the maxillary cast in a plaster bowl, but do not cover the teeth with water. Carefully seat the maxillary cast into the imprints in the baseplate wax on the bitefork.

Raise the upper member of the articulator and place a golf-ball-sized mound of thick, creamy mounting stone on the base of the cast. Swing the upper member of the cast down until the incisal pin is resting on the mounting guide or the anterior table, depending on the type of guide used. Be sure that stone is engaging the cutouts in the top of the mounting plate. Add more stone if necessary, and smooth off the top with a spatula. When the stone has set completely, remove the bitefork assembly and mounting guide from the articulator. Attach a clean mounting plate to the lower member of the articulator.

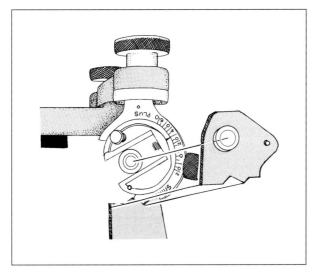

Fig 5-49 Before the facebow is attached, the condylar inclination is set at 30 degrees.

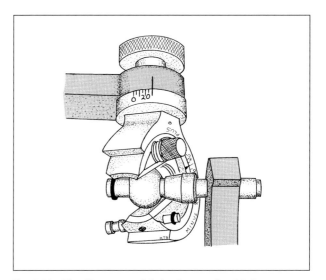

Fig 5-50 The "Bennett angle" ring is rotated to 30 degrees.

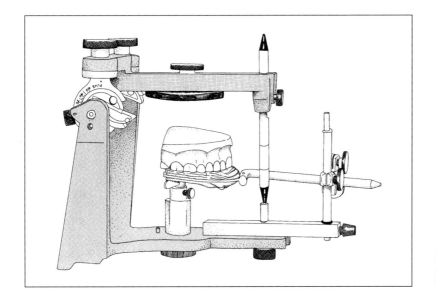

Fig 5-51 The maxillary cast is oriented to the articulator by the bitefork assembly in the mounting guide.

Mounting the Mandibular Cast

Extend the incisal guide pin 1 to 2 mm to compensate for the thickness of the interocclusal wax record. Tighten the centric lock on each enclosed condylar track mechanism to insure that the articulator is capable of nothing but a hinge opening.

Invert the articulator on the benchtop, resting it on the three thumbnuts protruding from the upper member of the articulator. Place the centric relation interocclusal wax record on the teeth of the maxillary cast. Be sure that the teeth seat completely into the wax record.

Place the mandibular cast into the interocclusal record and again confirm complete seating. There should be no contact between the maxillary and mandibular casts.

Remove the mandibular cast and soak it for about 2 minutes. To prevent any erosion of the teeth on the cast, make sure that they are not covered by water. Reseat the soaked mandibular cast into the record. Swing the lower member of the articulator up and back. Place a mound of thick, creamy mounting stone on the bottom of the cast. Apply enough to the mounting plate on the lower member to fill the cutout slots on either side of it. Hinge the lower member of the articulator back over into the soft mounting stone. The incisal guide pin should be resting firmly against the incisal guide table. Use your hand to steady the mandibular cast in the retruded position wax registration until the mounting stone has achieved an initial set (Fig 5-52).

Inspect the articulated casts:

1. The condyle is in the retruded position in its condylar track mechanism.
2. Both casts are seated completely in the interocclusal wax record.
3. Mounting stone is securely attached to both casts and mounting plates.

After the mounting stone has achieved a final set, corroborate the accuracy of the mounting. Open the articulator and raise the incisal guide pin so that it will not touch the incisal table when the teeth are contacting. Remove the interocclusal record and place a 2-inch piece of no. 10 red-inked silk ribbon between the posterior teeth on both sides. Tap the teeth together lightly, producing red marks on the teeth where they contact in the retruded position.

Retrieve the pieces of 28-gauge green wax and carefully position them on the teeth of the maxillary cast. If the cast mounting is correct, the red marks on the teeth will be visible through the perforations in the wax. If they are not visible, recheck the procedure step by step and then correct the error.

Unscrew the mounting plates and remove the casts from the articulator. Soak the plates and attached mounting stone in water. Add more mounting stone wherever it is needed to fill voids between the casts and the mounting plates. Smooth the additional stone as it sets to give it a neat appearance. Be careful not to leave any stone on the surface of the mounting plate that will contact the articulator frame. It has been said that sloppy cast mountings are not an indication of a poor operator; they are absolute proof.

Setting Condylar Guidance

Wax lateral or protrusive interocclusal records are used for setting the condylar inclination of this instrument. Loosen the thumbnut at the rear of each condylar track mechanism so that it can be easily rotated. At this time, however, leave the condylar inclination at 30 degrees. The incisal guide pin should still be raised out of contact with the incisal table.

Seat the right interocclusal record on the teeth of the mandibular cast. Gently lower the upper member of the articulator until the maxillary teeth engage the wax record. Adjust the left condylar guide by changing the condylar inclination with the thumbnut located at the rear of the guide. The teeth on the right side of the cast will rock in and out of the record. If the condylar path is too shallow, the anterior teeth will be drawn out of the wax record (Fig 5-53, A). When the path becomes too steep, the posterior teeth become unseated (Fig 5-53, B). The correct condylar inclination has been determined when the cast is seated completely in the wax record (Fig 5-53, C). Tighten the nut at the rear of the condylar guide.

Loosen the thumbnut on the top of each condylar

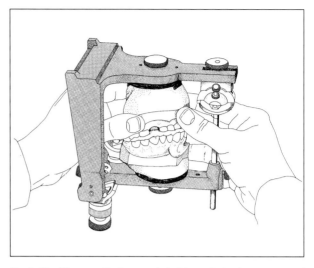

Fig 5-52 The mandibular cast is held steady in the wax record while the mounting stone sets.

guide of the articulator. Slowly rotate the "Bennett angle" ring outward (from 30 degrees toward 0 degrees) until the flat side on the outer aspect of the condylar ball contacts the inner surface of the sleeve on the condylar shaft, forming a "brass to brass" contact (Fig 5-54). Repeat the process on the right side.

If a protrusive interocclusal wax record is used to establish the condylar inclination, both condylar mechanisms are rotated simultaneously in the same manner described above for setting each condylar inclination separately. In this situation, the angle of mandibular lateral translation is estimated by use of the "Hanau Formula," $L = H/8 + 12$, where "H" is the condylar protrusive inclination. Since a change in condylar inclination from 20 to 50 degrees would produce less than a 4-degree change in the "Bennett angle" by this calculation, placing the "Bennett angle" ring at an arbitrary 15-degree angle would produce a minimal error.

Enter the condylar inclinations in the patient's record. Write the amount of condylar inclination for each condyle on the corresponding side of the cast. When teeth are prepared at some future time, it will not be necessary to make new interocclusal records to adjust the articulator. The settings developed during the diagnostic mounting can be reused.

Custom Anterior Guidance

A customized anterior guidance jig can be made for this articulator by using a round-end incisal pin and a flat anterior table or an incisal cup. Acrylic resin is molded by the end of the incisal pin in the same manner that the anterior guidance is recorded for the other articulators. Examine the mounted casts on the articulator and remove any nonworking interferences. The articulator

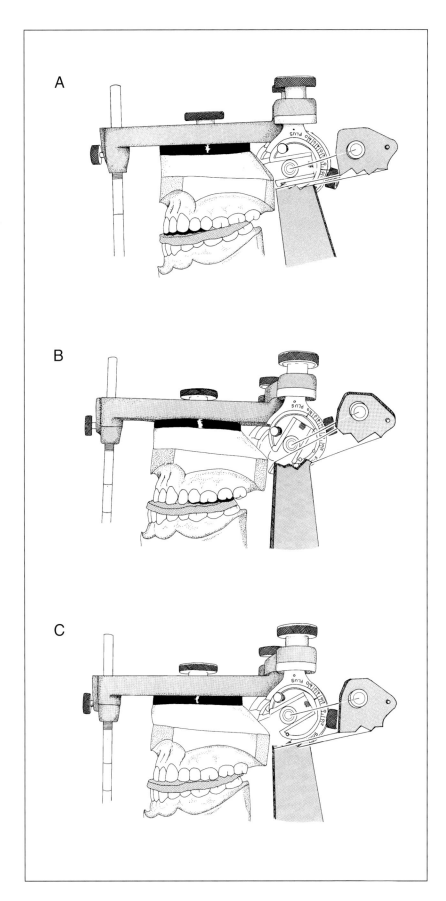

Fig 5-53 To use a protrusive interocclusal record to set the condylar guidance, the condylar inclination is rocked up and down. When the angle is too shallow, the anterior teeth lift out of the record (A). When the inclination is too steep, the posterior teeth lift out (B). When the cast is completely seated, the inclination is correct (C). When lateral interocclusal records are employed, the left record is used for the right condylar inclination and the right record for the left condylar inclination.

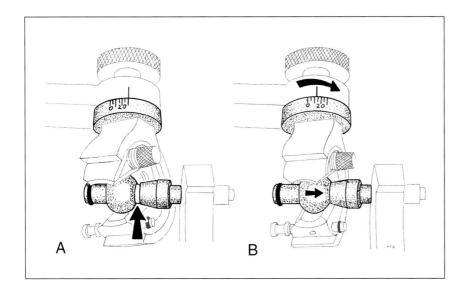

Fig 5-54 With the casts seated in a lateral interocclusal record, there is a gap between the condyle and sleeve (A). When the "Bennett angle" ring (and condylar track mechanism) are rotated, the condyle contacts the sleeve (B). The number on the scale is the angle of the lateral translation.

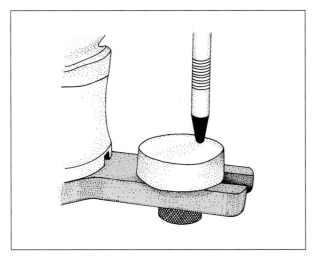

Fig 5-55 The incisal guide pin is raised 1.0 mm off the guide block.

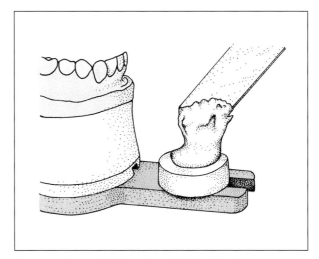

Fig 5-56 Tray resin is placed on the incisal block.

must be able to move freely with the anterior teeth in contact. If the guidance is inadequate, rebuild it to an optimum configuration with a diagnostic wax-up.

Raise the incisal guide pin at least 1.0 mm off the plastic incisal guide block in all excursions (Fig 5-55). Moisten the surface of the guide block with monomer. Mix one-half scoop of tray resin and, while it is still free-flowing, place a little on the incisal guide. As the polymerizing resin becomes stiffer, add more until there is about 6.0 mm (1/4 inch) of it covering the guide block (Fig 5-56). Lubricate the tip of the incisal guide pin and the

occluding surfaces of the anterior teeth with petrolatum. Close the articulator to complete contact between the casts. The guide pin should sink into the soft acrylic resin (Fig 5-57). Move the articulator through all excursions repeatedly, keeping the anterior teeth touching at all times (Fig 5-58). The pathways of all the movements will be imprinted by the tip of the guide pin in the acrylic resin as a permanent record (Fig 5-59). Continue moving the casts until polymerization is complete. Remove the excess.

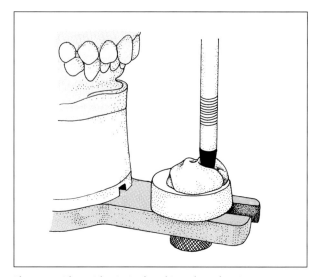

Fig 5-57 The guide pin is closed into the soft resin.

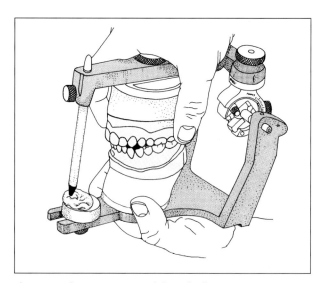

Fig 5-58 The casts are moved through all excursions.

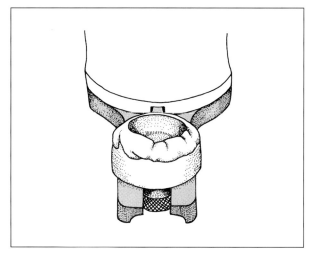

Fig 5-59 There is a custom anterior guidance record on the guide block.

Mechanical Anterior Guidance

The guidance of mandibular movement imparted by the anterior teeth also can be recorded on this instrument with a mechanical incisal guide. Examine the mounted casts. Remove any interferences from the casts that prevent the anterior teeth from remaining in contact in all excursions. Restore any inadequacies in the guidance by building up an optimum configuration in a diagnostic wax-up.

Loosen the lock nut under the incisal table at the front end of the lower member of the articulator. The incisal pin should be in contact with the incisal table.

Protect the casts from undue abrasion by lubricating contacting surfaces with petrolatum. Gently move the upper member of the articulator back to bring the maxillary and mandibular teeth into an end-to-end position. The incisal pin will be lifted off the incisal table. Rotate the incisal guide to raise it posteriorly. Stop when it makes contact with the pin (Fig 5-60, A). Tighten the lock nut to maintain this inclination of the table.

Move the casts into a right lateral excursion. The pin will move to the left side and will again be lifted off the table. Loosen the small thumbnut under the left side of the table and use the elevating screw to raise the left wing of the table into contact with the corner of the guide pin (Fig 5-60, B). Repeat the process by moving the casts into a left lateral excursion. Raise the right wing of the incisal table to contact the pin (Fig 5-60, C).

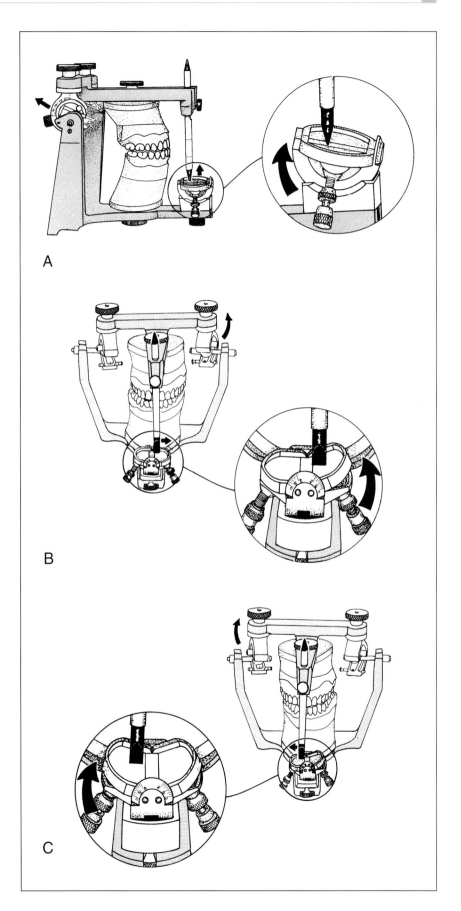

Fig 5-60 To set the mechanical incisal guide, the casts are moved into a protrusive relationship. The angulation of the table is increased to contact the pin (A). The casts are moved into a right lateral excursion and the left wing of the incisal table is raised (B). The casts are moved into a left lateral excursion and the right wing of the table is lifted to complete the recording (C).

References

1. Pruden WH: The role of study casts in diagnosis and treatment planning. *J Prosthet Dent* 1960; 10:707–710.

2. Hickey JC, Lundeen HC, Bohannan HM: A new articulator for use in teaching and general dentistry. *J Prosthet Dent* 1967; 18:425–437.

3. Teteruck WR, Lundeen HC: The accuracy of an ear facebow. *J Prosthet Dent* 1966; 16:1039–1045.

4. Gross MD, Gazit E: Articulators used in North American dental schools. *J Dent Educ* 1985; 49:710–711.

5. Cowan RD, Sanchez RA, Chappell RP, Glaros AG, Hayden WJ: Verifying the reliability of interchanging casts with semi-adjustable articulators. *Int J Prosthodont* 1991; 4:258–264.

6. Sokolow SM: Interchangeable quick-mounted study models. *J Clin Orthod* 1986; 20:779–781.

7. Weinberg LA: Physiologic objective of reconstruction techniques. *J Prosthet Dent* 1960; 10:711–724.

8. Schuyler CH: The function and importance of incisal guidance in oral rehabilitation. *J Prosthet Dent* 1963; 13:1011–1030.

9. Strohaver RA, Ryan JR: New face-bow simplifies use and dental laboratory cooperation. *J Prosthet Dent* 1988; 60:638–641.

Chapter 6

Treatment Planning for Single-Tooth Restorations

By using cast metal, ceramic, and metal-ceramic restorations, large areas of missing coronal tooth structure can be replaced while that which remains is preserved and protected. Function can be restored, and where required, a pleasing esthetic effect can be achieved. The successful use of these restorations is based on thoughtful treatment planning, which is manifested by choosing a restorative material and a restoration design that are suited to the needs of the patient. In a time when production and efficiency are heavily stressed, it should be restated that the needs of the patient take precedence over the convenience of the dentist.

In what circumstances should cemented restorations made from cast metal or ceramic be used instead of amalgam or composite resin restorations? The selection of the material and design of the restoration is based on several factors:

1. Destruction of tooth structure
2. Esthetics
3. Plaque control
4. Financial considerations
5. Retention

Destruction of tooth structure: If the amount of destruction previously suffered by the tooth to be restored is such that the remaining tooth structure must gain strength and protection from the restoration, cast metal or ceramic is indicated over amalgam or composite resin.

Esthetics: If the tooth to be restored with a cemented restoration is in a highly visible area, or if the patient is highly critical, the cosmetic effect of the restoration must be considered. Sometimes a partial veneer restoration will serve this function. Where full veneer coverage is required in such an area, the use of ceramic in some form is indicated. Metal-ceramic crowns can be used for single-unit anterior or posterior crowns, as well as for fixed partial dentures. All-ceramic crowns are most commonly used on incisors, although they can be used on posterior teeth when an adequate bulk of tooth structure has been removed and the patient is willing to accept the possibility of more frequent replacement.

Plaque control: The use of a cemented restoration demands the institution and maintenance of a good plaque-control program to increase the chances for suc-

cess of the restoration. Many teeth are seemingly prime candidates for cast metal or ceramic restorations, based solely on the amount of tooth destruction that has previously occurred. However, when these teeth are evaluated from the standpoint of the oral environment, they may, in fact, be poor risks for cemented restorations. If extensive plaque, decalcification, and caries are present in a mouth, the use of crowns of any kind should be carefully weighed. The design of a restoration should take into account those factors that will enable the patient to maintain adequate hygiene to make the restoration successful. The patient must be motivated to follow a regimen of brushing, flossing, and dietary regulation to control or eliminate the disease process responsible for destruction of tooth structure. It may be desirable to use pin-retained amalgam "temporary" restorations to save the teeth until the conditions responsible for the tooth destruction can be controlled. This will give the patient the time necessary to learn and demonstrate good oral self-care. It will also permit the dentist and staff to reinforce the skills required of the patient and to evaluate the patient's willingness and ability to cooperate. If these measures prove successful, cast metal, ceramic, or metal-ceramic restorations can be fabricated. Since these restorations are used to repair the damage caused by caries and do nothing to cure the condition responsible for the caries, they should not be used if the oral environment has not been brought under control.

Financial considerations: Finances are a factor in all treatment plans, because someone must pay for the treatment. That "someone" may be a government agency, a branch of the military, an insurance company, and/or the patient. If the patient is to pay, give your best advice and then allow the patient to make the choice. A conscientious dentist must walk a fine ethical line. On the one hand, you should not preempt the choice by selecting a less than optimum restoration just because you think that the patient cannot afford the preferred treatment. On the other hand, you also should be sensitive enough to the individual patient's situation to offer a sound alternative to the preferred treatment plan and not apply pressure.

Retention: Full veneer crowns are unquestionably the most retentive[1,2] (Fig 6-1). However, maximum retention is not nearly as important for single-tooth restorations as

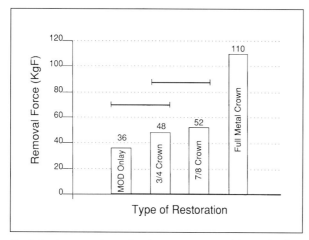

Fig 6-1 A comparison of resistance to removal forces for four types of crowns *(P* = .05).[1,2]

Glass Ionomer

Small lesions where extensions can be kept minimal and where preparation retention will be minimal can be restored with this material. It is useful for restoring class 5 lesions caused by erosion or abrasion (Fig 6-2). It also can be employed for incipient lesions on the proximal surfaces of posterior teeth by use of a "tunnel" preparation, which leaves the marginal ridge intact (Fig 6-3).

Glass ionomer has found a niche in the restoration of root caries in geriatric and periodontal patients (Fig 6-4). An occlusal approach may be precluded by the presence of an otherwise acceptable crown, or a conventional restoration at such an apical level might require the destruction of an unacceptable amount of tooth structure. However, handpiece access may be too restricted to create the needed retention for a small amalgam restoration. Glass ionomer also lends itself to rapid placement well enough to serve as an interim treatment restoration to assist in the control of a mouth with rampant caries (Fig 6-5). This is further enhanced by the release of fluoride by the material.

Composite Resin

This material can be used for minor to moderate lesions in esthetically critical areas (Fig 6-6). While it can be used in the restoration of incisal angles assisted by acid etching, a tooth that has received a class 4 resin restoration ultimately will require a crown.

Composite resin has been used in the restoration of posterior teeth with mixed results. Sufficient abrasion resistance to prevent occlusal wear has been a problem. Also, unless the resin is carefully applied in small increments, polymerization shrinkage will lead to leakage and ultimately to failure. Its use probably should be restricted to small occlusal and mesio-occlusal restorations on first premolars.

A technique devised to combat the problems of shrinkage and leakage is the fabrication of a composite resin inlay (Fig 6-7). This can be accomplished in the dental office, using a fast-setting gypsum cast, or in a dental laboratory. The resultant bench-polymerized inlay will have greater hardness, and the thin layer of resin used for affixing it to tooth structure will be less susceptible to significant shrinkage at the margin than a restoration that is bulk cured in situ.

it is for fixed partial denture retainers. It does become a special concern for short teeth and removable partial denture abutments.

Twelve restoration types are presented in the following pages to provide a frame of reference for making a decision whether to use a "plastic restoration" or a "cemented restoration." The "plastic restoration" is inserted as a soft, or plastic, mass into the cavity preparation, where it will harden and be retained by mechanical undercuts or adhesion. The "cemented restoration," made of cast metal, metal and ceramic, or ceramic material alone, is fabricated away from the operatory and is luted in or on the patient's tooth at a subsequent appointment. One type can be better suited for a particular application than the other, or their suitabilities may overlap.

Intracoronal Restorations

When sufficient coronal tooth structure exists to retain and protect a restoration under the anticipated stresses of mastication, an intracoronal restoration can be employed. In this circumstance, the crown of the tooth and the restoration itself are dependent upon the strength of the remaining tooth structure to provide structural integrity.

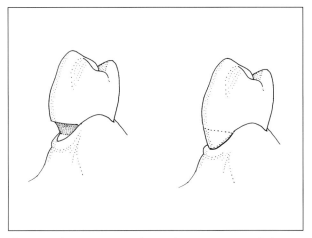

Fig 6-2 Glass ionomer can be used to restore gingival abrasion or erosion.

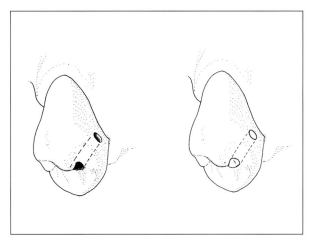

Fig 6-3 "Tunnel" preparation and glass ionomer can be used to restore an incipient lesion on the proximal surface of a posterior tooth.

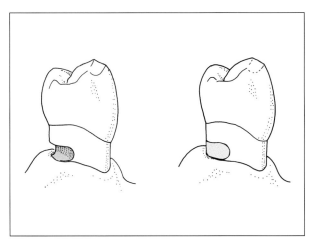

Fig 6-4 Root caries restored with glass ionomer.

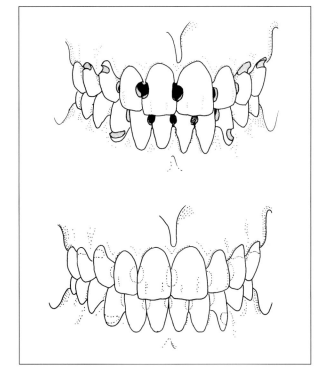

Fig 6-5 Rampant caries can be brought under control with glass ionomer.

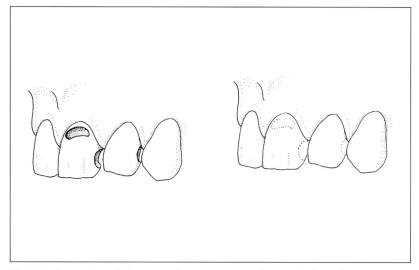

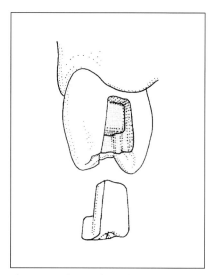

Fig 6-6 Composite resin is commonly used to restore class 3 and class 5 lesions on anterior teeth.

Fig 6-7 Indirect inlays of composite resin can be used for proximo-occlusal restorations on posterior teeth.

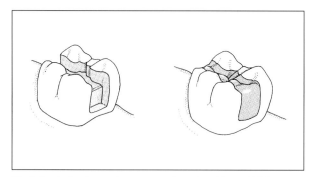

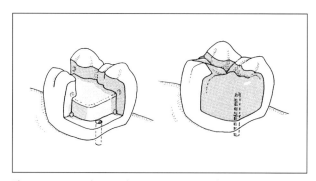

Fig 6-8 A simple amalgam restoration placed in an MOD preparation on a molar.

Fig 6-9 A complex amalgam restoration replaces a missing cusp on a molar.

Simple Amalgam

The simple amalgam, without pins or other means of auxiliary retention, for decades has been the standard one- to three-surface restoration for minor- to moderate-sized lesions in esthetically noncritical areas (Fig 6-8). It has received a "bum rap" from an ill-informed, sensationalizing press in recent years. Approximately 100 million or more simple amalgam restorations are placed annually.[3] They are best used where more than half of the coronal dentin is intact.

Tooth preparation size for incipient lesions has diminished in recent years as the concept of "extention for prevention" has waned. This move toward less destructive preparations has been augmented by the development of smaller instruments and stronger amalgams. Nonetheless, even a minimal preparation for an amalgam restoration significantly weakens the structural integrity of the tooth.[4]

Complex Amalgam

Amalgam augmented by pins or other auxiliary means of retention can be used to restore teeth with moderate to severe lesions in which less than half of the coronal dentin remains (Fig 6-9). Amalgam used in this manner can be employed as a final restoration when a crown is contraindicated because of limited finances or poor oral hygiene. It can be used in the restoration of teeth with missing cusps, or endodontically treated premolars and molars—teeth that ordinarily would be restored with mesio-occluso-distal (MOD) onlays or other extracoronal restorations. In such situations, amalgam is used to replace or overlay the cusp to provide the protection of occlusal coverage. It does produce good strength in the restored tooth.[5] Ideally, however, a crown should be constructed over the pin-retained amalgam, using it as a core, or foundation restoration.

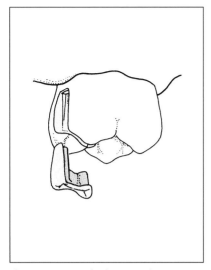

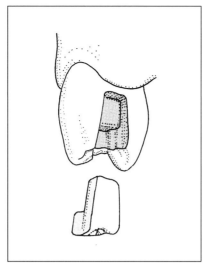

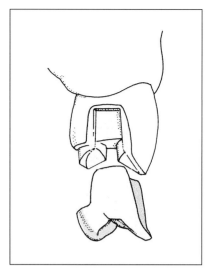

Fig 6-10 A metal inlay is used to restore a molar.

Fig 6-11 Ceramic inlays can be used to restore posterior teeth.

Fig 6-12 An MOD onlay for a maxillary premolar.

Metal Inlay

Minor to moderate lesions on teeth where the esthetic requirements are low can be restored with this restoration type (Fig 6-10). While usually made of softer gold alloys, metal inlays can also be fabricated of etchable base metal alloys if a bonding effect is desired.[6,7] The preparation isthmus should be narrow to minimize stress in the surrounding tooth structure. Premolars should have one intact marginal ridge to preserve structural integrity and minimize the possibility of coronal fracture.

The additional bulk of tooth structure found in a molar permits the use of this restoration type in an MOD configuration. The indications for this type of restoration are much the same as those for an amalgam, since this restoration only replaces lost tooth structure and will not protect remaining tooth structure. Because of the amount of destruction of tooth structure required by this restoration, it is not recommended for incipient lesions.

Ceramic Inlay

This restoration is utilized to restore teeth with minor- to moderate-sized lesions that will permit a narrow preparation isthmus in an area of the mouth where the esthetic demand is high (Fig 6-11). Premolars should have one intact marginal ridge, but MOD ceramic inlays can be used in molars. Because this type of restoration can also be etched to enhance bonding, there is some evidence that the structural integrity of the tooth cusps may be stabilized by bonding.[8] The relatively large size of the cavity preparation required for this restoration mitigates its use in the treatment of incipient lesions.

MOD Onlay

This design can be used for restoring moderately large lesions on premolars and molars with intact facial and lingual surfaces (Fig 6-12). It will accommodate a wide isthmus and up to one missing cusp on a molar. If a cast metal restoration is needed on a premolar with both marginal ridges compromised, it should include occlusal coverage to protect the remaining tooth structure. This restoration also can be considered an extracoronal restoration because of the occlusal coverage that overlays and protects the tooth cusps.

The MOD onlay does not have the necessary resistance to be used as a fixed partial denture retainer. Although ordinarily fabricated of a gold alloy, this restoration design has been used with cast glass and other types of ceramics. Ceramic MOD onlays should be used very cautiously. Without generous occlusal thickness, these restorations are susceptible to fracture.

Extracoronal Restorations

If insufficient coronal tooth structure exists to retain the restoration within the crown of the the tooth, an extracoronal restoration, or crown, is needed. It may also be used where there are extensive areas of defective axial tooth structure, or if there is a need to modify contours to refine occlusion or improve esthetics.

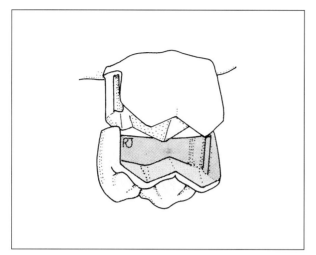

Fig 6-13 A three-quarter crown being seated on a molar.

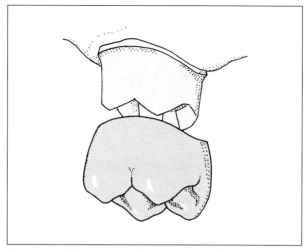

Fig 6-14 A full veneer metal crown on a maxillary second molar.

Partial Veneer Crown

This is a crown that leaves one or more axial surfaces unveneered (Fig 6-13). Therefore, it can be used to restore a tooth with one or more intact axial surfaces with half or more of the coronal tooth structure remaining. It will provide moderate retention and can be used as a retainer for short-span fixed partial dentures. If tooth destruction is not excessive, a partial veneer crown with a minimally extended preparation and carefully finished margins can satisfy moderate esthetic demands in the maxillary arch.

Full Metal Crown

The conventional full crown can be used to restore teeth with multiple defective axial surfaces (Fig 6-14). It will provide the maximum retention possible in any given situation, but its use must be restricted to situations where there are no esthetic expectations. This will usually limit it to second molars, some mandibular first molars, and occasionally mandibular second premolars. Because less tooth structure must be removed for its preparation than for crowns with a ceramic component, and its fabrication is the simplest of any crown, this restoration should remain among those designs considered in planning single-tooth restorations on molars as well as posterior fixed partial dentures.

Metal-Ceramic Crown

This crown can also be used to restore teeth with multiple defective axial surfaces (Fig 6-15). It too is capable of providing maximum retention, but it also will meet high esthetic requirements. It can be used as a fixed partial denture retainer where full coverage and a good cosmetic result must be combined.

All-Ceramic Crown

When full coverage and maximum esthetics must be combined, this crown is the choice (Fig 6-16). All-ceramic crowns are not as resistant to fracture as metal-ceramic crowns, so their use must be restricted to situations likely to produce low to moderate stress. They are usually used for incisors, although cast glass ceramics are also employed in the restoration of posterior teeth. Preparations for this type of restoration on premolars and molars do require the removal of large quantities of tooth structure.

Ceramic Veneer

Because all-ceramic and metal-ceramic crowns require the removal of such large quantities of tooth structure, there has been considerable interest in less destructive alternatives. The ceramic veneer has emerged as a means of producing a very cosmetic result on otherwise intact anterior teeth that are marred by severe staining or developmental defects restricted to the facial surface of the tooth (Fig 6-17). This restoration also can be used to restore moderate incisal chipping and small proximal lesions. The use of a veneer requires only a minimum tooth preparation, so it offers an alternative to crowns that is attractive to patient and dentist alike.

The features and capabilities of the 12 types of single-tooth restorations described in this chapter are shown in Table 6-1.

Table 6-1 Attributes of Single-Tooth Restorations

Restoration	Size of lesion	Longevity rating	FPD abutment	RPD abutment	Esthetics	Retention	Protects tooth	Replaces cusp	Occlusal restoration	Incisal restoration	Facial restoration	Endodontic restoration
Intracoronal												
Glass ionomer	Incipient	5	No	No	Adequate	—	No	No	Poor	Poor	Class 5	No
Composite resin	Incipient to Moderate	4	No	No	Good	—	No	No	Poor	Adequate	Class 5	No
Simple amalgam	Incipient to Moderate	1	No	Yes	Poor to Adequate*	—	No	No	Class 2	No	Class 5	No
Complex amalgam	Large	3	No	Yes	Poor to Adequate*	—	Some	Yes	Adequate	No	All†	Yes‡
Metal inlay	Moderate	2	No	Yes	Poor to Adequate*	Minimal	No§	No	Class 2	Poor	Class 5	No
Ceramic inlay	Moderate	3	No	No	Good	Minimal	No§	No	Class 2	Adequate	Class 5	No
MOD onlay	Moderate to Large	1	No	Yes	Poor to Adequate*	Moderate	Yes	Yes	Good	No	No	Yes
Extracoronal												
Partial veneer crown	Large	1	Yes	Yes	Poor to Adequate*	Moderate	Yes	Yes	Good	Poor	Rev 3/4; Prox 1/2†	Yes
Full metal crown	Large	1	Yes	Yes	Poor	Good	Yes	Yes	Good	Poor	All†	Yes
Metal-ceramic crown	Large	2	Yes	Yes	Good	Good	Yes	Yes	Good	Good	All	Yes
All-ceramic crown	Large	3	No	No	Good	Good	Yes	Yes‖	Adequate	Good	All	Yes
Ceramic veneer	Incipient	3	No	No	Good	Adequate	No	No¶	Poor	Good	All	No

*Dependent on tooth position, location of restoration (mesial or distal), and patient expectation.
†Structurally sound, but not esthetic.
‡An acceptable compromise treatment, if cusps are capped with amalgam.
§May offer some protection in conjunction with etching and bonding.
‖When used with a core or foundation restoration.
¶It can be used to replace an incisal corner, however.

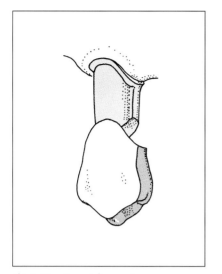

Fig 6-15 A metal-ceramic crown on a maxillary premolar.

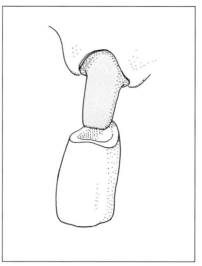

Fig 6-16 An all-ceramic crown for an incisor.

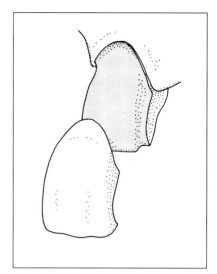

Fig 6-17 A ceramic veneer on a maxillary incisor.

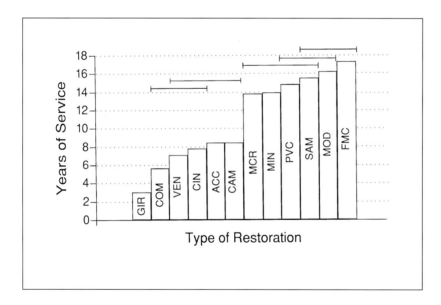

Fig 6-18 Comparison of the estimated longevity of 12 types of restorations, based on a survey of 36 dentists. ANOVA was performed, with $P = .05$. GIR = glass-ionomer restoration, COM = composite resin restoration, VEN = ceramic veneer, CIN = ceramic inlay, ACC = all-ceramic crown, CAM = complex amalgam restoration, MCR = metal-ceramic crown, MIN = metal inlay, PVC = partial veneer crown, SAM = simple amalgam restoration, MOD = metal MOD only, FMC = full metal crown.

Restoration Longevity

Every dentist would like to be able to answer the patient's question, "How long will my restoration last?" Logical though this question may be, unfortunately it is impossible to answer directly. We cannot predict the life span of a pair of shoes or a television set, and these everyday items are not custom made, nor do they perform their service in a hostile biological environment, submerged in water.

Clinical studies of restoration longevity have produced widely disparate figures. As a general rule, cast restorations will survive in the mouth longer than amalgam restorations, which in turn will last longer than composite resin restorations.[9] A compilation of five studies of 676 patients concluded that amalgam restorations exhibit a 50% failure rate between 5.5 and 11.5 years, with an extrapolated life expectancy of 10 to 14 years.[10]

Meeuwissen et al[11] reported a 10-year survival rate of 58% for amalgam restorations in Dutch military patients; Arthur et al[12] reported an 83% survival rate for the same time span in a US military population. Qvist et al[13] found that 50% of the amalgam restorations in a group of Danish patients had failed at 7.0 years. Christensen[14] estimated a 14-year longevity for amalgam restorations. In selected populations, amalgam restorations of unspecified types or sizes in one study[9] have shown 10-year survival rates as high as 72.0%. A 15-year survival rate of 72.8% was reported for simple amalgams in another study.[15]

A survey of 571 fixed prosthodontists, nonspecialist restorative dentists, and dental school faculty projected an average life span of 11.2 years for simple amalgams and 6.1 years for complex amalgams.[16] In fact, one group of 125 complex amalgams was reported to have a 76% survival rate at 15 years,[15] while another group of 171 complex amalgam restorations exhibited a 50% survival rate at 11.5 years.[17]

Composite resin restorations have not been included in many longevity studies. A study of dental school patients did incorporate them, reporting a 10-year survival rate of 55.9%.[9] Another report, done on a general patient population, described a shorter life span for composite resin restorations, with 50% of them having failed in 6.1 years.[18]

Mount[19] disclosed an overall success rate of 93% for 1,283 glass-ionomer restorations for up to 7 years, with the rate varying from 2% to 36% depending on the class of cavity and the brand of cement. In that study, the patients evaluated had been treated by only two dentists, and not all of the restorations had been in place for the full 7-year span of the study. While promising, these figures must be assessed cautiously until longer studies of a broader population have been completed.

Schwartz et al, after studying a group of 791 failed restorations, reported mean life spans, at failure, of 10.3 years for full crowns, 11.4 years for three-quarter crowns, and 8.5 years for porcelain jacket crowns (anterior all-ceramic crowns). The mean life span for all fixed prostho-dontic restorations was 10.3 years.[20] Walton and associates, evaluating a group of 424 restorations, found full crowns lasting 7.1 years, partial veneer crowns 14.3 years, metal-ceramic crowns 6.3 years, inlays and onlays 11.2 years, and porcelain jacket crowns 8.2 years.[21]

The dentists responding to Christensen's survey estimated the longevity of crowns to be from 21 to 22 years.[14] The estimates supplied by the respondents to a survey by Maryniuk and Kaplan were 12.7 years for metal-ceramic crowns and 14.7 years for all-gold restorations.[16] Kerschbaum, examining German insurance records, found 91.5% of gold crowns still in the mouth after 8 years.[22] In a review of records in 40 Dutch dental offices, Leempoel et al told of 10-year survival rates of 98% and 95.3% for full crowns and metal-ceramic crowns, respectively.[23]

Several of the restorations described in this chapter have not been in widespread use for a long enough period of time to have been included in longevity studies. Thirty-six restorative dentists and prosthodontists with a mean experience of 19.2 years were surveyed to provide a basis for estimates of the life expectancies of some of the newer restorations discussed in this chapter (Fig 6-18).[24] The longevities given are only opinions, based on extensive experience with some restoration types and only limited experience with others. A compilation of longevities from this survey and from other studies cited in this chapter is presented in Table 6-2.

The question of longevity is an important one to consider when deciding on treatment for a patient. The more destructive the preparation required for the restoration, the greater the potential risk for the tooth, and ultimately the greater expense. It has been estimated that if a crown were placed in a patient's mouth at age 22, at a fee of $425, attendant services and replacements of that crown will have cost the patient nearly $12,000 considering an average life expectancy of 75 years.[25]

Table 6-2 Longevity of Single-Tooth Restorations

Investigator(s)	Type of study	No. of respondents	Glass ionomer	Composite resin	Simple amalgam	Complex amalgam	Metal inlay	Ceramic inlay	MOD onlay	Partial veneer crown	Full metal crown	Metal-ceramic crown	All-ceramic crown	Ceramic veneer
Bentley and Drake[9]	Clinical	1207	—	55.9% at 10 years	72.0% at 10 years	—	87.3% at 10 years	—	87.3% at 10 years	—	86.3% at 10 years	—	—	—
Maryniuk[10]	Clinical*	1940	—	—	10 to 14 years	—	—	—	—	—	—	—	—	—
Meeuwissen et al[11]	Clinical	8492	—	—	58.0% at 10 years	—	—	—	—	—	—	—	—	—
Arthur et al[12]	Clinical	2200	—	—	83% at 10 years	—	—	—	—	—	—	—	—	—
Qvist et al[13,18]	Clinical	442	—	50% at 6.1 years	50% at 7.0 years	—	—	—	—	—	—	—	—	—
Christensen[14]	Survey	731	—	7.3 years	13.8 years	—	20.6 years	12.7 years	20.6 years	20.6 years	20.6 years	22.2 years	—	—
Smales[15]	Clinical	768	—	—	72.8% at 15 years	72.6% at 15 years	—	—	—	—	—	—	—	—
Maryniuk and Kaplan[16]	Survey	571	—	—	11.2 years	6.1 years	12.7 years	—	—	—	14.7 years	12.7 years	—	—
Robbins and Summit[17]	Clinical	128	—	—	—	50% at 11.5 years	—	—	—	—	—	—	—	—
Mount[19]	Clinical	1283	93% at 7 years	—	—	—	—	—	—	—	—	—	—	—
Schwartz et al[20]	Clinical	791	—	—	—	—	11 years	—	—	—	10.3 years	—	8.5 years	—
Walton et al[21]	Clinical	451	—	—	—	—	11.2 years	—	—	—	7.1 years	6.3 years	8.2 years	—
Kerschbaum[22]	Clinical	9737	—	—	—	—	—	—	—	—	91.5% at 8 years	—	—	—
Leempoel et al[23]	Clinical	10000†	—	—	—	—	—	—	—	—	98% at 10 years	95.3% at 10 years†	82% at 10 years	—
Shillingburg[24]	Survey	36	3.0 years	5.7 years	15.7 years	8.4 years	13.9 years	7.8 years	16.2 years	15.1 years	17.3 years	13.9 years	8.4 years	7.1 years

*A compilation and interpretation of five clinical studies.
†Average of survival rates for anterior, premolar, and molar crowns.

References

1. Potts RG, Shillingburg HT, Duncanson MG: Retention and resistance of preparations for cast restorations. *J Prosthet Dent* 1980; 43:303–307.

2. Kishimoto M, Shillingburg HT, Duncanson MG: Influence of preparation features on retention and resistance. Part I: MOD onlays. *J Prosthet Dent* 1983; 49:35–39.

3. Osborne, JW: In defense of amalgam. *Oper Dent* 1991; 16: 157–159.

4. Mondelli J, Steagall I, Ishikiriama A, Navarro MF, Soares FB: Fracture strength of human teeth with cavity preparations. *J Prosthet Dent* 1980; 43:419.

5. Reagan SE, Schwandt NW, Duncanson MG: Fracture resistance of wide-isthmus mesio-occulusal-distal preparations with and without amalgam cuspal coverage. *Quintessence Int* 1989; 20:469–472.

6. Kent WA, Shillingburg HT, Duncanson MG, Nelson EL: Fracture resistance of ceramic inlays with three luting materials. *J Dent Res* 1991; 70:561.

7. Livaditis GJ: Etched metal resin-bonded intracoronal cast restorations. Part II: Design criteria for cavity preparation. *J Prosthet Dent* 1986; 56:389–395.

8. Bodell RW, Kent WA, Shillingburg HT, Duncanson MG: Fracture resistance of intracoronal metallic restorations and three luting materials. *J Dent Res* 1991; 70:562.

9. Bentley C, Drake CW: Longevity of restorations in a dental school clinic. *J Dent Educ* 1985; 50:594–600.

10. Maryniuk GA: In search of treatment longevity—A 30-year perspective. *J Am Dent Assoc* 1984; 109:739–744.

11. Meeuwissen R, Elteren P, Eschen S, Mulder J: Durability of amalgam restorations in premolars and molars in Dutch servicement. *Community Dent Health* 1985; 2:293–302.

12. Arthur JS, Cohen ME, Diehl MC: Longevity of restorations in a U.S. military population. *J Dent Res* 1988; 67:388.

13. Qvist V, Thylstrup A, Mjor IA: Restorative treatment pattern and longevity of amalgam restorations. *Acta Odontol Scand* 1986; 44:343–349.

14. Christensen GJ: The practicability of compacted golds in general practice—A survey. *J Colo Dent Assoc* 1971; 49: 18–22.

15. Smales RJ: Longevity of cusp-covered amalgams: Survivals after 15 years. *Oper Dent* 1991; 16:17–20.

16. Maryniuk GA, Kaplan SH: Longevity of restorations: Survey results of dentists' estimates and attitudes. *J Am Dent Assoc* 1986; 112:39–45.

17. Robbins JW, Summitt JB: Longevity of complex amalgam restorations. *Oper Dent* 1988; 13:54–57.

18. Qvist V, Thylstrup A, Mjor IA: Restorative treatment pattern and longevity of resin restorations. *Acta Odontol Scand* 1986; 44:351–356.

19. Mount GJ: Longevity of glass ionomer cements. *J Prosthet Dent* 1986; 55:682–685.

20. Schwartz NL, Whitsett LD, Berry TG, Stewart JL: Unserviceable crowns and fixed partial dentures: life span and causes for loss of serviceability. *J Am Dent Assoc* 1970; 81:1395–1401.

21. Walton JN, Gardner FM, Agar JR: A survey of crown and fixed partial denture failures: Length of service and reasons for replacement. *J Prosthet Dent* 1986; 56:416–421.

22. Kerschbaum T: Uberlebenzeiten von kronen- und brucken zahneratz heute. *Zahnaertzl Mitt* 1986; 76:2315–2320.

23. Leempoel PJB, de Haan AFJ, Reintjes AGM: The survival rate of crowns in 40 Dutch practices. *J Dent Res* 1986; 65:565.

24. Shillingburg HT: Unpublished research.

25. Cohen BD, Milobsky SA: Monetary damages in dental-injury cases. *Trial Lawyers Quarterly* 1989; 20:80–81.

Chapter 7

Treatment Planning for the Replacement of Missing Teeth

The need for replacing missing teeth is obvious to the patient when the edentulous space is in the anterior segment of the mouth, but it is equally important in the posterior region. It is tempting to think of the dental arch as a static entity, but that is certainly not the case. It is in a state of dynamic equilibrium, with the teeth supporting each other (Fig 7-1). When a tooth is lost, the structural integrity of the dental arch is disrupted, and there is a subsequent realignment of teeth as a new state of equilibrium is achieved. Teeth adjacent to or opposing the edentulous space frequently move into it (Fig 7-2). Adjacent teeth, especially those distal to the space, may drift bodily, although a tilting movement is a far more common occurrence.

If an opposing tooth intrudes severely into the edentulous space, it is not enough just to replace the missing tooth (Fig 7-3). To restore the mouth to complete function, free of interferences, it is often necessary to restore the tooth opposing the edentulous space (Fig 7-4). In severe cases, this may necessitate the devitalization of the supererupted opposing tooth to permit enough shortening to correct the plane of occlusion.

Selection of the Type of Prosthesis

Missing teeth may be replaced by one of three prosthesis types: a *removable partial denture* (*RPD*), a *tooth-supported fixed partial denture* (*FPD*), or an *implant-supported fixed partial denture* (Table 7-1). Several factors must be weighed when choosing the type of prosthesis to be used in any given situation. Biomechanical, periodontal, esthetic, and financial factors, as well as the patient's wishes, are some of the more important ones. It is not uncommon to combine two types in the same arch, such as a removable partial denture and a tooth-supported fixed partial denture, or implant-supported and tooth-supported fixed partial dentures.

In treatment planning, there is one principle that should be kept in mind: *treatment simplification*. There are many times when certain treatments are technically possible but too complex. Something must be done to cut through the possibilities and come up with a recommendation

that will serve the patient's needs and still be reasonable to accomplish. At such times, the restorative dentist, or prosthodontist, is the one who should manage the sequencing and referral to other specialists. He or she will be finishing up the treatment and should act as "the quarterback." Communicate and be open to suggestions, but don't allow someone else to dictate the restorative phase of the treatment, leaving you with a treatment plan you do not think will work. You will be doing the restoration and the patient will return to you if it fails, so be sure you are comfortable with the planned treatment. The following guidelines are not "laws," and they are not absolute. However, when a preponderance of these items is used in the consideration of the planning for one arch or one mouth, a more compelling reason exists for the selection of the type of prosthesis described.

Removable Partial Denture

A removable partial denture is generally indicated for edentulous spaces greater than two posterior teeth, anterior spaces greater than four incisors, or spaces that include a canine and two other contiguous teeth; ie, central incisor, lateral incisor, and canine; lateral incisor, canine, and first premolar; or the canine and both premolars.

An edentulous space with no distal abutment will usually require a removable partial denture. There are exceptions in which a cantilever fixed partial denture can be used, but this solution should be approached cautiously. See the section on cantilevers later in the chapter for a more detailed description of this type of restoration. Multiple edentulous spaces, each of which may be restorable with a fixed partial denture, nonetheless may call for the use of a removable partial denture because of the expense and technical complexity. Bilateral edentulous spaces with more than two teeth missing on one side also may call for the use of a removable prosthesis instead of two fixed prostheses.

The requirements of an abutment for a removable partial denture are not as stringent as those for a fixed partial denture abutment. Tipped teeth adjoining edentulous spaces and prospective abutments with divergent align-

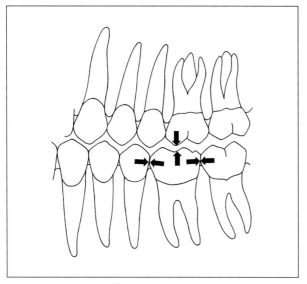

Fig 7-1 Tooth position and alignment are maintained, in part, by interaction between teeth *(arrows)*.

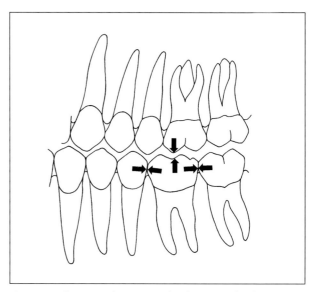

Fig 7-2 When a tooth is removed, adjacent teeth often migrate into the vacated space.

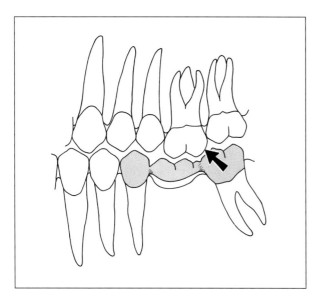

Fig 7-3 If a fixed partial denture is fabricated without first re-establishing the occlusal plane, an occlusal interference may be created *(arrow)*.

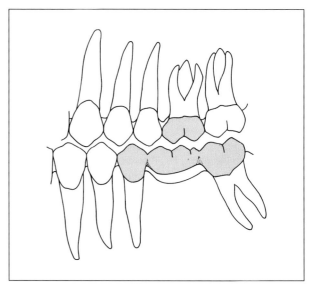

Fig 7-4 Occlusion is properly restored by correction of the occlusal plane in conjunction with placement of a fixed partial denture.

ments may lend themselves more readily to utilization as RPD rather than FPD abutments. Periodontally weakened primary abutments may serve better in retaining a well-designed removable partial denture than in bearing the load of a fixed partial denture. It is also possible to design the partial denture framework so that retentive clasps will be placed on teeth other than those adjacent to the edentulous space.

Teeth with short clinical crowns or teeth that are just generally short usually will not be good FPD abutments for anything other than a single pontic prosthesis. An insufficient number of abutments may also be a reason for selecting a removable rather than a fixed partial denture.

If there has been a severe loss of tissue in the edentulous ridge, a removable partial denture can more easily be used to restore the space both functionally and esthetically. For successful removable partial denture treatment, the patient should demonstrate acceptable oral hygiene and show signs of being a reliable recall candidate.

Table 7-1 Replacement of Missing Teeth

	Removable partial denture	Conventional tooth-supported fixed partial denture	Resin-bonded tooth-supported fixed partial denture	Implant-supported fixed partial denture
Span length	• Posterior spans longer than teeth • Anterior spans longer than 4 incisors • Canine + 2 or more contiguous teeth	• Posterior span: 2 or fewer teeth • Incisors: 4 or fewer	• Single tooth • Possible for 2 incisors	• Single tooth • 2- to 6-unit span
Span configuration	• No distal abutment • Multiple or bilateral edentulous spaces	• Usually has distal abutment but can be used with short cantilever pontic	• Abutments mesial and distal to pontic	• No distal abutment • Pier in 3 + pontic span • All abutments at ends and as pier(s) of long span
Abutment alignment	• Tipped abutments can be tolerated • Widely divergent abutment alignment	• Less than 25° inclination can be accommodated by preparation modification	• Less than 15° inclination mesiodistally • Should be in same faciolingual plane • Preparations are not easily modified because of minimal reduction	• Need for implant/abutment alignment requires close coordination between surgeon and restorative dentist
Abutment condition	• Short clinical crowns • Insufficient abutments	• Good if abutments need crowns • Nonvital teeth can be used if there is sufficient coronal tooth structure	• Defect-free abutments • Incisor, premolar replacements	• Defect-free abutments requiring no restoration
Occlusion	• More adaptable to irregularities in a healthy opposing natural dentition	• Favorable loading (magnitude, direction, frequency, duration)	• Cannot be used for incisor replacement in presence of deep vertical overlap	• Occlusal forces must be as nearly vertical as possible to prevent unfavorable lateral loading of implants
Periodontal condition	• Can use alternate (secondary abutments) when primary abutments are weakened	• Good alveolar bone support • Crown-root ratio 1:1 or better • No mobility • Favorable root morphology • Provides rigid stabilization	• No mobility • Periodontal splints (with auxiliary resistance in tooth preparation)	• Dense bone
Ridge form	• Gross tissue loss in residual ridge	• Moderate resorption • No gross soft tissue defects	• Moderate resorption • No gross soft tissue defects	• Broad, flat ridge
General features	• Dry mouth poor RPD risk • Limited patient finances • Acceptable oral hygiene • Reliable recall candidate • Treatment simplification • Advanced age • Systemic health problems • More adaptable to dentition in transition to edentulous state	• Dry mouth high caries risk with FPD • Muscular discoordination • Mandibular tori • Palatal soft tissue lesions • Large tongue • Exaggerated gag reflex • Unfavorable attitude toward RPD • Patient can't cope with aging, tooth loss • Favorable opposing occlusion: removable prosthesis or periodontally weakened natural dentition may permit FPD in less than optimal situations • Must be within dentist's skills	• Well suited for young patients • Can be used for replacing molars if masticatory muscles are not too well developed	• Able to survive in dry mouth • May be better choice if teeth will require extensive treatment and will still be weak, questionable abutments • Unfavorable attitude toward RPD • Must be within dentist's skills

Patients of advanced age who are on fixed incomes or have systemic health problems may require special treatment simplification efforts, either to cut down on the amount of appointment time required to restore the mouth or to make the treatment affordable. Cajoling patients of limited means into overinvesting their resources is not in their best interest.

A large tongue is a good reason to avoid a removable prosthesis if at all possible, as is muscular discoordination. An unfavorable attitude toward a removable partial denture also makes it a poor choice.

Conventional Tooth-Supported Fixed Partial Denture

When a missing tooth is to be replaced, a fixed partial denture is preferred by the majority of patients. The usual configuration for a fixed partial denture utilizes an abutment tooth on each end of the edentulous space to support the prosthesis. If the abutment teeth are periodontally sound, the edentulous span is short and straight, and the retainers are well designed and executed, the fixed partial denture can be expected to provide a long life of function for the patient. Several factors have an influence on the decision whether to fabricate a fixed partial denture, what teeth to use as abutments, and what retainer designs to use (see Table 7-1).

There should be no gross soft tissue defect in the edentulous ridge. If there is, it may be possible to augment the ridge with grafts to enable the construction of a fixed prosthesis. This treatment is reserved for patients who are both highly motivated and able to afford this special procedure. If this is not the case, a removable partial denture should be considered.

A dry mouth creates a poor environment for a fixed partial denture. The margins of the retainers will be at great risk from recurrent caries, limiting the life span of the prosthesis. However, an absence of moisture in the mouth also will hinder the successful wearing of a removable partial denture. In either case, the patient must be made aware of the high risk involved. The risk may be minimized through home fluoride application and frequent recall, but it cannot be eliminated.

Resin-Bonded Tooth-Supported Fixed Partial Denture

The resin-bonded fixed partial denture is a conservative restoration that is reserved for use on defect-free abutments in situations where there is a single missing tooth, usually an incisor or premolar. A single molar can be replaced by this type of prosthesis if the patient's muscles of mastication are not too well developed, thus assuring that a minimum load will be placed on the retainers. The resin-bonded fixed partial denture requires

an abutment both mesial and distal to the edentulous space.

This prosthesis utilizes a standard pontic form, accommodating an edentulous ridge with moderate resorption and no gross soft tissue defects. Because it requires a shallow preparation that is restricted to enamel, the resin-bonded fixed partial denture is especially useful in younger patients whose immature teeth with large pulps are poor risks for endodontic-free abutment preparations.

Tilted abutments can be accommodated only if there is enough tooth structure to allow a change in the normal alignment of axial reduction. This is limited by the need to restrict most of the reduction to enamel. Rarely can a mesiodistal difference in abutment inclination greater than 15 degrees be accommodated. There can be little or no difference in the inclination of the abutments faciolingually.

The resin-bonded prosthesis cannot be used for replacing missing anterior teeth where there is a deep vertical overlap. Reduction deep into the underlying dentin of the abutment teeth will be required in this situation, so a conventional fixed partial denture should be employed.

Although this type of prosthesis has been described for periodontal splints, it should be used with extreme care in those situations. Preparations will demand additional resistance features, such as long, well-defined grooves. Abutment mobility has been shown to be a serious hazard in the successful use of this type of restoration.

Implant-Supported Fixed Partial Denture

Fixed partial dentures supported by implants are ideally suited for use where there are insufficient numbers of abutment teeth or inadequate strength in the abutments to support a conventional fixed partial denture, and when patient attitude and/or a combination of intraoral factors make a removable partial denture a poor choice. Implant-supported fixed partial dentures can be employed in the replacement of teeth when there is no distal abutment. Span length is limited only by the availability of alveolar bone with satisfactory density and thickness in a broad, flat ridge configuration that will permit implant placement.

A single tooth can be replaced by a single implant, saving defect-free adjacent teeth from the destructive effects of retainer crown preparations. A span length of two to six teeth can be replaced by multiple implants, either as single-unit restorations or as implant-supported fixed partial dentures. An implant can be used as a pier in an edentulous span three or more teeth long. There is some risk involved in using an immovable implant abutment in the same rigid prosthesis with natural teeth. In such a situation, it is preferred that implants serve as the abutments at both ends and as the pier(s) of a long span. In fact, an entire arch can be replaced by an implant-supported complete prosthesis, but that type of restoration lies outside the realm of this discussion.

The retainers used for most implant systems require a greater degree of abutment alignment precision than do the retainers for a tooth-supported fixed partial denture. If implants are placed by someone other than the restoring dentist, implant/abutment alignment demands close coordination between surgeon and restorative dentist. The abutments should be positioned so that the occlusal forces will be as nearly vertical to the implants as possible to prevent destructive lateral forces.

Implants should be better able than natural teeth to survive in a dry mouth. Implants may be a better choice for FPD abutments if prospective tooth abutments will require endodontic therapy with or without dowel cores, periodontal surgery, and possibly root resections to support a long-span, complex, and expensive prosthesis whose success is dependent on "feet of clay."

No Prosthetic Treatment

If a patient presents with a long-standing edentulous space into which there has been little or no drifting or elongation of the adjacent or opposing teeth, the question of replacement should be left to the patient's wishes. If the patient perceives no functional, occlusal, or esthetic impairment, it would be a dubious service to place a prosthesis. This in no way contradicts the recommendation that a missing tooth routinely should be replaced. The teeth adjoining an edentulous space *usually* move, but they do not *always* move. When you meet the occasional patient who has beaten the odds, recognize it for what it is, congratulate the patient for being fortunate, and tend to his or her other needs.

Case Presentation

In cases where the choice between a fixed partial denture and a removable partial denture is not clear cut, two or more treatment options should be presented to the patient along with their advantages and disadvantages. The dentist is in the best position to evaluate the physical and biological factors present, while the patient's feelings should carry considerable weight on matters of esthetics and finances.

Both dentist and patient must agree on the definitive treatment plan. If the patient understands and is willing to accept the risks associated with treatment that is your second choice, it is prudent to make a notation to that effect and have it signed by the patient. If you are convinced that a particular type of treatment is absolutely wrong for a given situation, try to educate the patient to the reasons for your opinion. If the patient remains unconvinced, you would do well to refer the patient to someone else. Life is too short for the aggravation that may follow if you do not.

Abutment Evaluation

Every restoration must be able to withstand the constant occlusal forces to which it is subjected. This is of particular significance when designing and fabricating a fixed partial denture, since the forces that would normally be absorbed by the missing tooth are transmitted, through the pontic, connectors, and retainers, to the abutment teeth. Abutment teeth are therefore called upon to withstand the forces normally directed to the missing teeth, in addition to those usually applied to the abutments.

If a tooth adjacent to an edentulous space needs a crown because of damage to the tooth, the restoration usually can double as an FPD retainer. If several abutments in one arch require crowns, there is a strong argument for the selection of a fixed partial denture rather than a removable partial denture.

Whenever possible, an abutment should be a vital tooth. However, a tooth that has been endodontically treated and is asymptomatic, with radiographic evidence of a good seal and complete obturation of the canal, can be used as an abutment. However, the tooth must have some sound, surviving coronal tooth structure to insure longevity. Even then, some compensation must be made for the coronal tooth structure that has been lost. This can be accomplished through the use of a dowel core, or a pin-retained amalgam or composite resin core.

Teeth that have been pulp capped in the process of preparing the tooth should not be used as FPD abutments unless they are endodontically treated. There is too great a risk that they will require endodontic treatment later, with the resultant destruction of retentive tooth structure and of the retainer itself. This is a situation that is better handled before the fixed partial denture is made.

The supporting tissues surrounding the abutment teeth must be healthy and free from inflammation before any prosthesis can be contemplated. Normally, abutment teeth should not exhibit mobility, since they will be carrying an extra load. The roots and their supporting tissues should be evaluated for three factors:

1. Crown-root ratio
2. Root configuration
3. Periodontal ligament area

Crown-Root Ratio

This ratio is a measure of the length of tooth occlusal to the alveolar crest of bone compared with the length of root embedded in the bone. As the level of the alveolar bone moves apically, the lever arm of that portion out of bone increases, and the chance for harmful lateral forces is increased. The optimum crown-root ratio for a tooth to be utilized as a fixed partial denture abutment is 2:3. A ratio of 1:1 is the minimum ratio that is acceptable for a prospective abutment under normal circumstances (Fig 7-5).

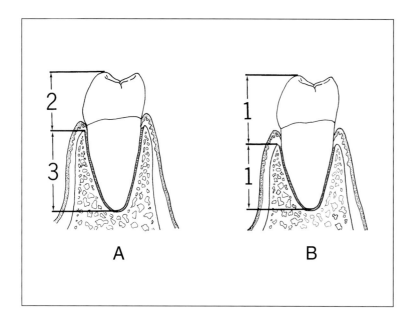

Fig 7-5 The optimum crown-root ratio for a fixed partial denture abutment is 2:3 (A). A ratio of 1:1 (B) is the minimum that is acceptable.

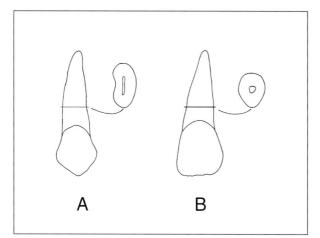

Fig 7-6 Although the root surface area of these teeth is similar, the root configuration of the maxillary premolar (A), with its greater faciolingual dimension, makes it a superior abutment to the maxillary central incisor (B), whose root is essentially circular in cross section.

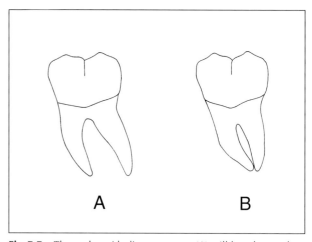

Fig 7-7 The molar with divergent roots (A) will be a better abutment tooth than one whose roots are fused (B).

However, there are situations in which a crown-root ratio greater than 1:1 might be considered adequate. If the occlusion opposing a proposed fixed partial denture is composed of artificial teeth, occlusal force will be diminished, with less stress on the abutment teeth. The occlusal force exerted against prosthetic appliances has been shown to be considerably less than that against natural teeth: 26.0 lb for removable partial dentures and 54.5 lb for fixed partial dentures versus 150.0 lb for natural teeth.[1]

For the same reasons, an abutment tooth with a less than desirable crown-root ratio is more likely to success-fully support a fixed partial denture if the opposing occlusion is composed of mobile, periodontally involved teeth than if the opposing teeth are periodontally sound. The crown-root ratio alone is not an adequate criteria for evaluating a prospective abutment tooth.[2]

Root Configuration

This is an important point in the assessment of an abutment's suitability from a periodontal standpoint. Roots

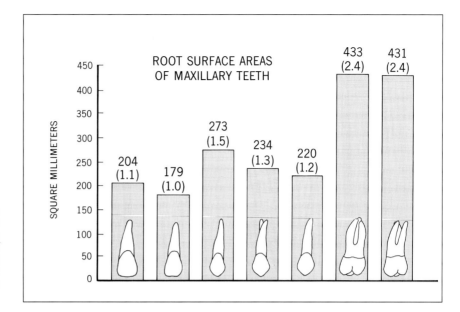

Fig 7-8 Comparative root surface areas of maxillary teeth. The figure in parentheses above each tooth is the ratio between the root surface area of the respective tooth and the root surface area of the smallest tooth in the arch, the lateral incisor (based on data by Jepsen[3]).

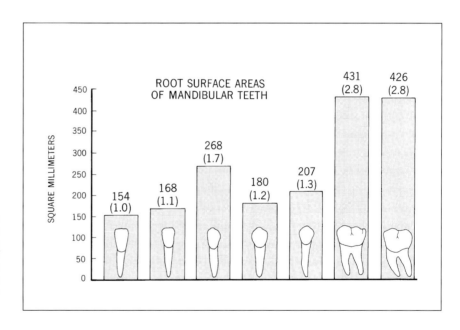

Fig 7-9 Comparative root surface areas of mandibular teeth. The figure in parentheses above each tooth is the ratio between the root surface area of the respective tooth and the root surface area of the smallest tooth in the arch, the central incisor (based on data by Jepsen[3]).

that are broader labiolingually than they are mesiodistally are preferable to roots that are round in cross section (Fig 7-6). Multirooted posterior teeth with widely separated roots will offer better periodontal support than roots that converge, fuse, or generally present a conical configuration (Fig 7-7). The tooth with conical roots can be used as an abutment for a short-span fixed partial denture if all other factors are optimal. A single-rooted tooth with evidence of irregular configuration or with some curvature in the apical third of the root is preferable to the tooth that has a nearly perfect taper.

Periodontal Ligament Area

Another consideration in the evaluation of prospective abutment teeth is the root surface area, or the area of periodontal ligament attachment of the root to the bone. Larger teeth have a greater surface area and are better able to bear added stress. The areas of the root surfaces of the various teeth have been reported by Jepsen,[3] and are shown in Figs 7-8 and 7-9. The actual values are not as significant as the relative values within a given mouth and the ratios between the various teeth in one arch. When supporting bone has been lost because of peri-

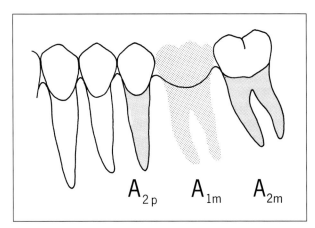

Fig 7-10 The combined root surface area of the second premolar and the second molar ($A_{2p}+A_{2m}$) is greater than that of the first molar being replaced (A_{1m}).

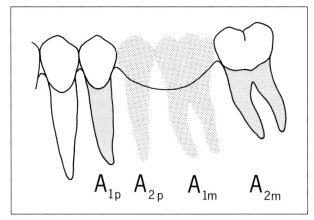

Fig 7-11 The combined root surface area of the first premolar and the second molar abutments ($A_{1p}+A_{2m}$) is approximately equal to that of the teeth being replaced ($A_{2p}+A_{1m}$).

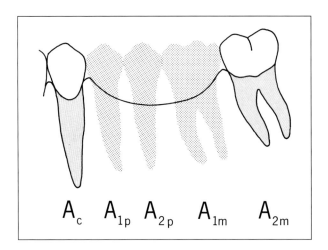

Fig 7-12 The combined root surface area of the canine and second molar (A_c+A_{2m}) is exceeded by that of the teeth being replaced ($A_{1p}+A_{2p}+A_{1m}$). A fixed partial denture would be a poor risk in this situation.

odontal disease, the involved teeth have a lessened capacity to serve as abutments. Millimeter per millimeter, the loss of periodontal support from root resorption is only one-third to one-half as critical as the loss of alveolar crestal bone.[4] The planned treatment should take this into account.

The length of the pontic span that can be successfully restored is limited, in part, by the abutment teeth and their ability to accept the additional load. Traditionally, there has been general agreement on the number of missing teeth that can be restored successfully. Tylman stated that two abutment teeth could support two pontics.[5] In a statement designated as "Ante's Law" by Johnston et al,[6] the root surface area of the abutment teeth had to equal or surpass that of the teeth being replaced with pontics.[7]

According to this premise, one missing tooth can be successfully replaced if the abutment teeth are healthy (Fig 7-10). If two teeth are missing, a fixed partial denture probably can replace the missing teeth, but the limit is being approached (Fig 7-11). When the root surface area of the teeth to be replaced by pontics surpasses that of the abutment teeth, a generally unacceptable situation exists (Fig 7-12).

It is possible for fixed partial dentures to replace more than two teeth, the most common examples being anterior fixed partial dentures replacing the four incisors. Canine to second molar fixed partial dentures also are possible (if all other conditions are ideal) in the maxillary arch, but not as often in the mandibular arch. However, any fixed prosthesis replacing more than two teeth should be considered a high risk.

As a clinical guideline, there is some validity in the concept referred to as "Ante's Law." Fixed partial dentures with short pontic spans have a better prognosis than do those with excessively long spans. It would be an oversimplification to attribute this merely to overstressing of the periodontal ligament, however. Failures from abnormal stress have been attributed to leverage and torque rather than overload.[1] Biomechanical factors and material failure play an important role in the potential for failure of long-span restorations.

There is evidence that teeth with very poor periodontal support can serve successfully as fixed partial denture abutments in carefully selected cases. Teeth with severe bone loss and marked mobility have been used as fixed partial denture and splint abutments.[8] Elimination of mobility is not the goal in such cases, but rather the stabilization of the teeth in a status quo to prevent an increase of mobility.[9]

Abutment teeth in these situations can be maintained free of inflammation in the face of mobility, if the patients are well motivated and highly proficient in plaque removal.[10] Crowns that anchor rigid prostheses to mobile teeth do require greater retention than do crowns attached to relatively immobile abutments, however.[11] Follow-up studies of these patients with "terminal dentitions" indicate a surprisingly low failure rate—less than 8% of 332 fixed partial dentures exhibited technical failure in a time span that averaged slightly more than 6 years.[12]

What is the impact of the success of this type of treatment on fixed partial dentures for the average patient? The successful restoration of mouths with severe periodontal disease does have significance in everyday practice. It emphasizes the extreme importance of carefully evaluating the strengths and weaknesses of the remaining dentition on an individual basis.

This should not be a signal for every dentist with a handpiece to start using severely periodontally involved teeth as abutments. Bear in mind that the successful treatments that have been cited are of the work of well-trained and highly skilled clinicians on selected, highly motivated patients.

This type of heroic treatment ("herodontics," if you will) is very demanding technically, and expensive as well. Performed by a well-trained, skilled clinician on an informed, motivated patient who dreads tooth loss, understands the patient's role in the success of the treatment, and accepts the risk (and expense) of failure, it can be a good service. "Sold" by a practitioner without special qualifications to an unmotivated and ill-informed patient, this type of treatment easily could result in a lawsuit.

Biomechanical Considerations

In addition to the increased load placed on the periodontal ligament by a long-span fixed partial denture, longer spans are less rigid. Bending or deflection varies directly with the cube of the length and inversely with the cube of the occlusogingival thickness of the pontic. Compared with a fixed partial denture having a single-tooth pontic span (Fig 7-13), a two-tooth pontic span will bend 8 times as much (Fig 7-14). A three-tooth pontic will bend 27 times as much as a single pontic (Fig 7-15).[13]

A pontic with a given occlusogingival dimension will bend (Fig 7-16) eight times as much if the pontic thickness is halved (Fig 7-17). A long-span fixed partial denture on short mandibular teeth could have disappointing results. Longer pontic spans also have the potential for producing more torquing forces on the fixed partial denture, especially on the weaker abutment. To minimize flexing caused by long and/or thin spans, pontic designs with a greater occlusogingival dimension should be selected. The prosthesis may also be fabricated of an alloy with a higher yield strength, such as nickel-chromium.

All fixed partial dentures, long or short, flex to some extent. Because of the forces being applied through the pontics to the abutment teeth, the forces on castings serving as retainers for fixed partial dentures are different in magnitude and direction from those applied to single restorations.[14] The dislodging forces on a fixed partial denture retainer tend to act in a mesiodistal direction, as opposed to the more common buccolingual direction of forces on a single restoration. Preparations should be modified accordingly to produce greater resistance and structural durability. Multiple grooves, including some on the buccal and lingual surfaces, are commonly employed for this purpose (Fig 7-18).

Double abutments are sometimes used as a means of overcoming problems created by unfavorable crown-root ratios and long spans. There are several criteria that must be met if a *secondary* (remote from the edentulous space) abutment is to strengthen the fixed partial denture and not become a problem itself. A secondary abutment must have at least as much root surface area and as favorable a crown-root ratio as the *primary* (adjacent to the edentulous space) abutment it is intended to bolster. As an example, a canine can be used as a secondary abutment to a first premolar primary abutment, but it would be unwise to use a lateral incisor as a secondary abutment to a canine primary abutment. The retainers on secondary abutments must be at least as retentive as the retainers on the primary abutments. When the pontic flexes, tensile forces will be applied to the retainers on the secondary abutments (Fig 7-19). There also must be sufficient crown length and space between adjacent abutments to prevent impingement on the gingiva under the connector.

Arch curvature has its effect on the stresses occurring in a fixed partial denture. When pontics lie outside the interabutment axis line, the pontics act as a lever arm, which can produce a torquing movement. This is a common problem in replacing all four maxillary incisors with a fixed partial denture, and it is most pronounced in the arch that is pointed in the anterior. Some measure must be taken to offset the torque. This can best be accomplished by gaining additional retention in the opposite direction from the lever arm and at a distance from the interabutment axis equal to the length of the lever arm (Fig 7-20).[15] The first premolars sometimes are used as secondary abutments for a maxillary four-pontic canine-to-canine fixed partial denture. Because of the tensile forces that will be applied to the premolar retainers, they must have excellent retention.

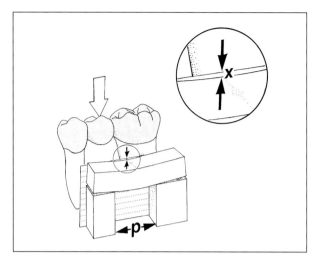

Fig 7-13   There is one unit of deflection (X) for a given span length (p).

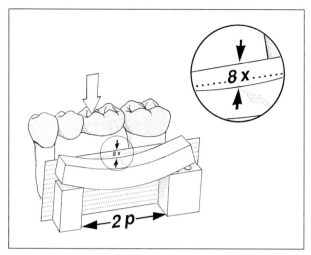

Fig 7-14   The deflection will be 8 times as great (8X) if the span length is doubled (2p).

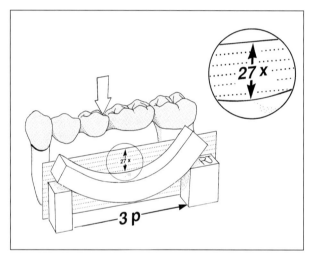

Fig 7-15   The deflection is 27 times as great (27X) when the span length is tripled (3p).

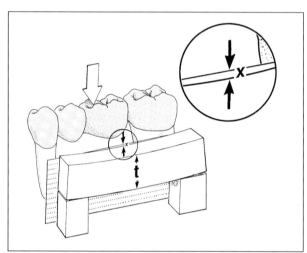

Fig 7-16   There is one unit of deflection (X) for a span with a given thickness (t).

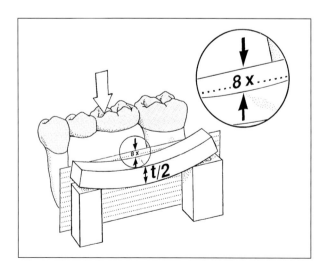

Fig 7-17   There will be 8 times as much deflection (8X) if the thickness is decreased by one-half (t/2).

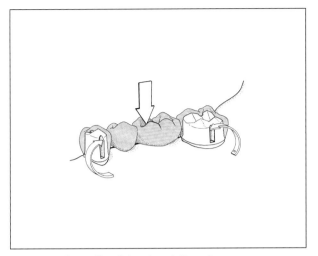

Fig 7-18 The walls of facial and lingual grooves counteract mesiodistal torque resulting from force applied to the pontic.

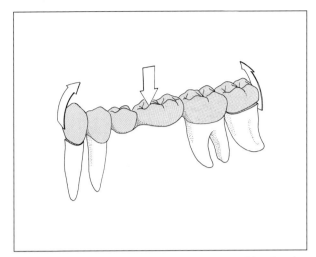

Fig 7-19 The retainers on secondary abutments will be placed in tension when the pontics flex, with the primary abutments acting as fulcrums.

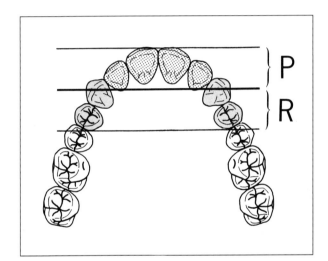

Fig 7-20 Secondary retention (R) must entend a distance from the primary interabutment axis equal to the distance that the pontic lever arm (P) extends in the opposite direction.

Special Problems

Some problem situations occur often enough to deserve mention. Some of the commonly used solutions to the problems are also presented.

Pier Abutments

Rigid connectors (eg, solder joints) between pontics and retainers are the preferred way of fabricating most fixed partial dentures. A fixed partial denture with the pontic rigidly fixed to the retainers provides desirable strength and stability to the prosthesis while minimizing the stresses associated with the restoration.

However, a completely rigid restoration is not indicated for all situations requiring a fixed prosthesis. An edentulous space can occur on both sides of a tooth, creating a lone, freestanding pier abutment (Fig 7-21). Physiologic tooth movement, arch position of the abutments, and a disparity in the retentive capacity of the retainers can make a rigid five-unit fixed partial denture a less than ideal plan of treatment.

Studies in periodontometry have shown that the faciolingual movement ranges from 56 to 108 μm,[16] and intrusion is 28 μm.[17] Teeth in different segments of the arch move in different directions.[18] Because of the curvature of the arch, the faciolingual movement of an anterior tooth occurs at a considerable angle to the faciolingual movement of a molar (Fig 7-22).

These movements of measurable magnitude and in divergent directions can create stresses in a long-span prosthesis that will be transferred to the abutments.

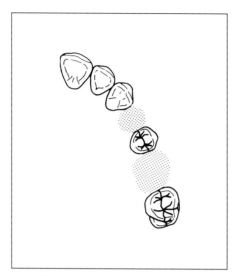

Fig 7-21 In this frequently occurring situation, the maxillary first premolar and molar are missing, leaving the second premolar as a pier abutment.

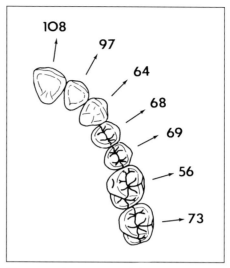

Fig 7-22 The amount of faciolingual movement (in μm) for each tooth in the maxillary arch (based on data by Rudd et al[16]). The direction of movement, indicated by arrows, varies considerably from the anterior to the posterior segment of the arch.

Because of the distance through which movement occurs, the independent direction and magnitude of movements of the abutment teeth, and the tendency of the prosthesis to flex, stress can be concentrated around the abutment teeth as well as between retainers and abutment preparations.

It has been theorized that forces are transmitted to the terminal retainers as a result of the middle abutment acting as a fulcrum, causing failure of the weaker retainer.[19] However, photoelastic stress analysis and displacement measurement indicate that the prosthesis bends rather than rocks. Standlee and Caputo suggest that tension between the terminal retainers and their respective abutments, rather than a pier fulcrum, is the mechanism of failure.[20] Intrusion of the abutments under the loading could lead to failure between any retainer and its respective abutment.

The loosened casting will leak around the margin, and caries is likely to become extensive before discovery. The retention on a smaller anterior tooth is usually less than that of a posterior tooth because of its generally smaller dimensions. Since there are limits to increasing a retainer's capacity to withstand displacing forces, some means must be used to neutralize the effects of those forces. The use of a nonrigid connector has been recommended to reduce this hazard.[19]

In spite of an apparently close fit, the movement in a nonrigid connector is enough to prevent the transfer of stress from the segment being loaded to the rest of the fixed partial denture (Fig 7-23). The nonrigid connector is a broken-stress mechanical union of retainer and pontic, instead of the usual rigid connector. The most commonly

used nonrigid design consists of a T-shaped key that is attached to the pontic, and a dovetail keyway placed within a retainer.

Use of the nonrigid connector is restricted to a short-span fixed partial denture replacing one tooth.[21] The magnification of force created by a long span is too destructive to the abutment tooth under the soldered retainer. Prostheses with nonrigid connectors should not be used if prospective abutment teeth exhibit significant mobility. There must be equal distribution of occlusal forces on all parts of the fixed partial denture.

A nonrigid fixed partial denture transfers shear stress to supporting bone rather than concentrating it in the connectors. It appears to minimize mesiodistal torquing of the abutments while permitting them to move independently.[22] A rigid fixed partial denture distributes the load more evenly than a nonrigid design, making it preferable for teeth with decreased periodontal attachment.[23] If the posterior abutment and pontic are either unopposed or opposed by a removable partial denture and if the three anterior units are opposed by natural teeth, the key and the posterior units that are subjected to little or no occlusal forces may supererupt.

The location of the stress-breaking device in the five-unit pier-abutment restoration is important. It usually is placed on the middle abutment, since placement of it on either of the terminal abutments could result in the pontic acting as a lever arm.

The keyway of the connector should be placed within the normal distal contours of the pier abutment, and the key should be placed on the mesial side of the distal pontic. The long axes of the posterior teeth usually lean

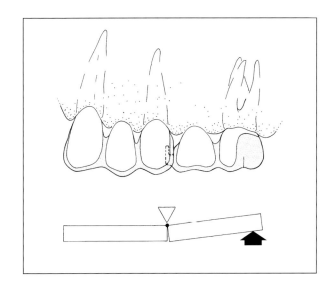

Fig 7-23 A nonrigid connector on the middle abutment isolates force to that segment of the fixed partial denture to which it is applied. (From Shillingburg and Fisher.[19])

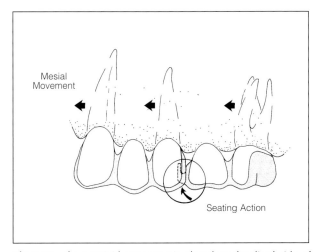

Fig 7-24 If a nonrigid connector is placed on the distal side of the retainer on a middle abutment, movement in a mesial direction will seat the key into the keyway. (From Shillingburg and Fisher.[19])

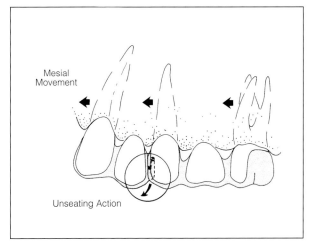

Fig 7-25 If a nonrigid connector is placed on the mesial side of the middle abutment, mesially directed movement will unseat the key. (From Shillingburg and Fisher.[19])

slightly in a mesial direction, and vertically applied occlusal forces produce further movement in this direction. Nearly 98% of posterior teeth tilt mesially when subjected to occlusal forces.[24] If the keyway of the connector is placed on the distal side of the pier abutment, mesial movement seats the key into the keyway more solidly (Fig 7-24).[19] Placement of the keyway on the mesial side, however, causes the key to be unseated during its mesial movements (Fig 7-25).[20] In time, this could produce a pathologic mobility in the canine or failure of the canine retainer.

Tilted Molar Abutments

A common problem that occurs with some frequency is the mandibular second molar abutment that has tilted mesially into the space formerly occupied by the first molar. It is impossible to prepare the abutment teeth for a fixed partial denture along the long axes of the respective teeth and achieve a common path of insertion (Fig 7-26).

There is further complication if the third molar is present. It will usually have drifted and tilted with the second molar. Because the path of insertion for the fixed partial denture will be dictated by the smaller premolar abut-

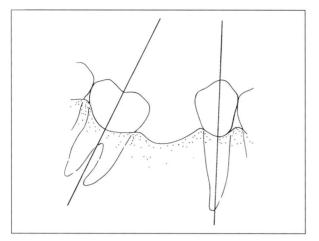

Fig 7-26 When a mandibular molar tilts mesially, there is a discrepancy between the long axis of the molar and that of the premolar.

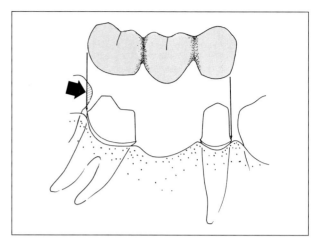

Fig 7-27 This fixed partial denture will not seat because the tooth distal to the fixed partial denture intrudes on the path of insertion *(arrow)*.

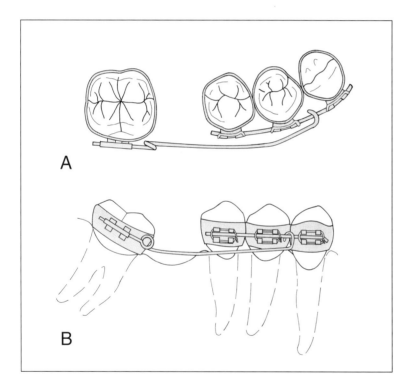

Fig 7-28 Orthodontic appliance for uprighting a tilted molar: (A) occlusal view; (B) buccal view.

ment, it is probable that the path of insertion will be nearly parallel to the former long axis of the molar abutment before it tilted mesially. As a result, the mesial surface of the tipped third molar will encroach upon the path of insertion of the fixed partial denture, thereby preventing it from seating completely (Fig 7-27).

If the encroachment is slight, the problem can be remedied by restoring or recontouring the mesial surface of the third molar. However, the overtapered second molar preparation must have its retention bolstered by the addition of facial and lingual grooves. If the tilting is

severe, more extensive corrective measures are called for. The treatment of choice is the uprighting of the molar by orthodontic treatment. In addition to placing the abutment tooth in a better position for preparation and for distribution of forces under occlusal loading, uprighting the molar also helps to eliminate bony defects along the mesial surface of the root.

Uprighting is best accomplished by the use of a fixed appliance.[25] Both premolars and the canine are banded and tied to a passive stabilizing wire (Fig 7-28). A helical uprighting spring is inserted into a tube on the banded

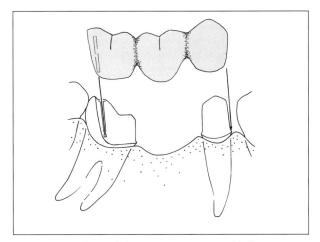

Fig 7-29 Fixed partial denture using a proximal half crown as a retainer on a tilted molar abutment.

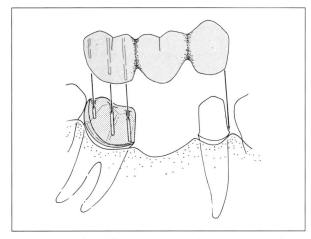

Fig 7-30 Fixed partial denture using a telescope crown and coping as a retainer on a tilted molar abutment.

molar and activated by hooking it over the wire on the anterior segment.[25,26] This is frequently followed by the use of an open coil spring to complete the uprighting and bring the tooth into the best possible alignment for fabrication of the fixed restoration. The average treatment time required is 3 months.[27]

The third molar, if present, is often removed to facilitate the distal movement of the second molar. The second molar will arc occlusally as it moves distally, so that it must be watched closely and ground out of occlusion to allow it to continue moving. Immediately upon removal of the appliance, the teeth are prepared and a temporary fixed partial denture is fabricated to prevent posttreatment relapse.[28]

If orthodontic correction is not possible, or if it is possible to achieve only a partial correction, a fixed partial denture can still be made. It has been suggested that the long axis of the prospective abutments should converge by no more than 25 to 30 degrees.[29] Photoelastic[30] and finite element[31] stress analyses have shown that a molar which has tipped mesially will actually exhibit less stress in the alveolar bone, along the mesial surface of its mesial root, with a fixed partial denture than without it. There will be an increase in stress along the premolar, however.

A proximal half crown sometimes can be used as a retainer on the distal abutment (Fig 7-29).[32] This preparation design is simply a three-quarter crown that has been rotated 90 degrees so that the distal surface is uncovered. This retainer can be used only if the distal surface itself is untouched by caries or decalcification and if there is a very low incidence of proximal caries throughout the mouth. The patient must also demonstrate an ability to keep the area exceptionally clean. If there is a severe marginal ridge height discrepancy between the distal of the second molar and the mesial of the third molar as a result of tipping, the proximal half crown is contraindicated.

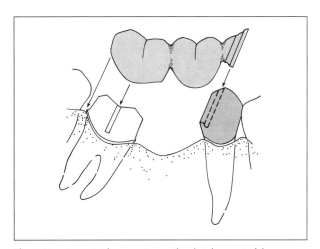

Fig 7-31 A nonrigid connector on the distal aspect of the premolar retainer compensates for the inclination of the tilted molar.

A telescope crown and coping can also be used as a retainer on the distal abutment.[33] A full crown preparation with heavy reduction is made to follow the long axis of the tilted molar. An inner coping is made to fit the tooth preparation, and the proximal half crown that will serve as the retainer for the fixed partial denture is fitted over the coping (Fig 7-30). This restoration allows for total coverage of the clinical crown while compensating for the discrepancy between the paths of insertion of the abutments. The marginal adaptation for this restoration is provided by the coping.

The nonrigid connector is another solution to the problem of the tilted fixed partial denture abutment (Fig 7-31). A full crown preparation is done on the molar, with its

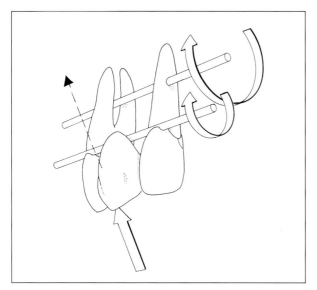

Fig 7-32 A fixed partial denture replacing a maxillary canine is subjected to more damaging stresses because the forces are directed outward and the pontic lies farther outside the interabutment axis.

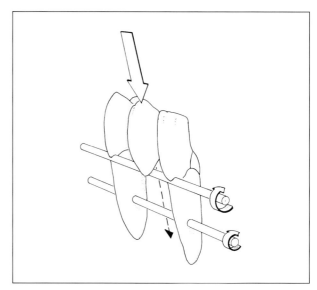

Fig 7-33 A fixed partial denture replacing a mandibular canine is more favorable because the forces are directed inward and the pontic will be closer to the interabutment axis.

path of insertion parallel with the long axis of that tilted tooth. A box form is placed in the distal surface of the premolar to accommodate a keyway in the distal of the premolar crown. It is tempting to place the connector on the mesial aspect of the tipped molar, but this could lead to even greater tipping of the tooth. A nonrigid connector for the tipped molar abutment is most useful when the molar exhibits a marked lingual as well as mesial inclination. Preparing a tooth with a combined mesial and lingual inclination as an abutment for a routine fixed partial denture can lead to a drastically overtapered preparation with no retention.

Because telescope crowns and nonrigid connectors both require tooth preparations that are more destructive than normal, the selection of one of these would be influenced by the nature of previous destruction of the prospective abutment teeth. The presence of a dowel core or a DO amalgam on the premolar, for example, would favor placement of a nonrigid connector on that tooth, while extensive facial and/or lingual restorations on the tilted molar would call for the use of a telescope crown.

Canine-Replacement Fixed Partial Dentures

Fixed partial dentures replacing canines can be difficult because the canine often lies outside the interabutment axis. The prospective abutments are the lateral incisor, usually the weakest tooth in the entire arch, and the first premolar, the weakest posterior tooth. A fixed partial denture replacing a maxillary canine is subjected to more stresses than that replacing a mandibular canine, since

forces are transmitted outward (labially) on the maxillary arch, against the inside of the curve (its weakest point) (Fig 7-32). On the mandibular canine the forces are directed inward (lingually), against the outside of the curve (its strongest point) (Fig 7-33). Any fixed partial denture replacing a canine should be considered a complex fixed partial denture. No fixed partial denture replacing a canine should replace more than one additional tooth. An edentulous space created by the loss of a canine and any two contiguous teeth is best restored with a removable partial denture.

Cantilever Fixed Partial Dentures

A cantilever fixed partial denture is one that has an abutment or abutments at one end only, with the other end of the pontic remaining unattached. This is a potentially destructive design with the lever arm created by the pontic, and it is frequently misused.

In the routine three-unit fixed partial denture, force that is applied to the pontic is distributed equally to the abutment teeth (Fig 7-34). If there is only one pontic and it is near the interabutment axis line, less leverage is applied to the abutment teeth or to the retainers than with a cantilever. When a cantilever pontic is employed to replace a missing tooth, forces applied to the pontic have an entirely different effect on the abutment tooth. The pontic acts as a lever that tends to be depressed under forces with a strong occlusal vector (Fig 7-35).

Prospective abutment teeth for cantilever fixed partial dentures should be evaluated with an eye toward lengthy roots with a favorable configuration, long clinical crowns,

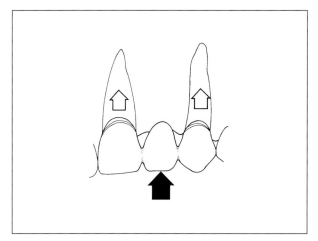

Fig 7-34 Forces applied to the pontic of a routine fixed partial denture are transmitted to both abutment teeth.

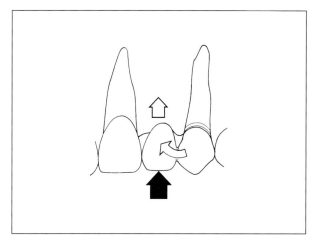

Fig 7-35 Forces on the pontic of a cantilever fixed partial denture tend to tip the fixed partial denture or the abutment tooth.

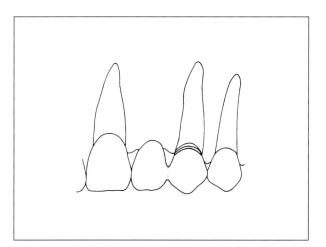

Fig 7-36 Cantilever fixed partial denture replacing a maxillary lateral incisor, using the canine as the abutment.

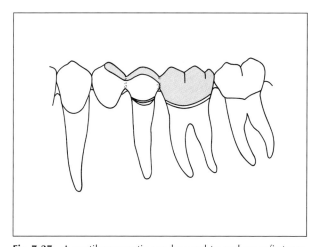

Fig 7-37 A cantilever pontic can be used to replace a first premolar, if full veneer retainers are used on the second premolar and first molar abutments.

good crown-root ratios, and healthy periodontium.[34] Generally, cantilever fixed partial dentures should replace only one tooth and have at least two abutments.[35,36]

A cantilever can be used for replacing a maxillary lateral incisor (Fig 7-36). There should be no occlusal contact on the pontic in either centric or lateral excursions.[37] The canine must be used as an abutment, and it can serve in the role of solo abutment only if it has a long root and good bone support. There should be a rest on the mesial of the pontic against a rest preparation in an inlay or other metallic restoration on the distal of the central incisor to prevent rotation of the pontic and abutment.

The mesial aspect of the pontic can be slightly "wrapped around" the distal portion of the uninvolved central incisor to stabilize the pontic faciolingually.[37] The root configuration of a central incisor does not make it a desirable cantilever abutment.

A cantilever pontic can also be used to replace a missing first premolar (Fig 7-37). This scheme will work best if occlusal contact is limited to the distal fossa. Full veneer retainers are required on both the second premolar and first molar. These teeth must exhibit excellent bone support. This design is attractive if the canine is unmarred and if a full veneer restoration is required for the first molar in any event.

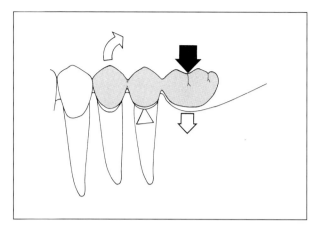

Fig 7-38 Forces on a full-size molar cantilever pontic place great stress on the mesial abutment.

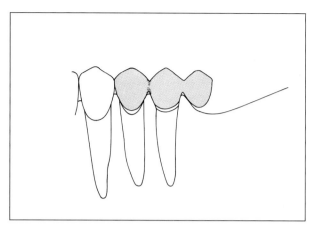

Fig 7-39 Cantilever fixed partial denture replacing a mandibular first molar, using both premolars as abutment teeth. To minimize stress on the abutments, the pontic is the size of a premolar rather than a molar.

Cantilever fixed partial dentures can also be used to replace molars when there is no distal abutment present. When used judiciously, it is possible to avoid the insertion of a unilateral removable partial denture.[34] Most commonly, this type of fixed partial denture is used to replace a first molar, although occasionally it is used to replace a second molar to prevent supereruption of opposing teeth.

When the pontic is loaded occlusally, the adjacent abutment tends to act as a fulcrum, with a lifting tendency on the farthest retainer (Fig 7-38).[38] To minimize the leverage effect, the pontic should be kept as small as possible, more nearly representing a premolar than a molar (Fig 7-39). There should be light occlusal contact with absolutely no contact in any excursion. The pontic should possess maximum occlusogingival height to ensure a rigid prosthesis.

A posterior cantilever pontic places maximum demands on the retentive capacity of the retainer.[39] Its use, therefore, should be reserved for those situations in which there is adequate clinical crown length on the abutment teeth to permit preparations of maximum length and retention. The success of cantilevers in the restoration of the periodontally compromised dentition is probably due at least in part to the fact that periodontally involved abutments do have extremely long clinical crowns. While cantilever fixed partial dentures appear to be a conservative restoration, the potential for damage to the abutment teeth requires that they be used sparingly.

References

1. Klaffenbach AO: Gnathodynamics. *J Am Dent Assoc* 1936; 23:371–382.

2. Penny RE, Kraal JH: Crown-to-root ratio: Its significance in restorative dentistry. *J Prosthet Dent* 1979; 42:34–38.

3. Jepsen A: Root surface measurement and a method for x-ray determination of root surface area. *Acta Odontol Scand* 1963; 21:35–46.

4. Kalkwarf KL, Krejci RF, Pao YC: Effect of root resorption on periodontal support. *J Prosthet Dent* 1986; 56:317–319.

5. Tylman SD: *Theory and Practice of Crown and Fixed Partial Prosthodontics (Bridge),* ed 6. St Louis, CV Mosby Co, 1970, p 17.

6. Johnston JF, Phillips RW, Dykema RW: *Modern Practice in Crown and Bridge Prosthodontics,* ed 3. Philadelphia, WB Saunders Co, 1971, p 11.

7. Ante IH: The fundamental principles of abutments. *Mich State Dent Soc Bull* 1926; 8:14–23.

8. Nyman S, Lindhe J: Prosthetic rehabilitation of patients with advanced periodontal disease. *J Clin Periodontol* 1976; 3:135–147.

9. Nyman S, Lindhe J, Lundgren D: The role of occlusion for the stability of fixed bridges in patients with reduced periodontal tissue support. *J Clin Periodontol* 1975; 2:53–66.

10. Lindhe J, Nyman S: The role of occlusion in periodontal disease and the biologic rationale for splinting in treatment of periodontics. *Oral Sci Rev* 1977; 10:11–43.

11. Jacobi R, Shillingburg HT, Duncanson MG: Effect of mobility, site, and angle of impact on retention of fixed partial dentures. *J Prosthet Dent* 1985; 54:178–183.

12. Nyman S, Lindhe J: A longitudinal study of combined periodontal and prosthetic treatment of patients with advanced periodontal disease. *J Periodontol* 1979; 50:163–169.

13. Smyd ES: Mechanics of dental structures: Guide to teaching dental engineering at undergraduate level. *J Prosthet Dent* 1952; 2:668–692.

14. Smyd ES: Advanced thought in indirect inlay and fixed bridge fabrication. *J Am Dent Assoc* 1944; 31:759–768.

15. Dykema RW: Fixed partial prosthodontics. *J Tenn Dent Assoc* 1962; 42:309–321.

16. Rudd KD, O'Leary TJ, Stumpf AJ: Horizontal tooth mobility in carefully screened subjects. *Periodontics* 1964; 2:65–68.

17. Parfitt GJ: Measurement of the physiological mobility of individual teeth in an axial direction. *J Dent Res* 1960; 39:608–618.

18. Chayes HES, cited in McCall JO, Hugel IM: Movable-removable bridgework: Principles and practice as developed by Herman ES Chayes, DDS. *Dent Items Interest* 1949; 71:512–525.

19. Shillingburg HT, Fisher DW: Nonrigid connectors for fixed partial dentures. *J Am Dent Assoc* 1973; 87:1195–1199.

20. Standlee JP, Caputo AA: Load transfer by fixed partial dentures with three abutments. *Quintessence Int* 1988; 19:403–410.

21. Markley MR: Broken-stress principle and design in fixed bridge prosthesis. *J Prosthet Dent* 1951; 1:416–423.

22. Sutherland JK, Holland GA, Sluder TB, White JT: A photoelastic analysis of the stress distribution in bone supporting fixed partial dentures of rigid and nonrigid designs. *J Prosthet Dent* 1980; 44:616–623.

23. Landry KE, Johnson PF, Parks VJ, Pelleu GB: A photoelastic study to determine the location of the nonrigid connector in a five-unit intermediate abutment prosthesis. *J Prosthet Dent* 1987; 57:454–457.

24. Picton DCA: Tilting movements of teeth during biting. *Arch Oral Biol* 1962; 7:151–159.

25. Khouw FE, Norton LA: The mechanism of fixed molar uprighting appliances. *J Prosthet Dent* 1972; 27:381–389.

26. Norton LA, Profitt WR: Molar uprighting as an adjunct to fixed prostheses. *J Am Dent Assoc* 1968; 76:312–315.

27. Simon RL: Rationale and practical technique for uprighting mesially inclined molars. *J Prosthet Dent* 1984; 52:256–259.

28. Norton LA, Parker WT: Management of repositioned teeth in preparation for fixed partial dentures. *J Am Dent Assoc* 1970; 81:916–922.

29. Reynolds JM: Abutment selection for fixed prosthodontics. *J Prosthet Dent* 1968; 19:483–488.

30. Hood JA, Farah JW, Craig RG: Modification of stresses in alveolar bone induced by a tilted molar. *J Prosthet Dent* 1975; 34:415–421.

31. Yang HS, Thompson VP: A two-dimensional stress analysis comparing fixed prosthodontic approaches to the tilted molar abutment. *Int J Prosthodont* 1991; 4:416–424.

32. Smith DE: Fixed bridge restorations with the tilted mandibular second or third molar as an abutment. *J South Calif Dent Assoc* 1939; 6:131–138.

33. Shillingburg HT: Bridge retainers for tilted abutments. *NM Dent J* 1972; 22:16–19.

34. Ewing JE: Re-evaluation of the cantilever principle. *J Prosthet Dent* 1957; 7:78–92.

35. Wright KWJ, Yettram AL: Reactive force distributions for teeth when loaded singly and when used as fixed partial denture abutments. *J Prosthet Dent* 1979; 42:411–416.

36. Wright WE: Success with the cantilever fixed partial denture. *J Prosthet Dent* 1986; 55:537–539.

37. Goldfogel MH, Lambert RL: Cantilever fixed prosthesis replacing the maxillary lateral incisor: Design consideration. *J Prosthet Dent* 1985; 54:477–478.

38. Schweitzer JM, Schweitzer RD, Schweitzer J: Free-end pontics used on fixed partial dentures. *J Prosthet Dent* 1968; 20:120–138.

39. Nyman S, Lindhe J: Considerations on the design of occlusion in prosthetic rehabilitation of patients with advanced periodontal disease. *J Clin Periodontol* 1977; 4:1–15.

Chapter 8

Fixed Partial Denture Configurations

Fixed partial dentures can be categorized as either simple or complex, depending on the number of teeth to be replaced and the position of the edentulous space in the arch. The classic simple fixed partial denture is one that replaces a single tooth. Longer spans generally place greater demands on the skills of the dentist, on the resistance of the retainers, and on the abutments and their periodontal support.

The maximum number of posterior teeth that can be safely replaced with a fixed partial denture is three, and this should be attempted only under ideal conditions. An edentulous space created by the loss of four adjacent teeth other than four incisors is usually best restored with either a removable partial denture or an implant-supported fixed partial denture. If more than one edentulous space exists in the same arch, even though each could be individually restored with a fixed partial denture, it may be desirable to use a removable partial denture. This is especially true when the spaces are bilateral and each involves two or more teeth.

Third molars are not shown in any of the examples, and no situation is shown in which a third molar would be a prospective abutment. Rarely can third molars be used as abutments, since they have been removed from the mouths of so many patients. Even when they are present, they frequently display incomplete eruption; short, fused roots; and a marked mesial inclination in the absence of a second molar.

If a third molar is to be considered as a potential abutment, it should be upright, with little or no mesial inclination; have long, distinctly separate roots; and be completely erupted. It must have a healthy cuff of attached, keratinized gingiva that completely surrounds the tooth.

The unattached mucosal tissue that frequently surrounds the distal 30% to 60% of third molars will become inflamed adjacent to even a well-fitting crown margin, and the abutment is likely to fail periodontally.

The following examples are given as a reference that will apply under ideal conditions. The abutment teeth that normally would be used are listed, along with the first choice of retainer designs based on adequate retention, esthetics, and conservation of tooth structure. Clinical situations vary widely, and less conservative designs will be required when caries, decalcification, or morphologic traits (such as short clinical crowns) dictate. These configurations assume that the prospective abutments are still in their original positions. If the abutments have drifted, the situation could become less demanding, and on occasion more demanding, depending on the current position of the tooth. Fewer or more abutments may be necessitated if there has been drifting, or if there has been bone loss. The ratios shown for root surface areas are intended as a general guideline. An abutment-pontic root ratio of 1.0 or greater is considered to be favorable.

Conventional partial veneer retainers could be used for many of the prostheses described. However, the reluctance of many patients to accept any display of metal and the lack of dentist familiarity with these preparations require that this design be used only on selected posterior abutments. Likewise, resin-bonded fixed partial dentures ("Maryland bridges") have replaced pin-modified three-quarter crown retainers because the skill level required for the pin-retained restoration, while attainable, lies outside the realm of basic, or "fundamental," fixed prosthodontics.

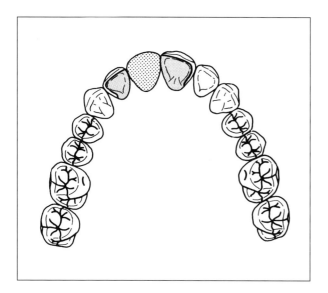

Simple Fixed Partial Dentures (one tooth)

Missing: Maxillary central incisor
Abutments: Central incisor and lateral incisor
Retainers: Resin-bonded retainers
Pontic: Metal-ceramic
Abutment-pontic root ratio: 1.9
Considerations: Abutment discoloration, rotated abutment, improper width of edentulous space, or proximal caries may require metal-ceramic retainers. If occlusal contact occurs on the gingival one-third of the lingual surfaces of the abutments, conventional retainers may be needed.

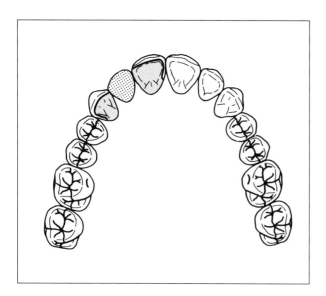

Missing: Mandibular central incisor
Abutments: Central incisor and lateral incisor
Retainers: Resin-bonded retainers
Pontic: Metal-ceramic
Abutment-pontic root ratio: 2.1
Considerations: Severely rotated, malposed, or mobile abutments will contraindicate the use of resin-bonded retainers. If metal-ceramic retainers are required, the preparations very easily could encroach on the pulp, and the patient should be so advised. Endodontic treatment and a dowel core would then be necessary.

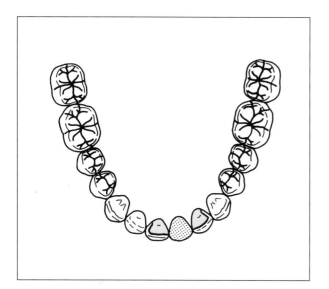

Missing: Maxillary lateral incisor
Abutments: Central incisor and canine
Retainers: Resin-bonded retainers
Pontic: Metal-ceramic
Abutment-pontic root ratio: 2.6
Considerations: Caries and/or restorations on the abutments would require metal-ceramic retainers. If the canine is long, well-supported periodontally, and in need of restoration, and if the pontic will not contact in centric or lateral excursions, a single-abutment cantilever fixed partial denture can be used. In that case, a metal-ceramic crown also should be used as a retainer. An untouched central incisor and a first premolar in need of restoration could call for a pontic cantilevered from metal-ceramic crowns on the canine and first premolar.

Missing: Mandibular lateral incisor
Abutments: Central incisor and canine
Retainers: Resin-bonded retainers
Pontic: Metal-ceramic
Abutment-pontic root ratio: 2.5
Considerations: Caries and/or restorations on the abutments would require metal-ceramic retainers. The patient should be warned of the potential for pulpal involvement with resultant endodontic treatment and dowel core. Even moderate bone loss around the central incisor will require that the other central incisor be used as a secondary abutment. Cantilever fixed partial dentures are not an option for the replacement of mandibular lateral incisors.

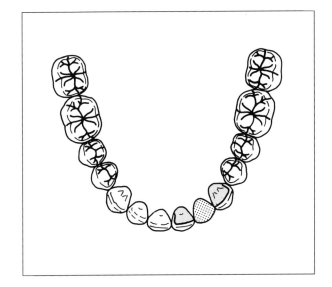

Missing: Maxillary first premolar
Abutments: Canine and second premolar
Retainers: Resin-bonded retainers, if teeth are unblemished
Pontic: Metal-ceramic
Abutment-pontic root ratio: 2.1
Considerations: Facial caries or any proximal caries other than incipient will necessitate metal-ceramic retainers. If the second premolar and first molar are restored or will need restoration, a cantilever prosthesis using metal-ceramic retainers on the second premolar and first molar is worthy of consideration. A canine-guided occlusal scheme would be necessary to prevent excessive forces on the cantilever pontic. If that is not possible, do not use a cantilever.

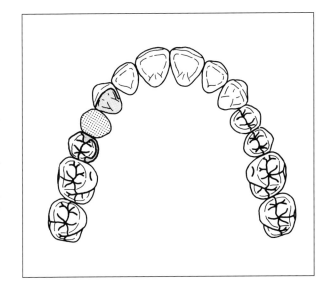

Missing: Mandibular first premolar
Abutments: Canine and second premolar
Retainers: Resin-bonded retainers, if teeth are unmarred
Pontic: Metal-ceramic
Abutment-pontic root ratio: 2.5
Considerations: Facial caries or any proximal caries other than incipient will necessitate metal-ceramic retainers. If the canine is intact and second premolar and first molar are restored or will need restoration, a cantilever fixed partial denture can be used, with metal-ceramic retainers on the second premolar and first molar abutments. If the patient does not object, an all-metal crown can be substituted on the molar.

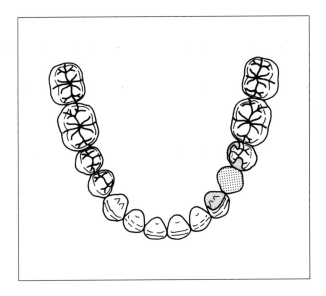

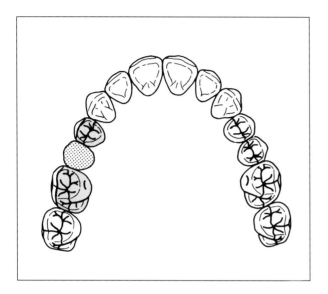

Missing: Maxillary second premolar
Abutments: First premolar and first molar
Retainers: Three-quarter crowns
Pontic: Metal-ceramic
Abutment-pontic root ratio: 3.1
Considerations: Facial defects or patient request will necessitate metal-ceramic retainers. Resin-bonded retainers can be used if the abutments are caries-free or very minimally affected by caries.

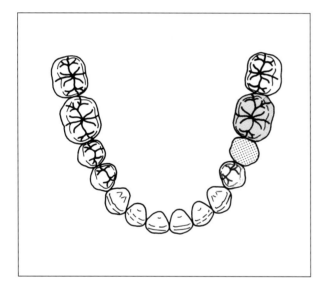

Missing: Mandibular second premolar
Abutments: First premolar and first molar
Retainers: Metal-ceramic crown on premolar and full crown on molar
Pontic: Metal-ceramic
Abutment-pontic root ratio: 3.1
Considerations: Esthetic requirements of the patient may necessitate a metal-ceramic retainer on the molar. A three-quarter crown can be suggested for the first premolar if it has an unusually large clinical crown. Patient acceptance is necessary but may not be forthcoming. Resin-bonded retainers can be used if the premolar is large and if the abutments are caries-free or only minimally affected by caries.

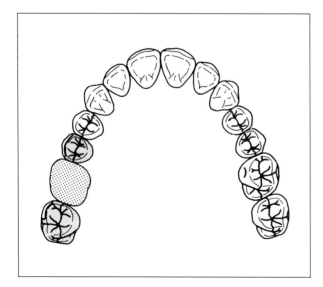

Missing: Maxillary first molar
Abutments: Second premolar and second molar
Retainers: Three-quarter crown on premolar and seven-eighths crown on molar
Pontic: Metal-ceramic
Abutment-pontic root ratio: 1.5
Considerations: If the clinical crown of the premolar is short, an additional set of grooves may be desirable to increase retention. Patient esthetic requirements can require a metal-ceramic crown on the premolar. A seven-eighths crown on the molar will not be objectionable in most mouths. Heavy occlusal forces and wider edentulous space of a first molar usually contraindicate resin-bonded retainers.

Missing: Mandibular first molar
Abutments: Second premolar and second molar
Retainers: Metal-ceramic crown on premolar and full veneer gold crown on molar
Pontic: All-metal hygienic
Abutment-pontic root ratio: 1.5
Considerations: A three-quarter crown is technically feasible on the second premolar if the clinical crown is longer than average and the patient is agreeable. A tilted molar may require orthodontic uprighting, a proximal half crown, or a telescope crown.

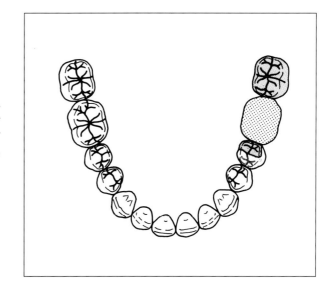

Complex Fixed Partial Dentures (one tooth)

Missing: Maxillary canine
Abutments: Central incisor, lateral incisor, and first premolar
Retainers: Metal-ceramic
Pontic: Metal-ceramic
Abutment-pontic root ratio: 2.3
Considerations: Restore the occlusion to group function. Use of the two premolars and the lateral incisor as abutments is not desirable because it places too heavy a burden on the smaller single abutment, the lateral incisor. A single implant supported metal-ceramic crown might be considered here.

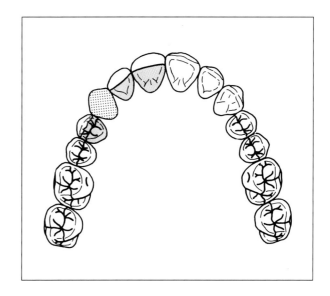

Missing: Mandibular canine
Abutments: Central incisor, lateral incisor, and first premolar
Retainers: Metal-ceramic
Pontic: Metal-ceramic
Abutment-pontic root ratio: 1.9
Considerations: Use group function to restore the occlusion. If there has been extensive bone loss around the lateral incisor, or if it is tilted to produce a line of draw discrepancy, remove the lateral incisor and use both central incisors as abutments. A single implant-supported metal-ceramic crown might be used here. Replacement of this tooth is not common.

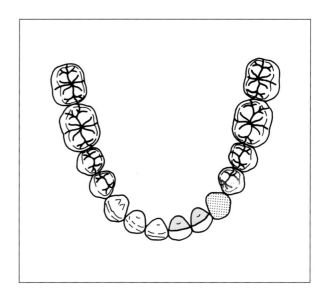

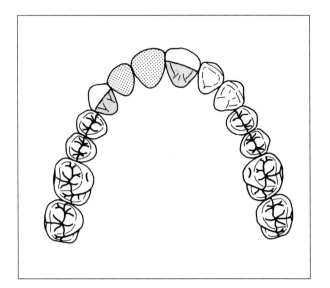

Simple Fixed Partial Dentures (two teeth)

Missing: Maxillary central incisor and lateral incisor
Abutments: Central incisor and canine
Retainers: Metal-ceramic
Pontic: Metal-ceramic
Abutment-pontic root ratio: 1.2
Considerations: If the central incisor and canine are unblemished and unusually large, conventional or pin-modified partial veneer crowns can be used. Patient acceptance and dentist skill are strong considerations.

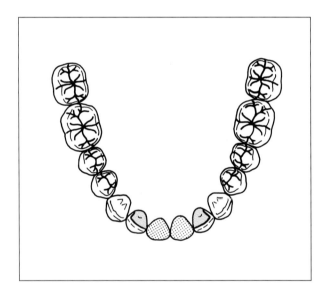

Missing: Mandibular central incisors
Abutments: Lateral incisors
Retainers: Resin-bonded
Pontics: Metal-ceramic
Abutment-pontic root ratio: 1.1
Considerations: If there has been any bone loss at all around the lateral incisors, the canines should be included as abutments and metal-ceramic retainers used. Malposition of the lateral incisors could dictate their removal.

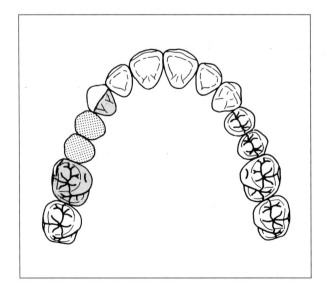

Missing: Maxillary first and second premolars
Abutments: Canine and first molar
Retainers: Metal-ceramic on canine and seven-eighths crown on molar
Pontics: Metal-ceramic
Abutment-pontic root ratio: 1.6
Considerations: A metal-ceramic crown may be used on the molar if the mesiofacial cusp is damaged or undermined, or if the patient requests it. If the canine is large enough, and the patient will accept a minimal display of metal, a three-quarter crown can be used.

Missing: Mandibular first and second premolars
Abutments: Canine and first molar
Retainers: Metal-ceramic crown on canine and full veneer gold crown on molar
Pontics: Metal-ceramic
Abutment-pontic root ratio: 1.8
Considerations: If the molar has tilted mesially, orthodontic uprighting or preparation modification may be required. The patient's esthetics expectations may require a metal-ceramic crown on the molar.

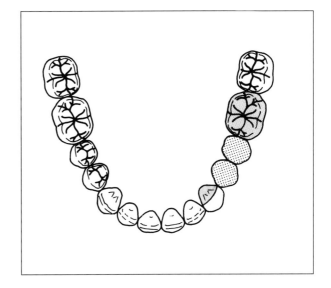

Missing: Maxillary second premolar and first molar
Abutments: First premolar and second molar
Retainers: Metal-ceramic crown on premolar and full veneer or seven-eighths crown on molar
Pontics: Metal-ceramic
Abutment-pontic root ratio: 1.0
Considerations: If the premolar has a long clinical crown and the patient will accept a minimal display of metal, a three-quarter crown with double grooves can be used.

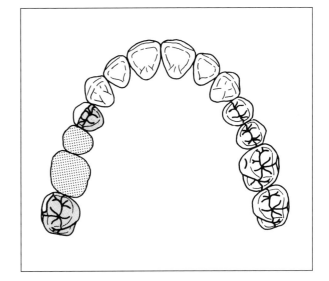

Missing: Mandibular second premolar and first molar
Abutments: First premolar and second molar
Retainers: Metal-ceramic crown on premolar and full veneer gold crown on molar
Pontics: Metal-ceramic
Abutment-pontic root ratio: 1.0
Considerations: If the premolar root is short or thin, or if the clinical crown is very small, the canine should be included as a secondary abutment.

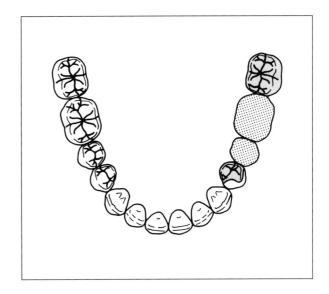

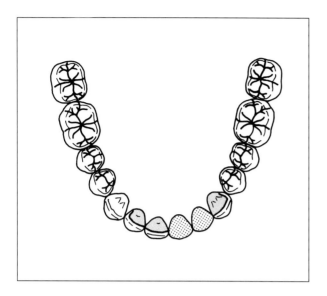

Complex Fixed Partial Dentures (two teeth)

Missing: Mandibular central incisor and lateral incisor
Abutments: Central incisor, lateral incisor, and canine
Retainers: Resin-bonded retainers
Pontics: Metal-ceramic
Abutment-pontic root ratio: 1.8
Considerations: Inadequate bone support around central and lateral incisors often requires their removal, with a resulting six-unit fixed partial denture with metal-ceramic retainers being required. Caries and/or restorations on the abutments would also require metal-ceramic retainers. The patient should be warned of the potential for pulpal involvement with resultant endodontic treatment and dowel core. Anterior guidance should be controlled carefully to avoid excessive lingually directed forces.

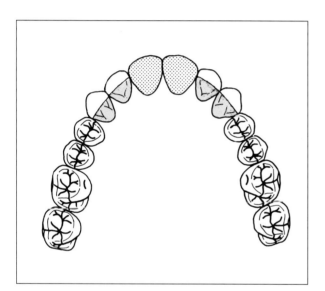

Missing: Maxillary central incisors
Abutments: Canines and lateral incisors
Retainers: Metal-ceramic
Pontics: Metal-ceramic
Abutment-pontic root ratio: 2.3
Considerations: When the bony support for the lateral incisors is poor, it is often best to extract them and lengthen the fixed partial denture. If the lateral incisors have long roots and crowns, they alone can be used as abutments. If the patient will accept a minimal display of metal, a skilled operator can use three-quarter crowns.

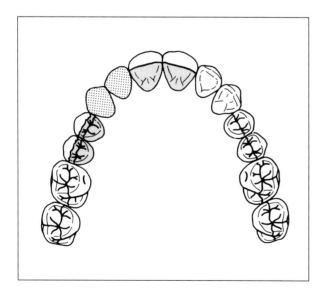

Missing: Maxillary lateral incisor and canine
Abutments: Both central incisors and both premolars
Retainers: Metal-ceramic
Pontics: Metal-ceramic
Abutment-pontic root ratio: 1.9
Considerations: Span length, abutment position, and root configuration make the use of four abutments desirable. All retainers must have good retention. If the premolars have drifted mesially, it may not be necessary to include the second premolar. Use group function to restore the occlusion.

Missing: Mandibular lateral incisor and canine
Abutments: Both central incisors and first premolar
Retainers: Metal-ceramic
Pontics: Metal-ceramic
Abutment-pontic root ratio: 1.1
Considerations: The short edentulous span and the direction of forces on the mandibular canine do not require the use of the second premolar as an abutment.

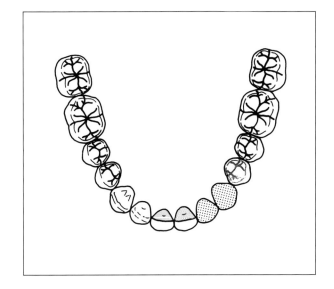

Missing: Maxillary canine and first premolar
Abutments: Central incisor, lateral incisor, second premolar, and first molar
Retainers: Metal-ceramic on incisors and second premolar, and seven-eighths crown on molar
Pontics: Metal-ceramic
Abutment-pontic root ratio: 2.0
Considerations: Group function should be used. This can be a difficult restoration.

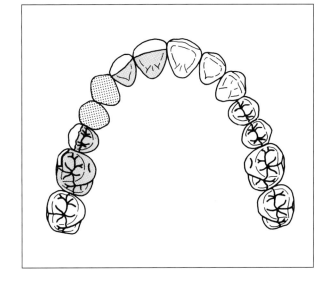

Missing: Mandibular canine and first premolar
Abutments: Central incisor, lateral incisor, and second premolar
Retainers: Metal-ceramic
Pontics: Metal-ceramic
Abutment-pontic root ratio: 1.5
Considerations: Use group function in restoring the occlusion. This also can be a difficult fixed partial denture, but fortunately it is rarely encountered.

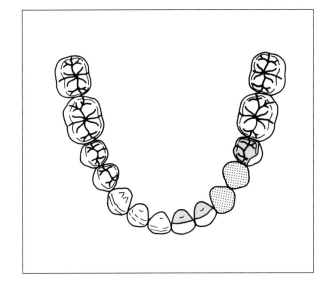

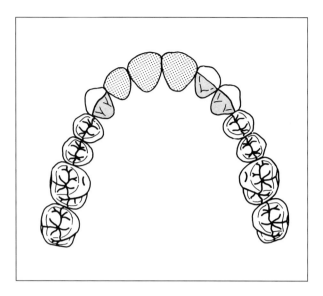

Complex Fixed Partial Dentures (more than two teeth)

Missing: Both maxillary central incisors and one lateral incisor
Abutments: Both canines and the remaining lateral incisor
Retainers: Metal-ceramic
Pontics: Metal-ceramic
Abutment-pontic root ratio: 1.3
Considerations: If the lateral incisor is questionable, it should be extracted and the fixed partial denture lengthened to include the first premolars. Standard three-quarter crowns can be used if the clinical crowns are long. Both patient approval of a minimal display of metal and a high degree of dentist skill are essential for this option to be considered.

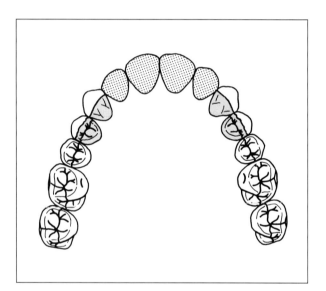

Missing: All maxillary incisors
Abutments: Canines and first premolars
Retainers: Metal-ceramic
Pontics: Metal-ceramic
Abutment-pontic root ratio: 1.3
Considerations: To counteract the lever arm created by the curve of the anterior segment of the arch, double abutments are often used with full veneer retainers to assure maximum retention. If the anterior curvature is slight and/or if the canines are exceptionally large, the premolars may be omitted as abutments.

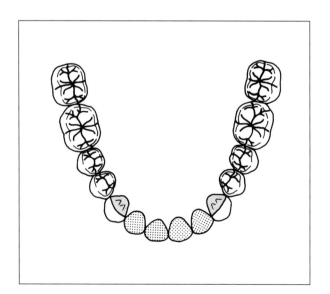

Missing: All mandibular incisors
Abutments: Canines
Retainers: Metal-ceramic
Pontics: Metal-ceramic
Abutment-pontic root ratio: 0.8
Considerations: There is no need to use double abutments on the mandibular canine to canine fixed partial denture, since the forces are less destructive. If a patient has a lone lateral or central incisor remaining, it is usually extracted. It would complicate the fixed partial denture without adding any appreciable support.

Missing: Maxillary first and second premolar and first molar
Abutments: Canine and second molar
Retainers: Metal-ceramic on canine and full veneer gold crown on molar
Pontics: Metal-ceramic
Abutment-pontic root ratio: 0.8
Considerations: This fixed partial denture can be made only if the clinical crowns of the abutments are long and perfectly aligned. The occlusogingival dimension of the edentulous space must be ample to provide adequate rigidity. This fixed partial denture has a much better prognosis if the opposing occlusion is on a removable partial denture. Canine guidance is important in this situation.

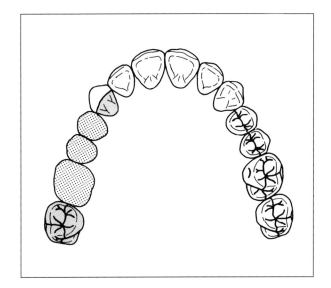

Complex Fixed Partial Dentures (pier abutment)

Missing: Maxillary central incisor and opposite-side lateral incisor
Abutments: Lateral incisor, central incisor, and canine
Retainers: Metal-ceramic
Pontics: Metal-ceramic
Abutment-pontic root ratio: 1.7
Considerations: A keyway is placed in the distal of the central incisor retainer to accommodate a key on the mesial of the lateral incisor pontic. If the central incisor is malpositioned or rotated, its extraction will simplify the restoration and improve its prognosis.

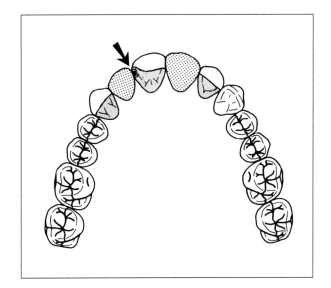

Missing: Mandibular central incisor and opposite-side lateral incisor
Abutments: Lateral incisor, central incisor, and canine
Retainers: Resin-bonded retainers
Pontics: Metal-ceramic
Abutment-pontic root ratio: 1.8
Considerations: A completely rigid fixed partial denture is used in this situation because of short span length and small teeth. If there are caries in any of the abutment teeth, metal-ceramic retainers are necessary. If either bone support or tooth alignment is poor, extract the central incisor and extend the fixed partial denture from canine to canine, again using metal-ceramic retainers. Metal-ceramic crowns on incisors may necessitate endodontic treatment and dowel cores.

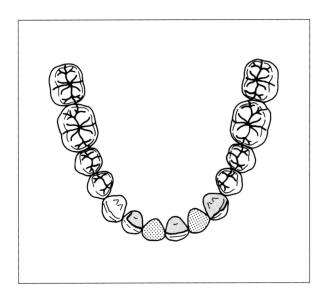

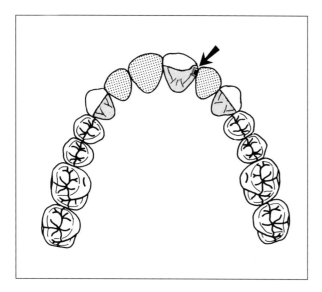

Missing: Both maxillary lateral incisors and one central incisor
Abutments: Central incisor and both canines
Retainers: Metal-ceramic
Pontics: Metal-ceramic
Abutment-pontic root ratio: 1.3
Considerations: There should be a nonrigid connector between the distal of the central incisor retainer and the mesial of the lone lateral incisor pontic. If the central incisor is malposed or periodontally compromised, it should be extracted. Three-quarter crowns can be used where the teeth are large and the patient will accept some display of metal.

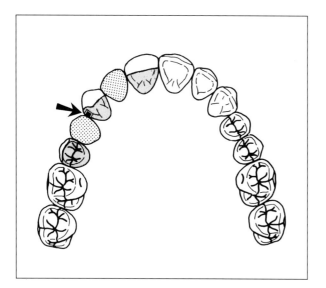

Missing: Maxillary lateral incisor and first premolar
Abutments: Central incisor, canine, and second premolar
Retainers: Metal-ceramic on central incisor and canine, and three-quarter crown on second premolar
Pontics: Metal-ceramic
Abutment-pontic root ratio: 1.7
Considerations: Nonrigid connector between canine and first premolar. A short clinical crown or esthetic concern will require a metal-ceramic crown on the second premolar. The corresponding mandibular situation would be restored in the same manner.

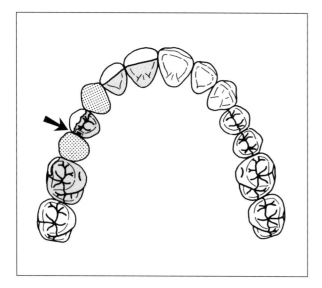

Missing: Maxillary canine and second premolar
Abutments: Central and lateral incisors, first premolar, and first molar
Retainers: Metal-ceramic on incisors and premolar, and seven-eighths crown on molar
Pontics: Metal-ceramic
Abutment-pontic root ratio: 2.1
Considerations: Nonrigid connector between first premolar retainer and second premolar pontic. The corresponding mandibular situation would be handled identically with the substitution of a full gold crown on the first molar, if the patient does not object. A metal-ceramic crown could be substituted.

Missing: All maxillary incisors and one first premolar
Abutments: Both canines, the first premolar on one side, and the second premolar on the other
Retainers: Metal-ceramic
Pontics: Metal-ceramic
Abutment-pontic root ratio: 1.0
Considerations: Nonrigid connector in the distal of the retainer on the canine "pier" abutment. A long second premolar or a lack of concern for esthetics by patient would permit the substitution of a three-quarter crown on the second premolar. The mandibular situation is handled similarly.

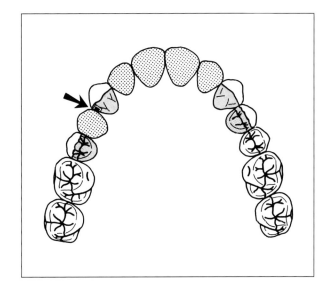

Missing: Maxillary lateral incisor, first and second premolars
Abutments: Canine and first molar
Retainers: Metal-ceramic
Pontics: Metal-ceramic
Abutment-pontic root ratio: 1.1
Considerations: Canine-guided posterior disocclusion. The short lever arm created by the lateral incisor cantilever should be adequately offset by the long span from first molar to canine. The mandibular situation is handled similarly.

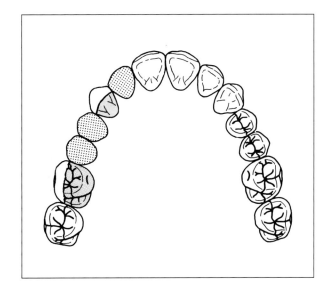

Missing: Maxillary first premolar and first molar
Abutments: Canine, second premolar, and second molar
Retainers: Metal-ceramic on canine and second premolar, with full veneer gold crown on second molar
Pontics: Metal-ceramic
Abutment-pontic root ratio: 1.4
Considerations: Nonrigid connector on distal of premolar retainer. If the canine and/or second premolar have long clinical crowns and the patient is amenable to a small display of metal, three-quarter crowns can be substituted. The corresponding mandibular situation can be treated similarly, with the substitution of an all-metal hygienic pontic for the molar.

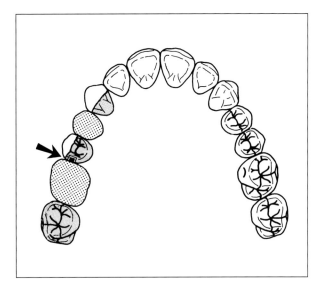

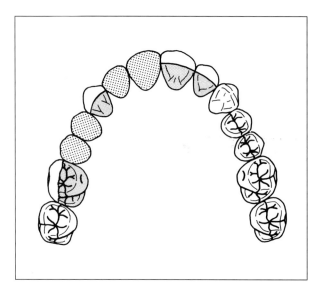

Missing: Maxillary central and lateral incisors, and first and second premolar on one side

Abutments: Central and lateral incisors, canine, and first molar

Retainers: Metal-ceramic

Pontics: Metal-ceramic

Abutment-pontic root ratio: 1.3

Considerations: This would be an extremely difficult fixed partial denture to undertake. The span lengths of both edentulous spaces are too great for nonrigid connectors with either pontic. The central and lateral incisors must have excellent retention. A removable partial denture or implant-supported segments should be considered. The corresponding mandibular configuration might use a full veneer gold crown on the molar.

Chapter 9

Principles of Tooth Preparations

The design of a preparation for a cast restoration and the execution of that design are governed by five principles:

1. Preservation of tooth structure
2. Retention and resistance
3. Structural durability
4. Marginal integrity
5. Preservation of the periodontium

Preservation of Tooth Structure

In addition to replacing lost tooth structure, a restoration must preserve remaining tooth structure. Intact surfaces of tooth structure that can be maintained while producing a strong, retentive restoration should be saved if patient acceptance and retention requirements will permit it. Whole surfaces of tooth structure should not be needlessly sacrificed to the bur in the name of convenience or speed.

Preservation of tooth structure in some cases may require that limited amounts of sound tooth structure be removed to prevent subsequent uncontrolled loss of larger quantities of tooth structure. This is the rationale for the removal of 1 to 1.5 mm of occlusal tooth structure when preparing a tooth for an MOD onlay. The metal on the occlusal surface can protect against dramatic failures, such as fracture of tooth structure, as well as the less obvious failures that may be occasioned by the flexing of tooth structure.

Retention and Resistance

For a restoration to accomplish its purpose, it must stay in place on the tooth. No cements that are compatible with living tooth structure and the biologic environment of the oral cavity possess adequate adhesive properties to hold a restoration in place solely through adhesion. The geometric configuration of the tooth preparation must place the cement in compression to provide the necessary retention and resistance.

Retention prevents removal of the restoration along the path of insertion or long axis of the tooth preparation. *Resistance* prevents dislodgment of the restoration by forces directed in an apical or oblique direction and prevents any movement of the restoration under occlusal forces. Retention and resistance are interrelated and often inseparable qualities.

The essential element of retention is two opposing vertical surfaces in the same preparation. These may be external surfaces, such as the buccal and lingual walls of a full veneer crown (Fig 9-1, A). An extracoronal restoration is an example of veneer, or sleeve, retention (Fig 9-1, B). The opposing surfaces can also be internal, such as the buccal and lingual walls of the proximal box of a proximo-occlusal inlay (Fig 9-2, A). An intracoronal restoration resists displacement by wedge retention (Fig 9-2, B). Many restorations are a combination of the two types.

Taper

Because a cast metal or ceramic restoration is placed on or in the preparation after the restoration has been fabricated in its final form, the axial walls of the preparation must *taper* slightly to permit the restoration to seat; ie, two opposing external walls must gradually converge or two opposing internal surfaces of tooth structure must diverge occlusally. The terms *angle of convergence* and *angle of divergence* can be used to describe the respective relationships between the two opposing walls of a preparation.

The relationship of one wall of a preparation to the long axis of that preparation is the *inclination* of that wall. A tapered diamond or bur will impart an inclination of 2 to 3 degrees to any surface it cuts if the shank of the instrument is held parallel to the intended path of insertion of the preparation. Two opposing surfaces, each with a 3-degree inclination, would give the preparation a 6-degree taper.

Theoretically, the more nearly parallel the opposing walls of a preparation, the greater should be the retention. The most retentive preparation should be one with

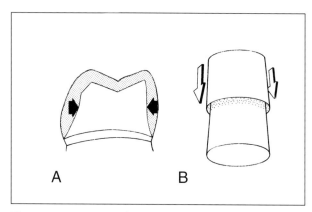

Fig 9-1 An extracoronal restoration (A) uses opposing external surfaces for retention (B).

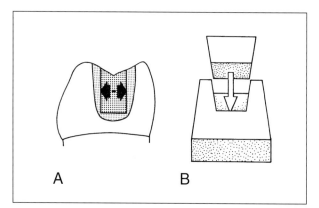

Fig 9-2 An intracoronal restoration (A) uses opposing internal surfaces for retention (B).

parallel walls. Indeed, parallel walls were advocated by some early authors.[1,2] However, parallel walls are impossible to create in the mouth without producing preparation undercuts. Preparation walls are tapered to visualize preparation walls, prevent undercuts, compensate for inaccuracies in the fabrication process, and permit more nearly complete seating of restorations during cementation.

Ward was one of the first to recommend taper as such, prescribing 5% to 20% per inch (3 to 12 degrees, respectively).[3] Jorgensen[4] and Kaufman et al[5] have demonstrated experimentally that retention decreases as taper is increased (Fig 9-3). In recent years, recommendations for optimum axial wall taper of tooth preparations for cast restorations have ranged from 3 to 5 degrees,[6] 6 degrees,[7] and 10 to 14 degrees.[8] To minimize stress in the cement interface between the preparation and restoration, a taper of 2.5 to 6.5 degrees has been suggested as optimum, but there is only a slight increase in stress as taper is increased from 0 to 15 degrees.[9] However, at 20 degrees, stress concentration was found to increase sharply.

Studies of actual crown preparations have shown average tapers that have been much greater than the values recommended. Ohm and Silness reported mean tapers of 19.2 degrees mesiodistally and 23.0 degrees faciolingually on vital teeth, and 12.8 degrees mesiodistally and 22.5 degrees faciolingually on nonvital teeth.[10] Mack found an average clinical taper of 16.5 degrees.[11] Weed et al found that dental students could produce full veneer crown preparations with a taper of 12.7 degrees on typodonts, but their clinical preparations had a mean taper of 22.8 degrees.[12] Noonan and Goldfogel, surveying 909 student-prepared full gold crown preparations, reported an overall mean taper of 19.2 degrees.[13] On proficiency examinations, preparation tapers were decreased by 20%. Dies taken at random from commercial laboratories by Eames et al were found to have an average overall taper of 20 degrees.[14]

Kent and associates evaluated the degree of taper of 418 preparations, cut over 12 years by one operator.[15] They found a mean of 15.8 degrees between mesial and distal walls and 13.4 degrees between facial and lingual walls for preparations in all areas of the mouth, with an overall mean of 14.3 degrees. The lowest combined taper (9.2 degrees) was seen on 145 anterior metal-ceramic crown preparations, while the greatest (22.2 degrees) was measured on 88 mandibular full crowns. Nordlander et al, analyzing 208 preparations done by 10 dentists, reported a low of 17.3 degrees for premolars and a high of 27.3 degrees for molars, with an overall mean of 19.9 degrees.[16]

Tooth preparation taper should be kept minimal because of its adverse effect on retention, but Mack estimates that a minimum taper of 12 degrees is necessary just to insure the absence of undercuts.[11] The tendency to overtaper preparations is one that must be guarded against constantly in order to produce preparations with the least possible taper and the greatest possible retention. Consciously attempting to cut a taper can easily result in an overtapered and nonretentive preparation. A taper or total convergence of 16 degrees has been proposed as being achievable clinically while still affording adequate retention.[17,18] This is probably an acceptable overall target. It can be as low as 10 degrees on preparations on anterior teeth and as high as 22 degrees on molars (Fig 9-4). Recommendations for degree of taper for specific teeth are given in Table 9-1.

Cement creates a weak bond, largely by mechanical interlocks, between the inner surface of the restoration and the axial wall of the preparation. Therefore, the greater the surface area of a preparation, the greater its retention.[5,19] Simply stated, preparations on large teeth are more retentive than preparations on small teeth (Fig 9-5). This is a factor that must be considered when a preparation is done on a small tooth, especially when it is an abutment for a fixed partial denture or a splint. Surface area can be increased somewhat by adding boxes and grooves. However, the benefits derived from such features may relate more to their limiting the freedom of movement than to the increase in surface area.

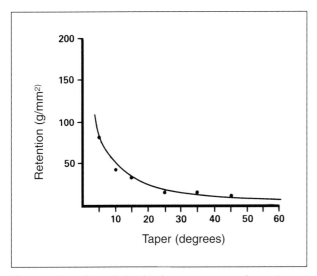

Fig 9-3 There is a relationship between taper and retention: as taper increases, retention decreases (after Jorgensen[4]).

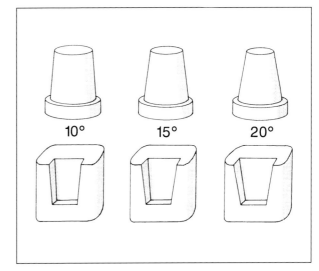

Fig 9-4 External *(top row)* and internal *(bottom row)* opposing surfaces demonstrate tapers of 10, 15, and 20 degrees.

Table 9-1 *Optimum Degree of Tooth Preparation Taper*

Arch	M/D	F/L	Overall
Maxillary			
Anterior tooth*	10	10	10
Premolar*	14	14	14
Molar*	17	21	19
Isthmus†	—	—	7
Box†	—	—	7
Mandibular			
Anterior tooth*	10	10	10
Premolar*	16	12	14
Molar*	24	20	22
Isthmus†	—	—	12
Box†	—	—	12

*Convergence angle.
†Divergence angle.
M/D = mesiodistal; F/L = faciolingual.

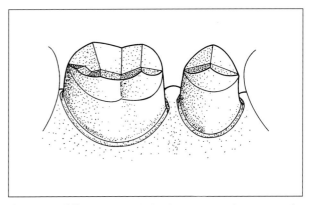

Fig 9-5 A full crown preparation is more retentive on a molar than on a premolar, because the molar preparation has greater surface area.

Freedom of Displacement

Retention is improved by geometrically limiting the numbers of paths along which a restoration can be removed from the tooth preparation.[20] Maximum retention is achieved when there is only one path. A full veneer preparation with long, parallel axial walls and grooves would produce such retention (Fig 9-6, A). On the opposite extreme, a short, overtapered preparation would be without retention because the restoration could be removed along an infinite number of paths (Fig 9-6, B). The best preparation, then, is one that approaches the ideal and can be achieved within the limits of operator skill, accessibility, and laboratory technology.

Limiting the freedom of displacement from torquing or twisting forces in a horizontal plane increases the resistance of a restoration. A groove whose walls meet the axial wall at an oblique angle does not provide the necessary resistance (Fig 9-7, A). V-shaped grooves produce roughly one-half as much resistance to lingual displacement as do grooves with a definite lingual wall.[21] Forces that produce rotating movement in the restoration can produce shear and eventual slippage along the surfaces oblique to the direction of the force. There must be a definite wall perpendicular to the direction of the force to sufficiently limit the freedom of displacement and provide adequate resistance (Fig 9-7, B).

A proximal box must be treated in a similar manner. If

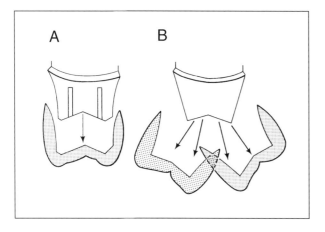

Fig 9-6 By limiting the paths of withdrawal, retention is improved (A). A preparation with unlimited freedom of displacement is much less retentive (B).

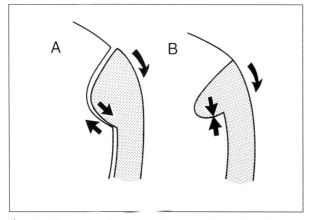

Fig 9-7 The walls of a groove that meet the axial wall at an oblique angle do not provide necessary resistance (A); the walls of a groove must be perpendicular to rotating forces to resist displacement (B).

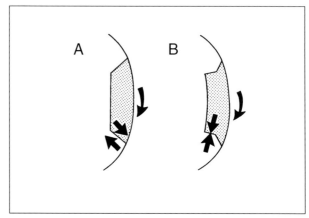

Fig 9-8 The buccal and lingual walls of a box will not resist rotational displacement if they form oblique angles with the pulpal wall (A); they must meet the pulpal wall at angles near 90 degrees (B).

its buccal and lingual walls form oblique angles with its pulpal wall, there will not be adequate resistance to rotating forces (Fig 9-8, A). The buccal and lingual walls must meet the pulpal wall at angles near 90 degrees so that these walls will be perpendicular to any forces which would tend to rotate the restoration (Fig 9-8, B). A flare is then added to the box so that there can be an acute edge of gold at the cavosurface margin of the restoration.

Length

Occlusogingival length is an important factor in both retention and resistance. Longer preparations will have more surface area and will therefore be more retentive. Because the axial wall occlusal to the finish line interferes

with displacement, the length and inclination of that wall become factors in resistance to tipping forces.

For the restoration to succeed, the length must be great enough to interfere with the arc of the casting pivoting about a point on the margin on the opposite side of the restoration (Fig 9-9, A).[22] The shorter wall does not afford this resistance (Fig 9-9, B). The shorter the wall, the more important its inclination. The walls of shorter preparations should have as little taper as possible to increase the resistance. Even this will not help if the walls are too short.

It may be possible to successfully restore a tooth with short walls if the tooth has a small diameter. The preparation on the smaller tooth will have a short rotational radius for the arc of displacement, and the incisal portion of the axial wall will resist displacement (Fig 9-10, A). The longer rotational radius on the larger preparation allows for a

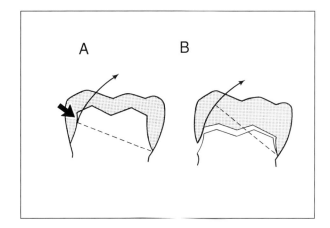

Fig 9-9 The preparation with longer walls (A) interferes with the tipping displacement of the restoration better than the short preparation (B).

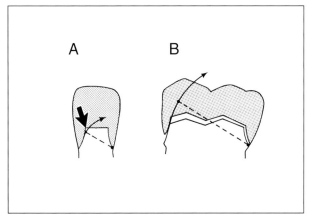

Fig 9-10 A preparation on a tooth with a smaller diameter (A) resists pivoting movements better than a preparation of equal length on a tooth of larger diameter (B).

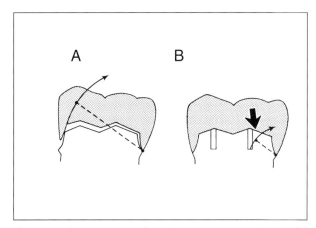

Fig 9-11 The resistance of a short preparation (A) can be improved by adding grooves (B).

more gradual arc of displacement, and the axial wall does not resist removal (Fig 9-10, B). Parker et al found that approximately 95% of anterior preparations analyzed had resistance form, while only 46% of those on molars did.[23]

Resistance to displacement for a short-walled preparation on a large tooth can be improved by placing grooves in the axial walls. In effect, this reduces the rotational radius, and that portion of the walls of the grooves near the occlusal surface of the preparation will interfere with displacement (Fig 9-11).

Substitution of Internal Features

The basic unit of retention for a cemented restoration is two opposing axial walls with a minimal taper. It may not always be possible to use opposing walls for retention: one may have been destroyed previously, or it may be desirable to leave a surface uncovered for a partial veneer restoration. It may also be that the walls are present, but with a greater than desirable inclination. Generally, internal features such as the groove, the box form, and the pin hole are interchangeable and can be substituted for an axial wall or for each other (Fig 9-12). Substitution is important, since conditions often preclude making an ideal preparation.

Kent et al reported a marked difference between the degree of taper of full crown preparations (18.4 to 22.2 degrees) and that of boxes and grooves in the axial surfaces of those preparations (7.3 degrees).[15] The taper of these internal features is nearly the same as the taper of the the instruments used to cut them (4 to 6 degrees). Apparently the widely separated axial walls of the prepa-

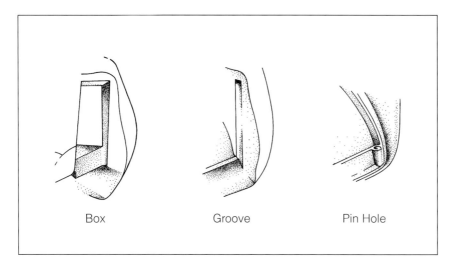

Box   Groove   Pin Hole

Fig 9-12 These preparation features are frequently substituted for each other.

rations are overinclined because of access, visibility, or both. In preparing an internal feature such as a groove or a box, however, the much shorter distance between the walls allows the dentist to prepare them more precisely. These features offer an excellent means of enhancing the overall retention and resistance of an otherwise over-inclined axial wall. Woolsey and Matich found that proximal grooves on short 15-degree dies provide complete resistance to faciolingual horizontal displacement.[24]

Path of Insertion

The *path of insertion* is an imaginary line along which the restoration will be placed onto or removed from the preparation. It is determined mentally by the dentist before the preparation is begun, and all features of the preparation are cut to coincide with that line. The path of insertion is not arbitrarily set at the completion of the preparation by adding some feature, such as grooves. It is of special importance when preparing teeth to be fixed partial denture abutments, since the paths of all the abutment preparations must parallel each other.

The correct technique must be used to survey a preparation visually, since this is the primary means of insuring that the preparation is neither undercut nor over-tapered. If the center of the occlusal surface of a preparation is viewed with one eye from a distance of approximately 30 cm (12 inches), it is possible to sight down the axial walls of a preparation with a minimum taper (Fig 9-13). However, it is possible to sight down the axial walls of a preparation with a reverse (ie, undercut) taper of 8 degrees when both eyes are open (Fig 9-14). This occurs because of the distance between the eyes, which is responsible for binocular vision. Therefore, it is important that preparations be viewed with one eye closed.

For a preparation to be surveyed in the mouth, where direct vision is rarely possible, a mouth mirror is used (Fig 9-15). It is held at an angle approximately 1/2 inch above the preparation, and the image is viewed with one eye. If fixed partial denture abutment preparations are being evaluated for a common path of insertion, a firm finger rest is established and the mirror is maneuvered until one preparation is centered. Then, pivoting on the finger rest, the mirror is moved, without changing its angulation, until it is centered over the second preparation.

The path of insertion must be considered in two dimensions: faciolingually and mesiodistally. The facio-lingual orientation of the path can affect the esthetics of metal-ceramic or partial veneer crowns. For metal-ceramic crowns, the path is roughly parallel with the long axis of the teeth (Fig 9-16). A facially inclined path of insertion on a preparation for a metal-ceramic crown will leave the facio-occlusal angle too prominent, resulting in overcontouring of the restoration, "opaque show-through," or both.

Leaning the path to the facial will force the overcutting of the mesiofacio-occlusal corner of a three-quarter crown preparation, leading to an unnecessary display of gold. For three-quarter crowns on anterior teeth, the path of insertion should parallel the incisal one-half of the labial surface (Fig 9-17). If it is inclined more facially, short grooves and an unnecessary display of gold will result.

The mesiodistal inclination of the path must parallel the contact areas of adjacent teeth. If the path is inclined mesially or distally, the restoration will be held up at the proximal contact areas and be "locked out" (Fig 9-18). This is a particular problem when restoring a tilted tooth. In this situation, making the path of insertion parallel with the long axis of the tooth will cause the contacts of the adjacent teeth to encroach on the path of insertion.

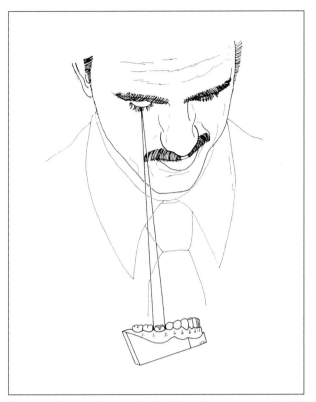

Fig 9-13 To examine a preparation for undercuts, one eye should be closed.

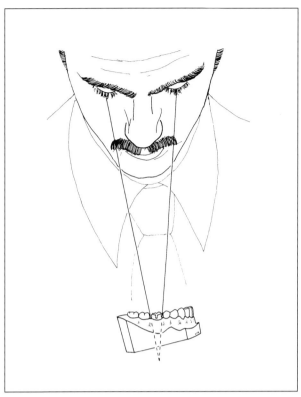

Fig 9-14 If both eyes are open when the preparation is viewed, undercuts may remain undetected.

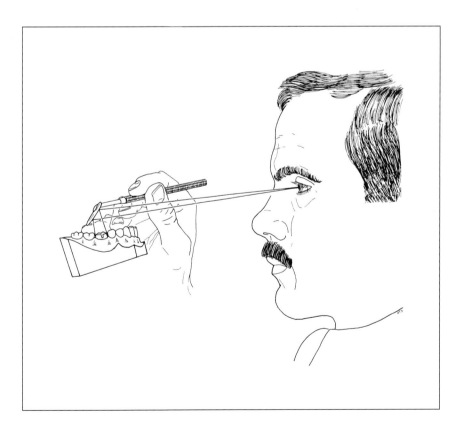

Fig 9-15 Preparations in the mouth are viewed through a mouth mirror using one eye.

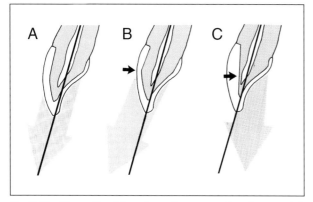

Fig 9-16 The path of insertion of a preparation for a metal-ceramic crown should parallel the long axis of the tooth (A). If the path is directed facially, the prominent facioincisal angle may create esthetic problems of overcontouring or "opaque show-through" (B). However, if the path is directed lingually, the facial surface will intersect the lingual surface, creating a shorter preparation. It also may encroach on the pulp (C).

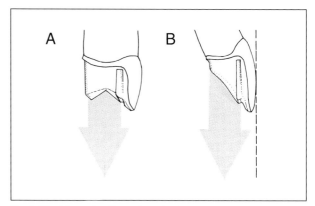

Fig 9-17 The path of insertion of a three-quarter crown on a posterior tooth parallels the long axis of the tooth (A), while it parallels the incisal one-half to two-thirds of the labial surface of an anterior tooth (B).

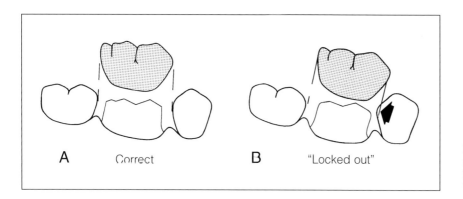

A   Correct   B   "Locked out"

Fig 9-18 The path of insertion of a preparation must parallel the adjacent proximal contacts (A), or it will be prevented from seating (B).

Structural Durability

A restoration must contain a bulk of material that is adequate to withstand the forces of occlusion. This bulk must be confined to the space created by the tooth preparation. Only in this way can the occlusion on the restoration be harmonious and the axial contours normal, preventing periodontal problems around the restoration.

Occlusal Reduction

One of the most important features for providing adequate bulk of metal and strength to the restoration is occlusal clearance (Fig 9-19). For gold alloys, there should be 1.5 mm of clearance on the functional cusps (lingual of maxillary molars and premolars and buccal of mandibular molars and premolars). Not quite as much is required on the nonfunctional cusp, where 1.0 mm is sufficient.

Metal-ceramic crowns will require 1.5 to 2.0 mm on functional cusps that will be veneered with porcelain and 1.0 to 1.5 mm on nonfunctional cusps to receive ceramic coverage. There should be 2.0 mm of clearance on preparations for all-ceramic crowns. Malposed teeth may have occlusal surfaces that are not parallel with the occlusal table. Therefore, it may not be necessary to reduce the occlusal surface by 1.0 mm to achieve 1.0 mm of clearance.

The basic inclined plane pattern of the occlusal surface should be duplicated to produce adequate clearance without overshortening the preparation (Fig 9-20). A flat occlusal surface may overshorten a preparation whose length is already minimal to provide adequate retention. Inadequate clearance makes a restoration weaker. In addition, inadequate reduction under the anatomic grooves of the occlusal surface will not provide adequate space to allow good functional morphology. The restoration also will be much more easily perforated by finishing procedures or by wear in the mouth.

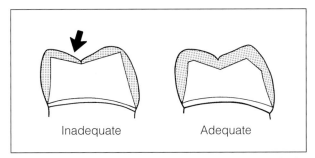

Fig 9-19 Inadequate occlusal reduction does not provide the needed space for a cast restoration of adequate thickness.

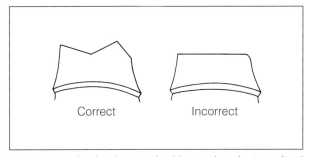

Fig 9-20 Occlusal reduction should reproduce basic inclined planes rather than being cut as one flat plane.

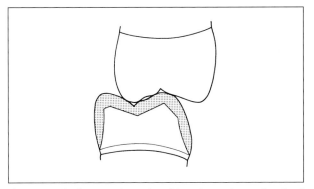

Fig 9-21 The functional cusp bevel is an integral part of occlusal reduction.

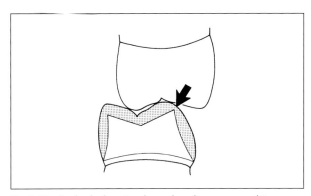

Fig 9-22 Lack of a functional cusp bevel can cause a thin area or perforation in the casting.

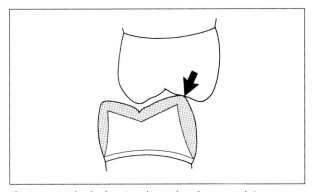

Fig 9-23 Lack of a functional cusp bevel may result in overcontouring and poor occlusion.

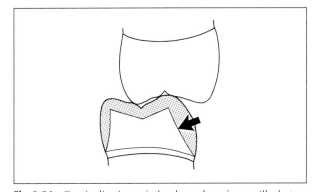

Fig 9-24 Overinclination of the buccal surface will destroy excessive tooth structure while lessening retention.

Functional Cusp Bevel

An integral part of the occlusal reduction is the functional cusp bevel (Fig 9-21). A wide bevel on the lingual inclines of the maxillary lingual cusps and the buccal inclines of mandibular buccal cusps provides space for an adequate bulk of metal in an area of heavy occlusal contact.

If a wide bevel is not placed on the functional cusp, several problems may occur. If the crown is waxed and cast to normal contour, the casting will be extremely thin in the area overlying the junction between the occlusal and axial reduction (Fig 9-22). To prevent a thin casting when there is no functional cusp bevel, an attempt may be made to wax the crown to optimal thickness in this area. An overcontoured restoration will result and a deflective occlusal contact is likely to occur unless the opposing tooth is reduced (Fig 9-23).

If an attempt is made to obtain space for an adequate bulk in a normally contoured casting without a bevel, the result will be an overcut axial surface (Fig 9-24). In addition to the unnecessary destruction of tooth structure, the severe inclination of the surface renders it useless for retention.

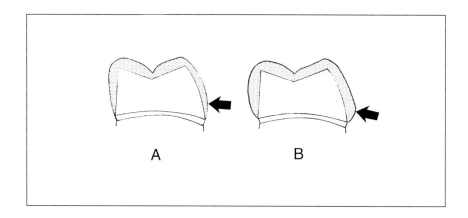

Fig 9-25 Inadequate axial reduction can cause thin walls and a weak restoration (A) or a bulbous, overcontoured restoration (B).

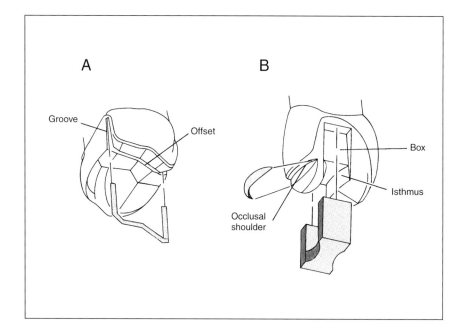

Fig 9-26 The three-quarter crown is reinforced by the bulk of gold that fills the offset and grooves (A). The occlusal shoulder strengthens the lingual margin, and the isthmus and boxes reinforce the main body of an MOD onlay (B).

Axial Reduction

Axial reduction also plays an important role in securing space for an adequate thickness of restorative material (Fig 9-25). If restorations are made with normal contours over preparations with inadequate axial reduction, they will have thin walls that will be subject to distortion. Frequently laboratory technicians attempt to compensate for this by overcontouring the axial surfaces. While this "solution" to the problem strengthens the restoration, it can have a disastrous effect on the periodontium.

There are other features that serve to provide space for metal that will improve the rigidity and durability of the restoration: the offset, the occlusal shoulder, the isthmus, the proximal groove, and the box (Fig 9-26). The isthmus connects the boxes, and the offset ties the grooves together to enhance the reinforcing "truss effect."[25]

Marginal Integrity

The restoration can survive in the biological environment of the oral cavity only if the margins are closely adapted to the cavosurface finish line of the preparation. The configuration of the preparation finish line dictates the shape and bulk of restorative material in the margin of the restoration. It also can affect both marginal adaptation and the degree of seating of the restoration.

To Bevel, or . . .

Cast metal restorations can be made to fit preparations with a high degree of precision, but even in well-fitting

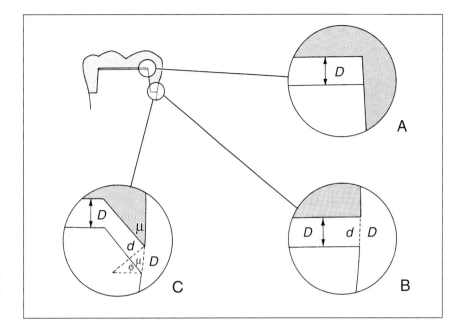

Fig 9-27 Any failure of the restoration to seat (*D* in inset A) is reflected as a marginal opening of the same dimension on a shoulder perpendicular to the path of insertion (B). As the angle of the margin (μ) approximates 0 degrees (C), the distance between the margin and the tooth (*d*) approaches 0, based on the assumption that the gap can be closed completely (after Rosner[26]).

castings there is some discrepancy between the margin of the restoration and the preparation. Bevels have been advocated as a means of diminishing marginal discrepancy.[26] If the vertical discrepancy in fit is designated as *D*, the distance between the restoration and preparation (Fig 9-27, A) occurs unchanged between the margin, *M*, and the finish line, *P* (Fig 9-27, B). However, the closest distance between the margin and the surface of the preparation is a line, *d*, that is perpendicular to the surface of the tooth (Fig 9-27, C). It can be stated as a function of *D* and the sine of angle μ, or the cosine of angle φ:

$$d = D \sin \mu \qquad (1)$$
or
$$d = D \cos \phi \qquad (2)$$

As angle μ becomes smaller (more acute), the sine of μ becomes smaller (Table 9-2); or as angle φ becomes larger (more obtuse), the cosine of φ becomes smaller. By either computation, *d* diminishes by the same amount. The more acute the angle of the margin, μ, or the more obtuse the angle of the finish line, φ, the shorter the distance between the restoration margin and the tooth. This argument is based on the premise that the distance between the margin and tooth structure is infinitely closeable, and as long as there is no cement between the restoration and the preparation, that is true.

. . . Not to Bevel

However, as shown so convincingly by Ostlund,[27] the presence of cement changes the scenario completely. The film thickness of the cement will prevent the com-

Table 9-2 *Trigonometric Functions of Angles 0 to 90 Degrees*

Angle (degrees)	Sine	Cosine
0	0	1.000
15	0.259	0.966
30	0.500	0.866
45	0.707	0.707
60	0.866	0.500
75	0.966	0.259
90	1.000	0

plete seating of a casting with bevels that are nearly parallel with the path of insertion, just as Jorgensen,[4] Kaufman et al,[5] and Eames and associates[14] found that crowns did not seat completely on dies with minimal taper.

The film thickness of the cement imposes a limit on the reduction of the perpendicular distance from the margin to the tooth, *d*. The distance, *d*, therefore becomes a constant, and the previous equation is solved for *D* instead of *d*:

$$D = d/\sin \mu \qquad (3)$$
or
$$D = d/\cos \phi \qquad (4)$$

As the angle of the margin bevel becomes more acute, its sine becomes smaller, and as the angle of the finish line becomes more obtuse, its cosine becomes smaller, and *D* becomes larger. The more nearly the bevel parallels the path of insertion, the greater the distance by which the restoration fails to seat (Fig 9-28).

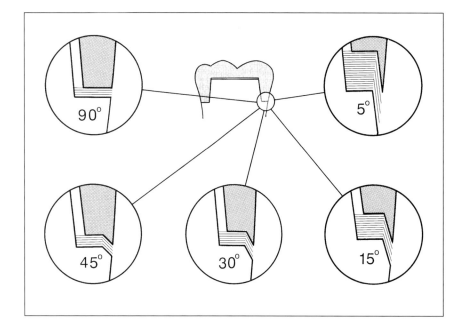

Fig 9-28 The cement film thickness prevents complete closure of the marginal gap. If a bevel of 45 degrees is added to a shoulder, the crown will be prevented from seating by a factor of 1.4. However, as the margin is decreased to an angle of 30 degrees, the crown is displaced twice as much as it would be with a shoulder. Margins of 15 and 5 degrees would prevent seating by factors of 3.9 and 11.5, respectively. If the marginal gap for the shoulder were 25 μm, the ADA specification for cement film thickness, the addition of a 5-degree bevel could keep the casting from seating by nearly 0.3 mm. All spaces in the insets are drawn to scale.

McLean and Wilson have disputed the use of bevels for metal-ceramic crowns because the bevel margin must be 10 to 20 degrees to noticeably improve adaptation.[28] The finish line must also be placed too far subgingivally to hide the resultant metal collar. Pascoe demonstrated that slightly oversized castings with shoulders exhibit the least marginal discrepancy.[29] Gavelis et al found a better marginal seal with acute-edged margins, but they found that shoulders permitted the most complete seating of a crown.[30] Panno and associates reported no better adaptability of crowns with highly acute 80-degree bevels than those with less acute 45-degree bevels.[31]

Empirical clinical results dictate that the acute angle margin should continue to be used on metal restorations but that the angle should be in the 30- to 45-degree range. The tapered edge in a wax pattern margin produced by a bevel is more readily adapted to a die than is a butt joint, and a gold margin can be burnished to slightly improve its adaptation after casting.

Finish Line Configurations

Wide, shallow bevels that are nearly parallel with the outer surface of the tooth should be avoided. They are likely to lead to overcontouring. Even if the axial surfaces of the overlying crown are not overcontoured, the resultant thin, unsupported wax at the margin potentially will break or distort when the wax pattern is withdrawn from the die and invested. The optimum margin for a gold alloy casting is an acute edge with a nearby bulk of metal.

The preferred gingival finish line for veneer metal restorations is the *chamfer* (Fig 9-29). This finish line has been shown experimentally to exhibit the least stress, so that the cement underlying it will have less likelihood of failure.[32,33] It can be cut with the tip of a round-end diamond, while the axial reduction is being done with the side of that instrument. However, a torpedo diamond is less likely to produce a butt joint. The margin of the cast restoration that fits against it combines an acute edge with a nearby bulk of metal.

A *heavy chamfer* is used to provide a 90-degree cavo-surface angle with a large-radius rounded internal angle (Fig 9-30). It is created with a round-end tapered diamond. In the hands of an unskilled operator, this instrument can create an undesirable fragile "lip" of enamel at the cavo-surface. The heavy chamfer provides better support for a ceramic crown than does a conventional chamfer, but it is not as good as a shoulder. A bevel can be added to the heavy chamfer for use with a metal restoration.

The *shoulder* has long been the finish line of choice for the all-ceramic crown (Fig 9-31). The wide ledge provides resistance to occlusal forces and minimizes stresses that might lead to fracture of the porcelain. It produces the space for healthy restoration contours and maximum esthetics. However, it does require the destruction of more tooth structure than any other finish line. The sharp, 90-degree internal line angle associated with the classic variety of this finish line concentrates stress in the tooth and is conducive to coronal fracture. The shoulder generally is not used as a finish line for cast metal restorations.

The *radial shoulder* is a modified form of shoulder finish line (Fig 9-32). The initial instrumentation of the ledge is accomplished with the same flat-end tapered diamond

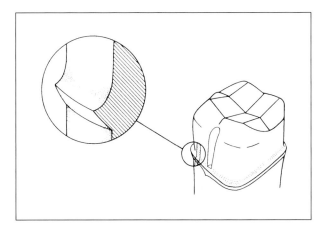

Fig 9-29 Chamfer finish line demonstrated on a full veneer crown preparation.

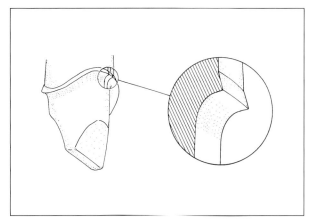

Fig 9-30 Heavy chamfer on a preparation for an all-ceramic crown.

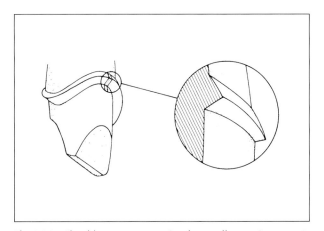

Fig 9-31 Shoulder on a preparation for an all-ceramic crown (a traditional porcelain jacket crown).

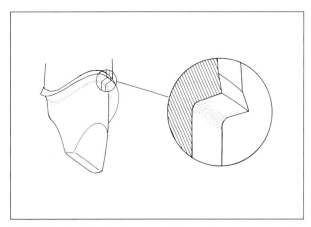

Fig 9-32 A radial shoulder on an all-ceramic crown preparation combines maximum support of the ceramic with a stress-reducing, rounded gingivoaxial "angle."

used for the classic shoulder. A small-radius rounded internal angle is instrumented by an end-cutting parallel-sided carbide finishing bur, and finishing is completed with a specially modified bin-angle chisel. The cavosurface angle is 90 degrees, and shoulder width is only slightly lessened by the rounded internal angle. Stress concentration is less in the tooth structure than with a classic shoulder, and support for ceramic restoration walls is good. Destruction of tooth structure required for this configuration is not significantly less than that required for a classic shoulder, however.

The *shoulder with a bevel* is used as a finish line in a variety of situations (Fig 9-33). It is utilized as the gingival finish line on the proximal box of inlays and onlays, and for the occlusal shoulder of onlays and mandibular three-quarter crowns. This design can also be used for the facial finish line of metal-ceramic restorations where gingival esthetics are not critical. It can be used in those situations where a shoulder is already present, either because of destruction by caries or the presence of previous restorations. It is also a good finish line for preparations with extremely short walls, since it facilitates axial walls that are nearly parallel.[34]

By adding a bevel to an existing shoulder, it is possible to create an acute edge of metal at the margin. The shoulder with a bevel should not be used routinely for full

131

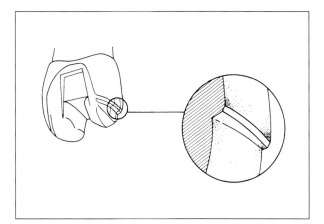

Fig 9-33 Shoulder with a bevel on the occlusal shoulder of an MOD onlay.

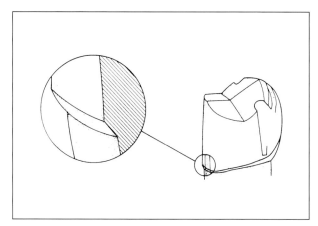

Fig 9-34 Knife edge on the lingual of a mandibular three-quarter crown.

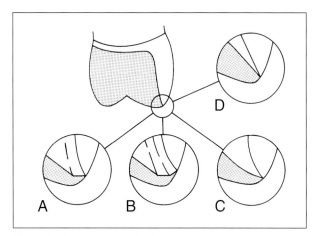

Fig 9-35 Bucco-occlusal finish lines on a maxillary three-quarter crown. A flat bevel (A), a contrabevel (B), and, when the cusp is bulky, a knife edge (C), are acceptable finish lines. The knife edge is not an acceptable finish line on small, sharp cusps (D). (After Ingraham et al[36] and Richter and Veno.[51])

veneer restorations because the axial reduction required to obtain it is unnecessarily destructive of tooth structure. Some variation of a shoulder, with or without a bevel, may afford some resistance against distortion during porcelain firing.[35]

The ultimate in finish lines that permit an acute margin of metal is the *knife edge* (Fig 9-34). Unfortunately, its use can create problems. Unless it is carefully cut, the axial reduction may fade out instead of terminating in a definite finish line. The thin margin of the restoration that fits this finish line may be difficult to accurately wax and cast. It is also more susceptible to distortion in the mouth when the casting is subjected to occlusal forces.

The use of the knife edge can result in overcontoured restorations when an attempt is made to obtain adequate bulk by adding to the external axial contours of the restoration. In spite of its drawbacks, it is sometimes nec-

essary to use the knife edge. It may have to be used on the lingual surface of mandibular posterior teeth, on teeth with very convex axial surfaces, and on the surface toward which a tooth may have tilted.

The finish line used for the bucco-occlusal margin of maxillary partial veneer and MOD onlay restorations is worthy of attention. It too must meet the requirement of providing an acute edge with a nearby bulk of metal. The enamel must also be protected by a finishing bevel that will leave the tooth structure at the cavosurface angle with sufficient bulk to resist fracture and chipping.[36] The most commonly used form is a narrow (0.3 to 0.5 mm) finishing bevel perpendicular to the path of insertion of the restoration (Fig 9-35, A). A contrabevel may also be used where function is heavy and esthetic requirements are minimal (Fig 9-35, B). There are a few situations in which no bevel is required (Fig 9-35, C), but this can only be accomplished on a cusp that is bulky enough to allow the acute edge of metal and still be able to finish the enamel at the cavosurface angle. A bevel is mandatory if its elimination will create an unsupported edge of enamel (Fig 9-35, D).

Preservation of the Periodontium

The placement of finish lines has a direct bearing on the ease of fabricating a restoration and on the ultimate success of the restoration. The best results can be expected from margins that are as smooth as possible and are fully exposed to a cleansing action.[37] Whenever possible, the finish line should be placed in an area where the margins of the restoration can be finished by the dentist and kept clean by the patient. In addition, finish lines must be placed so that they can be duplicated by the impression, without tearing or deforming the impression when it is removed past them.

Finish lines should be placed in enamel when it is possible to do so. In the past, the traditional concept has been to place margins as far subgingivally as possible, based on the mistaken concept that the subgingival sulcus is caries-free.[38] The practice of routinely placing margins subgingivally is no longer acceptable. Subgingival restorations have been described as a major etiologic factor in periodontitis.[39–46] The deeper the restoration margin resides in the gingival sulcus, the greater the inflammatory response.[47–50]

Although Richter and Ueno reported no difference between subgingival and supragingival margins in a 3-year clinical study, they recommended that placement be supragingival whenever possible.[51] Eissmann et al made a similar recommendation.[37] Koth also failed to find a link between margin location and gingival health in a selected patient population on a strict hygiene regimen.[52]

These studies do not refute the evidence that subgingival margins are likely to cause gingival inflammation. They merely demonstrate that margin location is not as crucial when placed by a highly skilled dentist in the mouth of a motivated, cooperative patient. Ego may tempt a dentist to believe that he or she is one of the "good guys" who can handle the "simple" task of achieving well-fitting albeit subgingival margins on a crown. However, subgingival margins can be very difficult to evaluate.

Christensen demonstrated that experienced restorative dentists can miss marginal defects as great as 120 µm when the margins are subgingival.[53] In a radiographic study, Bjorn et al found that more than half of the proximal margins of gold crowns had defects greater than 0.2 mm and more than 40% of the proximal margins of ceramic crowns had defects that exceeded 0.3 mm.[54]

Nonetheless, there will be many situations in which subgingival margins are unavoidable. Because preparation length is such an important factor in resistance and retention, preparations are frequently extended subgingivally to increase retention.[45,55–58] The placement of finish lines can also be altered from ideal locations by caries,[45,55–58] the extensions of previous restorations,[45,55–57] trauma,[45,57] or esthetics.[45,55–58]

Exercise caution if conditions require that the finish line be placed any closer to the alveolar crest than 2.0 mm, which is the combined dimension of the epithelial and connective tissue attachments.[59] Placement of a restoration margin in this area probably will result in gingival inflammation, loss of alveolar crest height, and formation of a periodontal pocket.[60] "Crown lengthening" may be done to surgically move the alveolar crest 3.0 mm apical to the location of the proposed finish line to guarantee the biologic width and prevent periodontal pathology. This will allow space for the connective and epithelial attachments and a healthy gingival sulcus. If the deep finish line is located interproximally and will require extensive removal of bone between the tooth being restored and the adjacent tooth, it may be better to extract the tooth in question rather than periodontally compromise its healthy neighbor.

Instrumentation

The preparation of teeth to receive cast metal or ceramic restorations does not require an extensive armamentarium (Table 9-3). The excavation of caries should be accomplished with sharp spoon excavators and round burs (no. 4 or no. 6) mounted in a contra-angle handpiece. Hand chisels may be used to accentuate the facial and lingual walls of proximal boxes. All other procedures usually are accomplished with a high-speed air turbine handpiece.

Small diamond points, used with a water-air spray in a high-speed handpiece, will remove precisely controlled amounts of tooth structure. The surface that remains can be easily smoothed. There is no indication for the use of large diamond cutting discs in low-speed contra-angle or straight handpieces. They frequently overextend preparations, and their potential for injury to the patient is great.

It is important that the cavosurface finish line be smooth and continuous to facilitate the fabrication of restorations with well-adapted margins. Gross reduction is most efficiently accomplished with coarse diamonds. However, they leave irregular cavosurface finish lines,[61,62] and some other instrument should be used to obtain a smooth finish line. By using diamonds and carbide finishing burs of the same size and shape, as developed by Lustig et al,[63,64] it is possible to maintain the finish line configuration developed by the diamond instrument. Torpedo diamonds are followed by torpedo carbide burs to produce chamfers; flat-end tapered diamonds by H158 carbide finishing burs for radial shoulders; and flame diamonds by flame burs for gingival bevels and conservative proximal flares. Acceptable finish lines on vertical flares can be obtained by the use of abrasive paper discs,[65] but they should be used with a rubber dam to protect soft tissue.

Nondentate tapered burs (169L, 170L, and 171L) are used for grooves, boxes, isthmuses, and offsets where they are needed. They are also used for smoothing any surface that will not terminate in a curved finish line, which they would nick, and for creating occlusal and incisal bevels. Cross-cut or dentate burs are employed for removal of old restorations, but the horizontal ridges they leave on tooth structure make them unacceptable for planing tooth surfaces.

Table 9-3 Rotary Instruments for Tooth Preparations

Shape	Use	Manufacturer*										
		Brasseler	Busch	Densco	Horico	Midwest	Miltex	Premier	SS White	Star	Union	Vantage
Round-end tapered diamond	1. Depth orientation grooves 2. Occlusal reduction 3. Functional cusp	856-016	—	775	199-016	198-016	—	770.8	854-016	770-8	D-18	850/018
Flat-end tapered diamond	1. Axial reduction (MCR, PJC) 2. Shoulder (MCR, PJC)	847-016	—	770	172-016	172-018	—	701.7	847-016	700-7	117	848/018
Torpedo diamond	1. Axial reduction 2. Chamfer finish line	877-010	—	232	130-012	289-012	—	251.8	884-012	250-7 ½	124	884/012
Short needle	1. Initial proximal axial reduction (posterior teeth)	852-012	—	715	164-012	161.016	—	209.6	845-010	769-5	D11	849/010
Long needle	1. Initial proximal axial reduction (anterior teeth)	30006-012	—	703	167-011	161.021	—	700.9	852-011	769T-9	D3	852/011
Flame diamond	1. Proximal flare 2. Gingival bevel	862-010	—	216	249-010	249-012	—	260.8	862-012	260-8	205L	862/012
Small wheel diamond	1. Lingual reduction (anterior teeth)	909-040	—	825	068-040	068-040	—	863	909-035	110	11A	909/035
Tapered fissure bur	1. Seating groove 2. Proximal groove (posterior teeth) 3. Offset 4. Occlusal shoulder 5. Isthmus 6. Proximal box 7. Smoothing and finishing 8. Occlusal and incisal bevels	171L-012	171L-012	171L-012	—	171L-012	171L	71L-012	171L	—	171L-012	—
Tapered fissure burs	1. Initial groove alignment 2. Angles of proximal boxes 3. Smoothing and finishing 4. Occlusal and incisal bevels	170L-010 169L-009	170L-010 —	170L-010 169L-009	— —	170L-010 169L-009	170L 169L	70L-009 69L-008	170L 169L	— —	170L-010 169L-009	— —

Table 9-3 *Continued*

Shape	Use	Brasseler	Busch	Densco	Horico	Midwest	Miltex	Premier	SS White	Star	Union	Vantage
											Manufacturer*	
End cutting bur	1. Conventional shoulder finishing	957-010	957-010	957-010	—	—	957	—	957	—	957-010	—
Torpedo bur	1. Axial wall finishing 2. Chamfer finishing	282-010	243-010	—	—	—	—	—	—	—	—	—
Flame bur	1. Flare and bevel finishing	H48L-010	—	—	—	—	—	—	—	—	—	—
Radial fissure bur	1. Radial shoulder finishing	H158-012	—	—	—	—	—	—	—	—	—	—

*Brasseler USA Inc, Savannah, GA
Busch, Pfingst & Co, Inc, South Plainfield, NJ
Densco, Teledyne Getz, Elk Grove Village, IL
Horico, Pfingst & Co, Inc, South Plainfield, NJ
Midwest Dental Products Corporation, Des Plaines, IL
Miltex Instrument Co, Inc, Lake Success, NY
Premier Dental Products Co, Norristown, PA
SS White Burs, Inc, Lakewood, NJ
Star Dental Products, Lancaster, PA
Union Broach Division of Moyco Industries, Emigsville, PA
Vantage, Miltex Instrument Co, Inc, Lake Success, NY

References

1. Conzett JV: The gold inlay. *Dent Cosmos* 1910; 52:1339.

2. Ferrier WI: Cavity preparation for gold foil, gold inlay, and amalgam operations. *J Natl Dent Assoc* 1917; 4:441.

3. Ward ML: *The American Textbook of Operative Dentistry*, ed 6. New York, Lea & Febiger, 1926, pp 381–395.

4. Jorgensen KD: The relationship between retention and convergence angle in cemented veneer crowns. *Acta Odontol Scand* 1955; 13:35–40.

5. Kaufman EG, Coelho DH, Colin L: Factors influencing the retention of cemented gold castings. *J Prosthet Dent* 1961; 11:487–502.

6. Dykema RW, Goodacre CJ, Phillips RW: *Johnston's Modern Practice in Crown and Bridge Prosthodontics*, ed 4. Philadelphia, WB Saunders Co, 1986, p 24.

7. Shillingburg HT, Hobo S, Fisher DW: *Preparations for Cast Gold Restorations*. Chicago, Quintessence Publ Co, 1974, p 16.

8. Tylman SD, Malone WFP: *Tylman's Theory and Practice of Fixed Prosthodontics*, ed 7. St Louis, CV Mosby Co, 1978, p 103.

9. El-Ebrashi MK, Craig RG, Peyton FA: Experimental stress analysis of dental restorations. Part IV. The concept of parallelism of axial walls. *J Prosthet Dent* 1969; 22:346–353.

10. Ohm E, Silness J: The convergence angle in teeth prepared for artificial crowns. *J Oral Rehabil* 1978; 5:371.

11. Mack PJ: A theoretical and clinical investigation into the taper achieved on crown and inlay preparations. *J Oral Rehabil* 1980; 7:255.

12. Weed RM, Suddick RP, Kleffner JH: Taper of clinical and typodont crowns prepared by dental students. *J Dent Res* 1984; 63:286 (abstr no. 1036).

13. Noonan JE, Goldfogel MH: Convergence of the axial walls of full veneer crown preparations in a dental school environment. *J Prosthet Dent* 1991; 66:706–708.

14. Eames WB, O'Neal SJ, Monteiro J, Roan JD, Cohen KS: Techniques to improve the seating of castings. *J Am Dent Assoc* 1978; 96:432.

15. Kent WA, Shillingburg HT, Duncanson MG: Taper of clinical preparations for cast restorations. *Quintessence Int* 1988; 19:339–345.

16. Nordlander J, Weir D, Stoffer W, Ochi S: The taper of clinical preparations for fixed prosthodontics. *J Prosthet Dent* 1988; 60:148–151.

17. Weed RM: Determining adequate crown convergence. *Tex Dent J* 1980; 98:14.

18. Dodge WW, Weed RM, Baez RJ, Buchanan RN: The effect of convergence angle on retention and resistance form. *Quintessence Int* 1985; 16:191.

19. Lorey RE, Myers GE: The retentive qualities of bridge retainers. *J Am Dent Assoc* 1968; 76:568–572.

20. Rosenstiel E: The retention of inlays and crowns as a function of geometrical form. *Br Dent J* 1957; 103:388–394.

21. Kishimoto M, Shillingburg HT, Duncanson MG: Influence of preparation features on retention and resistance. Part II: Three-quarter crowns. *J Prosthet Dent* 1983; 49:188–192.

22. Smyd ES: Advanced thought in indirect inlay and fixed bridge fabrication. *J Am Dent Assoc* 1944; 31:759–768.

23. Parker MH, Malone KH, Trier AC, Striano TS: Evaluation of resistance form for prepared teeth. *J Prosthet Dent* 1991; 66:730–733.

24. Woolsey GD, Matich JA: The effect of axial grooves on the resistance form of cast restorations. *J Am Dent Assoc* 1978; 97:978–980.

25. Willey RE: The preparation of abutments for veneer retainers. *J Am Dent Assoc* 1956; 53:141–154.

26. Rosner D: Function, placement and reproduction of bevels for gold castings. *J Prosthet Dent* 1963; 13:1160–1166.

27. Ostlund LE: Cavity design and mathematics: Their effect on gaps at the margins of cast restorations. *Oper Dent* 1985; 10:122–137.

28. McLean JW, Wilson AD: Butt joint versus bevelled gold margin in metal ceramic crowns. *J Biomed Mater Res* 1980; 14:239–250.

29. Pascoe DF: Analysis of the geometry of finishing lines for full crown restorations. *J Prosthet Dent* 1978; 40:157–162.

30. Gavelis JR, Morency JD, Riley ED, Sozio RB: The effect of various finish line preparations on the marginal seal and occlusal seat of full crown preparations. *J Prosthet Dent* 1981; 45:138–145.

31. Panno FV, Vahidi F, Gulker I, Ghalili KM: Evaluation of the 45-degree labial bevel with a shoulder preparation. *J Prosthet Dent* 1986; 56:655–661.

32. El-Ebrashi MK, Craig RG, Peyton FA: Experimental stress analysis of dental restorations. Part III. The concept of the geometry of proximal margins. *J Prosthet Dent* 1969; 22:333–345.

33. Farah JW, Craig RG: Finite element stress analysis of a restored axisymmetric first molar. *J Dent Res* 1974; 53:859–866.

34. Gage JP: Rationale for bevelled shoulder veneer crown preparations. *Aust Dent J* 1977; 22:432–435.

35. Shillingburg HT, Hobo S, Fisher DW: Preparation design and margin distortion in porcelain-fused-to-metal restorations. *J Prosthet Dent* 1973; 29:276–284.

36. Ingraham R, Bassett RW, Koser JR: *An Atlas of Cast Gold Procedures*, ed 2. Buena Park, CA, Uni-Tro College Press, 1969, p 34.

37. Eissmann HF, Radke RA, Noble WH: Physiologic design criteria for fixed dental restorations. *Dent Clin North Am* 1971; 15:543–568.

38. Black GV: The management of enamel margins. *Dent Cosmos* 1891; 33:85–100.

39. Waerhaug J: Histologic considerations which govern where the margins of restorations should be located in relation to the gingiva. *Dent Clin North Am* 1960; 4:161–176.

40. Mormann W, Regolati B, Renggli HH: Gingival reaction to well-fitted subgingival proximal gold inlays. *J Clin Periodontol* 1974; 1:120–125.

41. Janenko C, Smales RJ: Anterior crowns and gingival health. *Aust Dent J* 1979; 24:225–230.

42. Romanelli JH: Periodontal considerations in tooth preparation for crowns and bridges. *Dent Clin North Am* 1980; 24:271–284.

43. Wilson RD: Intracrevicular restorative dentistry. *Int J Periodont Rest Dent* 1981; 1(4):35–49.

44. Silness J: Periodontal conditions in patients treated with dental bridges. III. The relationship between the location of the crown margin and the periodontal condition. *J Periodont Res* 1970; 5:225–229.

45. Larato DC: Effect of cervical margins on gingiva. *J Calif Dent Assoc* 1969; 45:19–22.

46. Reeves WG: Restorative margin placement and periodontal health. *J Prosthet Dent* 1991; 66:733–736.

47. Silness J: Fixed prosthodontics and periodontal health. *Dent Clin North Am* 1980; 24:317–329.

48. Karlsen K: Gingival reactions to dental restorations. *Acta Odontol Scand* 1970; 28:895–904.

49. Newcomb GM: The relationship between the location of subgingival crown margins and gingival inflammation. *J Periodontol* 1974; 45:151–154.

50. Jameson LM, Malone WFP: Crown contours and gingival response. *J Prosthet Dent* 1982; 47:620–624.

51. Richter WA, Ueno H: Relationship of crown margin placement to gingival inflammation. *J Prosthet Dent* 1973; 30:156–161.

52. Koth DL: Full crown restorations and gingival inflammation in a controlled population. *J Prosthet Dent* 1982; 48:681–685.

53. Christensen GJ: Marginal fit of gold inlay castings. *J Prosthet Dent* 1966; 16:297–305.

54. Bjorn AL, Bjorn H, Grkovic B: Marginal fit of restorations and its relation to periodontal bone level. Part II. Crowns. *Odontol Rev* 1970; 21:337–346.

55. Berman MH: The complete coverage restoration and the gingival sulcus. *J Prosthet Dent* 1973; 29:301–304.

56. Stein RS, Kuwata M: A dentist and a dental technologist analyze current ceramo-metal procedures. *Dent Clin North Am* 1977; 21:729–749.

57. Behend DA: Ceramometal restorations with supragingival margins. *J Prosthet Dent* 1982; 47:625–632.

58. Gardner FM: Margins of complete crowns—Literature review. *J Prosthet Dent* 1982; 48:396–400.

59. Garguilo AW, Wentz FM, Orban B: Dimensions of the dentogingival junction in humans. *J Periodontol* 1961; 32:261–267.

60. Ingber JS, Rose LF, Coslet JG: The "biologic width"—A concept in periodontics and restorative dentistry. *Alpha Omegan* 1977; 10:62–65.

61. Barnes IE: The production of inlay cavity bevels. *Br Dent J* 1974; 137:379–390.

62. Kinzer RL, Morris C: Instruments and instrumentation to promote conservative operative dentistry. *Dent Clin North Am* 1976; 20:241–257.

63. Lustig LP, Perlitsh MJ, Przctak C, Mucko K: A rational concept of crown preparation. *Quintessence Int* 1972; 3:35–44.

64. Lustig LP: A rational concept of crown preparation revised and expanded. *Quintessence Int* 1976; 7:41–48.

65. Tronstad L, Leidal TI: Scanning electron microscopy of cavity margins finished with chisels or rotating instruments at low speed. *J Dent Res* 1974; 53:1167–1174.

Chapter 10

Preparations for Full Veneer Crowns

There are numerous situations that call for the use of a full veneer restoration. Clinicians have long considered it to be the most retentive of the veneer preparations.[1] Controlled laboratory studies have shown that when compared with partial veneer designs, the full veneer crown exhibits superior retention[2,3] and resistance.[4] This does not mean that a full veneer design must be used on every tooth. Instead, it should be used on those teeth whose restoration demands maximum retention.

A requirement for maximum retention is not commonly seen in the placement of single restorations. This need is more likely to be manifested in the design of retainers for fixed partial dentures, where additional demands are placed on the preparation and restoration. The selection of a full veneer crown retainer becomes mandatory when the abutment tooth is small or when the edentulous span is long.

Variations of the full veneer crown, the metal-ceramic crown or the all-ceramic crown, are used in situations that require a good cosmetic result. The full veneer crown should be used when less extensive and less destructive designs have been considered and found lacking in retention, resistance, coverage, or esthetics to properly restore the tooth.

Full coverage in the right circumstances can be excellent treatment, but it is overused. A report of dental insurance data in 1979 indicated that nearly 93% of the cast restorations done by dentists submitting claims to that company were of a full-coverage design.[5] Undoubtedly the percentage would be greater today. The removal of all morphologic form of the tooth is radical treatment, and restoring it properly can be difficult.[6] The dentist should be sure it is necessary.

Full Metal Crown Preparation

When all of the axial surfaces of a posterior tooth have been attacked by decalcification or caries, or when those surfaces have been previously restored, the tooth is a candidate for a full metal crown. By tying together the remaining tooth structure, a full metal crown can strengthen and support the tooth.[7] It should be used judiciously, though, because it does require a destructive preparation. It may weaken rather than strengthen the remaining tooth structure when there has been extensive destruction previously in the center of the tooth. However, the preparation for a full metal crown is less destructive than that required for either metal-ceramic or all-ceramic crowns.

Full coverage should not be used in mouths with uncontrolled caries. The full veneer crown is a restoration that replaces lost tooth structure and imparts some measure of structural support to the tooth. However, it does not protect the tooth against the biological causes of the caries. These processes must be controlled by other means before any restoration can be successful.

Armamentarium

1. Handpiece
2. No. 171L bur
3. Round-end tapered diamond
4. Short needle diamond
5. Torpedo diamond
6. Torpedo bur
7. Red utility wax

The preparation for a full veneer crown is begun with occlusal reduction, creating about 1.5 mm of clearance on the functional cusps and 1.0 mm on the nonfunctional cusps. By accomplishing this step first, the occlusogingival length of the preparation can be determined. The potential retention of the preparation can then be assessed, and auxiliary features can be added if necessary.

Depth-orientation grooves are placed on the occlusal surface of the tooth to provide an easy reference to determine when reduction is sufficient. If reduction is begun without orientation marks, time will be wasted in repeated checks for adequate clearance. A round-end tapered diamond is used to place the grooves on the ridges and the primary grooves of the occlusal surface. If there is already some clearance with the opposing tooth because

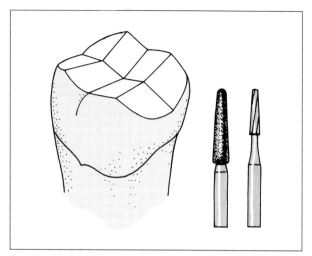

Fig 10-1 Occlusal reduction: Round-end tapered diamond and no. 171L bur.

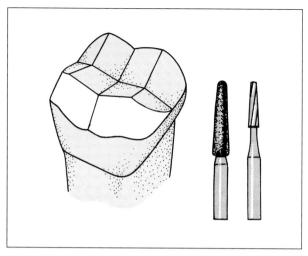

Fig 10-2 Functional cusp bevel: Round-end tapered diamond and no. 171L bur.

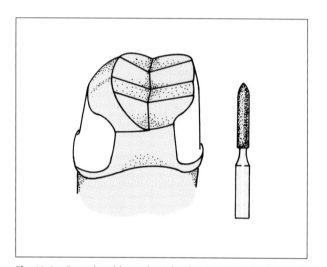

Fig 10-3 Buccal and lingual axial reduction: Torpedo diamond.

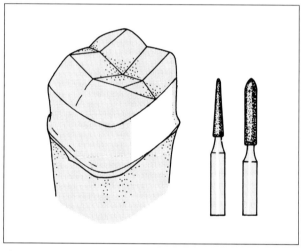

Fig 10-4 Proximal axial reduction: Short needle and torpedo diamonds.

of malpositioning or fracture of the tooth being prepared, the grooves should not be made as deep.

The tooth structure remaining between the orientation grooves is removed to accomplish the occlusal reduction (Fig 10-1). Any roughness left by the grooves should be removed, keeping the occlusal surface in the configuration of the geometric inclines that make up the occlusal surface of any posterior tooth.

A wide bevel is placed on the functional cusp, again using the round-end tapered diamond (Fig 10-2). Depth-orientation grooves are also helpful in obtaining this reduction. The functional cusp bevel, placed on the buccal inclines of mandibular buccal cusps and the lingual inclines of maxillary lingual cusps, is an integral part of the occlusal reduction. Failure to place this bevel can produce a thin casting or poor morphology in the restoration.

Occlusal clearance is checked by having the patient close on a 2.0-mm-thick strip of red utility wax held over the preparation. The wax is then held up to a light to determine the adequacy of the occlusal clearance. Any part of the preparation that has insufficient occlusal clearance will be readily detectable as a thin spot in the wax. Additional tooth structure should be removed from the indicated areas and rechecked.

The occlusal reduction and functional cusp bevel are planed smooth with a no. 171L bur now or when the bur is used to instrument the seating groove. There should not be sharp angles or ridges where the planes or bevel join. If there are, they should be removed with the tapered fissure bur.

The buccal and lingual walls are reduced with a torpedo diamond, whose sides will produce the desired axial

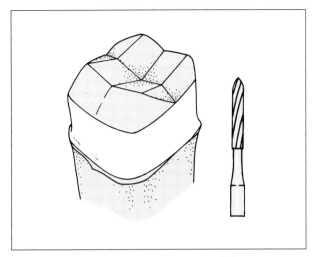

Fig 10-5   Chamfer and axial finishing: Torpedo bur.

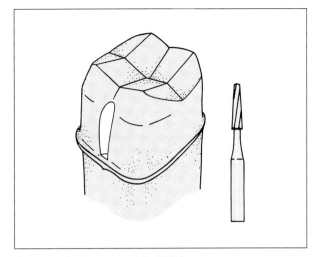

Fig 10-6   Seating groove: No. 171L bur.

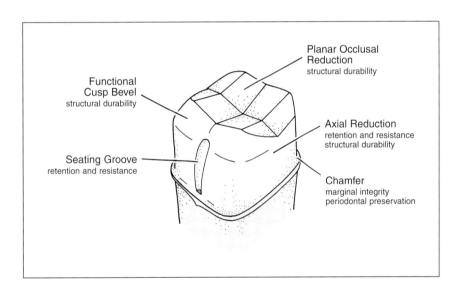

Fig 10-7   Features of a mandibular full metal crown preparation and the function served by each.

reduction while its tapered tip forms a chamfer finish line (Fig 10-3). A definite, even finish line is necessary to enable the fabrication of a well-fitting restoration,[8] and the chamfer is the best for providing the bulk needed for strength while still allowing good adaptation.[1]

The initial proximal cuts are made with a short needle diamond (Fig 10-4). The thin diamond is worked through the proximal area in an occlusogingival or buccolingual "sawing" motion, carefully avoiding the adjacent teeth. Once sufficient maneuvering room has been obtained, the torpedo diamond is introduced to plane the walls while simultaneously forming a chamfer as the interproximal gingival finish line.

All of the axial surfaces are smoothed with a torpedo carbide finishing bur whose size and shape enable it to finish the chamfer finish line as well (Fig 10-5). Special

care should be taken in rounding the corners from the buccal or lingual surfaces to the proximal surfaces to insure that the finish line will be smooth and continuous. The final step in the full veneer preparation is the placement of a seating groove (Fig 10-6). It will prevent any rotational tendencies during cementation, and it will help guide the casting to place. The groove is formed with a no. 171L bur and is placed in the axial surface with the greatest bulk. This usually will be on the buccal surface of mandibular preparations and on the lingual surface of maxillary preparations. On preparations for long-span fixed partial dentures, there should be a buccal and a lingual groove to increase the resistance to mesiodistal movement. The features of a preparation for a full veneer metal crown and the function served by each are shown in Fig 10-7.

Metal-Ceramic Crowns

The *metal-ceramic restoration*, also called a porcelain-fused-to-metal restoration, consists of a ceramic layer bonded to a thin cast metal coping that fits over the tooth preparation. Such a restoration combines the strength and accurate fit of a cast metal crown with the cosmetic effect of a ceramic crown. With a metal understructure, metal-ceramic restorations have greater strength than restorations made of the ceramic alone. Friedlander et al found the metal-ceramic restoration to be 2.8 times as strong.[9] As a result, the longevity of metal-ceramic restorations is greater, and it can be used in a wider variety of situations, including the replacement of missing teeth with fixed partial dentures.

Since the restoration is a combination of metal and ceramic, it is not surprising that the tooth preparation for it is likewise a combination. There is deep reduction on the facial surface to provide space for the coping and a ceramic layer thick enough to achieve the desired cosmetic result. On the lingual surface and the lingual aspects of the proximal surfaces, there is shallower reduction similar to that used for a full metal crown. There may be a wing on each proximal surface where the deep facial reduction ends and the shallower proximal reduction begins.[10]

Adequate reduction is essential to achieving a good cosmetic result. Without the space for a sufficient thickness of ceramic material, two things can happen: *(1)* the restoration will be poorly contoured, adversely affecting both the cosmetic effect of the crown and the health of the surrounding gingiva, and *(2)* the shade and translucency of the restoration will not match adjacent natural teeth.

Anterior Metal-Ceramic Crowns

A uniform reduction of approximately 1.2 mm is needed over the entire facial surface. To achieve adequate reduction without encroaching upon the pulp, the facial surface must be prepared in two planes that correspond roughly to the two geometric planes present on the facial surface of an uncut tooth (Fig 10-8). If the facial surface is reduced in one plane that is an extension of the gingival plane, the incisal edge will protrude, resulting in a bad shade match or an overcontoured "block." If the facial surface is prepared in one plane that has adequate facial reduction in the incisal aspect, the facial surface will be overtapered and too close to the pulp.

Armamentarium

1. Laboratory knife with no. 25 blade
2. Silicone putty and accelerator
3. Handpiece
4. Flat-end tapered diamond
5. Small wheel diamond
6. Long needle diamond
7. Torpedo diamond
8. Torpedo bur
9. H158–012 radial fissure bur
10. RS-1 binangle chisel

If an index is made before the preparation is begun, it will be possible to have a positive check on reduction produced by the preparation. If the contours of the existing tooth are correct, the index can be made intraorally while waiting for the anesthetic to take effect. However, if the tooth is badly broken down, or if contours are to be changed in the finished restoration, the index should be made from a preoperative wax-up on the diagnostic cast.

One-half scoop of putty is mixed with the appropriate amount of accelerator and kneaded in the palm of the hand until all streaks of the accelerator have disappeared. The putty is then adapted with a thumb and forefinger over the tooth to be prepared (Fig 10-9). It should be allowed to polymerize on the tooth, which should take about 2 minutes. The index should cover the entire labial and lingual surface of the tooth to be prepared, plus the corresponding surfaces of at least one adjacent tooth (Fig 10-10).

The index is then removed from the teeth. A laboratory knife with a no. 25 blade is used to cut along the incisal edges of the tooth imprints to separate the index into a labial and a lingual half (Fig 10-11). The lingual half is set aside for the time being. The labial portion of the index is cut from mesial to distal across the imprints of the labial surfaces of the teeth to produce an incisal and a gingival half (Fig 10-12).

The gingival half of the labial portion is positioned on the teeth to insure that it is closely adapted to the labial surfaces (Fig 10-13). After removing the labial index, the lingual index is put in position and its adaptation to the incisal edges of the teeth is checked (Fig 10-14).

The labial and lingual indices are set aside until the preparation is completed. Then the gingival half of the labial index is positioned and checked for adequate labial clearance for a metal coping and porcelain (Fig 10-15). If the reduction is inadequate, the index is removed from the mouth and more tooth structure must be removed. The incisal clearance is checked by putting the lingual index in place and evaluating the distance between the incisal edge of the prepared tooth and the incisal edge of the tooth imprint on the index (Fig 10-16).

The initial step in the preparation for a metal-ceramic crown is the placement of depth-orientation grooves on the labial and incisal surfaces with a flat-end tapered diamond. These orientation cuts, recommended by Preston[10] and Miller,[11] are a means of judging the amount

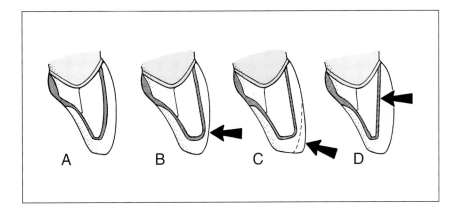

Fig 10-8 It is important to reduce the labial surface in two planes to receive a metal-cearmic restoration (A). If only one plane is produced, opaque porcelain may show through (B), the labial surface may be overcontoured (C), or the pulp may be encroached upon (D).

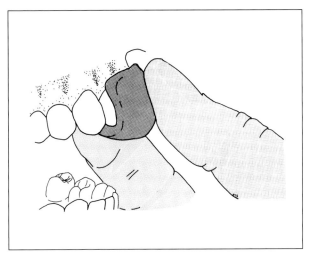

Fig 10-9 Mold silicone putty on the labial and lingual surfaces of the tooth to be prepared and the teeth adjacent to it.

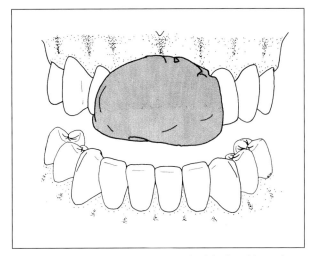

Fig 10-10 The index should contact the labial and lingual surfaces of the tooth on either side of the tooth to be prepared.

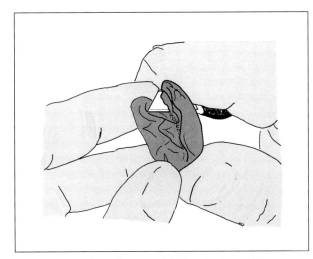

Fig 10-11 Cut the index into a labial and a lingual half.

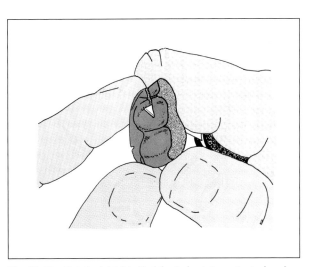

Fig 10-12 Cut the labial half of the index into a gingival and an incisal half.

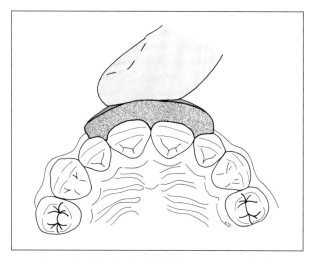

Fig 10-13 Place the gingival half of the index on the teeth to see if it fits accurately.

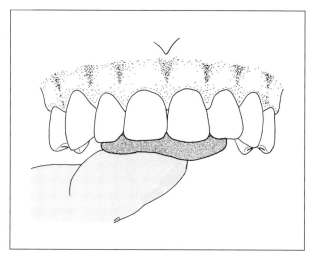

Fig 10-14 Place the lingual index in position to check its accuracy.

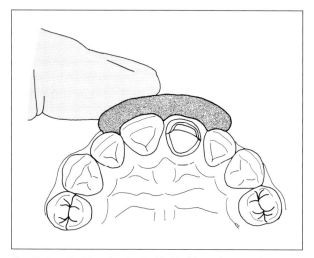

Fig 10-15 Position the gingival half of the index over the preparation to check the labial reduction.

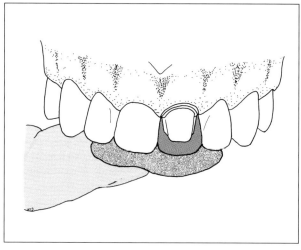

Fig 10-16 Place the lingual index in position to evaluate the incisal reduction.

of tooth structure to be removed. The full diameter of an instrument of known dimension is sunk into the tooth. The depth of reduction can be measured using the uncut outer surface of the remaining tooth structure as a reference point.[11] If reduction is done without grooves, time will be wasted in repeatedly rechecking reduction with the index.

The labial grooves should be cut in two sets: one set parallel with the gingival half of the labial surface and one set parallel with the incisal half of the labial surface (Fig 10-17). These grooves should be 1.2 mm deep. The incisal grooves should be cut all the way through the incisal edge and should extend 2.0 mm gingivally.

Incisal reduction is done with the flat-end tapered diamond so that it parallels the inclination of the unprepared incisal edge (Fig 10-18). This is done first to allow easy instrument access to the axial surfaces and the gingival finish line. Inadequate incisal reduction results in poor incisal translucency in the finished restoration.

Reduction of the incisal portion of the labial surface is done with the same flat-end tapered diamond. All tooth structure is planed off to the depth of the orientation grooves (Fig 10-19). The gingival portion of the labial surface is likewise reduced to the depth of the grooves with the flat-end tapered diamond. The reduction is carried around the labioproximal line angles to a point 1.0

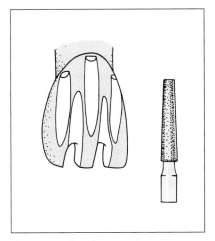

Fig 10-17 Depth-orientation grooves: Flat-end tapered diamond.

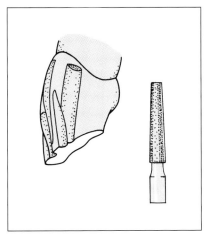

Fig 10-18 Incisal reduction: Flat-end tapered diamond.

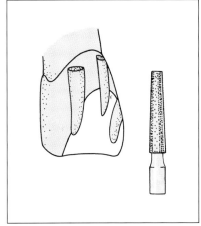

Fig 10-19 Labial reduction (incisal half): Flat-end tapered diamond.

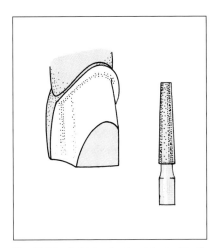

Fig 10-20 Labial reduction (gingival half): Flat-end tapered diamond.

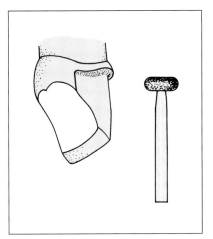

Fig 10-21 Lingual reduction: Small wheel diamond.

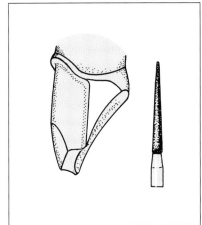

Fig 10-22 Initial proximal reduction: Long needle diamond.

mm lingual to the proximal contacts (Fig 10-20). Although the resulting wings of tooth structure can provide some resistance to rotation, that is not the primary reason for their existence. They conserve tooth structure, if in fact there is still sound tooth structure left on the proximal surfaces. It is important that the portion of each wing that faces labially has the same inclination as the gingival portion of the labial surface.

The lingual surface is reduced with a small wheel diamond to obtain a minimum of 0.7 mm of clearance with the opposing teeth (Fig 10-21). Those portions of the lingual surface that will have a ceramic veneer should have 1.0 mm of clearance. The junction between the cingulum

and the lingual wall must not be overreduced. Overshortening the lingual wall will reduce retention.

A long needle diamond is used to complete access through the proximal areas to minimize the chances of nicking the adjacent teeth (Fig 10-22). Much of the axial reduction in the region of the proximal contact will have been accomplished already by the flat-end tapered diamond. The lingual aspect of the proximal axial walls, as well as the lingual surface, are reduced with the torpedo diamond (Fig 10-23). The lingual and proximal axial surfaces are smoothed with the torpedo bur, accentuating the chamfer on the lingual and proximal surfaces at the same time (Fig 10-24).

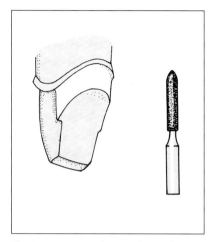

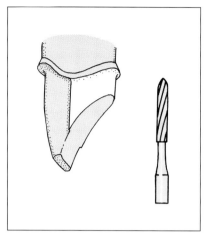

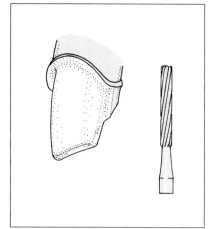

Fig 10-23 Lingual axial reduction: Torpedo diamond.

Fig 10-24 Axial finishing: Torpedo bur.

Fig 10-25 Axial and shoulder finishing: Radial fissure bur.

An H158–012 radial fissure bur is used to smooth the labial surface (Fig 10-25). All angles and edges on the preparation are rounded with the sides of the bur to facilitate seating of the restoration later. At the same time that the labial surface is being planed by the side of the bur, the end is forming a radial shoulder finish line.

Shoulders have been advocated for gingivofacial finish lines of metal-ceramic preparations alone[12-16] or with narrow bevels.[10,17-20] Some investigators have reported that metal-ceramic crowns with metal gingivofacial margins made over shoulder finish lines distort less during porcelain firing.[21,22] A possible explanation is that the shoulder configuration provides space for an internal rib of metal to buttress the margin.[10,23] Other investigators have reported not finding a difference in marginal fit. They hypothesize that marginal gaps following ceramic firing may be caused either by technical difficulties in forming a knife edge of metal and ceramic[24] or by differences in metal/ceramic combinations.[25]

However, there is a compelling reason for not using a metal margin at all. The metal collar that accompanies a bevel on a shoulder[26] often requires the finish line to be placed deep in the gingival sulcus to hide the metal.[27] If some form of shoulder without a bevel is used, an all-ceramic margin can be fabricated. This eliminates a metal collar at the faciogingival margin of the finished metal-ceramic restoration, and there is no need to bury the margin beneath the gingiva.

Quantitative evaluations of the marginal fit of all-ceramic shoulders on metal-ceramic crowns have found satisfactory adaptation of the ceramic to the preparation finish line. Belser et al reported in vivo marginal discrepancies of 46 μm on cemented metal-ceramic crowns with all-ceramic facial margins.[28] They found no significant differences among crowns with all-ceramic margins and those with metal collar margins over shoulder and beveled shoulder finish lines. In vitro studies by West and associates[29] and Hunt et al[30] found minimal marginal discrepancies in all-ceramic shoulder margins on metal-ceramic crowns. Of course, a dentist can use all-ceramic margins on metal-ceramic crowns only if the technician is capable of producing restorations with accurate ceramic margins.

Zena et al demonstrated that all-ceramic margins made over hand-planed shoulders fit significantly better than margins made over finish lines cut solely with rotary instruments.[31] However, if a conventional enamel chisel is used for planing a radial shoulder, the sharp angles at the ends of the cutting blade will destroy the rounded internal angle of the finish line (Fig 10-26).

A modified 15-8-8 binangle chisel, the RS-1 (Suter Dental Mfg, Chico, CA), is recommended to avoid this problem (Fig 10-27). This instrument has a hoe (pull stroke) blade at both ends, unlike a conventional 15-8-8 binangle chisel, which has a hoe (pull stroke) blade at one end and a chisel (push stroke) blade at the other (Fig 10-28). One corner of one RS-1 blade is rounded with a mounted Arkansas stone (Fig 10-29, A), and the opposite corner is rounded on the other end (Fig 10-29, B).

One end, with the rounded corner against the gingivoaxial "angle," is used to instrument the radial shoulder on one-half of the preparation (Fig 10-30). The other end, with its modified corner also against the rounded gingivoaxial junction, is used to smooth the finish line on the other half of the preparation. The 1.5-mm-wide blade will extend over the actual finish line, which is 1.2 to 1.5 mm wide. This will remove any lip of enamel that might extend occlusally from the cavosurface angle.

The features of a preparation for an anterior metal-ceramic restoration and the function served by each are shown in Fig 10-31.

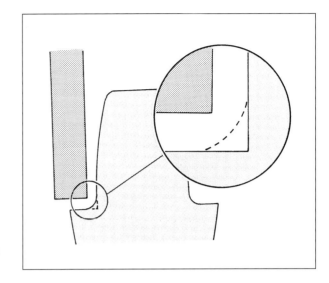

Fig 10-26 The sharp corners of a conventional chisel will gouge the gingivoaxial angle *(inset)* of a radial shoulder.

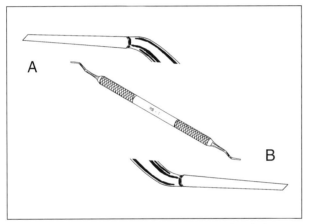

Fig 10-27 The RS-1 is a modified 15-8-8 chisel with the same hoe (pull stroke) blade on both ends (A and B).

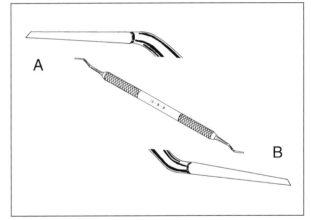

Fig 10-28 A conventional 15-8-8 binangle chisel has a hoe (pull stroke) blade on one end (A) and a chisel (push stroke) blade at the other (B).

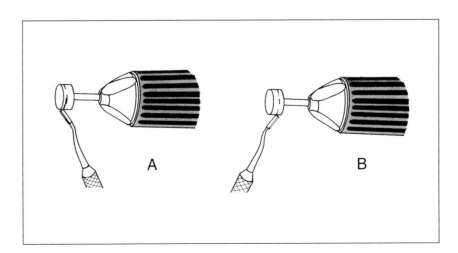

Fig 10-29 Round an angle at one end of the RS-1 (A) and the opposite angle on the other end (B).

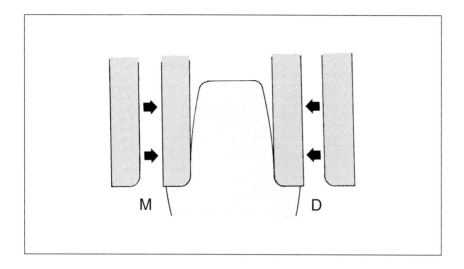

Fig 10-30 The rounded corner of one end of the RS-1 is placed against the gingivoaxial angle while planing the mesial half of the shoulder (M). The other end is used to instrument the distal half of the finish line (D).

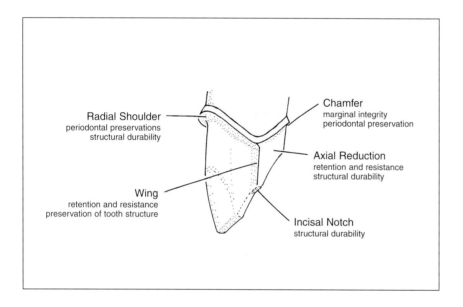

Radial Shoulder
periodontal preservations
structural durability

Chamfer
marginal integrity
periodontal preservation

Axial Reduction
retention and resistance
structural durability

Wing
retention and resistance
preservation of tooth structure

Incisal Notch
structural durability

Fig 10-31 Features of an anterior metal-ceramic preparation and the function served by each.

Posterior Metal-Ceramic Crowns

The use of metal-ceramic crowns on posterior teeth allows the creation of an esthetic restoration on a posterior tooth needing a full crown in the appearance zone. Maxillary premolars, maxillary first molars, and mandibular first premolars are almost always in the appearance zone. Mandibular second premolars also can fall into this category. Maxillary second molars and mandibular molars may require metal-ceramic crowns if a patient will not accept all-metal crowns on those teeth.

Routinely placing metal-ceramic crowns on all premolars and molars is overtreatment because of the additional tooth structure that must be destroyed to accommodate the combined thickness of metal and ceramic. Often there is added expense for the patient because of higher laboratory fees, as well as an increased risk of failure from ceramic veneer fracture.

The routine use of all-ceramic occlusal surfaces has been criticized.[32] This restoration design offers maximum cosmetic effect when required by location in a highly visible area or by patient preference. Patients who demand ceramic occlusal surfaces should know of the potential problems. The use of all-ceramic occlusal surfaces requires the removal of more tooth structure, and the completed restorations pose a threat to the structural integrity of opposing occlusal surfaces. Conventional glazed dental porcelain is approximately 40 times as abrasive as gold to tooth enamel.[33] Preparations for metal-ceramic crowns should be done with a plan for the extent of ceramic coverage in mind, since the areas to be veneered with ceramic require deeper reduction than those portions of the tooth that will be overlaid with metal alone.

Armamentarium

1. Laboratory knife with no. 25 blade
2. Silicone putty and accelerator
3. Handpiece
4. Flat-end tapered diamond
5. Short needle diamond
6. Torpedo diamond
7. Torpedo bur
8. H158–012 radial fissure bur
9. RS-1 binangle chisel

Before the preparation is begun, silicone putty is adapted to the facial, lingual, and occlusal surfaces of the tooth to be prepared as well as to one tooth on each side. After polymerization, a midsagittal index can be formed by cutting the silicone in half along the faciolingual midline of the tooth to be prepared. The putty is placed back on the tooth to insure good adaptation. If the clinical crown of the tooth being restored is severely damaged, the index should be made from a diagnostic wax-up.

A facial index is made by cutting through the silicone along the facial cusps of the teeth. The facial piece is divided along a line midway between the cervical lines of the teeth and the facial cusp tips. The occlusal portion is discarded and the gingival portion is used as an index. The occlusal reduction is begun by making depth-orientation grooves with a round-end tapered diamond. In the areas where there will be ceramic coverage, reduction should be 1.5 mm[34] to 2.0 mm.[10,17,35] The occlusal reduction is completed by removing the strips of intact enamel between the depth-orientation grooves with the same diamond. The reduction should take the form of definite planes reproducing the general occlusal morphology[36] or the basic geometric shape of the occlusal surface (Fig 10-32).

The functional cusp bevel, which allows a uniform bulk of restorative material on the lingual inclines of maxillary lingual cusps and the facial inclines of mandibular facial cusps, is also begun with depth-orientation grooves (Fig 10-33). The depth required will be 1.5 mm if the coverage will be metal only, and 2.0 mm if the metal will be veneered with ceramic. The functional cusp bevel is completed by removing the tooth structure between the depth-orientation grooves. The angulation of the bevel approximates the inclination of the opposing cusps.

A no. 171L bur is used to smooth the planes of the occlusal reduction to remove any roughness or pits that might interfere with the complete seating of the finished restoration. Any sharp corners or edges on the preparation that might cause problems in impression pouring,

investing, casting, and ultimately in the seating of the completed crown should be rounded over.

The flat-end tapered diamond is aligned with the occlusal segment of the facial surface and three vertical grooves are cut in the occlusal portion of the facial surface. These are nearly the full diameter of the instrument, fading out gingivally (Fig 10-34). The same diamond is aligned with the gingival component of the facial surface, and the side of the instrument is used to cut into the tooth surface. The full diameter of the instrument must cut into the tooth. The instrument tip should be slightly supragingival at this point, even if the intended location of the finish line is flush with or slightly below the gingival crest. At least two more orientation grooves should be placed near the line angles of the tooth.

All tooth structure remaining between the depth-orientation grooves in the occlusal segment of the facial surface is removed with the flat-end tapered diamond (Fig 10-35). The gingival portion of the facial surface is then reduced, extending it well into the proximal surface (Fig 10-36). If facial reduction of less than 1.2 mm is done for a base metal–ceramic crown or 1.4 mm for a noble metal–ceramic crown, the restoration will be either opaque or overcontoured.

The proximal axial reduction is begun with a short needle diamond (Fig 10-37). Its narrow diameter allows interproximal reduction without nicking adjacent teeth. The instrument can be used with an up-and-down motion on the facial aspect of the interproximal tooth structure, or it can be used on the occlusal portion with a faciolingual movement. Initially, the objective is to achieve separation between the teeth without overtapering the prepared walls or mutilating the adjacent tooth. The proximal axial surfaces are then planed with the needle diamond. The lingual axial wall is reduced with a torpedo diamond (Fig 10-38). Enough tooth structure is removed on both the lingual and proximal axial walls to create a distinct chamfer finish line wherever there will not be a ceramic veneer. The chamfer finish line and the axial surfaces adjacent to it are smoothed with a torpedo carbide finishing bur. All axial surfaces that will be veneered only with metal are finished in this way.

The facial surface and those parts of the proximal surfaces to be veneered with ceramic are smoothed with an H158–012 radial fissure bur (Fig 10-39). At the lingual-most extension of the facial reduction, lingual to the proximal contact, the transition from the deeper facial reduction to the relatively shallower lingual axial reduction results in a vertical wall or "wing" of tooth structure. The wings must not be undercut with the facial or lingual axial walls of the preparation.

If the shoulder and wings are not lingual to the proximal contact, the proximal area of the ceramic veneer will lack translucence. If there was an amalgam restoration in the tooth prior to this preparation, the wing is made to coincide with the lingual wall of the amalgam's proximal box. If the entire proximal surface is to be veneered with ceramic, the shoulder is extended across the proximal surface with no wing.

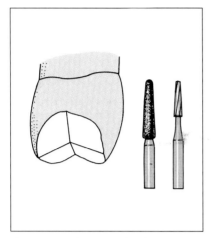

Fig 10-32 Planar occlusal reduction: Round-end tapered diamond and no. 171L bur.

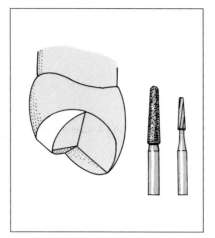

Fig 10-33 Functonal cusp bevel: Round-end tapered diamond and no. 171 bur.

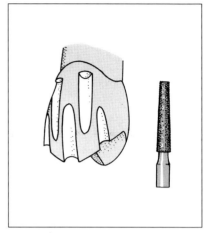

Fig 10-34 Depth-orientation grooves: Flat-end tapered diamond.

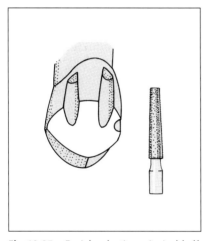

Fig 10-35 Facial reduction, gingival half: Flat-end tapered diamond.

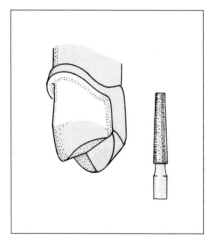

Fig 10-36 Facial reduction, gingival half: Flat-end tapered diamond.

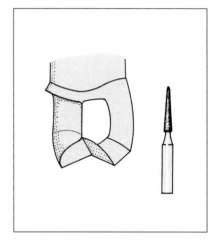

Fig 10-37 Proximal axial reduction: Short needle diamond.

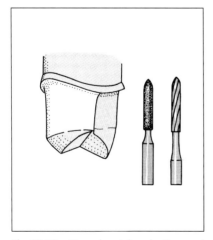

Fig 10-38 Lingual axial reduction and finishing: Torpedo diamond and bur.

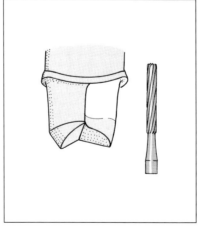

Fig 10-39 Facial axial and radial shoulder finishing: Radial fissure bur.

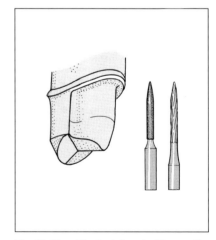

Fig 10-40 Gingival bevel: Flame diamond and finishing bur.

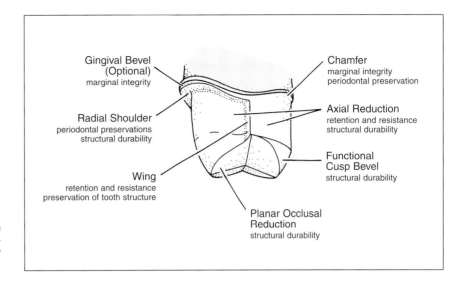

Fig 10-41 Features of a preparation for a metal-ceramic crown on a posterior tooth and the function served by each.

The radial shoulder, started with the flat-end tapered diamond at the time the facial reduction was accomplished, is finished now with the radial fissure bur. On highly visible posterior teeth, such as the maxillary premolars, an all-ceramic margin is frequently used to achieve a good esthetic result without intruding into the gingival sulcus. The 1.0-mm-wide shoulder is smoothed by planing it with the RS-1 modified binangle chisel, which will preserve the rounded internal angle created by the radial fissure bur. Any "lip" or reverse bevel of enamel at the cavosurface angle should be removed. Small, sharp edges in this area may not be reproduced when the impression is poured, and they are susceptible to fracture on the cast or on the tooth in the mouth.

There are occasions when a shoulder with a bevel is the finish line of choice: when esthetic needs are not as critical or the dental technician is unable to consistently produce a precise all-ceramic margin. A narrow bevel, no wider than 0.3 mm, can be placed on the shoulder with the tip of a flame-shaped diamond (Fig 10-40). The bevel should be kept narrow, since the metal collar on the resulting crown must be as wide as the bevel. The bevel is easier to wax and cast to if the diamond is leaned toward the center of the tooth as much as possible. The bevel is finished with an H48L-010 flame-shaped carbide finishing bur to create a finish line that is as clear as possible. The features of a preparation for a posterior metal-ceramic restoration and the function served by each are shown in Fig 10-41.

All-Ceramic Crowns

The all-ceramic crown differs from other cemented veneer restorations because it is not cast in gold or some other metal. It is capable of producing the best cosmetic effect of all dental restorations. However, since it is made entirely of ceramic, a brittle substance, it is more susceptible to fracture. The development of dental porcelain reinforced with alumina in the 1960s created renewed interest in the restoration.[37] Dicor cast glass ceramic, Hi-ceram, In-ceram, and IPS Empress restorations have maintained the interest of the profession over the past decade.

Preparations for this type of crown should be left as long as possible to give maximum support to the porcelain. An overshortened preparation will create stress concentrations in the labiogingival area of the crown,[38] which can produce a characteristic "half-moon" fracture in the labiogingival area of the restoration.[38–40] A shoulder of uniform width (approximately 1 mm) is used as a gingival finish line to provide a flat seat to resist forces directed from the incisal.[38,41] The incisal edge is flat and placed at a slight inclination toward the linguogingival to meet forces on the incisal edge and prevent shearing.[42,43] Finally, all sharp angles of the preparation should be slightly rounded to reduce the danger of fracture caused by points of stress concentration.[38,42,43]

The position of the tooth in the arch, factors relating to occlusion, and morphologic features of the tooth all should be weighed when an all-ceramic crown is considered for a restoration. All-ceramic crowns are best suited for use on incisors. If they are used on other teeth, patients should know that there is an increased risk of fracture.

Use of the all-ceramic crown should be avoided on teeth with an edge-to-edge occlusion that will produce stress in the incisal area of the restoration. It likewise should not be used when the opposing teeth occlude on the cervical fifth of the lingual surface. Tension will be produced, and a "half-moon" fracture is likely to occur. Teeth with short cervical crowns also are poor risks for all-ceramic crowns because they do not have enough preparation length to support the lingual and incisal surfaces of the restoration.

Armamentarium

1. Handpiece
2. Flat-end tapered diamond
3. Small wheel diamond
4. H158–012 radial fissure bur
5. RS-1 binangle chisel

Depth-orientation grooves are placed on the labial and incisal surfaces with the flat-end tapered diamond before any reduction is done (Fig 10-42). Without grooves it is impossible to accurately gauge the depth of reduction done on the labial surface. The grooves are 1.2 to 1.4 mm deep on the labial and 2.0 mm deep on the incisal. Three labial grooves are cut with the diamond held parallel to the gingival one-third of the labial surface. A second set of two grooves is made parallel to the incisal two-thirds of the uncut labial surface. The labial surface of an all-ceramic preparation is done in two planes to achieve adequate clearance for good esthetics without encroaching on the pulp.[42]

Incisal reduction is done with the flat-end tapered diamond so that it will be possible for instruments to reach the finish line area of the preparation in subsequent steps. From 1.5 to 2.0 mm of tooth structure is removed (Fig 10-43).

The tooth structure remaining between the depth-orientation grooves on the incisal portion of the labial surface is planed away (Fig 10-44). The gingival portion of the labial surface is reduced with the flat-end tapered diamond to a depth of 1.2 to 1.4 mm. This reduction extends around the labioproximal line angles and fades out on the lingual aspects of the proximal surfaces (Fig 10-45). The end of the flat-end tapered diamond bur will form the shoulder finish line, while the axial reduction is done with the sides of the diamond. The shoulder should be a minimum of 1.0 mm wide. Lingual reduction is done with the small wheel diamond, being careful not to overreduce the junction between the cingulum and the lingual wall (Fig 10-46). Overshortening the lingual wall will reduce the retention of the preparation.

Reduction of the lingual axial surface is done with the flat-end tapered diamond (Fig 10-47). The wall should form a minimum taper with the gingival portion of the labial wall. The radial shoulder is at least 1.0 mm wide and should be a smooth continuation of the labial and proximal radial shoulders. All-ceramic crowns made over shoulder finish lines exhibit greater strength than those made over chamfers.[9,44] All of the axial walls should be smoothed with an H158–012 radial fissure bur, accentuating the shoulder at the same time (Fig 10-48). All sharp angles should be rounded over at this time. The RS-1 modified binangle chisel is used to smooth the shoulder, removing any loose enamel rods at the cavosurface angle. Care must be taken not to create undercuts in the axial walls where they join the shoulder. The features of a preparation for an all-ceramic crown and the purpose served by each are shown in Fig 10-49.

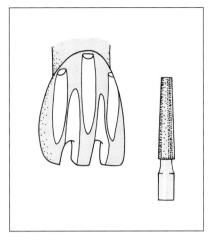

Fig 10-42 Depth-orientation grooves: Flat-end tapered diamond.

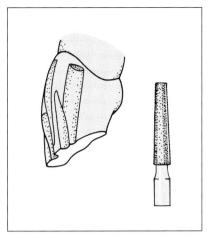

Fig 10-43 Incisal reduction: Flat-end tapered diamond.

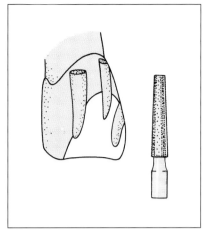

Fig 10-44 Labial reduction (incisal half): Flat-end tapered diamond.

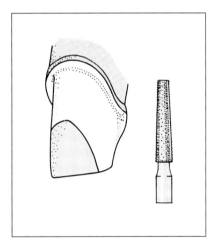

Fig 10-45 Labial reduction (gingival half): Flat-end tapered diamond.

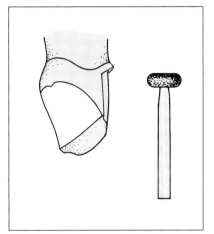

Fig 10-46 Lingual reduction: Small wheel diamond.

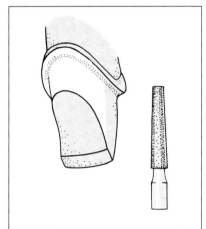

Fig 10-47 Lingual axial reduction: Flat-end tapered diamond.

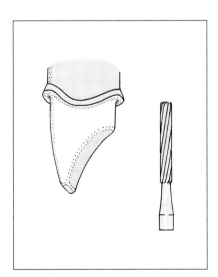

Fig 10-48 Axial wall and radial shoulder finishing: Radial fissure bur.

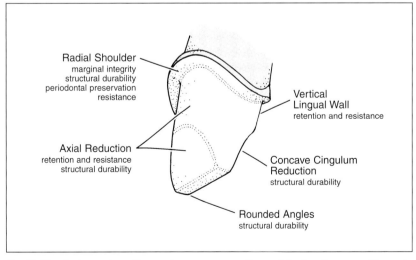

Radial Shoulder
marginal integrity
structural durability
periodontal preservation
resistance

Vertical
Lingual Wall
retention and resistance

Axial Reduction
retention and resistance
structural durability

Concave Cingulum
Reduction
structural durability

Rounded Angles
structural durability

Fig 10-49 Features of an all-ceramic crown preparation and the function served by each.

References

1. Thom LW: Principles of cavity preparation in crown and bridge prostheses: I. The full crown. *J Am Dent Assoc* 1950; 41:284–289.

2. Lorey RE, Myers GE: The retentive qualities of bridge retainers. *J Am Dent Assoc* 1968; 76:568–572.

3. Reisbick MH, Shillingburg HT: Effect of preparation geometry on retention and resistance of cast gold restorations. *J Calif Dent Assoc* 1975; 3:50–59.

4. Potts RG, Shillingburg HT, Duncanson MG: Retention and resistance of preparations for cast restorations. *J Prosthet Dent* 1980; 43:303–308.

5. Howard WW: Full coverage restorations: Panacea or epidemic? *Gen Dent* 1979; 27:6–7.

6. Wheeler RC: The implications of full coverage restorative procedures. *J Prosthet Dent* 1955; 5:848–851.

7. Smith GP: What is the place of the full crown in restorative dentistry? *Am J Orth Oral Surg* 1947; 33:471–478.

8. Smith GP: The marginal fit of the full cast shoulderless crown. *J Prosthet Dent* 1957; 7:231–243.

9. Friedlander LD, Munoz CA, Goodacre CJ, Doyle MG, Moore BK: The effect of tooth preparation design on the breaking strength of Dicor crowns: Part 1. *Int J Prosthodont* 1990; 3:159–168.

10. Preston JD: Rational approach to tooth preparation for ceramo-metal restorations. *Dent Clin North Am* 1977; 21:683–698.

11. Miller L: A clinician's interpretation of tooth preparations and the design of metal substructures for metal-ceramic restorations, in McLean JW (ed): *Dental Ceramics: Proceedings of the First International Symposium on Ceramics.* Chicago, Quintessence Publ Co, 1983, pp 173–206.

12. Johnston JF, Mumford G, Dykema RW: The porcelain veneered gold crown. *Dent Clin North Am* 1963; 7:853–864.

13. Shelby DS: Practical considerations and design of porcelain fused to metal. *J Prosthet Dent* 1962; 12:542–548.

14. Romanelli JH: Periodontal considerations in tooth preparation for crown and bridge. *Dent Clin North Am* 1977; 21:683–698.

15. Grundy JR: *Color Atlas of Conservative Dentistry.* Chicago, Year Book Medical Publishers, 1980, pp 68–75.

16. Behrend DA: Ceramometal restorations with supragingival margins. *J Prosthet Dent* 1982; 47:625–632.

17. Brecker SC: Porcelain baked to gold—A new medium in prosthodontics. *J Prosthet Dent* 1956; 6:801–810.

18. Silver M, Howard MC, Klein G: Porcelain bonded to a cast metal understructure. *J Prosthet Dent* 1961; 11:132–145.

19. Hobo S, Shillingburg HT: Porcelain fused to metal: Tooth preparation and coping design. *J Prosthet Dent* 1973; 30:28–36.

20. Goldstein RE: Esthetic principles for ceramo-metal restorations. *Dent Clin North Am* 1977; 21:803–822.

21. Shillingburg HT, Hobo S, Fisher DW: Preparation design and margin distortion in porcelain fused to metal restorations. *J Prosthet Dent* 1973; 29:276–284.

22. Faucher RR, Nicholls JI: Distortion related to margin design in porcelain-fused-to-metal restorations. *J Prosthet Dent* 1980; 43:149–155.

23. Engleman MA: Simplified esthetic ceramo-metal restorations. *NY J Dent* 1971; 49:252–261.

24. Hamaguchi H, Cacciatore A, Tueller VM: Marginal distortion of the porcelain-bonded-to-metal complete crown: An SEM study. *J Prosthet Dent* 1982; 47:146–153.

25. DeHoff PH, Anusavice KJ: Effect of metal design on marginal distortion of metal-ceramic crowns. *J Dent Res* 1984; 63:1327–1331.

26. Strating H, Pameijer CH, Gildenhuys RR: Evaluation of the marginal integrity of ceramo-metal restorations. Part I. *J Prosthet Dent* 1981; 46:59–65.

27. Wilson RD: Intracrevicular restorative dentistry. *Int J Periodont Rest Dent* 1981; 1:35–49.

28. Belser UC, MacEntee MI, Richter WA: Fit of three porcelain-fused-to-metal marginal designs in vivo: A scanning electron microscope study. *J Prosthet Dent* 1985; 53:24–29.

29. West AJ, Goodacre CJ, Moore BK, Dykema RW: A comparison of four techniques for fabricating collarless metal-ceramic crowns. *J Prosthet Dent* 1985; 54:636–642.

30. Hunt JL, Cruickshanks-Boyd DW, Davies EH: The marginal characteristics of collarless bonded porcelain crowns produced using a separating medium technique. *Quint Dent Technol* 1978; 2:21–25.

31. Zena RB, Khan Z, von Fraunhofer JA: Shoulder preparations for collarless metal ceramic crowns: Hand planing as opposed to rotary instrumentation. *J Prosthet Dent* 1989; 62:273–277.

32. Nabers CL, Christensen GJ, Markely MR, Miller EF, Pankey LD, Potts JW, Pugh CE: Porcelain occlusals–To cover or not to cover? *Tex Dent J* 1983; 100:6–10.

33. Jacobi R, Shillingburg HT, Duncanson MG: A comparison of the abrasiveness of six ceramic surfaces and gold. *J Prosthet Dent* 1991; 66:303–309.

34. Johnston JF, Dykema RW, Mumford G, Phillips RW: Construction and assembly of porcelain veneer gold crowns and pontics. *J Prosthet Dent* 1962; 12:1125–1137.

35. Goldstein RE: *Esthetics in Dentistry.* Philadelphia, JB Lippincott, 1976, pp 65–85, 332–341.

36. Tjan AH: Common errors in tooth preparation. *Gen Dent* 1980; 28:20–25.

37. McLean JW, Hughes TH: The reinforcement of dental porcelain with ceramic oxides. *Br Dent J* 1965; 119:251–267.

38. Pettrow JN: Practical factors in building and firming characteristics of dental porcelain. *J Prosthet Dent* 1961; 11:334–344.

39. Nuttal EB: Factors influencing success of porcelain jacket restorations. *J Prosthet Dent* 1961; 11:743–748.

40. Bartels JC: Preparation of the anterior teeth for porcelain jacket crowns. *J South Calif Dent Assoc* 1962; 30:199–205.

41. Bastian CC: The porcelain jacket crown. *Dent Clin North Am* 1959; 3:133–146.

42. Bartels JC: Full porcelain veneer crowns. *J Prosthet Dent* 1957; 7:533–540.

43. Fairley JM, Deubert LW: Preparation of a maxillary central incisor for a porcelain jacket restoration. *Br Dent J* 1958; 104:208–212.

44. Sjogren G, Bergman M: Relationship between compressive strength and cervical shaping of the all-ceramic Cerestore crown. *Swed Dent J* 1987; 11:147–152.

Chapter 11

Preparations for Partial Veneer Crowns

The partial veneer crown is a conservative restoration that requires less destruction of tooth structure than does a full veneer crown. Its use is based on the premise that an intact surface of tooth structure should not be covered by a crown if its inclusion is not essential to the retention, strength, or cosmetic result of the final restoration. No technician can exactly duplicate the texture and appearance of untouched enamel. Gingival health near a partial veneer crown is protected by the supragingival margin,[1–4] and a tooth with a full veneer crown is about 2.5 times as likely to have a pulpal problem as one with a partial veneer crown.[5]

A partial veneer restoration should be considered first when a cast restoration is needed. A full veneer crown should be chosen only when the coverage or retention afforded by a partial veneer crown is found wanting. Reluctance to use a three-quarter crown because it has more margin than a full crown is unfounded; the additional margin is vertical, which fits better than a horizontal margin.[6]

There are many advantages to the use of partial veneer restorations:

1. Tooth structure is spared.
2. Much of the margin is accessible to the dentist for finishing and to the patient for cleaning.
3. Less restoration margin is in proximity to the gingival crevice, lowering the possibility of periodontal irritation.
4. An open-faced partial veneer crown is more easily seated completely during cementation, while a full veneer crown tends to act like a hydraulic cylinder containing a highly viscous fluid.[7]
5. With some of the margin visible, complete seating of a partial veneer crown is more easily verified.
6. If an electric pulp test ever needs to be conducted on the tooth, a portion of enamel is unveneered and accessible.[8]

A partial veneer crown is not as retentive as a full veneer crown,[9–11] but it has adequate retention for single restorations and retainers for short-span fixed partial dentures. Some preparation feature must be substituted to compensate for the retention and resistance lost when an axial surface is not covered. The most commonly used feature is a groove.

To achieve maximum effectiveness, grooves must have definite lingual walls.[12] Resistance to torquing is produced by achieving a "lingual hook"[8] or a "lock effect"[13] by directing the bur (and groove) slightly to the opposite corner of the tooth (Fig 11-1, A). A V-shaped groove, without a definite lingual wall, provides only 68% of the retention and 57% of the resistance of a concave groove with a lingual wall (Fig 11-1, B).[14]

Maxillary Posterior Three-quarter Crowns

The standard three-quarter crown is a partial veneer crown in which the buccal surface is left uncovered. It is the most commonly used partial veneer crown. The occlusal finish line on a maxillary tooth terminates near the bucco-occlusal angle. If designed skillfully, the three-quarter crown can be very esthetic.[15] It can be used successfully on maxillary posterior teeth, where esthetic demands are moderate and reasonable. Metal will not be invisible, but it will not be seen in normal conversation.

Armamentarium

1. Handpiece
2. Round-end tapered diamond
3. Short needle diamond
4. Torpedo diamond
5. Torpedo bur
6. No. 169L bur
7. No. 171L bur
8. Flame diamond
9. Flame bur
10. Enamel hatchet

Occlusal reduction is the first step in preparing a tooth for a three-quarter crown. Depth-orientation grooves are cut on the anatomic ridges and grooves of the occlusal surface with a round-end tapered diamond. Clearance should be 1.5 mm on the functional cusp (lingual on maxillary teeth) and 1.0 mm on the nonfunctional cusp

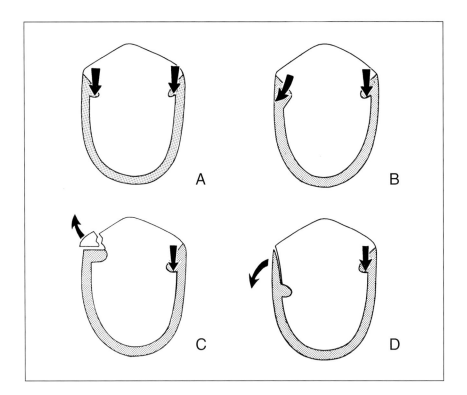

Fig 11-1 A: Definite lingual walls resist displacement. B: An oblique lingual wall offers poor resistance. C: An undermined buccal enamel plate may fracture. D: A groove that is too far lingual does not provide bulk of metal to support the margin.

(facial). The depth-orientation grooves should be made that deep on the respective cusps. The grooves do extend through the occlusobuccal line angle, but they will be only 0.5 mm deep there.

Occlusal reduction is completed by removing the tooth structure between the grooves (Fig 11-2), reproducing the geometric inclined plane pattern of the cusps. The depth decreases at the occlusobuccal line angle to minimize the display of metal.[15,16]

Next the functional cusp bevel is made. Holding the round-end tapered diamond at a 45-degree angle to the long axis of the preparation, three to five depth-orientation grooves are placed on the lingual or outer incline of the lingual cusp. The grooves are 1.5 mm deep at the cusp tip and fade out at their apical end.

The functional cusp bevel is completed by removing the tooth structure between the grooves with the same diamond (Fig 11-3). The bevel extends from the central groove on the mesial to the central groove on the distal. It makes space for metal on the lingual-facing incline of the lingual cusp to match the space on the buccal-facing incline created by the occlusal reduction. The occlusal reduction and functional cusp bevel are smoothed with a no. 171L bur.

Axial reduction is begun by reducing the lingual surface with a torpedo diamond, taking care not to overincline the lingual wall. The cut is extended interproximally on each side as far as possible without nicking the adjacent teeth (Fig 11-4). As the axial reduction is done, a chamfer finish line is formed. A smooth, continuous transition should be made from the lingual to the proximal surface with no sharp angles in the axial reduction or in the chamfer.

Proximal access is gained by using a short needle diamond in an up and down "sawing" motion. This is continued facially until contact with the adjacent tooth is broken and maneuvering space is produced for larger instruments. Final extension to the buccal is achieved with the short needle diamond or, in esthetically critical areas, with an enamel hatchet. The gingivofacial angle should not be underextended; it is the most likely area of a three-quarter crown to fail.[17]

A flame diamond, with its long, thin tip, can be used as an intermediate instrument where there is minimal proximal clearance. It is followed by the torpedo diamond to complete the axial reduction and form a chamfer (Fig 11-5). The axial wall and chamfer are finished with the torpedo bur of the same size and configuration (Fig 11-6).

Proximal grooves are approximately the size of a no. 171L bur (Fig 11-7), but an inexperienced student may find it easier to begin the groove with a no. 169L bur, leaving room for minor adjustment. A groove must be cut into the tooth to the full diameter of the bur to create a definite lingual wall.

The outline form of the finished groove is drawn on the occlusal surface with a sharp pencil (Fig 11-8). The pencil outline is followed to cut a "template" approximately 1.0 mm deep (Fig 11-9, A). This template is used as a guide to extend the groove to half its length, keeping the bur aligned with the path of insertion (Fig 11-9, B). If examination of the groove shows it to be properly aligned and directed, it should be extended to its full length, ending it

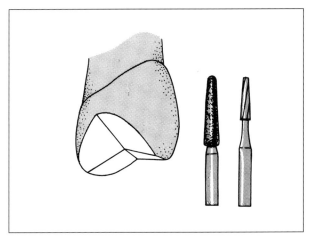

Fig 11-2 Occlusal reduction: Round-end tapered diamond and no. 171L bur.

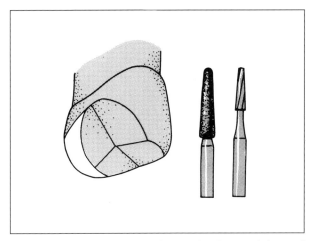

Fig 11-3 Functional cusp bevel: Round-end tapered diamond and no. 171L bur.

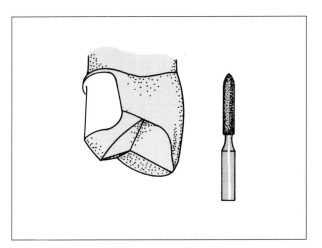

Fig 11-4 Lingual axial reduction: Torpedo diamond.

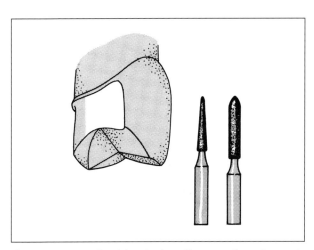

Fig 11-5 Proximal axial reduction: Short needle and torpedo diamonds.

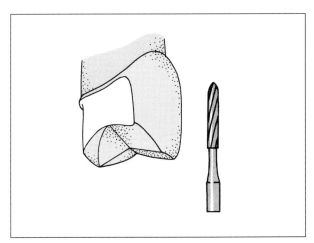

Fig 11-6 Axial finishing: Torpedo bur.

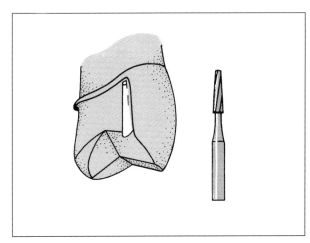

Fig 11-7 Proximal grooves: No. 171L bur.

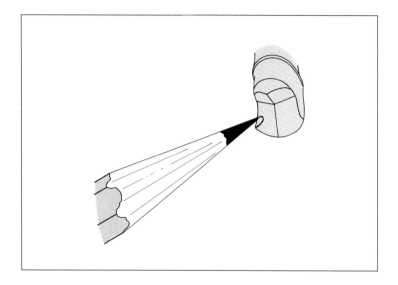

Fig 11-8   The outline of the groove is drawn on the occlusal surface of the tooth.

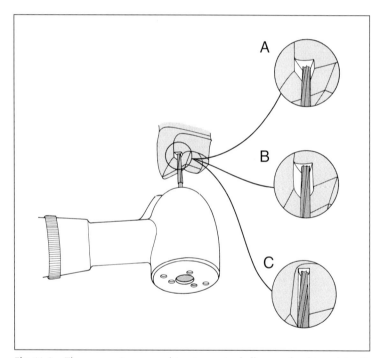

Fig 11-9   The groove is prepared in stages: A, shallow occlusal template; B, extension to half length; C, completion to full length.

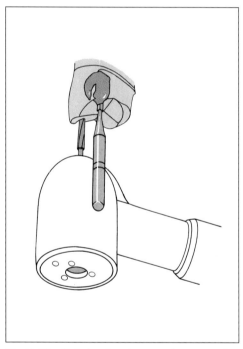

Fig 11-10   To help align the second groove, a bur may be held in the first groove with utility wax.

about 0.5 mm occlusal to the chamfer[18] (Fig 11-9, C).

Grooves should be placed as far facially as possible without undermining the facial surface, paralleling the long axis of a posterior tooth. Grooves are done first on the more inaccessible proximal surface of molars (the distal) and the more esthetically critical surface of premolars (the mesial). If a problem is encountered in placing the first groove, alignment of the second can be altered in a more accessible area or without adversely affecting the cosmetic result. The first few times that

grooves are prepared, it may help to place a bur in the first groove as an alignment guide while the second groove is made (Fig 11-10).

A flare is a flat plane that removes equal amounts of the facial wall of the groove and the outer surface of the tooth. It is cut from the groove outward with the tip of a flame diamond to prevent overextension (Fig 11-11). The flare is reachable by explorer and toothbrush, but there should not be a noticeable display of metal. The flare should be smoothed with a carbide bur matching the

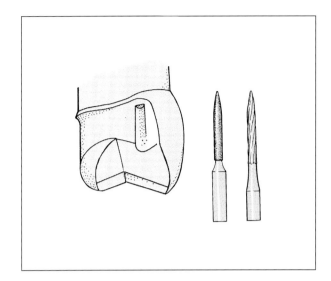

Fig 11-11   Proximal flares: Flame diamond and bur.

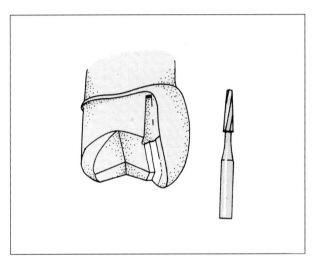

Fig 11-12   Occlusal offset: No. 171L bur.

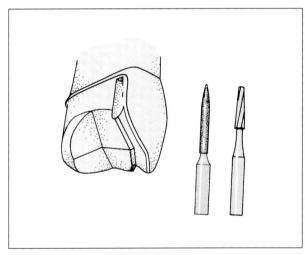

Fig 11-13   Buccal bevel: Flame diamond and no. 171L bur.

configuration of the flame diamond. Short, crisp strokes of the bur in one direction prevent rounding of the finish line. Where facial extension is critical, the flare can be formed with a wide enamel chisel.

The occlusal offset, a 1.0-mm-wide ledge on the lingual incline of the facial cusp, is made with a no. 171L bur (Fig 11-12). It forms an inverted "V" that lies a uniform distance from the finish line. It provides space for a truss of metal that ties the grooves together to form a reinforcing staple.[15–22] The angle between the upright wall of the

offset and the lingual slope of the facial cusp is rounded. Any sharp corners between the lingual inclines of the facial cusp and the flares are removed.

A flame diamond and a no. 170 bur are used to place a 0.5-mm bevel along the bucco-occlusal finish line, perpendicular to the path of insertion (Fig 11-13). It rounds over the mesial and distal corners and blends into the proximal flares. The function served by each of the features of the maxillary posterior three-quarter crown preparation is shown in Fig 11-14.

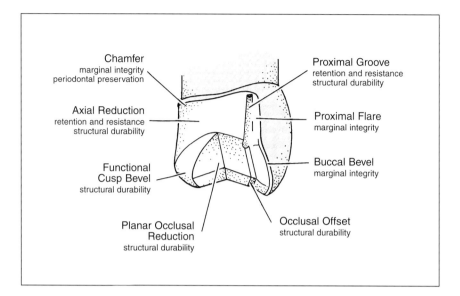

Chamfer
marginal integrity
periodontal preservation

Axial Reduction
retention and resistance
structural durability

Functional
Cusp Bevel
structural durability

Planar Occlusal
Reduction
structural durability

Proximal Groove
retention and resistance
structural durability

Proximal Flare
marginal integrity

Buccal Bevel
marginal integrity

Occlusal Offset
structural durability

Fig 11-14 Features of a maxillary three-quarter crown preparation and the function served by each.

Posterior Partial Veneer Variations

There are several modifications of posterior partial veneer crowns that can be used. A three-quarter crown preparation with proximal boxes (Fig 11-15) is more retentive than a standard preparation with grooves,[10,23] but boxes are very destructive. They can be justified only if there has been proximal caries or previous restorations. A less destructive way to augment retention and resistance uses four grooves,[24] which is not significantly less retentive than two boxes.[23]

A three-quarter crown preparation on a mandibular molar or premolar has many features found in the preparation of a maxillary tooth (Fig 11-16). The biggest difference is the location of the occlusal finish line on the facial surface, gingival to occlusal contacts. The occlusal shoulder on the buccal aspect of the buccal cusp(s) serves the same purpose as the offset on the maxillary preparation, tying the grooves together and strengthening the nearby bucco-occlusal margin. There is no need for an offset on the lingual inclines of the buccal cusps.

The seven-eighths crown is a three-quarter crown whose vertical distobuccal margin is positioned slightly mesial to the middle of the buccal surface (Fig 11-17). Esthetics are good because the veneered distobuccal cusp is obscured by the mesiobuccal cusp. With more of the tooth encompassed, resistance is better than that of the three-quarter crown.[11] The accessible location of the distobuccal finish line makes the preparation easy to do. Margin finishing by the dentist and cleaning by the patient are also facilitated.

The seven-eighths crown can be used on any posterior tooth needing a partial veneer restoration where the distal cusp must be covered.[25,26] It is most commonly used on maxillary molars, but it also can be placed on mandibular premolars and molars.[27] It is good for restoring teeth with caries or decalcification on the distal aspect of the buccal surface, and it is an excellent fixed partial denture retainer.

The reverse three-quarter crown is used on mandibular molars[22] to preserve an intact lingual surface. It is useful on fixed partial denture abutments with severe lingual inclinations, preventing the destruction of large quantities of tooth structure that would occur if a full veneer crown were used. The grooves at the linguoproximal line angles are joined by an occlusal offset on the buccal slope of the lingual cusps. This preparation closely resembles a maxillary three-quarter crown preparation because the axial surface of the nonfunctional cusp is uncovered (Fig 11-18).

The proximal half crown is a three-quarter crown that is rotated 90 degrees, with the distal rather than the buccal surface left intact (Fig 11-19). It can be a retainer on a tilted mandibular molar fixed partial denture abutment.[28,29] This design can be used only in mouths with excellent hygiene and a low incidence of interproximal caries. It is contraindicated if there is a blemish on the distal surface.

The mesial surface parallels the path of insertion of the mesial abutment preparation. Clearance of 1.5 mm is obtained from occlusal reduction that terminates at the distal marginal ridge, with little or no reduction of the mesial cusps. Grooves paralleling the mesial surface are placed in the buccal and lingual axial walls. A heavy channel or occlusal offset connects the grooves to strengthen the disto-occlusal margin. An occlusal isthmus augments retention and rigidity. A countersink in the distal channel helps resist mesial displacement.

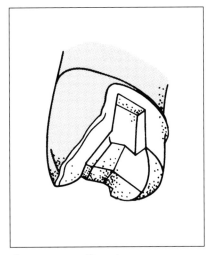

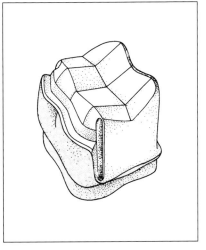

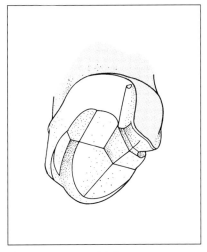

Fig 11-15 Maxillary three-quarter crown preparation with proximal boxes.

Fig 11-16 Three-quarter crown preparation on a mandibular molar.

Fig 11-17 Seven-eighths crown preparation on a maxillary molar.

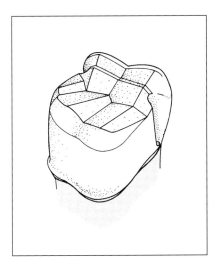

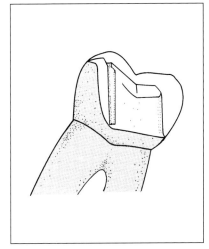

Fig 11-18 Reverse three-quarter crown preparation on a mandibular molar.

Fig 11-19 Proximal half crown preparation on a tilted mandibular molar.

Anterior Three-quarter Crowns

Demands for the avoidance of any display of metal, coupled with the ease of preparing a tooth for a metal-ceramic crown, have led to the near total demise of the anterior three-quarter crown. Unsightly, unnecessary displays of metal in poor examples of this restoration made it unpopular with both the public and the profession. When a partial veneer is used, it is usually a pin-modified three-quarter crown in which metal coverage is minimized by using pins.

However, a well-executed standard three-quarter crown on a maxillary incisor or canine need not show much metal. It can be used as a retainer for short-span fixed partial dentures on restoration- and caries-free abutments.[30,31] Well-aligned, thick, square anterior teeth with a large faciolingual bulk of tooth structure are the best candidates for three-quarter crowns.[13]

Two factors must be controlled successfully to produce a restoration with a minimal display of metal: *(1)* path of insertion and groove placement, and *(2)* placement and instrumentation of extensions. The path of insertion of an anterior three-quarter crown parallels the incisal one-half to two-thirds of the labial surface, not the long axis of the tooth.[13] This gives the grooves a slight lingual inclination, placing their bases more apically and labially, and making the grooves longer. If the grooves incline labially, the labioincisal corners are overcut, displaying metal. The bases of the grooves then move lingually, becoming shorter and less retentive.[32]

Proximal extensions are done with thin diamonds or hand instruments with a lingual approach to minimize the display of metal. Use of a large instrument or a labial approach will result in overextension and an unsightly display of metal.

Armamentarium

1. Handpiece
2. Small round diamond
3. Small wheel diamond
4. Long needle diamond
5. Torpedo diamond
6. Torpedo bur
7. No. 169L bur
8. No. 170L bur
9. Flame diamond
10. Flame bur
11. Enamel hatchet

A small wheel diamond is used to create a concave lingual reduction incisal to the cingulum (Fig 11-20). It is necessary to create 0.7 mm or more clearance with opposing teeth. To ensure adequate reduction, depth-orientation cuts are made on the lingual surface with a small round diamond whose head has a diameter 1.4 mm larger than its shaft. Buried in enamel to the shaft, the diamond penetrates 0.7 mm. Reduction is done to the depth of the orientation cuts. The lingual reduction of a canine is done in two planes, with a slight ridge extending incisogingivally down the middle of the lingual surface. On incisors, the entire surface is smoothly concave. The junction between the cingulum and the lingual wall must not be overreduced. If excessive tooth structure is removed, the lingual wall will be too short to provide retention.

Incisal reduction is done with the small wheel diamond (Fig 11-21). It parallels the inclination of the uncut incisal edge and barely breaks through the labioincisal line angle. Near the junction between the incisal edge and the lingual surface, it is about 0.7 mm deep. On a canine, the natural mesial and distal inclines of the incisal edge are followed. On an incisor, a flat plane is cut from mesial to distal.

The lingual axial wall is reduced with a torpedo diamond, creating a chamfer finish line at the same time (Fig 11-22). The diamond is kept parallel with the incisal two-thirds of the labial surface to initiate the path of insertion of the preparation.

The vertical lingual wall is essential to retention. If the cingulum is short, wall length can be increased with a lingual beveled shoulder that moves the wall farther into the tooth. A 3.0-mm-deep pin hole can be placed in the cingulum to compensate for a very short lingual wall. This common variation of the anterior three-quarter crown is frequently used on abutments for fixed partial dentures.

Proximal reduction is started with a long needle diamond (Fig 11-23). The instrument comes from the lingual, to minimize the display of metal later. An up and down motion is used, with care not to nick the adjacent tooth or lean the diamond too far into the center of the prepared tooth. The labial proximal extensions are completed, and contact with the adjacent tooth should be barely broken with an enamel hatchet, not with the diamond.

The axial reduction is completed and the finish line is accentuated with a torpedo diamond. To prevent binding between the prepared proximal axial wall and the adjacent tooth, it may be necessary to use a flame diamond before the torpedo diamond. The axial surface and chamfer are then planed with the torpedo carbide bur (Fig 11-24).

The grooves are placed as far labially as possible without undermining the labial enamel plate. To implement groove placement, outlines of the grooves are drawn on the lingual incisal area of the preparation. The first groove is begun by cutting a 1.0-mm-deep "template" within the penciled outline using a no. 170L bur. The groove is extended gingivally in increments to its full length. A novice may want to use a no. 169L bur initially to allow adjustment of the groove without overcutting it.

The second groove is cut parallel with the first, ending both just short of the chamfer (Fig 11-25). Remember that grooves in an anterior three-quarter crown preparation parallel the incisal one-half to two-thirds of the facial surface, unlike those in a posterior tooth, which parallel the long axis of the tooth. Boxes may be substituted for grooves if there are existing proximal restorations or caries. Boxes must be narrow to be resistant, because the lingual wall of a box shortens as it moves lingually.

On the facial aspect of each groove, a flare is started at the gingival end with the thin tip of a flame diamond (Fig 11-26). It is finished with the flame bur to make a smooth flare and a sharp, definite finish line. If a very minimal extension is desired, a wide enamel chisel should be used instead.

Using a no. 170L bur, the grooves are connected with an incisal offset, staying a uniform distance from the incisal edge (Fig 11-27). The offset is a definite step on the sloping lingual surface, placed near the opposing occlusal contact. The metal that occupies the space reinforces the margin.[15,25,33,34] On a canine it forms a V, but on an incisor it is a straight line.

The angles between the incisal edge and the upright wall of the offset and between the incisal reduction and each flare are rounded. A 0.5-mm-wide bevel is placed on the labioincisal finish line using a no. 170L bur (Fig 11-28). This can also be done with a flame diamond and bur, but finishing is still done with a bur to create the sharpest

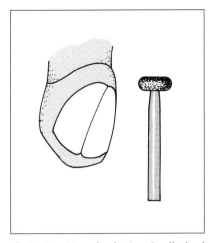

Fig 11-20 Lingual reduction: Small wheel diamond.

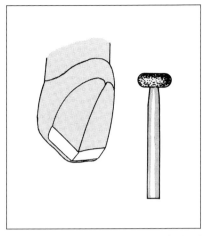

Fig 11-21 Incisal reduction: Small wheel diamond.

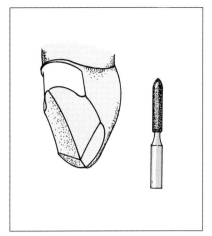

Fig 11-22 Lingual axial reduction: Torpedo diamond.

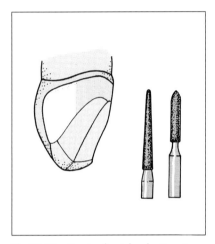

Fig 11-23 Proximal axial reduction: Long needle and torpedo diamonds.

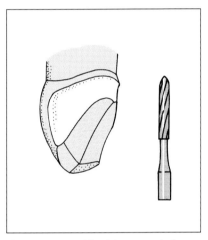

Fig 11-24 Axial finishing: Torpedo bur.

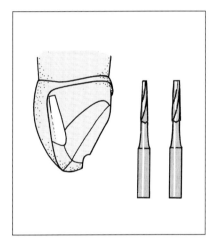

Fig 11-25 Proximal grooves: No. 169L and 170L burs.

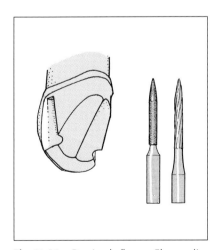

Fig 11-26 Proximal flares: Flame diamond and bur.

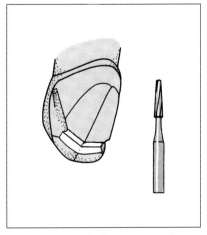

Fig 11-27 Incisal offset: No. 171L bur.

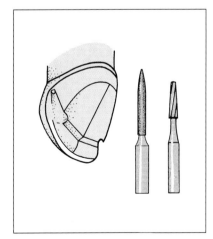

Fig 11-28 Incisal bevel: Flame diamond and no. 170L bur.

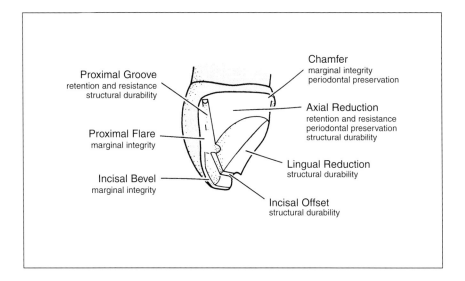

Proximal Groove
retention and resistance
structural durability

Chamfer
marginal integrity
periodontal preservation

Axial Reduction
retention and resistance
periodontal preservation
structural durability

Proximal Flare
marginal integrity

Lingual Reduction
structural durability

Incisal Bevel
marginal integrity

Incisal Offset
structural durability

Fig 11-29 Features of an anterior three-quarter crown preparation and the function served by each.

finish line. The bevel is perpendicular to the path of insertion along the mesial incline. A contrabevel can be placed on the distal incline, where esthetic considerations are not as critical. A contrabevel should never be used on an incisor.

Conservative extension and careful finishing of the gold incisal margin will cause light to be reflected downward, making the incisal edges appear dark rather than metallic to the viewer.[15] As a result, it will blend in with the dark background of the oral cavity. The functions served by each of the features of the anterior three-quarter crown preparation are shown in Fig 11-29.

Pin-modified Three-quarter Crowns

There are situations calling for a partial veneer crown that will not permit the use of a "classic" preparation design. The pin-modified three-quarter crown is an esthetic modification that has long been considered the retainer of choice on unblemished teeth used as fixed partial denture abutments in esthetically critical areas.[35] Although resin-bonded retainers gained popularity in such situations in the 1980s, the pin-modified three-quarter crown is still an excellent retainer for short-span fixed partial dentures.

The pin-modified three-quarter crown preserves the facial surface and one proximal surface. With minimal subgingival margins, it is periodontally preferable to a full crown. An unsightly display of metal is avoided without resorting to a destructive full veneer metal-ceramic restoration. The pin-modified three-quarter crown is good for repairing incisors and canines with severe lingual abrasion.[35–37] It should not be used on teeth with caries

or restorations, on surfaces that are not to be covered, or in mouths with extensive caries.

Although this restoration design is conservative in the amount of enamel that is untouched, a variety of factors could place the pin holes near or even in the pulp. Therefore, pin-modified three-quarter crowns should not be used on teeth that are small,[38] thin,[39,40] possessed of large pulps,[41] or malpositioned. They should not be used by unskilled dentists.

Pins are likely to produce less retention, and pin-retained castings are less retentive than standard three-quarter crowns.[9] However, the greater the number, depth, or diameter of pins, the greater the retention.[42] The pin-modified three-quarter crown is an old restoration that was revived in the 1960s by the development of small twist drills to make pin holes and nylon bristles to accurately reproduce them.[43]

Pin holes are usually made with a 0.6-mm drill.[37,38,43–45] Nylon bristles, 25 to 50 microns smaller in diameter than the drill, are placed in the pin holes[43,44] because the pin holes are too small to be reproduced by impression material. Impression material surrounds the pin and incorporates it into the impression. When the impression is poured, the nylon bristles protruding from it reproduce the pin holes.

Serrated pins produce more retention than smooth pins,[42,46,47] so serrated iridioplatinum pins 25 to 50 microns smaller than the pin holes in the stone cast[43] are used in the wax pattern (Fig 11-30). The resulting pins in the casting are 50 to 100 microns smaller than the original pin holes in the preparation.

Pins should be 2.0 to 3.0 mm long.[38,43,44,48] Adequate pin length is essential to retention, and short pins will cause the failure of a conservative fixed partial denture. These are very destructive failures, because the pin holes become channels for oral fluids and microorganisms to penetrate deep into the tooth. Considerable damage may occur before a loose retainer is detected. If ade-

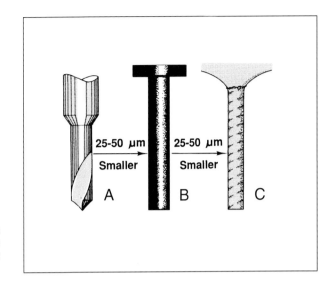

Fig 11-30 Retentive pins are made by using a drill for the pin hole (A), a smaller diameter nylon bristle for the impression (B), and an even smaller diameter iridioplatinum pin as part of the restoration (C).

quate pin hole depth is not possible, a different retainer design should be used.

Armamentarium

1. Handpieces
2. Small round diamond
3. Small wheel diamond
4. Long needle diamond
5. Torpedo diamond
6. Torpedo bur
7. No. 169L bur
8. No. 170L bur
9. Flame diamond
10. Flame bur
11. Enamel hatchet
12. No. 1/2 round bur
13. 0.6-mm drill
14. Nylon bristle

Concave reduction of the the lingual aspect of the tooth is done with a small wheel diamond to produce a minimum clearance of 0.7 mm with adjacent teeth (Fig 11-31). Depth-orientation cuts can be made using a small round diamond with a head diameter 1.4 mm greater than its shaft diameter. It is sunk into enamel down to the shaft to make a cut approximately 0.7 mm deep. Excessive shortening of the vertical wall of the cingulum should be avoided.

A lingual incisal bevel paralleling the uncut surface of the incisal edge is also prepared with the wheel diamond. This bevel is approximately 1.5 mm wide, but it may vary on teeth with unusually thick or thin incisal edges. It should stop lingual to the labioincisal line angle to prevent a display of metal.

Using a torpedo diamond, the lingual axial wall is reduced to parallel the incisal two-thirds of the labial sur-

face (Fig 11-32), simultaneously forming a chamfer finish line. Care should be taken not to extend too far labially into the lingual proximal embrasure on the proximal surface opposite the retentive feature. The finish line must be far enough lingual to the proximal contact so that the restoration margin can be finished by the dentist and cleaned by the patient. If the cingulum is short, a beveled shoulder should be used to move the lingual wall toward the center of the tooth, making it longer.

The torpedo diamond is used to continue the axial reduction to its most facial extension near the labioproximal line angle (Fig 11-33). The reduction is diminished at the finish line. The location of this finish line is critical. If it is not far enough facial, it can cause an undersized, weak connector,[37] and a margin that would be impossible to finish properly. The axial reduction and the chamfer finish line should be smoothed with a torpedo carbide bur (Fig 11-34).

The primary axial retention/resistance features, two grooves, are placed next to the edentulous space (Fig 11-35). If the proximal surface is carious or has been restored previously, a box form is used. The box is too destructive to use routinely on unblemished proximal surfaces. Kishimoto et al demonstrated that two grooves are equal to a box on a premolar.[14] On an anterior tooth, they are probably superior. Since the lingual surface slopes linguogingivally, moving the lingual wall a slight distance lingually shortens it and decreases resistance.[49] By using two grooves, there will be *two* lingual walls. The wall of the more facially positioned groove will be longer and more resistant than the single, shorter lingual wall of a box.

The facial groove is placed with a no. 170L bur. An inexperienced dentist may want to start the grooves with a no. 169L bur to avoid overcutting. Shallow pilot grooves are made and checked for location and direction. Then a no. 170L bur is sunk into the track of the trial groove to the full diameter of the bur.

The lingual groove is placed next, paralleling it with the

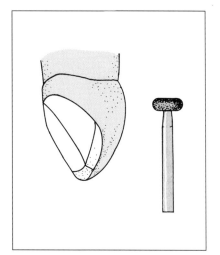

Fig 11-31 Lingual reduction: Small wheel diamond.

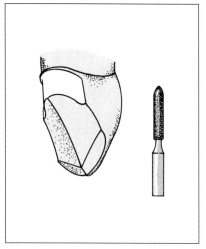

Fig 11-32 Lingual axial reduction: Torpedo diamond.

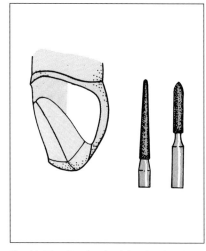

Fig 11-33 Proximal axial reduction: Long needle and torpedo diamonds.

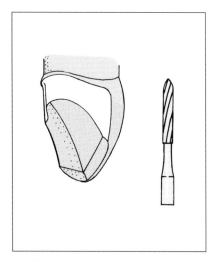

Fig 11-34 Axial finishing: Torpedo bur.

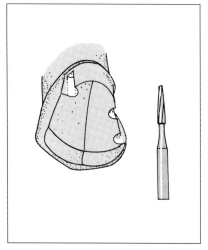

Fig 11-35 Proximal grooves: No. 169L and 170L burs.

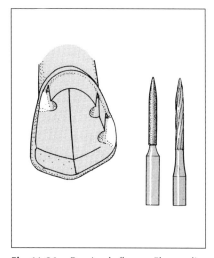

Fig 11-36 Proximal flares: Flame diamond and bur.

first. A third, much shorter groove is placed on the opposite side of the cingulum near the vertical finish line on that surface. This groove enhances the restoration resistance slightly, and it accommodates a bulk of metal to reinforce the margin.

Proximal flares are formed with a flame diamond (Fig 11-36). For the flare to draw, it must be wider incisally than it is gingivally. It nearly eliminates the facial wall of the groove at its incisal end. A slight flare is placed on the mesial groove. The distal and mesial flares are reinstrumented with a matching flame carbide bur. Care should be taken not to round over the finish line.

A flat ledge or countersink is cut in the incisal corner opposite the site of the proximal grooves using a no. 170L bur. It must be gingival to the incisal edge, in

dentin, and lingual to the finish line. A ledge is also placed in the middle of the cingulum. These flat areas on the sloping lingual surface provide easy starts for precise pin hole placement (Fig 11-37), and they create space for a reinforcing bulk of metal at the base of the pins.[50]

The no. 170L bur is used to connect the incisal ledge and the facialmost proximal groove with an incisal offset. A V-shaped trough is cut along the side of the lingual surface from the incisal ledge to the short cingulum groove. The metal in the trough will reinforce the linguoproximal margin of the restoration (Fig 11-38).

A shallow depression to begin a pin hole in the center of each ledge is made using a no. 1/2 round bur. To initiate the first pin hole, a low-speed contra-angle 0.6-mm (0.024-inch) drill is carefully aligned with the grooves.

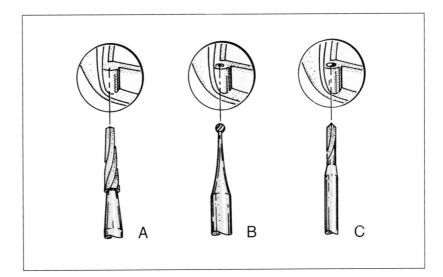

Fig 11-37 Instrument sequence for cutting pin holes: Form the ledge with a tapered fissure bur (A); start the pin hole with a small round bur (B); and finish the pin hole with a twist drill (C).

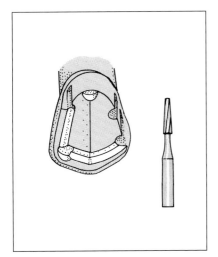

Fig 11-38 Ledge, offset and trough: No. 170L bur.

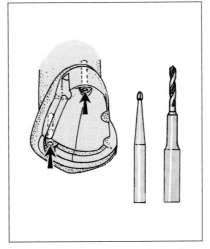

Fig 11-39 Pin holes: No. 1/2 bur and 0.6-mm drill.

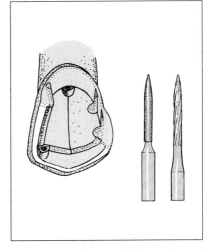

Fig 11-40 Incisal bevel: Flame diamond and bur.

The handpiece is started before touching the tooth and should not be stopped while the drill is in the pin hole, as it will snap off. When the first pin hole is approximately 3.0 mm deep, the handpiece is withdrawn and a nylon bristle is placed in the pin hole. Using the bristle and grooves as guides, a 3.0-mm-deep pin hole is made in the other ledge (Fig 11-39).

The angle between the facial wall of the offset and the incisal edge of uncut tooth structure is beveled. Care should be taken not to extend this bevel too far facially, as metal will show. A finishing bevel is placed on the functional area of the incisal edge using a flame diamond (Fig 11-40). Care is taken to prevent an unnecessary display of metal, but it may be necessary to extend the

bevel on the distal incline of the incisal edge of a canine onto the labial surface. This is not likely to be unacceptable cosmetically, since it is usually hidden from view. This should not be done on an incisor. The incisal bevel is blended into the flare and the bevel is redefined on the marginal ridge next to the incisocingulum trough.

The areas just described are smoothed with a flame bur. Acute angles between the lingual and proximal surfaces are blunted, and any sharp corners at the incisal ends of the grooves are eliminated. The functions served by each of the features of a pin-modified three-quarter crown preparation on a maxillary canine are shown in Fig 11-41.

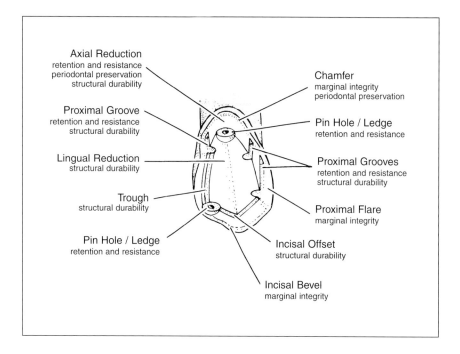

Axial Reduction
retention and resistance
periodontal preservation
structural durability

Proximal Groove
retention and resistance
structural durability

Lingual Reduction
structural durability

Trough
structural durability

Pin Hole / Ledge
retention and resistance

Chamfer
marginal integrity
periodontal preservation

Pin Hole / Ledge
retention and resistance

Proximal Grooves
retention and resistance
structural durability

Proximal Flare
marginal integrity

Incisal Offset
structural durability

Incisal Bevel
marginal integrity

Fig 11-41 Features of a pin-modified three-quarter crown preparation and the function served by each.

References

1. Kahn AE: Partial versus full coverage. *J Prosthet Dent* 1960; 10:167–178.

2. Maxwell EL, Wasser VE: Debate: Full vs. partial coverage as the abutment of choice in fixed bridgework. *J DC Dent Soc* 1961; 36:9–11.

3. Miller LL: Partial coverage in crown and bridge prosthesis with the use of elastic impression materials. *J Prosthet Dent* 1963; 13:905–910.

4. Silness J: Periodontal conditions in patients treated with dental bridges. II. The influence of full and partial crowns on plaque accumulation, development of gingivitis and pocket formation. *J Periodont Res* 1970; 5:219–224.

5. Felton D, Madison S, Kanoy E, Kantor M, Maryniuk G: Long-term effects of crown preparation on pulp vitality. *J Dent Res* 1989; 68:1008, abstr no. 1139.

6. Kishimoto M, Hobo S, Duncanson MG, Shillingburg HT: Effectiveness of margin finishing techniques on cast gold restorations. *Int J Periodont Rest Dent* 1981; 1(5):21–29.

7. Jorgensen KD: Structure of the film of zinc phosphate cements crowns. *Acta Odontol Scand* 1960; 18:491–501.

8. Ho G: Lecture notes, School of Dentistry, University of Southern California, 1959.

9. Lorey RE, Myers GE: The retentive qualities of bridge retainers. *J Am Dent Assoc* 1968; 76:568–572.

10. Reisbick MH, Shillingburg HT: Effect of preparation geometry on retention and resistance of cast gold restorations. *J Calif Dent Assoc* 1975; 3:50–59.

11. Potts RG, Shillingburg HT, Duncanson MG: Retention and resistance of preparations for cast restorations. *J Prosthet Dent* 1980; 43:303–308.

12. Shillingburg HT, Fisher DW: The partial veneer restoration. *Aust Dent J* 1972; 17:411–417.

13. Cowger GT: Retention, resistance, and esthetics of the anterior three-quarter crown. *J Am Dent Assoc* 1961; 62:167–171.

14. Kishimoto M, Shillingburg HT, Duncanson MG: Influence of preparation features on retention and resistance. Part II: Three-quarter crowns. *J Prosthet Dent* 1983; 49:188–192.

15. Ingraham R, Bassett RW, Koser JR: *An Atlas of Cast Gold Procedures*, ed 2. Buena Park, CA, Uni-Tro College Press, 1969, pp 161–165.

16. Racowsky LP, Wolinsky LE: Restoring the badly broken-down tooth with esthetic partial coverage restorations. *Compend Contin Educ Dent* 1981; 11:322–335.

17. Tinker HA: The three-quarter crown in fixed bridgework. *J Can Dent Assoc* 1950; 16:125–129.

18. Tjan AHL, Miller GD: Biometric guide to groove placement on three-quarter crown preparations. *J Prosthet Dent* 1979; 42:405–410.

19. Willey RE: The preparation of abutments for veneer retainers. *J Am Dent Assoc* 1956; 53:141–154.

20. Guyer SE: Multiple preparations for fixed prosthodontics. *J Prosthet Dent* 1970; 23:529–553.

21. Smith DE: Abutment preparations. *J Am Dent Assoc* 1931; 18:2063–2075.

22. Rhoads JE: Preparation of the teeth for cast restorations. In Hollenback GM: *Science and Technic of the Cast Restoration*. St Louis, CV Mosby Co, 1964, p 66.

23. Kishimoto M, Shillingburg HT, Duncanson MG: Influence of preparation features on retention and resistance. Part I. MOD onlays. *J Prosthet Dent* 1983; 49:35–39.

24. Tanner H: Ideal and modified inlay and veneer crown preparations. *Ill Dent J* 1957; 26:240–244.

25. Willey RE: The preparation of abutments for veneer retainers. *J Am Dent Assoc* 1956; 53: 141–154.

26. Ingraham R, Bassett RW, Koser JR: *An Atlas of Cast Gold Procedures,* ed 2. Buena Park, CA, Uni-Tro College Press, 1969, p 34.

27. Kessler JC, Shillingburg HT: The seven-eighths crown. *Gen Dent* 1983; 31:132–133.

28. Smith DE: Fixed bridge restorations with the tilted mandibular second or third molar as an abutment. *J South Calif Dent Assoc* 1939; 6:131–138.

29. Shillingburg HT: Bridge retainers for tilted abutments. *New Mexico Dent J* 1972; 22:16–18, 32.

30. Hughes HJ: Are there alternatives to the porcelain fused to gold bridge? *Aust Dent J* 1970; 15:281–287.

31. Leander CT: Preparation of abutments for fixed partial dentures. *Dent Clin North Am* 1959; 3:59–72.

32. Tinker ET: Fixed bridgework. *J Natl D A* 1920; 7:579–595.

33. Smith DE: Abutment preparations. *J Am Dent Assoc* 1931; 18:2063–2075.

34. Tjan AHL, Miller GD: Biometric guide to groove placement on three-quarter crown preparations. *J Prosthet Dent* 1979; 42:405–410.

35. Baum L: New cast gold restorations for anterior teeth. *J Am Dent Assoc* 1960; 61:15–22.

36. Arbo MA: A simple technique for castings with pin retention. *Dent Clin North Am* 1970; 14:19–29.

37. Clyde JS, Sharkey SW: The pin ledge crown. A re-appraisal. *Br Dent J* 1978; 144:239–245.

38. Baum L, Contino RM: Ten years of experience with cast pin restorations. *Dent Clin North Am* 1970; 14:81–91.

39. Hughes HJ: Are there alternatives to the porcelain fused to gold bridge? *Aust Dent J* 1970; 15:281–287.

40. Crispin BJ: Conservative alternatives to full crowns. *J Prosthet Dent* 1979; 42:392–397.

41. Bruce RW: Parallel pin splints for periodontally involved teeth. *J Prosthet Dent* 1964; 14:738–745.

42. Moffa JP, Phillips RW: Retentive properties of parallel pin restorations. *J Prosthet Dent* 1967; 17:387–400.

43. Shooshan ED: A pin-ledge casting technique—its application in periodontal splinting. *Dent Clin North Am* 1960; 4:189–206.

44. Mosteller JH: Parallel pin castings. *Practical Dental Monographs.* Chicago, Year Book Medical Publishers, Inc, 1963, pp 5–29.

45. Burns BB: Pin retention of cast gold restorations. *J Prosthet Dent* 1965; 15:1101–1108.

46. Lorey RE, Embrell KA, Myers GE: Retentive factors in pin-retained castings. *J Prosthet Dent* 1967; 17:271–276.

47. Courtade GL, Timmermans JJ: *Pins in Restorative Dentistry.* St Louis, CV Mosby Co, 1971, p 6.

48. Mann AW, Courtade GL, Sanell C: The use of pins in restorative dentistry. Part I. Parallel pin retention obtained without using paralleling devices. *J Prosthet Dent* 1965; 15:502–516.

49. Welk DA: Personal communication.

50. Pruden WH: Partial coverage retainers: A critical evaluation. *J Prosthet Dent* 1966; 16:545–548.

Chapter 12

Preparations for Intracoronal Restorations

The intracoronal inlay is the simplest of the cast restorations and has been used for the restoration of occlusal, gingival, and proximal lesions. Intracoronal restorations utilize "wedge" retention, which exerts some outward pressure on the tooth. This pressure is exerted first during try-in and cementation, but it occurs again when occlusal force is applied. For the restoration to be successful, there must be some form of counteraction. When an inlay is placed in a tooth with ample bulk of tooth structure, the tooth structure itself resists the force.

The use of cast metal inlays, at one time considered the mark of quality restorative care, has declined in recent years. A group of US dental educators concluded in 1979 that: "Cast gold restorations should be limited to those teeth which need cusp coverage for protection and reinforcement of the tooth. The true cast gold inlay is no longer a reasonable consideration in the conservative treatment of unrestored teeth."[1] A survey of North American dental faculty in the early 1980s indicated that nearly one-third of their schools taught limited use of inlays, or none at all.[2]

The indications for an inlay are virtually the same as for an amalgam restoration. The inlay simply replaces missing tooth structure without doing anything to reinforce that which remains.[3] If the tooth requires protection from occlusal forces, the protection must be gained by the use of some other type of restoration that incorporates a veneer of casting alloy over the occlusal surface.[4] Inlays tend to wedge cusps apart,[5] and a lone-standing unsupported cusp is at risk of fracture.[6]

Mechanical cusp height is normally equal to anatomic cusp height, measured from cusp tip to the bottom of the central groove. An occlusal intracoronal preparation increases mechanical cusp height to a hazardous extent,[7] as it becomes the distance from the cusp tip to the gingival extension of the preparation. In premolars, this elongation of the lever arm can increase stress.

Stress concentrations can manifest themselves in various forms of clinical failure. The most dramatic and the most evident is the loss of a whole cusp because of fracture. Failure also may occur in less obvious ways. The cement seal can rupture, with ensuing marginal leakage, when tooth structure flexes in weakened cusps and preparation walls bend without actually fracturing[8] or spring away from the restoration.[7] This may not become apparent for some period of time, but it would eventually surface as an open margin, possibly with recurrent caries. This type of failure may escape being identified as an ill-designed restoration that did not protect the tooth from destructive, occlusally generated stresses.

Analysis has detected greater stress when intracoronal preparations are wide.[9,10] Because a wider isthmus can lead to failure,[8,11,12] and an inlay that is one-third the faciolingual width of the occlusal surface can wedge the cusps apart,[13] the recommended isthmus width has been reduced to one-fourth the intercuspal distance.[14]

Vale[15] found a 35% decrease in the fracture resistance of a maxillary premolar when the isthmus of a proximo-occlusal preparation was widened from one-fourth to one-third the intercuspal distance. Mondelli et al[16] reported decreases of 42%, 39%, and 29% with similar isthmus widening of proximo-occlusal, occlusal, and MOD preparations, respectively.

Depth, combined with width, decreased the fracture strength of teeth in studies by Blaser and associates[11] and Re et al.[17] This corroborates clinical observations of inlays acting as wedges between the facial and lingual cusps of teeth.[5,7] Deepening an isthmus to increase resistance, or inlay strength, is not a good practice.

Proximo-occlusal Inlays

A proximo-occlusal inlay is indicated for premolars or molars, with minimal caries or previous restoration, that need a mesio-occlusal or disto-occlusal restoration. It offers a superior material and margins that will not deteriorate with time. The restoration will be visible on premolars, although careful extensions on mesiobuccal flares should keep the display minimal. MOD inlays that can be kept narrow are acceptable for molars. If a premolar is damaged badly enough to warrant even a conservative MOD cast restoration, that restoration should be an onlay. Class 2 inlays should be used in mouths that have shown a low caries rate for some time preceding the placement of the restoration. It is a dubious service to place a two-surface restoration in a tooth that has a high likelihood of requiring that the third surface be restored in the not-too-

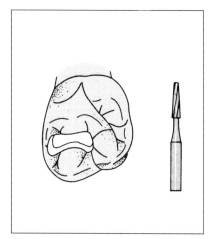

Fig 12-1 Occlusal outline: No. 170 bur.

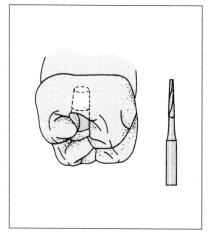

Fig 12-2 Undermining marginal ridge: No. 169L bur.

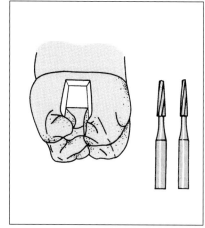

Fig 12-3 Proximal box: No. 169L and 170L burs.

distant future. Patients with accumulations of plaque or a recent history of caries, or those who are still in adolescence, are poor candidates for inlays.

Armamentarium

1. Handpiece
2. No. 170L bur
3. No. 169L bur
4. Flame diamond
5. Flame bur
6. Enamel hatchet
7. Binangle chisel
8. Gingival margin trimmer

Use a no. 170L bur to make the occlusal outline (Fig 12-1). Initial penetration is made in a fossa with the edge of the bur tip. The isthmus is then cut to its final extension by following the central groove and any deep or faulty grooves leading to it. The extension should be conservative because an occlusal bevel will widen it later.

A distinct dovetail extends facially, enhancing resistance and retention. The pulpal floor should be flat, at an even depth of approximately 1.5 mm, and perpendicular to the path of insertion for maximum resistance.[7] The outline should avoid occlusal contacts marked with articulating paper. The initial cut extends far enough to undermine the marginal ridge, which will be removed shortly. The walls of the isthmus will be slightly inclined by the bur used to cut them. Check the walls to make sure there are no undercuts. Do not err in the opposite direction by overtapering the walls.

If the tooth being prepared has not been previously restored, complete the undermining of the marginal ridge with a no. 169L bur. Do not cut all the way through the enamel to the outer surface at this time. Penetrate in an apical direction with the bur, with the tip apical to the con-

tact (Fig 12-2). Do not be too conservative with the gingival extension, since box length is an important factor in inlay retention.[14] Cut buccally and lingually to the approximate width of the proposed box, just inside the cementoenamel junction.

Break through the undermined enamel to rough out the proximal box, using either the no. 169L bur or an enamel chisel. Use the 169L bur to finish smoothing the box. Extend it buccally and lingually just far enough to barely break contact with the adjacent tooth (Fig 12-3). The final extension will be achieved when the facial and lingual flares are placed. Widen the isthmus where it joins the box, rounding any angle in the area where they meet.

The buccoaxial and linguoaxial line angles of the box are accentuated with a no. 169L bur. The same bur is also used to form the facial and lingual walls of the box, and they are smoothed with an enamel chisel. The box walls, not the angles, resist displacement.[14] Those walls should have a minimum degree of divergence of the facial and lingual walls to promote optimum retention and resistance. As taper increases, stress rises and retention decreases.

The pulpal floor of the isthmus and the gingival floor of the box should be flat. A gingival margin trimmer is used to form a V-shaped groove at the junction of the axial wall and the gingival floor of the box (Fig 12-4). This groove, sometimes referred to as the "Minnesota ditch,"[18] is placed to enhance resistance to displacement by occlusal forces.[19]

Flares are flat planes added to the buccal and lingual walls of the box using a flame diamond or an enamel hatchet (Fig 12-5). The hatchet is reserved for use in those areas where esthetics is an important consideration. The flares provide for the acute angle of gold to meet the finish line on the preparation. Check the flares to make sure that they "draw." The buccal flare leans slightly to the buccal; the lingual flare, slightly to the lingual; and both flares, slightly to the center of the tooth. A

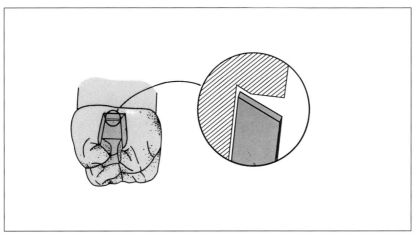

Fig 12-4 Gingivoaxial groove: Gingival margin trimmer.

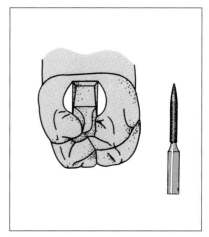

Fig 12-5 Proximal flares: Flame diamond.

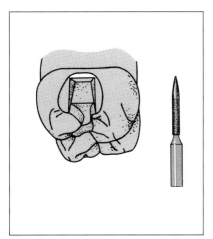

Fig 12-6 Gingival bevel: Flame diamond.

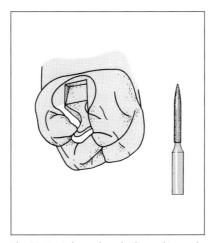

Fig 12-7 Isthmus bevel: Flame diamond.

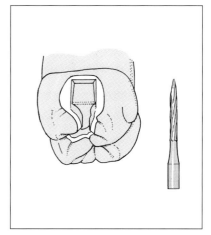

Fig 12-8 Bevel and flare finishing: Flame bur.

flare is cut equally at the expense of the wall of the box and of the outer enamel surface of the tooth. As a result, a flare is narrow at its gingival end and much wider at its occlusal end.

To start the flare, place the flame diamond in the proximal box and use the small-diameter tip to cut the cavo-surface angle of the box from the gingival floor up. Continue the occlusally directed sweep of the diamond tip without changing the angle or direction of the instrument. The diamond should be cutting only when it is moving in the occlusal direction. If it is moved back and forth, the finish line may be rounded over.

The flame diamond is carried across the gingival cavo-surface angle of the box, forming a gingival bevel on the box that is a smooth continuation of the buccal and lingual flares (Fig 12-6). Avoid creating undercuts where the gingival bevel joins the flares. Lean the flame diamond against the pulpal axial line angle. The bevel

should lay between 30 and 45 degrees to provide an optimum blend of strength and marginal fit.[20] A gingival margin trimmer is unacceptable because it will produce a ragged finish line.

The inlay preparation is finished by placing a bevel on the occlusal isthmus with a flame diamond (Fig 12-7). If a shallow bevel is used in this location, the result will be a thin flash of gold that will probably extend into areas of occlusal contact. The bevel on the isthmus begins at the junction of the occlusal one-third and the gingival two-thirds of the isthmus walls, and should extend outward at an angle of 15 to 20 degrees.[21]

The bevel must be minimal, because compressive stress increases as the inclination of the bevel increases.[10] The bevel is likely to produce some stress, but it is a necessary risk to produce a finishable casting. Blend the occlusal bevel into the proximal flares to produce a smooth, continuous finish line. Use a flame carbide bur

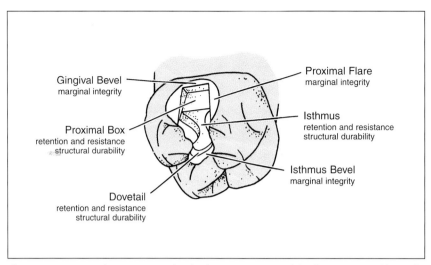

Fig 12-9 Features of a proximo-occlusal inlay preparation and the function served by each.

to go over the flares and the bevels (Fig 12-8). The flame bur produces the most consistent bevel,[22] and carbide finishing burs will produce the smoothest finish lines.[23]

A torpedo diamond can be used to create the bevel; it will produce one that is slightly concave, as suggested by Tucker.[24] The finish line is much more easily read. The features of the class 2 inlay preparation and the function served by each feature are shown in Fig 12-9.

Metal Inlay Variations

Other types of metal inlays are used even less frequently than the class 2 restoration. A class 1 inlay can be used to restore a moderately sized occlusal lesion in the mouth of a patient with predominantly gold restorations in other teeth. The 1.0-mm-wide isthmus follows the central groove, ending short of the marginal ridges or transverse ridge, if there is one on the tooth.

The outline extends moderately into the facial and lingual grooves, with small "barbell" dovetails at each end (Fig 12-10). Besides increasing retention and resistance, these extensions place the finish line on the slopes of the triangular and marginal ridges, where the inlay margins can be finished more easily. A 15- to 20-degree bevel extends a third of the way down the sides of the isthmus wall. Overextending the bevel will make the restoration too wide, and the finish line will form such an obtuse angle with the enamel surface that it will be difficult to identify during margin finishing .

The class 3 inlay shows metal, making it unacceptable for incisors. However, it is useful for restoring the distal surface of canines if a slight display of metal is acceptable to the patient.[25] A well-done inlay in a canine will

look better than an amalgam restoration, last longer than a composite resin restoration, and be much less destructive than a porcelain crown. It is not commonly used, but the restoration does have a place.

The class 3 inlay preparation has a 1.0-mm-deep lingual dovetail at the incisal end of the cingulum that resists displacement (Fig 12-11).[26] The proximal box is prepared with a lingual approach to minimize the display of metal.[27] An incisal approach will destroy excessive tooth structure as well as create an unesthetic restoration.

The class 5 inlay is used to restore severe abrasion[28] or erosion as well as large caries on the gingivofacial aspect of molars (Fig 12-12). It cannot tie into other restorations without producing a poor marginal seal. The preparation should be 1.0 mm deep axially and extend to the line angles. The gingival finish line is supragingival, if damage permits, and approximately 0.5 mm above the jaw of the cervical rubber dam clamp placed for preparing the tooth.[29] The height of contour is the occlusal limit of the preparation.

To enhance retention and resistance,[30,31] drill 0.6-mm-diameter pin holes to a depth of 3.0 mm at the proximal edges of the outline form. Place a 0.5-mm-wide, 45-degree bevel around the periphery of the preparation. For the impression, use a custom tray that draws buccally.

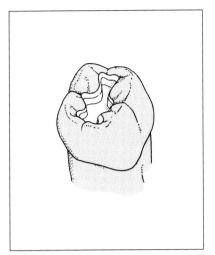

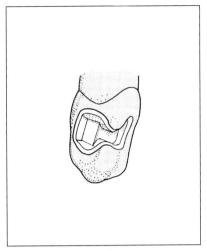

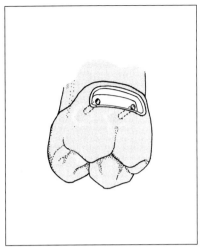

Fig 12-10 Class 1 inlay preparation on a mandibular molar.

Fig 12-11 Class 3 inlay preparation on a maxillary canine.

Fig 12-12 Class 5 inlay preparation on a maxillary molar.

MOD Onlays

The use of inlays to restore mesio-occluso-distal lesions in premolars is questionable. Occlusal force on an inlay produces stress along the sides of the restoration and at its base, as the inlay pushes against the tooth structure surrounding it. This could fracture the tooth,[32] so the inlay must be modified to distribute the load evenly over a wide surface. Stress analysis has shown that covering the occlusal surface with metal will do much to minimize the potentially damaging effects of stress in an intracoronal restoration (Fig 12-13).[10,33]

The MOD onlay is indicated for a variety of situations[3]:

1. Broken down teeth with intact buccal and lingual cusps.
2. MOD restorations with wide isthmuses.
3. Endodontically treated posterior teeth with sound buccal and lingual tooth structure. (Access for root canal therapy weakens a tooth structurally, and the crown of the tooth must be protected after treatment is complete.)

There has been a renewed interest in the MOD onlay, based on an occlusion-centered approach to restorative dentistry rather than one that is solely tooth oriented. MOD onlays are significantly less retentive and resistant than three-quarter crowns[34] and should not be used as fixed partial denture retainers. They lack sufficient retention to successfully resist the additional forces placed on an abutment tooth by a fixed partial denture.

Fisher et al[31] showed that onlays protect teeth from the high stress concentrations at the walls and line angles of the isthmus that are found under inlays. Studies by Craig et al[35] and Farah and associates[10] also showed the superiority of MOD onlays in protecting teeth from stress.

Armamentarium

1. Handpiece
2. Round-end tapered diamond
3. No. 171L bur
4. No. 170L bur
5. No. 169L bur
6. Flame diamond
7. Flame bur
8. Enamel hatchet

The previous restoration should be removed at this point. The occlusal reduction is done with a round-end tapered diamond to establish preparation length. About 1.5 mm of clearance is gained on the functional cusp and 1.0 mm on the nonfunctional cusp (Fig 12-14). Orientation grooves are used to gauge the depth of reduction. There should be one on the crest of each triangular ridge and one in each major developmental groove.

On a maxillary tooth where the nonfunctional facial cusp will be highly visible, do not overreduce the facio-occlusal angle or the restoration will show metal unnecessarily. The depth of the orientation grooves and the occlusal reduction should be about 0.5 mm at the line angle.

Occlusal reduction is accomplished by removing the tooth structure left between the depth-orientation grooves with the round-end tapered diamond. The reduction follows the original contours of the cusp,[36] reproducing the geometric inclined planes of the occlusal surface.[37] It has been hypothesized that this corrugated multiplanar design enhances restoration strength.[38]

A wide bevel is placed on the outer-facing inclines of the functional cusp with the round-end tapered diamond to insure an adequate bulk of metal on the functional

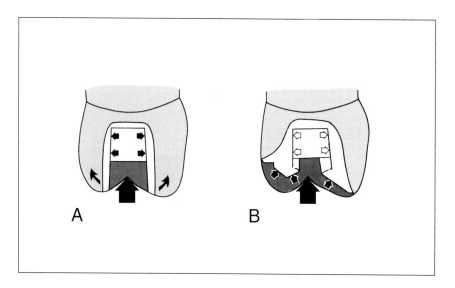

Fig 12-13 Occlusal forces applied to an MOD inlay produce stresses that tend to separate the cusps (A), while the same force applied to an MOD onlay is dissipated over a wide area in less destructive patterns (B).

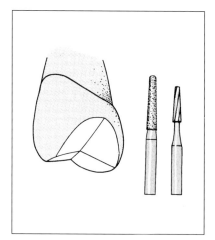 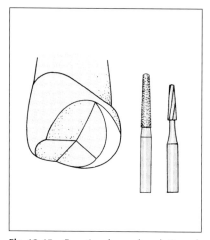 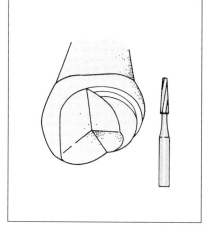

Fig 12-14 Planar occlusal reduction: Round-end tapered diamond and no. 171L bur.

Fig 12-15 Functional cusp bevel: Round-end tapered diamond and no. 171L bur.

Fig 12-16 Occlusal shoulder: No. 171L bur.

cusp (Fig 12-15). The functional cusp bevel approximates the inclination of the cusps in the opposing arch, extending from the central groove on the mesial to the central groove on the distal surface.

Begin with depth-orientation cuts that are 1.5 mm deep at the cusp tip. They fade out along a line that will later be the occlusal shoulder, 1.0 mm apical to the lowest occlusal contact. Remove the tooth structure left between the orientation grooves. Smooth the occlusal reduction and funtional cusp bevel with the no. 171L bur. The inclined planes should be well defined, but there should be no sharp angles where they meet. Check the occlusal reduction visually in the facial half of the occlusal surface and with red utility wax on the lingual cusp.

Cut an occlusal shoulder on the nonfunctional cusp with a no. 171L bur at the level of the axial termination of the functional cusp bevel (Fig 12-16). The shoulder is 1.0 mm wide and extends from the central groove on the mesial to the central groove on the distal surface. It provides space for metal to reinforce the occlusal margin on the funtional cusp.

There are two acceptable occlusal finish lines for the functional cusp of an MOD onlay: an occlusal shoulder or a heavy chamfer (Fig 12-17).[39] Both configurations provide an acute edge of gold at the cavosurface angle, with a nearby bulk of metal for strength. The shoulder with a bevel is easier to prepare properly and should be used by the novice.

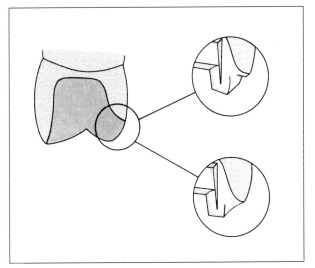

Fig 12-17 Functional cusp finish lines for MOD onlay: Occlusal shoulder *(top)* and chamfer *(bottom)*. (After Ingraham.[7])

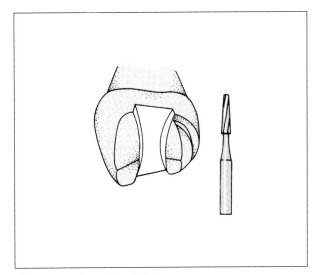

Fig 12-18 Isthmus: No. 171L bur.

The isthmus is made next with the no. 171L bur (Fig 12-18). If an old restoration was removed earlier, the isthmus is retouched to smooth the walls and impart a minimum taper. Besides removing caries and old restorations, the isthmus reinforces the restoration. It provides some retention and a great deal of resistance.[40] Because the occlusal surface already has been reduced, the isthmus of an onlay is shallower than that of an inlay.

The no. 170L bur is used to begin the proximal boxes (Fig 12-19). If the proximal surface is intact, it is easier to start with a no. 169L bur. The walls of the boxes are carried far enough buccally and lingually to barely break contact with the adjacent teeth. The facial extension of the mesial box is usually more conservative than that of the distal box. Extensions will be finalized with a flame diamond on the flares later.

Redefine the buccoaxial and linguoaxial line angles of each box with the no. 169L bur. Then use an enamel chisel to plane the facial and lingual walls. Flat walls perpendicular to the direction of rotating forces, not box angles, give a restoration resistance. Be sure the boxes have a common path of insertion. Smooth the pulpal floor of the isthmus, the 1.0-mm-wide occlusal shoulder on the functional cusp bevel, and the gingival floors of the proximal boxes, which are also 1.0 mm wide.

Proximal flares are added after the boxes have been formed (Fig 12-20). If the flares were cut first, facial and lingual box walls will be poorly defined, and retention will suffer. Flares are usually cut with the tip of the flame diamond, starting from within the box. A wide enamel hatchet can be used for mesiobuccal flares in areas where the cosmetic result is important.

Use a flame diamond to add a bevel 0.5 to 0.7 mm wide to the gingival cavosurface angle of each box (Fig 12-21). It provides for an acute edge of metal in these areas. The instrument is leaned against the pulpal-axial

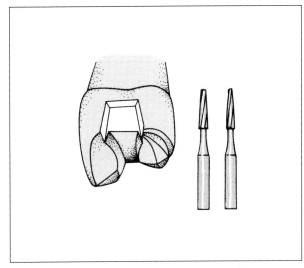

Fig 12-19 Proximal box: No. 169L and no. 170L burs.

line angle to prevent the bevel from being too long and having too sharp an angle. This may round the proximo-occlusal line angle, which is acceptable. Blend the bevel into the facial and lingual flares without creating an undercut. Smooth the flares and gingival bevel with a flame carbide bur. This produces a sharp, distinct finish line that will facilitate marginal adaptation of the restoration.

Occlusal finishing bevels 0.5 to 0.7 mm wide are placed at the buccal and lingual occlusal finish lines with a flame diamond followed by a no. 170L carbide bur (Fig 12-22). The buccal bevel is perpendicular to the path of insertion where esthetics are important, and forms a heavier contrabevel where they are not. The bevels are blended into the respective flares. If the bevel on the

177

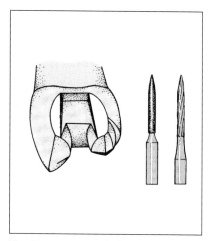

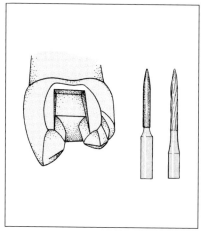

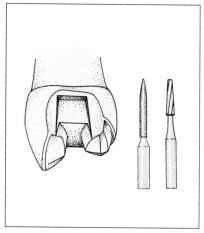

Fig 12-20 Proximal flares: Flame diamond and flame bur.

Fig 12-21 Gingival bevel: Flame diamond and flame bur.

Fig 12-22 Facial and lingual bevels: Flame diamond and no. 170 bur.

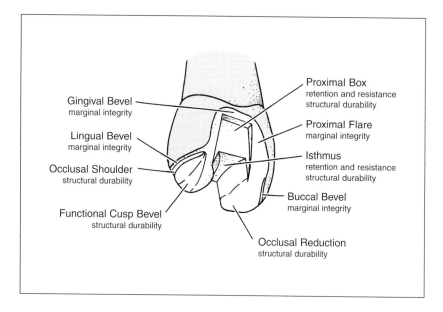

Fig 12-23 Features of a maxillary MOD onlay preparation and the function served by each.

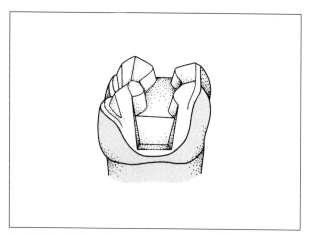

Fig 12-24 MOD onlay preparation on a mandibular molar.

occlusal shoulder is too wide, a thin, unsupported margin will result in the wax pattern and the casting. Figure 12-23 identifies the features of an MOD onlay preparation on a maxillary premolar and the function served by each feature.

The preparation on a mandibular molar differs from that on a maxillary tooth in that the functional cusp bevel and occlusal shoulder are located on the buccal cusp (Fig 12-24). In addition, the lingual bevel is wider and it can be a definite contrabevel, since esthetics is not a consideration on the lingual cusp of a mandibular tooth and structural durability is. These bevels should blend into the proximal flares, with the cavosurface line of the bevel continuous with the cavosurface line of the flare. There should not be a sharp occlusoproximal corner where the bevel and flare meet.

References

1. Nuckles DB: Inlay vs. amalgam restorations. *S C Dent J* 1980; 38:23-25.

2. Clark NP, Smith GE: Teaching gold castings in North American dental schools. *Oper Dent* 1984; 9:26-31.

3. Shillingburg HT, Fisher DW: The MOD onlay—A rational approach to a restorative problem. *N M Dent J* 1970; 21:12-14.

4. Tanner H: Ideal and modified inlay and veneer crown preparations. *Ill Dent J* 1957; 26:240-244.

5. Smith DE: Twenty-five years of fixed bridgework. *J South Calif Dent Assoc* 1936; 7:794-799.

6. McCollum BB: Tooth preparation and its relation to oral physiology. *J Am Dent Assoc* 1940; 27:701-707.

7. Ingraham R: The application of sound biomechanical principles, in the design of inlay, amalgam, and gold foil restorations. *J Am Dent Assoc* 1950; 40:402-413.

8. Mahler DB, Terkla LG: Relationship of cavity design to restorative materials. *Dent Clin North Am* 1965; 9:149-157.

9. Granath LE: Photoelastic studies on certain factors influencing the relation between cavity and restoration. *Odontol Revy* 1963; 14:278-293.

10. Farah JW, Dennison JB, Powers JM: Effects of design on stress distribution in intracoronal gold restorations. *J Am Dent Assoc* 1977; 94:1151-1154.

11. Blaser PK, Lund MR, Cochran MA, Potter RH: Effects of designs of class 2 preparations on resistance of teeth to fracture. *Oper Dent* 1983; 8:6-10.

12. Larson TD, Douglas WH, Gustfeld RE: Effect of prepared cavities on the strength of teeth. *Oper Dent* 1981; 6:2-5.

13. Werrin SR, Jubach TS, Johnson BW: Inlays and onlays: Making the right decision. *Quintessence Int* 1980; 11:13-18.

14. Smith GE, Grainger DA: Biomechanical design of extensive cavity preparations for cast gold. *J Am Dent Assoc* 1974; 89: 1152-1157.

15. Vale WA: Cavity preparation. *Ir Dent Rev* 1956; 2:33-41.

16. Mondelli J, Steagall L, Ishikiriama A, Navarro MF, Soares FB: Fracture strength of human teeth with cavity preparations. *J Prosthet Dent* 1980; 43:419-422.

17. Re GJ, Norling BK, Draheim RN: Fracture resistance of lower molars with varying faciocclusolingual amalgam restorations. *J Prosthet Dent* 1982; 47:518-521.

18. Frates FE: Inlays. *Dent Clin North Am* 1967; 11:163-173.

19. Gabel AB: Present-day concepts of cavity preparation. *Dent Clin North Am* 1957; 1:3-17.

20. Rosenstiel E: To bevel or not to bevel. *Br Dent J* 1975; 138:389-392.

21. Ingraham R, Bassett RW, Koser JR: *An Atlas of Cast Gold Procedures,* ed 2. Buena Park, CA, Uni-Tro College Press,1969, p 12.

22. Barnes IE: The production of inlay cavity bevels. *Br Dent J* 1974; 137:379-390.

23. Christensen GJ: Clinical and research advancements in cast-gold restorations. *J Prosthet Dent* 1971; 25:62-68.

24. Tucker RV: Variation of inlay cavity design. *J Am Dent Assoc* 1972; 84:616-620.

25. Redfern ML: The dovetail class III inlay. *Oper Dent* 1983; 8:67-72.

26. Thom LW: Principles of cavity preparation in crown and bridge prosthesis. III. The inlay abutment. *J Am Dent Assoc* 1950; 41:541-544.

27. Gerson IV: Invisible gold restorations for anterior teeth. *J Prosthet Dent* 1961; 11:749-764.

28. Mack AO, Allan DN: Reconstruction of a severe case of attrition and abrasion. *Br Dent J* 1974; 137:379-390.

29. Ingraham R, Bassett RW, Koser JR: *An Atlas of Cast Gold Procedures,* ed 2. Buena Park, CA, Uni-Tro College Press,1969, p 209.

30. Finger, EM: Restorations for class V cavities. *J Prosthet Dent* 1960; 10:775-778.

31. Howard WW: *Atlas of Operative Dentistry,* ed 2. St Louis, CV Mosby Co, 1973, p 73.

32. Maxwell EH, Braly BV: Incomplete tooth fracture: Prediction and prevention. *J Calif Dent Assoc* 1977; 5:51-55.

33. Fisher DW, Caputo M, Shillingburg HT, Duncanson MG: Photoelastic analysis of inlay and onlay preparations. *J Prosthet Dent* 1975; 33:47-53.

34. Kishimoto M, Shillingburg HT, Duncanson MG: Influence of preparation features on retention and resistance. Part II: Three-quarter crowns. *J Prosthet Dent* 1983; 49:188-192.

35. Craig RG, El-Ebrashi MK, LePeak PJ, Peyton FA: Experimental stress analysis of dental restorations. Part I. Two-dimensional photoelastic stress analysis of inlays. *J Prosthet Dent* 1967; 17:277-291.

36. Draheim RN: Current concepts in intracoronal casting preparations: A new look at the gold casting preparation. *Compend Contin Educ Dent* 1985; 6:373-379.

37. Shillingburg HT: Conservative preparations for cast restorations. *Dent Clin North Am* 1976; 20:259-271.

38. Racowsky LP, Wolinsky LE: Restoring the badly broken-down tooth with esthetic partial coverage restorations. *Compend Contin Educ Dent* 1981; 2:322-333.

39. Ingraham R, Bassett RW, Koser JR: *An Atlas of Cast Gold Procedures,* ed 2. Buena Park, CA, Uni-Tro College Press,1969, p 35.

40. Kishimoto M, Shillingburg HT, Duncanson MG: Influence of preparation features on retention and resistance. Part I: M.O.D. onlays. *J Prosthet Dent* 1983; 49:35-39.

Chapter 13

Preparations for Extensively Damaged Teeth

One of the criteria for the use of a cast metal, metal-ceramic, or all-ceramic restoration is a tooth that has been damaged to the extent that it must be reinforced and protected. It should not be surprising that unmodified classic preparation designs are used infrequently. They are applicable only on intact fixed partial denture abutments and on severely damaged teeth following the replacement of coronal bulk with an amalgam or resin core, or with a dowel core.

Most individual teeth requiring cemented restorations, as well as many fixed partial denture abutments, have been damaged enough to require modification of a classic preparation design. The amount of tooth structure destroyed is only one factor to consider in selecting a restorative material and designing a preparation. Equally important is the location of the destruction and the amount of tooth surface involved. Location can be classified as *peripheral,* occurring on the axial surfaces of the tooth; *central,* in the center of the tooth; or *combined,* with destruction in both sites.[1]

Peripheral destruction, even when it does not threaten the pulp, may require an extensive restoration such as a full crown because of the wide expanses of enamel that have been affected (Fig 13-1). A large central lesion that has undermined much of the enamel may require the placement of an amalgam core followed by a crown (Fig 13-2). However, less extensive damage in the central region, with or without proximal involvement, may be better restored with a less destructive MOD onlay that gains retention from peripheral tooth structure rather than destroying it (Fig 13-3). Combined destruction of severe dimensions may also require the placement of a core or foundation restoration followed by a crown (Fig 13-4).

Principle of Substitution

When it is necessary to compensate for mutilated or missing cusps, inadequate length, and in extreme cases even a missing clinical crown, the *principle of substitution* is used. For those teeth with moderate to severe damage that test a dentist's ingenuity, a preparation may

be modified by squaring the walls of defects left by caries and old restorations, and by adding features to enhance retention and resistance. Boxes may be substituted where grooves might ordinarily be utilized. Grooves may be used to augment retention and resistance where axial walls have been shortened. Pins may be employed where much of the supragingival tooth structure has been destroyed. More than one of these auxiliary features may be employed where damage is severe.

Two rules should be observed to avoid excessive tooth destruction while creating retention in an already weakened tooth:

1. The central "core" (the pulp and the 1.0-mm-thick surrounding layer of dentin) must not be invaded in vital teeth.[2] No retentive features should extend farther into the tooth than 1.5 mm at the cervical line or down 1.5 mm from the central fossa (Fig 13-5). If caries removal results in a deeper cavity, any part lying within the vital core should be filled with glass ionomer cement. Any preparation feature added for mechanical retention is kept in the safe area of the tooth, peripheral to the vital core.
2. No wall of dentin should be reduced to a thickness less than its height for the sake of retention. This may preclude the use of a full veneer crown, or if one must be used, it might first require the placement of a core or foundation restoration.

Box Forms

Small to moderate interproximal carious lesions or prior restorations can be incorporated into a preparation as a box form. This substitute for grooves serves the dual purpose of caries removal and retention form[3-5] (Fig 13-6). Because large quantities of tooth structure must be removed for it, the box is not usually used on an intact surface.

Opposing upright surfaces of tooth structure adjacent to a damaged area can be used to create a box form if at least half the circumference (180 degrees) remains in the area outside the lingual walls of the boxes. The walls of the box, and not the line angles, will resist displacement.[6] If the mesial and distal surfaces are extensively

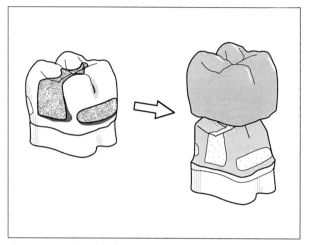

Fig 13-1 Teeth with large areas of enamel involvement may require full-coverage restorations regardless of the amount of dentin that has been destroyed.

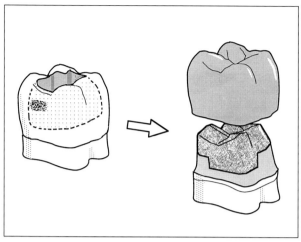

Fig 13-2 A large central lesion may require a full-coverage restoration, but only after the tooth is built up with a core.

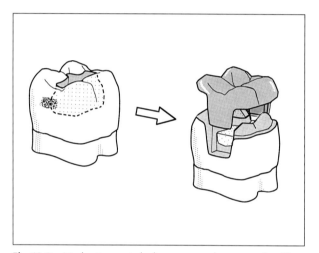

Fig 13-3 Moderate central damage can be restored with a restoration that preserves and uses sound peripheral tooth structure rather than destroying it.

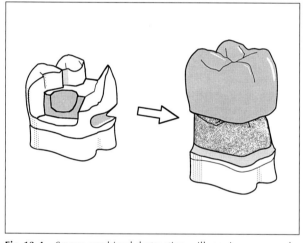

Fig 13-4 Severe combined destruction will require a core and a full-coverage restoration.

involved, another means must be used to compensate for the diminished lingual tooth structure (Fig 13-7). This situation may require a crown placed over a pin-retained amalgam core.

Grooves

Grooves placed in vertical walls of bulk tooth structure must be well formed, at least 1.0 mm wide and deep, and as long as possible to improve retention and resistance. Multiple grooves are as effective as box forms in providing resistance,[7] and they can be placed in axial walls without excessive destruction of tooth structure. They may also be added to the angles of oversized box forms to augment the resistance provided by the box walls.

This is particularly helpful when the facial and lingual walls of a box are a considerable distance apart. However, too many grooves in a crown preparation can adversely affect the seating of a full veneer crown.[8]

Pins

Pins effectively increase retention[9,10] by generating additional length internally and apically rather than externally.[11] They do not require vertical, supragingival tooth structure for their placement, and they can be used where there is insufficient axial wall length. They can extend apically beyond the gingival attachment without harming it.

Pins are commonly used in two ways: *(1)* Pin holes parallel the path of insertion of the preparation, receiving

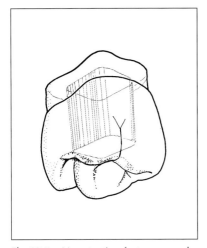

Fig 13-5 No retentive features may be cut into the "vital core" of the tooth *(center)*.

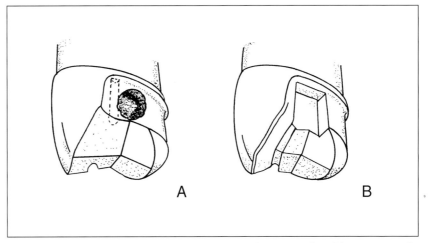

Fig 13-6 Interproximal caries may preempt the use of a groove *(dotted line)* (A). Use of a box in this situation accommodates caries removal and provides retention (B).

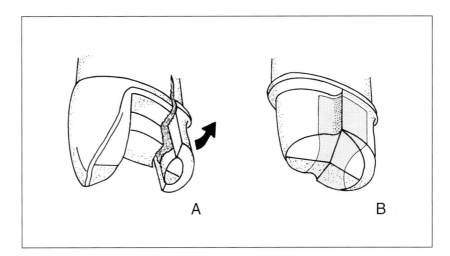

Fig 13-7 If significantly less than 180 degrees of the tooth's circumference remains between two boxes, the lingual cusp is susceptible to fracture during function, upon removal of the provisional restoration, or at try-in of the permanent restoration (A). A core with a different preparation design will minimize the risk of fracture and provide better longevity for the crown (B).

pins that are an integral part of the cast restoration (Fig 13-8, A), or *(2)* nonparallel pins are placed in the tooth to retain an amalgam or composite resin core in which a classic preparation for a cast restoration can be formed (Fig 13-8, B).

Careful pin hole placement is critical for restoration success. Four guidelines should be followed in drilling pin holes[12]:

1. Place them in sound dentin.
2. Do not undermine enamel.
3. Avoid perforation into the periodontal membrane.
4. Do not encroach upon the pulp.

Pin holes should be placed vertically in shoulders or ledges halfway between the outer surface of the tooth and the pulp, surrounded by at least 0.5 mm of dentin.[13] The safest locations for pin holes are the line angles or corners of the teeth (Fig 13-9).[14] The least desirable area for placing pin holes is midway between the corners,[14] especially in regions overlying the furcations.[15]

To avoid problems, the location and direction of the drill must be carefully controlled. After studying a radiograph, gently place a probe,[14] or the drill itself,[16] into the gingival sulcus, against the side of the tooth, to get a clear picture of the direction of the outer tooth surface in the area of the pin hole. This limits the use of parallel pins that are part of the casting, because the preparation path of insertion may dictate a pin direction that could cause pulpal or periodontal complications.

If bleeding occurs while drilling a pin hole, determine whether the misdirected drill has gone into the pulp or the periodontal membrane. If it is in the pulp, perform endodontic therapy before proceeding. If the hole exits the root surface, measure the pin before insertion so that

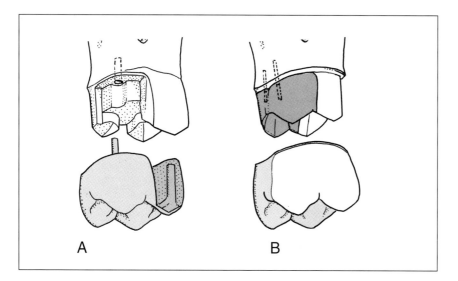

Fig 13-8 A pin can be incorporated into a crown to augment retention and resistance (A); or pins can be used to retain a core, which in turn will help to retain a crown (B).

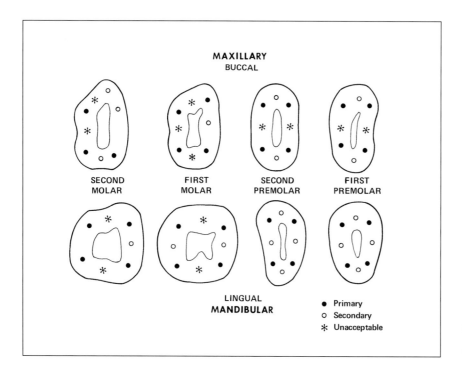

Fig 13-9 Areas for the placement of retentive pin holes in posterior teeth (after Fisher).

it neither overfills nor underfills the hole. Healing is then possible, although not guaranteed. A pin that extends into the periodontium coronal to the alveolar crest should be exposed with a surgical flap and trimmed flush with the root surface.

The technique used for placing the pin holes and reproducing them in the impression is that described by Shooshan.[17] It uses a 0.6-mm (0.024-inch) drill to cut the pin hole, a nylon bristle to reproduce the pin hole in the impression, and a nylon bristle or iridioplatinum pin to produce a pin in the restoration. The pin hole is counter-sunk slightly to form a funnel-shaped opening. This strengthens the pin where it joins the casting[18] and guides the pin into the hole during seating.

Although retention increases as the number, depth, and diameter of pins increases,[19,20] a point of diminishing returns occurs after four or five pins are placed.[21] This experimental finding confirms the clinical recommendations that one pin should be used for each missing cusp,[22] line angle,[23] or axial wall.[24] Self-threading pins are nearly five times more retentive than cemented pins and need be placed to a depth of only 2.0 mm. However, cemented pins that are an integral part of the restoration need to extend 4.0 mm into the tooth.[25]

Bases and Cores

When the destruction of tooth structure is more extensive, a decision must be made whether to augment the retention and resistance by adding auxiliary features or to build up the tooth preparation with a pin-retained core (Fig 13-10).

Bases

Cement bases are used only to protect the pulp and to eliminate undercuts in defects in tooth structure produced by the removal of caries or old restorations. They are used if there is adequate bulk of tooth structure to resist occlusal forces and enough axial wall surface to provide retention for the final restoration.

Glass ionomer and polycarboxylate cements are excellent materials for this purpose. They are nonirritating to the pulp and have some adhesive properties that make them less likely to become dislodged during subsequent preparation of the tooth. Deep areas of the preparation near the pulp may be covered with calcium hydroxide. Cement bases do not have sufficient strength to effectively replace weakened dentinal walls, unless there are two walls of tooth structure remaining.[26] Amalgam or composite resin should be used for that purpose.

An undercut left by caries removal often can be eliminated by creating a box, if the additional retention is needed. However, if creation of a box will destory excessive sound tooth structure, it is better to fill the defect with cement. If the defect is very close to a finish line, amalgam should be used because it is strong and insoluble.

Cores

If half or more of the clinical crown has been destroyed, an amalgam or composite resin core should be placed in the tooth. The core is then treated as though it were tooth structure, and a classic full veneer preparation is used. If less than half of a clinical crown has been destroyed, a preparation design that will employ auxiliary features for added retention in the area of missing cusps can be used.

All cusps thinner than half their height should be shortened or removed. Cavity floors and walls are flattened for increased resistance, taking care not to traumatize the pulp or weaken the remaining walls. A core must be anchored firmly to the tooth and not just placed to fill the void. Otherwise, it offers no advantage over allowing the bulk of the casting to occupy the space.

Pin-retained cores have been utilized to retain cast restorations on severely damaged teeth for nearly 40 years.[16,27,28] Both amalgam and composite resin have been used for this purpose. Composite resins are favored by some because they are easily molded into large cavities and they polymerize quickly, allowing the crown preparation to be done at the same appointment.

However, composite resin cores exhibit greater microleakage than do amalgam cores,[29] and they are not as dimensionally stable as amalgam. In an in vitro study, crowns made for teeth with composite resin cores failed to seat by 226 μm more than crowns made for teeth with amalgam cores after immersion in body-temperature normal saline solution for 1 week.[30] The surface of a composite resin core is affected adversely by exposure to zinc oxide–eugenol temporary cement,[31] although that does not seem to have a negative effect on the tensile strength of the final crown.[32]

Single-phase, copper-rich amalgams attain sufficient hardness to allow a crown preparation to be made after only 10 minutes.[33] Retention devices other than pins can be used for amalgam cores. Slots that are the width and depth of a no. 33$^1/_2$ bur can be placed around the periphery of the preparation.[34] "Dentin chambers," or pot holes, 2 to 3 mm deep can be placed with no. 1156, 1157, or 1158 burs. When amalgam is condensed into these holes, they become "amalgapins."[35]

Retentive features for the core must be deep enough not to be removed by the axial reduction done in the crown preparation. A properly contoured amalgam core can serve as a temporary restoration for several weeks, giving the tissue an opportunity to recover while more urgent treatment is being performed.

The preparation finish line for the cast restoration should extend beyond the core into tooth structure.[36] The farther the core extends subgingivally, the more likely it is to have voids and overhangs that will make it unsuitable to remain exposed beyond the margin of the final restoration. If the core is amalgam, dissimilar metals in contact with it are more prone to corrosion when exposed to the oral environment. If the core is composite resin, it is susceptible to leakage.

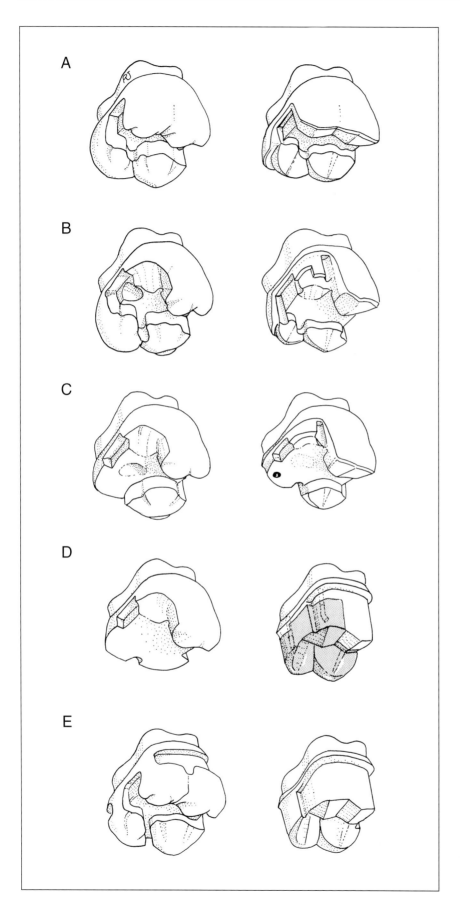

A

B

C

D

E

Fig 13-10 If the tooth to be prepared for a cast restoration has been only moderately damaged (eg, an old MOD amalgam), a standard MOD onlay preparation or a three-quarter crown preparation with boxes can be used (A). If one cusp has been destroyed, a widened box with groove augmentation can be used (B). When half of the crown has been destroyed, grooves may provide sufficient retention if the supragingival tooth structure in which they are placed has sufficient length. Pin holes may be added to the preparation (C). If three or more cusps have been destroyed, a pin-retained core should be fabricated before proceeding to a full-coverage cast restoration (D). Extensive peripheral destruction often requires a full-coverage cast restoration if caries has been controlled (E).

Modifications for Damaged Vital Teeth

In preparing a damaged tooth (Fig 13-11, A), follow an orderly sequence to take full advantage of remaining tooth structure to attain the most retentive preparation possible.

1. *Evaluate pulpal health.* If it is questionable, or if there is an exposure, however small, endodontic therapy should be done before placing a cast restoration.[37] Otherwise, the restoration later may be compromised by the endodontic access. Nonetheless, make every effort to maintain the vitality of the pulp. Endodontic treatment is usually successful, but nothing is perfect. Even if it is successful, it weakens the tooth and increases the cost of restoring it.
2. *Assess the periodontal condition.* Examine periodontal tissues for deep subgingival extensions of caries, fractures, or previous restorations. Finish line extensions that violate the "biologic width" of 2.0 mm of tissue attachment may require periodontal surgery before a restoration is made.[38,39]
3. *Make a preliminary preparation design.* A general concept can be formulated beforehand, but the specific features to be used and their location cannot be ascertained until the initial phases of the preparation have been completed.
4. *Remove previous restorations and bases, all caries, and any unsupported enamel* (Fig 13-11, B). Even if an existing restoration appears sound, it may conceal caries or a pulp exposure. Remove it. Concave, roughened areas from which caries and previous restorations have been removed, or sloping surfaces remaining after cuspal fracture, must be oriented to enhance resistance and retention. They should be formed into vertical and horizontal components, or steps, with essentially vertical surfaces made parallel with the path of insertion (Fig 13-11, C). They must be kept at the periphery of the preparation, with gingival shoulders and floors no wider than 1.5 mm. Horizontal surfaces are made perpendicular to the path of insertion to increase resistance to occlusal forces (Fig 13-11, D). No flat horizontal surface in the central portion of the tooth should be any deeper than the level of the pulpal floor of a classic isthmus.
5. *Evaluate the strength of the remaining walls.* Decide whether to incorporate remaining defects into the preparation or to fill them in. If more than 50% of the coronal tooth structure of a posterior tooth is sound, and the tooth will not be an abutment, sufficient retention can be achieved by adding supplemental features to the preparation. Internal features such as isthmuses or box forms must have surrounding walls of dentin that are at least as wide as they are high. If the thickness-to-height ratio of a wall lies between 1:1 and 1:2, it should be supported. Any wall with a thickness-to-height ratio of less than 1:2 is subject to fracture and should be shortened.
6. *Finalize the preparation design.* Begin with occlusal reduction (Fig 13-11, D) and then proceed with axial reduction (Fig 13-11, E). With a base, fill in the central areas of the tooth that were too deep to be included in the orientation of horizontal and vertical surfaces. Do not bother to mold a large bulk of base to a classic preparation configuration, since no retention is gained from a cement base.

The preparation is ready for the placement of its retention features. Only after all other portions of the preparation are complete can a decision be made about the type, number, and location of retentive features that will be used. The preparation is completed by their addition (Fig 13-11, F).

Placement of grooves, pin holes, and box walls in a base is the same as not using them at all (Fig 13-12, A). Retention and resistance forms must be placed in solid tooth structure, not in base, if they are to provide any resistance to dislodgment (Fig 13-12, B). Since retentive features can be formed no more than 1.5 mm from the outer surface of the tooth, deep destruction of tooth structure requires that the axial wall of a box be placed in a nonretentive base rather than in dentin. If the buccal and lingual walls are in dentin, the box will provide significant retention. The danger to the pulp from extending the box closer to the pulp would be an unacceptable risk for the little retention that might be added.

An important aspect of restoring damaged teeth is the protection of remaining tooth structure. Teeth already weakened by the loss of large amounts of tooth structure are ill-equipped to withstand occlusal forces unassisted. Protection can be provided by capping cusps with the cast restoration.[40,41] The occlusal thickness in metal should be 1.0 mm over the nonfunctional cusps and 1.5 mm over the functional cusps.

The choices for anterior teeth are more limited because of esthetic requirements and the smaller bulk of dentin in which supplemental features can be placed. Modifications of classic anterior preparations are limited to substitution of a box for a groove to encompass a carious lesion, or addition of extra grooves or pin holes. If more than one-third of the coronal structure is lost, placement of a pin-retained core followed by a metal-ceramic crown is usually indicated.

There will be times when it is necessary to devitalize a tooth to obtain retention. If a crown is to be placed on a narrow, single-rooted tooth with little or no coronal tooth structure, a core may not have sufficient resistance to dislodgment without a dowel that extends into the root.

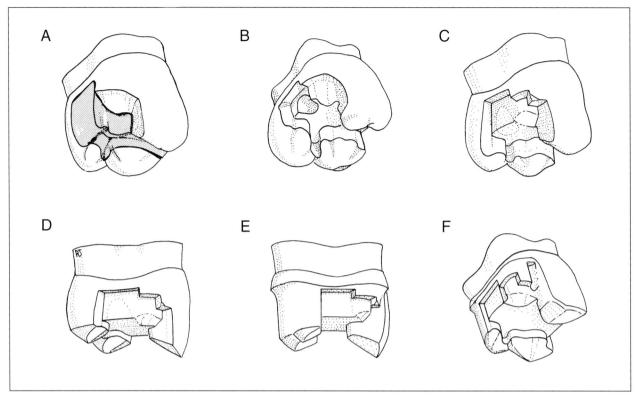

Fig 13-11 Maxillary molar with a missing distobuccal cusp and a defective MOD amalgam (A). All caries, previous restorations, bases, and undermined enamel are removed (B). Steps are formed in sloping areas with vertical surfaces made parallel with the path of insertion and horizontal surfaces perpendicular to it (C). Occlusal reduction (D) and axial reduction (E) are done on the remaining tooth structure. Addition or refinement of auxiliary retention features completes the preparation (F).

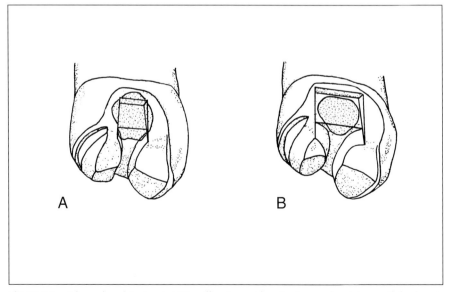

Fig 13-12 A box placed in cement (A) will not provide retention and resistance. If the box is widened buccolingually and lengthened gingivally so that the facial and lingual walls are in solid tooth structure, retention will be improved (B).

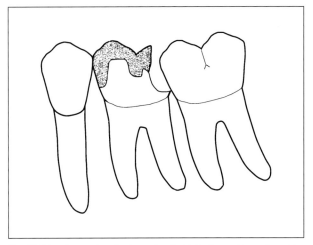

Fig 13-13   Second molar has migrated into the void produced by caries.

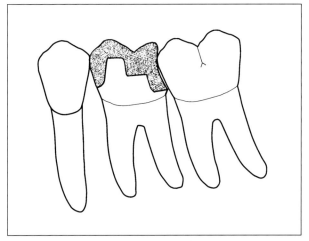

Fig 13-14   The tooth is first built up with a core.

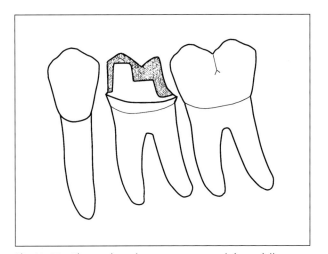

Fig 13-15   The tooth and core are prepared for a full veneer crown.

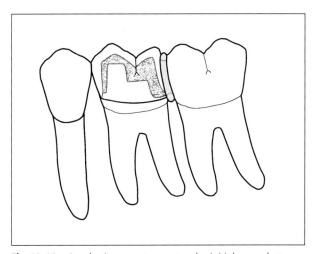

Fig 13-16   An elastic separator creates the initial space between the provisional crown and the adjacent tooth.

Orthodontic Adjuncts to Restoring Damaged Teeth

Caries or trauma may produce tooth destruction of a magnitude or in a location that makes it difficult or impossible to restore the tooth without serious esthetic or periodontal compromise. Simple orthodontic procedures can be employed in some of these situations to make it possible to restore the teeth in a manner that will improve the prognosis for long-term success and provide a more pleasing esthetic result where required.

Regaining Interproximal Space

A long-standing carious lesion on the proximal surface of a molar often will result in migration of the adjacent molar into the void created by the caries (Fig 13-13). It is not enough just to excavate the caries and place a restoration in such a situation. The teeth frequently contact at, or apical to, the cementoenamel junction. Simply placing a restoration in these circumstances would result in a concave proximal contour and a closed embrasure space that would wreak havoc on the periodontium. Instead, the space should be regained by separating the teeth with the brass wire technique described by Reagan.[42]

A core or foundation restoration is placed in the tooth requiring restoration (Fig 13-14) and then it is prepared for a full crown (Fig 13-15). An acrylic resin provisional crown is fabricated using the technique described in

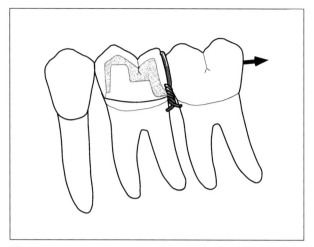

Fig 13-17 Brass wire is wrapped around the contact and twisted to further separate the teeth.

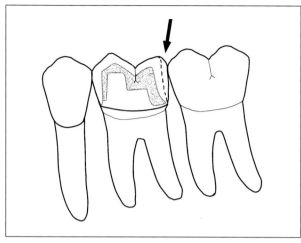

Fig 13-18 The contact is closed by adding resin to the distal aspect of the provisional restoration *(arrow)*.

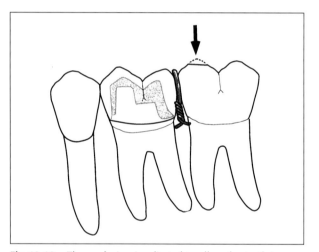

Fig 13-19 The occlusion is adjusted to allow the tooth to continue moving distally *(arrow)*.

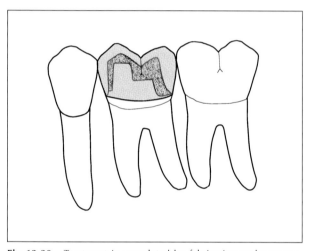

Fig 13-20 Treatment is completed by fabrication and cementation of the final crown.

Chapter 15. After adjusting and polishing the provisional crown, it is cemented. An elastic orthodontic separator is inserted into the proximal surface to initiate the movement of the adjacent tooth (Fig 13-16).

At a subsequent appointment, the elastic is removed and a piece of 0.6-mm (0.025-inch) brass wire is threaded between the teeth from the facial side, apical to the contact. The wire is wrapped around the contact, bringing the two ends together on the facial side. There the wire is twisted together until the patient feels pressure. The twisted end of the wire is cut off, leaving a 5- to 6-mm tail. The cut end is bent over so that it will not stab the patient's cheek (Fig 13-17).

At approximately 1-week intervals, the wire is tightened by twisting until the tooth shows no movement from the previous appointment. At this point the provisional restoration is removed and the crown is built back into contact with the adjacent tooth by adding acrylic resin (Fig 13-18). The crown is repolished and recemented, and the brass wire is reapplied. As the adjacent tooth is tipped distally, it may move upward into the occlusal plane. If it does, adjust it occlusally to permit it to continue to move distally (Fig 13-19).

Caries extensive enough to require orthodontic movement often extends far enough apically that some type of surgical crown-lengthening procedure will be required. This will not only facilitate successful completion of the crown, but it will also prevent subsequent periodontal inflammation around the crown margin. Then the full crown that will serve as the final restoration is fabricated and cemented (Fig 13-20).

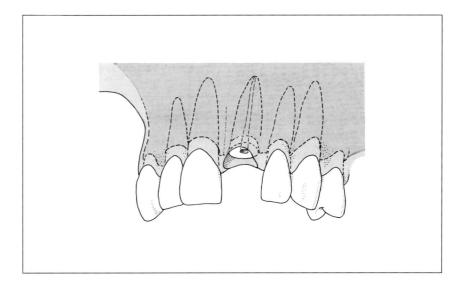

Fig 13-21 This central incisor is fractured to the level of the alveolar crest.

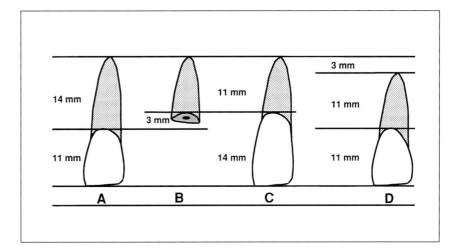

Fig 13-22 Extrusion vs surgical crown lengthening. The normal anatomic crown-root ratio for an average central incisor is 11:14 (A). In this example, the tooth is fractured 3.0 mm beyond the cementoenamel junction (B). Surgical crown lengthening alone would produce an unstable and unesthetic crown-root ratio of 14:11 (C). Extrusion followed by crown lengthening produces a more stable crown-root ratio of 11:11 with a more esthetic, normal crown length (D).

Extrusion of Teeth

When all tooth structure has been lost to the level of the alveolar crest or beyond, because of either fracture or caries, the tooth cannot be satisfactorily restored without some extraordinary measure (Fig 13-21). Even if a dowel core is placed in the tooth, the root will remain susceptible to fracture without the crown encircling the tooth apical to the core. This *ferrule effect* around the tooth protects it from fracture by the dowel from within.[36] In fact, if tooth structure is lost "only" to the level of the epithelial attachment, minor extrusion may be desirable to permit access to enough tooth structure apical to the finish line to produce a ferrule effect.

Burying the finish line subgingivally will not solve the problem. Rather, it will create new ones: the increased possibility of an ill-fitting crown and placement of the margin in an area that would violate the "biologic width" of soft tissue attachment. This particular problem can be overcome by surgical crown lengthening alone, but the result will be most unesthetic. Surgery shortens the root and also increases the crown-root ratio (Fig 13-22).

Orthodontic extrusion has been used to move solid root structure into an accessible area.[43] The use of orthodontic brackets has been described for this purpose.[44-47] However, they are bulky and unesthetic, and they may be difficult to place far enough apically to permit sufficient space for extrusion. Furthermore, their use may cause unwanted movement of the abutment teeth.[48] Removable appliances also can be used to extrude teeth,[49] but they require a high degree of patient compliance. The technique presented below utilizes an anchorage wire bonded to adjacent teeth as described by Oesterle and Wood.[48]

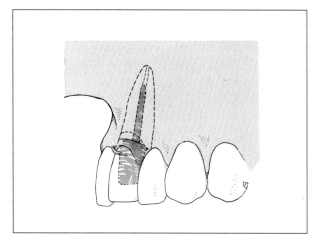

Fig 13-23 A bent pin is placed in the gingival area of the facial surface of the provisional crown.

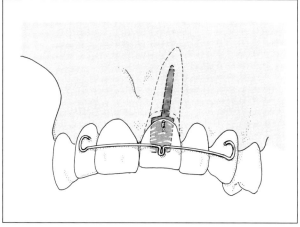

Fig 13-24 Arch wire extends two teeth on either side of the tooth to be extruded. There is a loop in the wire over both terminal abutments, to aid retention by resin, and a loop in the middle over the tooth to be extruded.

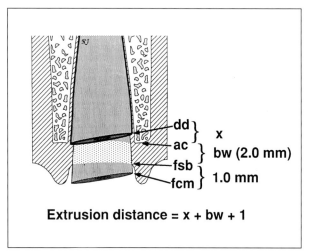

Extrusion distance = x + bw + 1

Fig 13-25 The amount of extrusion needed is determined by adding the distance the destruction extends beyond the alveolar crest, the biologic width of 2.0 mm, and 1.0 mm between the bottom of the sulcus and the crown margin. If the destruction extends 1.0 mm beyond the alveolar crest, 4.0 mm of extrusion would be necessary. ac = alveolar crest, bw = biologic width, dd = deepest extent of destruction, fcm = final crown margin, and fsb = final bottom of sulcus.

The tooth first must be endodontically treated. The extrusion can be done with either a permanent or a temporary dowel core in the tooth. In either case, place a provisional crown on the tooth to be extruded. This maintains space and provides an esthetic appearance during treatment. If the permanent dowel core is fabricated before extrusion, make it at least 3.0 mm short of its normal incisal length to allow space for extrusion.

Embed a TMS pin (Coltene-Whaledent, New York, NY) in the mesiodistal center of the facial surface of the provisional crown, as near the gingiva as possible. The pin

is either directed slightly gingivally or bent to facilitate retention of the elastic that will be placed on it later (Fig 13-23).

Bend a facial 0.018 x 0.025-inch stainless steel orthodontic arch wire, with a small loop opposite the middle of the tooth to be extruded. The loop, an attachment for the elastic, is bent in an incisal direction to prevent the elastic from slipping off. The base of the loop should touch the facial surface of the tooth to prevent the tooth from moving lingually as it erupts. The arch wire should extend for two teeth on either side of the tooth to be extruded with a loop in each end of the wire for retention (Fig 13-24). The use of this number of abutments minimizes the possibility of moving them rather than the intended tooth.

Place the arch wire at the incisogingival level to which the TMS pin will be moved, equaling the amount of extrusion to be accomplished. The distance that the tooth is to be extruded is calculated by adding *(1)* the distance from the most apical point of fracture or caries to the alveolar crest (if the damage extends subcrestally); *(2)* 2.0 mm for the biologic width[38]; and *(3)* at least 1.0 mm to prevent placement of the crown margin too far subgingivally (Fig 13-25). If the damage is flush with the alveolar crest, a minimum of 3.0 mm of extrusion would be required.[48]

Affix the arch wire to each of the four abutment teeth, using a light-activated resin. Create an occlusal clearance of 1.0 mm on the provisional crown, and attach an elastic to the pin on the crown and the loop on the wire (Fig 13-26). Check the patient weekly.[45] The tooth will elongate at a rate of 1.0 to 1.5 mm per week.[44,48,49] Relieve the occlusion again and replace the elastic.

When the TMS anchorage pin in the facial surface of the provisional crown is even with the arch wire, the extrusion is completed. Remove the elastic and replace it with a ligature wire, tying the pin on the crown to the loop in the arch wire (Fig 13-27). Check the occlusion to

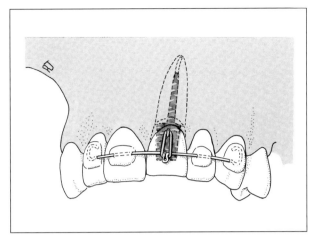

Fig 13-26 An elastic extends from the pin on the crown to the loop in the arch wire.

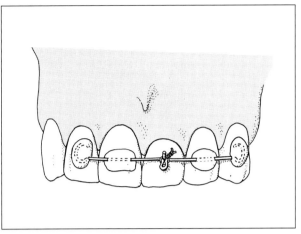

Fig 13-27 When the tooth has been extruded so that the pin on the crown contacts the loop in the arch wire, it should be stabilized with ligature wire. The descended level of the gingiva makes the clinical crown shorter.

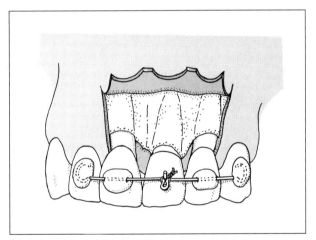

Fig 13-28 An elevated flap reveals that the alveolar level has descended with the tooth.

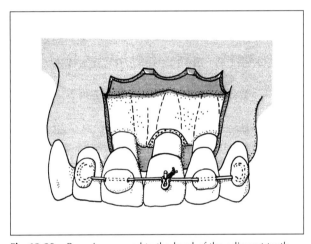

Fig 13-29 Bone is removed to the level of the adjacent teeth.

insure that there are no interferences. Traumatic occlusal contacts will interfere with healing and stabilization of the tooth. The teeth should remain ligated for at least 1 month before proceeding to the next phase of the treatment.[48]

The alveolar bone and gingival attachment frequently will descend with the tooth (Fig 13-28). If there was a preexisting periodontal defect, it may be lessened or eliminated.[47,50-52] However, if the periodontium was normal before the extrusion was undertaken, surgery may be necessary to bring the levels of the bone and the gingival crest into line with those of the adjacent teeth.[48,52-54] A flap is reflected over the extruded tooth, and bone is removed to match the osseous level of the adjacent teeth (Fig 13-29). The final restoration can be started approximately 4 weeks after the surgery (Fig 13-30).[48]

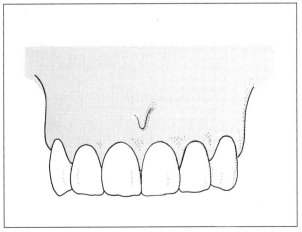

Fig 13-30 Final restoration on a tooth with a clinical crown whose length is similar to that of the adjacent teeth.

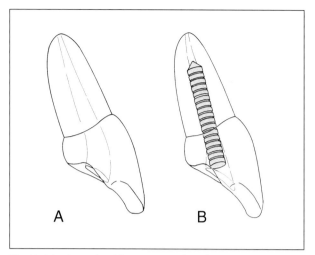

Fig 13-31 A tooth with an intact clinical crown can be adequately restored with composite resin (A). A dowel provides unnecessary "reinforcement" that may weaken the tooth instead (B). (From Shillingburg and Kessler.[58])

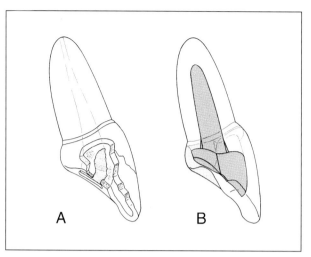

Fig 13-32 A single-rooted pulpless tooth with a severely damaged crown (A) usually will require a dowel core before placement of a crown (B). (From Shillingburg and Kessler.[58])

Restoration of Endodontically Treated Teeth

The restoration to be used on an endodontically treated tooth is dictated by the extent of coronal destruction and by the type of tooth. Traditionally, a pulpless tooth received a dowel to "reinforce" it and a crown to "protect" it. Retrospective clinical surveys in recent years have caused a reappraisal of this thinking. In a study of 220 endodontically treated teeth, Ross[55] found that nearly 61% of the teeth that had been in service for 5 years or longer had not been restored with dowels. Sorensen and Martinoff[56] reported almost identical success rates for endodontically treated anterior teeth restored with and without dowels.

Rationale

In that same study by Sorensen and Martinoff,[56] there also was no significant difference between the success achieved with anterior pulpless teeth that had received crowns and those that had not. It is then obvious that endodontically treated anterior teeth do not automatically require crowns.[57-59] If a moderate-sized anterior tooth is intact except for the endodontic access and one or two small proximal lesions, composite resin restorations will suffice. Placement of a dowel in such a tooth is more likely to weaken it than to strengthen it (Fig 13-31).

Lovdahl and Nicholls[60] found that intact endodontically treated central incisors were three times as resistant to fracture as teeth that had been restored with dowel cores.

For a tooth that has become discolored following devitalization, bleaching is preferable to crown placement if the tooth is relatively intact.[57] A laminate veneer offers a less destructive alternative if the facial surface of a reasonably intact tooth must be masked by a restoration.

However, the axial reduction for a crown preparation (peripheral destruction) combined with an endodontic access preparation (central destruction) frequently leaves insufficient sound dentin to support a crown unaided. If a metal-ceramic crown is required because of extensive coronal destruction, a *dowel core* probably is needed (Fig 13-32). A dowel is placed to provide the retention for a crown that ordinarily would have been gained from coronal tooth structure.[61,62] The use of a dowel requires that the canal be obturated with gutta-percha. It is difficult to ream out a canal filled with a silver point or other hard material. Lateral perforation of the root becomes a distinct possibility. If a dowel is used, its extension into the root must at least equal the length of the crown for optimum stress distribution[63] and maximum retention, or the dowel should be two-thirds the length of the root, whichever is greater (Fig 13-33). A minimum length of 4.0 mm of gutta-percha, and more if possible, should remain at the apex to prevent dislodgment and subsequent leakage. If it is not possible to meet these criteria, the prognosis for the restoration will be compromised and some alternative should be explored.

The longer a dowel, the greater its retention.[64-67] A tooth with a dowel that is three-quarters the length of the crown or shorter has less chance for success than a tooth that has no dowel at all.[68] However, the success rate of dowel-treated teeth can increase to more than 97.5% when dowel length equals or exceeds the length of the crown.[68]

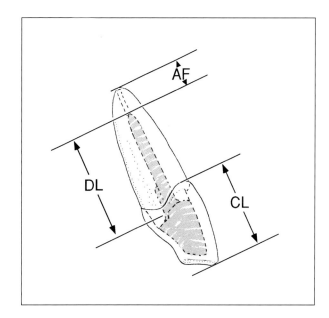

Fig 13-33 The length of the dowel (DL) should equal the crown length (CL) or two-thirds the length of the root, whichever is greater. The length of the remaining apical fill (AF) should be at least 4.0 mm.

Posterior teeth must be treated differently. Because of their naturally divided occlusal surface, even caries-free teeth can fracture vertically under occlusal forces. The minimum treatment indicated for an endodontically treated molar or premolar is the placement of a cast restoration with occlusal coverage, such as an MOD onlay.[69] Sorensen and Martinoff[68] found that 94% of endodontically treated molars and premolars that subsequently received coronal coverage were successful, while only 56% of occlusally unprotected endodontically treated posterior teeth survived.

Those endodontically treated posterior teeth with sufficient sound tooth structure to be restored with an MOD onlay are in a distinct minority. Many teeth that require endodontic therapy have been so damaged by caries, previous restorations, and the endodontic access, that limited coronal tooth structure remains to be used for retaining the final restoration.

Frequently a core must be substituted for the supragingival axial walls and auxiliary features that are customarily used. Maxillary premolars often have drastically tapering roots, thin root walls, and proximal root concavities or invaginations, all of which are predisposing factors to perforation or fracture.[70] In a study of 468 teeth that had fractured in vivo, 78% were premolars, with 62% being maxillary premolars.[71] A dowel core should be utilized on premolars only if the roots are adequately long, bulky, and straight (Fig 13-34).

Care must be exercised in the selection of restorations for teeth that have no remaining coronal tooth structure. The encirclement of 1.0 to 2.0 mm of vertical axial tooth structure within the walls of a crown creates a ferrule effect around the tooth to protect it from fracture (Fig 13-35).[36] If the crown margin is not placed onto solid tooth

structure, the risk of root fracture is greatly increased (Fig 13-36). Orthodontic extrusion and crown lengthening surgery may be needed to prevent encroachment on periodontal tissues (Fig 13-37).

Rosen[72] advocated a subgingival collar to act as an extracoronal brace. Hoag and Dwyer[73] determined that the type of dowel core was not as important as the presence of a full crown with margins that extended beyond the core. Having 1.0 mm of vertical tooth wall between the margin of the core and the shoulder of the preparation was found by Sorensen and Engleman[74] to provide a ferrule effect, enhancing fracture resistance by 80% to 139%. Milot and Stein[75] demonstrated that a steep,1.0-mm-wide bevel that is nearly parallel with the long axis of the preparation also strengthens the tooth against fracture.

If a minimum of 1.0 mm of vertical axial wall cannot be covered by a crown on a premolar that is to serve as an abutment, the tooth should be extracted. Endodontically treated teeth should not be used as abutments for distal extension removable partial dentures.[76] They are more than four times as likely to fail than pulpless teeth not serving as abutments.[77] Pulpless fixed partial denture abutment teeth fail nearly twice as often as single teeth.

Even with a ferrule effect, it is questionable whether a pulpless tooth should be used as an abutment for a fixed partial denture with a span longer than one pontic. The tooth is structurally compromised and susceptible to fracture if overloaded. The more extensive the restoration required for an endodontically treated tooth, the more time-consuming and technique-sensitive the restoration will be.[78] If a fixed partial denture must be used in such circumstances, strong consideration should be given to the use of an implant-supported prosthesis.

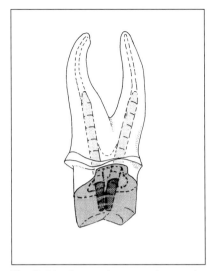

Fig 13-34 Roots of a premolar require bulk and length for the successful use of a dowel core. Both canals of a two-canal tooth are used if possible.

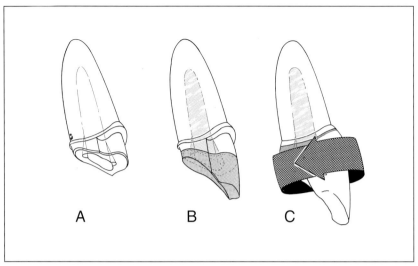

Fig 13-35 The preparation for a dowel core should preserve solid tooth structure (A). The crown preparation finish line should be apical to the dowel-core margin (B), enabling the crown to girdle the tooth *(arrow)* and brace it externally (C). (From Shillingburg and Kessler.[58])

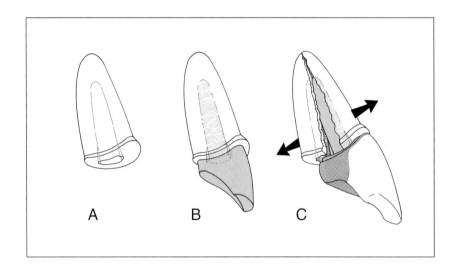

Fig 13-36 If a tooth is flush with the gingiva (A), fabrication of a dowel core and a crown without encirclement of tooth structure by the crown walls (B) could result in root fracture (C). (From Shillingburg and Kessler.[58])

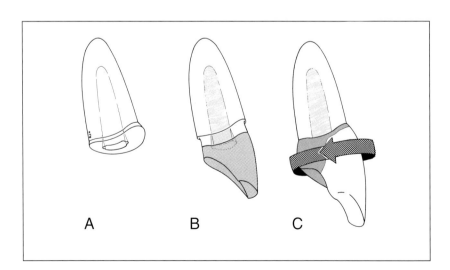

Fig 13-37 A tooth without coronal tooth structure (A) can be protected by moving the crown preparation finish line apically (B) to brace the tooth *(arrow)* against root fracture (C). (From Shillingburg and Kessler.[58])

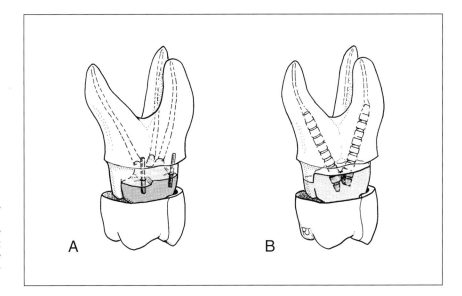

Fig 13-38 A core retained by pins, slots, amalgapins, or extension into the pulp chamber is used to build up a molar with some coronal tooth structure (A). However, if there is insufficient coronal tooth structure to support the core, two dowels are added for resistance (B).

A pulpless molar with a moderately damaged clinical crown can be built up with an amalgam or composite resin core prior to placement of an artificial crown (Fig 13-38, A). If there is one sound cusp, the core may be retained by gross extension of the amalgam into the pulpal chamber alone,[79] or in conjunction with pins,[80] peripheral slots,[34] or dentinal wells (amalgapins).[35] A variation, usually employing two dowels, is used for molars that have little or no remaining coronal tooth structure (Fig 13-38, B).

The core and its attachment(s) are made separately from the final restoration. The crown is then fabricated and cemented over the core just as a restoration would be placed over a preparation done in tooth structure. This two-unit system offers several advantages over a one-piece dowel crown. The marginal adaptation and fit of the restoration are independent of any dowel that must be used. The restoration can be replaced at some future time, if necessary, without disturbing the dowel core. If a dowel is necessary, the choice is not limited to a custom cast device. Prefabricated systems can be used if the dowel does not have to be incorporated into the crown. If the endodontically treated tooth must serve as a fixed partial denture abutment, it is not necessary to make the root canal preparation parallel with the path of insertion of other preparations.

Prefabricated Dowel With Amalgam or Resin Core

Numerous techniques have been described for the fabrication of dowel cores. Prefabricated dowels with amalgam or composite resin cores are the most commonly used dowel cores today, and there is a wide variety of dowel systems available. Kits for prefabricated dowels utilize special reamers or drills for canal preparations that are the same size and configuration as the dowels. Through the use of one of these systems, it is possible to complete the entire procedure in a single appointment.[81]

Amalgam provides greater strength. Kovarik et al[82] found that 67% of the amalgam cores tested in an in vitro study survived 1,000,000 cycles of 75-lb loading, while only 17% of the composite resin cores survived. In that same study, all of the glass ionomer cores had failed within the first 220,000 cycles. Composite resin remains popular because it is easily placed, polymerizing in minutes and allowing work on the core preparation to progress almost immediately. Resin requires less bulk of material than does amalgam, which makes it useful on small teeth.

A dowel increases resistance to lateral forces applied to the crown from 15%[83] to 48%.[84] Dowels can be made of stainless steel, titanium, brass, or a chromium-containing alloy. The preferred materials in light of current knowledge of galvanism and corrosion are titanium, high platinum, and cobalt-chromium-molybdenum alloys.[85] The least desirable are brass and chromium-nickel steel.[85] Prefabricated dowels are made in both parallel-sided and tapered configurations.

Dowel systems can be classified by their mechanism of retention: *passive* (cemented) or *active* (threaded). The threaded dowels are more retentive than the cemented, but they also produce more stress in the tooth.[67,86,87] The techniques for all of these systems are similar, except for the final dowel space (canal) preparation instrumentation, which is usually specific for the particular dowel system being used.

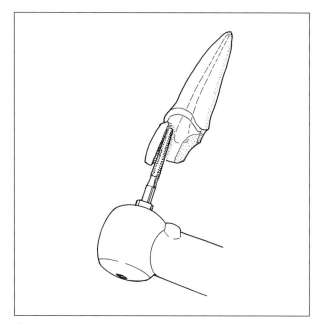

Fig 13-39 The initial step in a dowel-core preparation is reduction for the crown preparation.

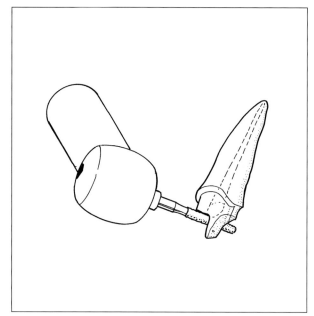

Fig 13-40 Unsupported tooth structure is removed next.

Armamentarium

1. Handpiece
2. Flat-end tapered diamond
3. Small wheel diamond
4. Flame diamond
5. No. 171L bur
6. No. 4 round bur
7. Endodontic condenser
8. Set of six Peeso reamers
9. Dowel kit, including dowel, special reamer, pin(s), and drill
10. Cement spatula and glass slab
11. Amalgam
    a. Copper band and wedges
    b. Capsule(s) and amalgamator
    c. Carrier
    d. Condenser
    e. Carver(s)
12. Composite resin
    a. Crown form (clear or polycarbonate)
    b. Resin kit
    c. Plastic filling instrument

The preparation for a dowel core is begun by preparing the coronal tooth structure for the crown that will be the final restoration for the tooth (Fig 13-39). Remove existing restorations, caries, bases, and thin or unsupported walls of tooth structure (Fig 13-40). Preserve as much coronal tooth structure as possible, to enable the axial walls of the crown to externally brace the tooth.

Measure a Peeso reamer (Union Broach Div of Moyco Industries, Philadelphia, PA) against a radiograph of the tooth being restored to determine the length to which the instrument (and later, the dowel) will be inserted into the canal (Fig 13-41). Slide a silicone rubber endodontic stop onto the shank of the reamer, aligning it with a landmark such as the incisal edge of the adjacent tooth to insure insertion of the instrument to the proper depth in the tooth. Place a rubber dam to prevent contamination of the canal and to protect nearby tissues. Begin the dowel space preparation by first removing gutta-percha in the canal with a hot endodontic condenser.[80] Start enlarging the canal with the largest Peeso reamer or Gates Glidden drill (Union Broach) that will fit into the canal (Fig 13-42).

Even if a specific reamer or drill is prescribed for a particular dowel system, begin with safety-tipped instruments that will follow the path of least resistance, the gutta-percha in the canal (Fig 13-43). With a series of successively larger reamers, enlarge the canal to a diameter slightly smaller than that of the specific instrument required for the system being used. Enlarging a previously instrumented canal in 0.2-mm increments diminishes the possibility of the instrument straying from the canal. Conventional drills used without any prior enlargement of the canal are more prone to stray from the original canal pathway than either Peeso reamers[88] or Gates Glidden drills.[89] Complete the preparation of the dowel space with the prescribed drill or reamer for the system being used (Fig 13-44). General guidelines for the final dowel diameter are shown in Fig 13-45, but individual teeth may require smaller dowels.

In the area of greatest bulk between the canal and the periphery of the tooth, drill one or two 0.6-mm pin holes to a depth of 2.0 mm. Place the pins in these holes to pro-

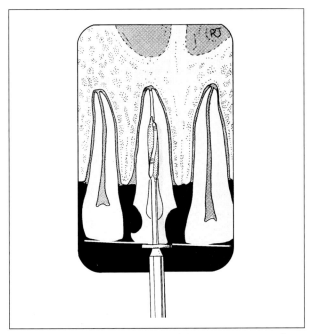

Fig 13-41 The depth of insertion of the Peeso reamer is determined by superimposing it over a radiograph of the tooth being restored.

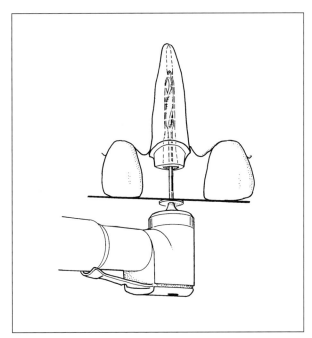

Fig 13-42 The canal is prepared with Peeso reamers.

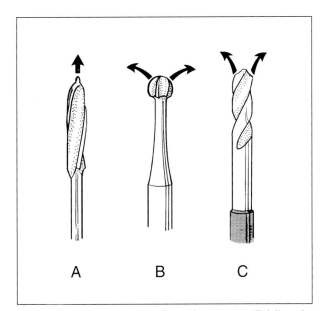

Fig 13-43 A Peeso reamer with a safety tip (A) will follow the path of least resistance, staying within the previously instrumented root canal. A bur (B) or a drill (C) can cut in any direction that it is pushed.

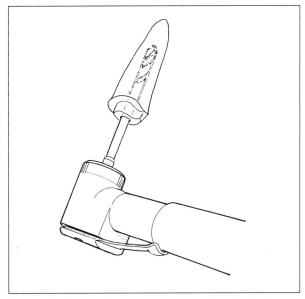

Fig 13-44 The dowel space preparation is finished with the specific drill or reamer for the dowel system being used.

vide antirotational resistance against forces transmitted from the incisal edge of the crown to the core under it. Try in the dowel to confirm fit and length (Fig 13-46). When it is necessary to shorten the dowel, do it at the apical end if the dowel has a special shape to the head, such as the Parapost (Coltene/Whaledent, Brooklyn, NY). On the other

hand, if the dowel has a specially shaped tip, such as the BCH, do any needed shortening at the coronal end.

Make a thin mix of cement, and coat the dowel with it. Introduce cement into the dowel space with a plastic instrument. Use a lentulo spiral (LD Caulk, Milford, DE) to insure that the walls of the canal are completely coated

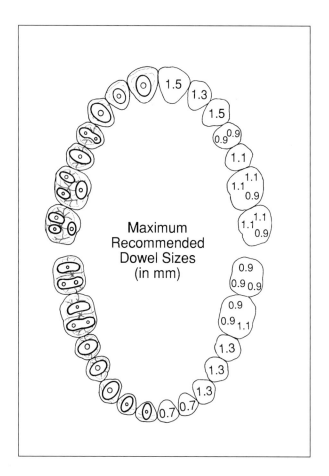

Maximum
Recommended
Dowel Sizes
(in mm)

Fig 13-45 The outlines of the roots *(pictured at midroot)* and the dowels are shown superimposed on the occlusal surfaces of the right teeth *(on the reader's left)*. The recommended dowel diameters are shown on the left teeth *(the reader's right)*.

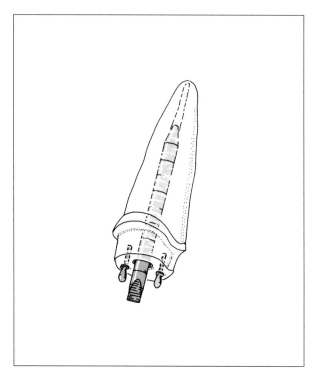

Fig 13-46 The prefabricated dowel will retain the core, and the pin(s) will give it resistance to rotation.

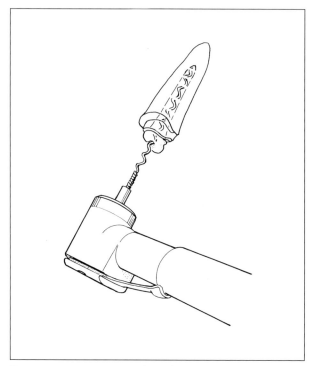

Fig 13-47 Cement is carried into the canal with a lentulo spiral.

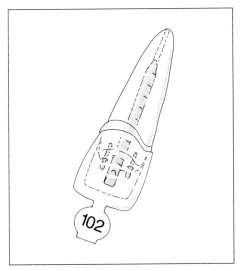

Fig 13-48 The gingival portion of a crown form is cut to follow the contours of the gingiva surrounding the tooth.

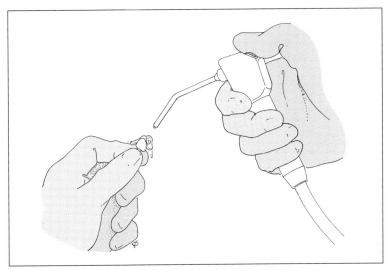

Fig 13-49 Excess separating material (impression material) is blown out of the crown form.

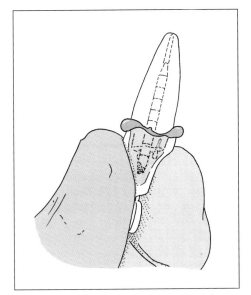

Fig 13-50 The crown form is held while the resin polymerizes.

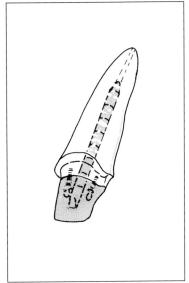

Fig 13-51 The tooth preparation for the final crown is completed.

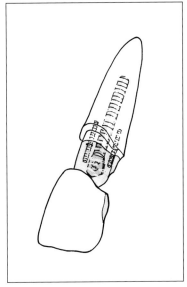

Fig 13-52 The crown is cemented over the the prefabricated dowel and core.

with cement (Fig 13-47). Retention can be increased by as much as 90% if a lentulo spiral is used.[90] Push the dowel slowly to place, allowing the excess cement to escape. Hold the dowel in place with finger pressure until initial set occurs. Then remove excess cement from around the dowel head and pins.

If amalgam will be used for the core, select a copper band of correct diameter to fit the tooth and festoon the gingival end to follow the gingival contours. If the core is to be composite resin, a copper band can be used, but it is easier and faster to use a crown form. A clear crown form permits the use of a light-activated resin, while a

polycarbonate form can be used with autopolymerizing resins (Fig 13-48).

If a polycarbonate crown form is used, place a separating medium in it. Fill it with light-bodied impression material and blow out the excess with an air syringe, leaving a thin film lining the walls of the crown (Fig 13-49). Then fill the crown form with resin and hold it in position over the protruding dowel until the resin core material has polymerized (Fig 13-50). Remove the matrix and shape the core with diamonds and burs to the form of a crown preparation (Fig 13-51). Be sure that the gingival finish line is on tooth structure.

Fabricate a provisional restoration and make the impression for the crown. If a polycarbonate crown was used as a matrix, it can be used as the provisional crown after the elastomeric material is peeled out and the margins are refined. The final restoration will be cemented at the return appointment (Fig 13-52).

Custom Cast Dowel Cores

Prefabricated noble-metal dowels have been combined with wax cores.[91,92] Direct wax patterns have been fabricated using either a fissure bur[72] or a paper clip[93] as reinforcement. A direct technique can be used to fabricate a dowel-core pattern from acrylic resin.[94-96]

The direct acrylic dowel-core technique can be used for teeth with single or multiple roots. When a dowel core is made for a premolar with two canals, a dowel of optimal length is made for the most desirable canal, and the second canal accommodates a short key that serves as an antirotational device. It adds little or no retention.

The direct method for fabrication of a dowel core is accomplished in three steps:

1. Canal preparation
2. Resin pattern fabrication
3. Finishing and cementation of the dowel core

Armamentarium

1. Handpiece
2. Flat-end tapered diamond
3. Small wheel diamond
4. Flame diamond
5. No. 170 bur
6. No. 4 round bur
7. Endodontic condenser
8. Set of six Peeso reamers
9. Straight handpiece
10. Coarse garnet disc on a Moore mandrel
11. Fine sandpaper disc on a Moore mandrel
12. Large green stone
13. Burlew wheel on mandrel
14. 14-gauge solid plastic sprue
15. Dappen dish
16. Cement spatula
17. Cotton pellets
18. Petrolatum
19. Resin monomer and polymer
20. Medicine dropper
21. IPPA plastic filling instrument

Canal Preparation

The preparation for the final restoration is roughly approximated. For an anterior tooth, the final restoration will probably be a metal-ceramic crown. Axial reduction and

Table 13-1 *Instrument Sizes*

	Diameter (in mm)						
	0.6	0.7	0.9	1.1	1.3	1.5	1.7
Peeso Reamer	—	1	2	3	4	5	6
Gates Glidden	1	2	3	4	5	6	—

incisal reduction of 2.0 mm are accomplished with a flat-end tapered diamond (Fig 13-53). Labial reduction should be 1.0 to 1.2 mm deep axially. Lingual reduction is done with a small wheel diamond.

All caries, bases, and previous restorations are removed, and the remaining tooth structure is evaluated to determine that which is sound enough to be incorporated into the final preparation. Thin walls of unsupported tooth structure should be removed at this time (Fig 13-54). It is neither necessary nor desirable to remove all supragingival coronal tooth structure unless it is weak and undermined.

The tooth is now ready for preparation of the canal. The instruments of choice for removing the gutta-percha and enlarging the canal are Peeso reamers. They are available in sets of six graduated sizes ranging from 0.7 to 1.7 mm in diameter (Table 13-1), with noncutting tips that follow the path of least resistance, the gutta-percha in the canal.

Begin the removal of gutta-percha in the canal with a hot endodontic condenser. Measure as large a Peeso reamer as will fit in the obturated canal against a radiograph of the tooth being restored to determine the length to which the reamer will be inserted into the canal (Fig 13-55). Use a landmark, such as the incisal edge of an adjacent tooth, to locate a stop on the shank of the reamer. Slide a small square of rubber dam material to the place on the reamer that will correspond with the landmark when the reamer is inserted to the proper depth in the canal.

Place the reamer in the tooth to the predetermined depth and expose a radiograph to check the accuracy of the length. Use this radiograph to establish the final length. Continue enlarging the canal with the graduated sizes of reamers until reaching the size that has been decided upon for that tooth. The size of reamer used will depend upon the diameter of the tooth. As a general rule, it will be no greater than one-third the diameter of the root at the cementoenamel junction, and there should be a minimum thickness of 1.0 mm of tooth structure around the dowel at midroot and beyond (Fig 13-56).

After the canal has been prepared for the dowel, use a no. 170 bur to make a *keyway,* or groove, in the orifice of the canal. Place it in the area of the tooth where there is the greatest bulk (Fig 13-57). The keyway should be cut to the depth of the diameter of the bur (approximately 0.6 mm) and up the canal to the length of the cutting blades of the bur (approximately 4 mm). On a premolar, the second canal serves the same antirotational function.

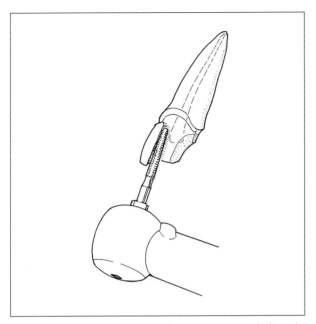

Fig 13-53 The tooth is prepared for a crown as a prelude to the dowel-core preparation.

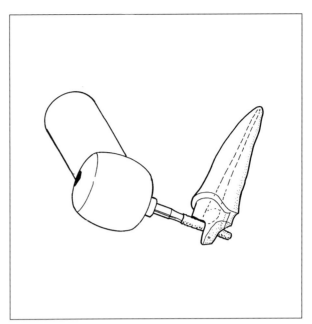

Fig 13-54 Unsupported tooth structure is removed next.

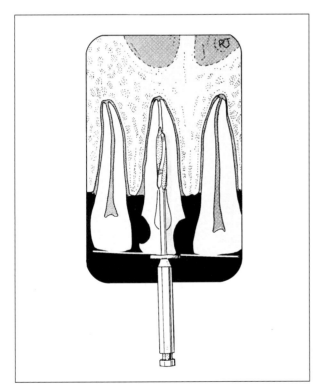

Fig 13-55 A Peeso reamer is superimposed over a radiograph of the tooth being restored to determine the depth of insertion.

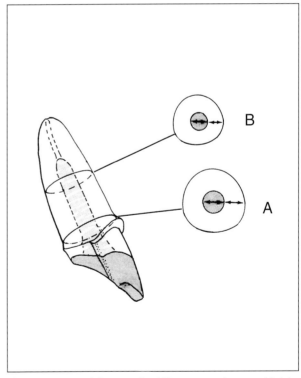

Fig 13-56 Dowel diameter should be no more than one-third the root diameter at the cementoenamel junction (A). It should be at least 2.0 mm less than the crown diameter at midroot (B).

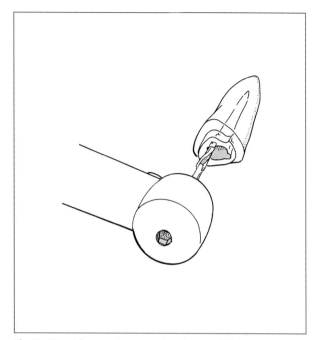

Fig 13-57   A keyway is prepared with a no. 170 bur.

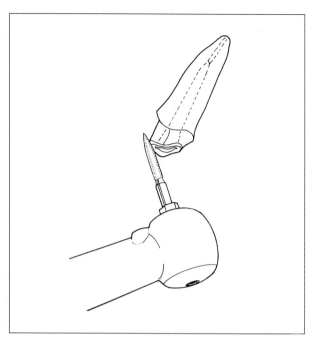

Fig 13-58   A flame diamond is used to place the contrabevel.

If there is supragingival tooth structure, use a flame diamond to place a contrabevel around the external periphery of the preparation (Fig 13-58). This feature provides a metal collar around the occlusal circumference of the preparation to aid in bracing the tooth against fracture of the remaining tooth structure.

Resin Pattern Fabrication

Trim a 14-gauge solid plastic sprue (Williams Dental, Buffalo, NY) so that it will slide easily into the canal to the apical end of the dowel preparation. It must not bind in the canal. Cut a small notch on the facial portion of the occlusal end of the plastic sprue to aid in orienting the dowel-core pattern when it is reseated in subsequent steps (Fig 13-59).

In a dappen dish, mix acrylic resin monomer and polymer to a runny consistency. Lubricate the canal with petrolatum on a small piece of cotton on a Peeso reamer. Fill the orifice of the canal as full as possible with acrylic resin (Duralay, Reliance Dental, Worth, IL) applied with an IPPA plastic filling instrument. Coat the sprue with monomer and seat it completely in the canal. Make sure that the external bevel is covered at this time (Fig 13-60). Trying to cover the bevel later may disturb the fit of the dowel in the canal.

When the acrylic resin has become tough and doughy, pump the pattern in and out to insure that it will not lock into any undercuts in the canal. As the resin polymerizes, remove the dowel from the canal and make sure that it extends to the apical end of the prepared canal. If there

are any voids, they can be filled with a soft, dead wax, such as utility wax. Reinsert the dowel into the canal and move it up and down to insure that it can be withdrawn easily at a later time.

After the resin in the dowel portion has polymerized, relubricate the canal and reseat the dowel. Make a second mix of acrylic resin and place it around the exposed sprue to provide the bulk from which to fashion a preparation for the final restoration (Fig 13-61). While the resin is polymerizing, the coronal portion can be roughly molded on the facial and lingual aspects by holding it between the thumb and forefinger.

The core can be roughly shaped in the hand with green stones and coarse garnet discs. The preparation for the final restoration is completed with the dowel-core pattern in place (Fig 13-62). It is desirable to complete reduction and contouring in resin, because it is both difficult and time-consuming to shape the metal after the dowel core has been cast. The finished pattern should be smoothed with fine sandpaper discs and a Burlew wheel (JF Jelenko, Armonk, NY). There should be no roughness or undercuts.

Wipe the dowel-core pattern with an alcohol sponge to remove any residual lubricant that could displace investment or promote bubble formation. Either could result in metal projections that would interfere with complete seating of the cast metal dowel core.

Finishing and Cementation of the Dowel Core

The dowel-core pattern is sprued on the incisal or occlusal end (Fig 13-63). Add 1.0 to 2.0 cc of extra water

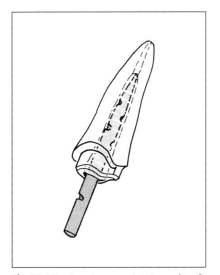

Fig 13-59 A resin sprue is trimmed to fit loosely in the canal.

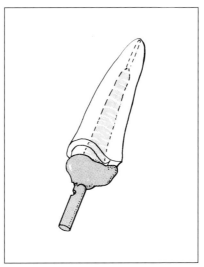

Fig 13-60 The first mix of resin in the canal should cover the contrabevel.

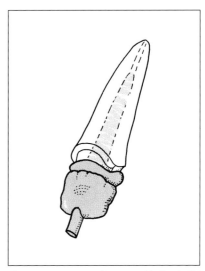

Fig 13-61 A second mix is added to build up the coronal portion of the dowel core.

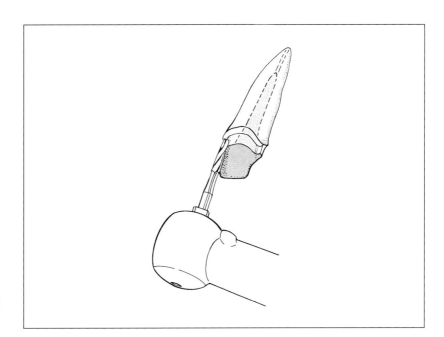

Fig 13-62 Coronal portion of the resin pattern is prepared to receive the final restoration.

to 50 g of investment, and do not use a liner in the ring. These measures will result in a slightly smaller dowel core that should have less tendency to bind in the canal. The invested pattern should remain in the burnout oven for 30 minutes longer to insure complete elimination of the resin. After the casting is removed from the investment, it is pickled and the sprue is cut off.

Check the fit of the dowel core in the tooth by seating it with light pressure. If it binds in the canal or will not seat completely, air abrade the dowel and reinsert it in the canal. Relieve any shiny spots. The core portion of the casting should be polished to a satin finish with a Burlew wheel. Cut a groove on the side of the dowel from apical end to contrabevel to provide an escape vent for cement (Fig 13-64).

Mix the cement and insert some of it in the canal with a lentulo spiral. Slowly insert the dowel core into the canal so that the excess cement may escape, allowing the dowel core to seat completely. Touch up the preparation for the final restoration, if necessary, and make the impression for it. The crown will be cemented at a subsequent appointment (Fig 13-65).

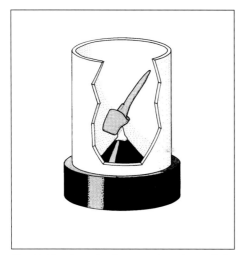

Fig 13-63   Sprued resin pattern in a ring ready for investing.

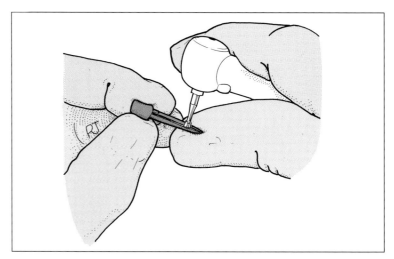

Fig 13-64   A groove is cut in the side of the dowel to allow cement to escape during cementation.

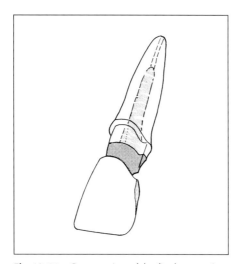

Fig 13-65   Cementation of the final restoration.

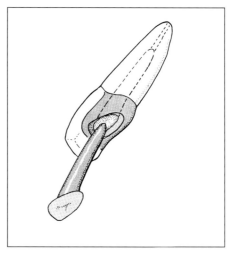

Fig 13-66   A dowel inlay is cemented through the access opening in the crown of an endodontically treated central incisor.

Cast dowel cores can be used on premolars. Mandibular premolars with a single root require no variations in procedure from dowel cores for anterior teeth. On maxillary premolars with two canals, one canal is employed for the dowel preparation, and a stabilizing keyway is placed in the other. Cast dowel-cores are very rarely done on molars, because they have divergent canals that require elaborate, interlocking multipiece castings.

A parallel pin may be added to a prefabricated resin post for antirotational stabilization and some minimal additional retention (Parapost). The canal is prepared with a special drill that is the same diameter as the dowel, and 0.6- or 0.7-mm pin holes are drilled parallel with the canal.[97] A resin core is fabricated over the parallel-sided, serrated, preformed resin post in the canal, with iridio-

platinum pins or nylon bristles in the pin holes. The pattern is invested, cast, and cemented in the same manner as a custom pattern.

If endodontic therapy must be done on a tooth after it has received a crown, the access opening will diminish crown retention by approximately 61%.[98] Placement of a *dowel inlay* has been described for stabilizing the crown.[99] A cast dowel is fabricated on a cast of the prepared tooth, with a slightly flared segment at the coronal end seating into the beveled orifice of the canal (Fig 13-66). If a tooth preparation fractures under a crown, a *retrofit dowel core* can be fabricated under the dislodged crown. The crown is cleaned out, lubricated, and used as a matrix for forming the core portion after the dowel segment of the pattern has been completed in the usual manner.[100]

References

1. Shillingburg HT, Jacobi R, Brackett SE: Preparation modifications for damaged vital posterior teeth. *Dent Clin North Am* 1985; 29:305–326.

2. Shillingburg HT, Jacobi R, Dilts WE: Preparing severely damaged teeth. *J Calif Dent Assoc* 1983; 11:85–91.

3. Rhoads JE: Preparation of the teeth for cast restorations. In Hollenback GM: *Science and Technic of the Cast Restoration.* St Louis, CV Mosby Co, 1964, pp 34–67.

4. Ingraham R, Bassett RW, Koser JR: *An Atlas of Cast Gold Procedures,* ed 2. Buena Park, CA, Uni-Tro College Press, 1969, pp 161–165.

5. Guyer SE: Multiple preparations for fixed prosthodontics. *J Prosthet Dent* 1970; 23:529–553.

6. Smith GE, Grainger DA: Biomechanical design of extensive cavity preparations for cast gold. *J Am Dent Assoc* 1974; 89:1152–1157.

7. Kishimoto M, Shillingburg HT, Duncanson MG: Influence of preparation features on retention and resistance. Part II. Three-quarter crowns. *J Prosthet Dent* 1983; 49:188–192.

8. Tjan AHL, Sarkissian R, Miller GD: Effect of multiple axial grooves on the marginal adaptation of full cast gold crowns. *J Prosthet Dent* 1981; 46:399–403.

9. Lorey RE, Myers GE: The retentive qualities of bridge retainers. *J Am Dent Assoc* 1968; 76:568–572.

10. Pruden WH: Full coverage, partial coverage, and the role of pins. *J Prosthet Dent* 1971; 26:302–306.

11. Gilboe DB, Teteruck WR: Fundamentals of extra-coronal tooth preparation. Part I. Retention and resistance form. *J Prosthet Dent* 1974; 32:651–656.

12. Ingraham R, Bassett RW, Koser JR: *An Atlas of Cast Gold Procedures,* ed 2. Buena Park, CA, Uni-Tro College Press, 1969, p 176.

13. Clyde JS, Sharkey SW: The pin ledge crown. A re-appraisal. *Br Dent J* 1978; 144:239–245.

14. Gourley JV: Favorable locations for pins in molars. *Oper Dent* 1980; 5:2–6.

15. Dilts WE, Mullaney TP: Relationship of pinhole location and tooth morphology in pin-retained silver amalgam restorations. *J Am Dent Assoc* 1968; 76:1011–1015.

16. Markley MR: Pin retained and reinforced restorations and foundations. *Dent Clin North Am* 1967; 11:229–244.

17. Shooshan ED: A pin-ledge casting technique—Its application in periodontal splinting. *Dent Clin North Am* 1960; 4:189–206.

18. Racowsky LP, Wolinsky LE: Restoring the badly broken-down tooth with esthetic partial coverage restorations. *Compend Contin Educ Dent* 1981; 2:322–335.

19. Lorey RE, Embrell KA, Myers GE: Retentive factors in pin-retained castings. *J Prosthet Dent* 1967; 17:271–276.

20. Moffa JP, Phillips RW: Retentive properties of parallel pin restorations. *J Prosthet Dent* 1967; 17:387–400.

21. Fujimoto J, Norman RD, Dykema RW, Phillips RW: A comparison of pin-retained amalgam and composite resin cores. *J Prosthet Dent* 1978; 39: 512–519.

22. Courtade GL: Pin pointers. III. Self-threading pins. *J Prosthet Dent* 1968; 20:335–338.

23. Roberts EW: Crown construction with pin reinforced amalgam. *Tex Dent J* 1963; 81:10–14.

24. Caputo AA, Standlee JP: Pins and posts—Why, when, and how. *Dent Clin North Am* 1976; 20:299–311.

25. Dilts WE, Welk DA, Stovall J: Retentive properties of pin materials in pin-retained silver amalgam restorations. *J Am Dent Assoc* 1968; 77:1085–1089.

26. DeWald JP, Arcoria CJ, Ferracane JL: Evaluation of glass-cermet cores under cast crowns. *Dent Mater* 1990; 6:129–132.

27. Shooshan ED: The full veneer cast crown. *J South Calif Dent Assoc* 1955; 23:27–38.

28. Markely MR: Pin reinforcement and retention of amalgam foundations and restorations. *J Am Dent Assoc* 1958; 56:675–679.

29. Hormati AA, Denehy GE: Microleakage of pin-retained amalgam and composite resin bases. *J Prosthet Dent* 1980; 44:526–530.

30. Oliva RA, Lowe JA: Dimensional stability of silver amalgam and composite used as core materials. *J Prosthet Dent* 1987; 57:554–559.

31. DeWald JP, Moody CR, Ferracane JL: Softening of composite resins by moisture and cements. *Quintessence Int* 1988; 19:619–621.

32. Gabryl RS, Mayhew RB, Haney SJ, Wilson AH: Effects of a temporary cementing agent on the retention of castings for composite resin cores. *J Prosthet Dent* 1985; 54:183–187.

33. Nitkin DA, Goldberg AJ: Another look at placing and polishing amalgam in one visit. *Quintessence Int* 1983; 14:507–512.

34. Outhwaite WC, Twiggs SW, Fairhurst CW, King GE: Slots vs. pins: A comparison of retention under simulated chewing stresses. *J Dent Res* 1982; 61:400–402.

35. Shavell HM: The amalgapin technique for complex amalgam restorations. *J Calif Dent Assoc* 1980; 8:48–55.

36. Eissmann HF, Radke RA: Post-endodontic restoration. In Cohen S, Burns RC: *Pathways of the Pulp.* St Louis, CV Mosby Co, 1976, pp 537–575.

37. Dilts WE: Pulpal considerations with fixed prosthodontic procedures. *Quintessence Int* 1982; 13:1287–1294.

38. Ingber JS, Rose LF, Coslet JG: The "biologic width"—A concept in periodontics and restorative dentistry. *Alpha Omegan* 1977; 10:62–65.

39. Murrin JR, Barkmeier WW: Restoration of mutilated posterior teeth: Periodontal, restorative, and endodontic considerations. *Oper Dent* 1981; 6:90–94.

40. Ingraham R: The application of sound biomechanical principles in the design of inlay, amalgam, and gold foil restorations. *J Am Dent Assoc* 1950; 40:402–413.

41. Holland CS: Cast gold restorations for teeth with large carious lesions. *Br Dent J* 1971; 131:16–21.

42. Reagan SE: Correcting space loss caused by severe decay: Report of a case. *J Am Dent Assoc* 1988; 116:878–879.

43. Heithersay GS: Combined endodontic-orthodontic treatment of transverse root fractures in the region of the alveolar crest. *Oral Surg Oral Med Oral Pathol* 1973; 36: 404–415.

44. Ingber JS: Forced eruption. Part II. A method of treating nonrestorable teeth—Periodontal and restorative considerations. *J Periodontol* 1976; 47:203–216.

45. Simon JHS, Kelly WH, Gordon DG, Ericksen GW: Extrusion of endodontically treated teeth. *J Am Dent Assoc* 1978; 97:17–23.

46. Ivey DW, Calhoun RL, Kemp WB, Dorfman HS, Wheless JE: Orthodontic extrusion: Its use in restorative dentistry. *J Prosthet Dent* 1980; 43: 401–407.

Preparations for Extensively Damaged Teeth

47. Ross S, Dorfman HS, Palcanis KG: Orthodontic extrusion: A multidisciplinary treatment approach. *J Am Dent Assoc* 1981; 102:189–191.

48. Oesterle LJ, Wood LW: Raising the root—A look at orthodontic extrusion. *J Am Dent Assoc* 1991; 122:193–198.

49. Reis BJ, Johnson GK, Nieberg LG: Vertical extrusion using a removable orthodontic appliance. *J Am Dent Assoc* 1988; 116:521–523.

50. Ingber JS: Forced eruption. Part II. A method of treating isolated one or two wall infrabony osseous defects—Rationale and case report. *J Periodontol* 1974; 45:199–206.

51. Garrett GB: Forced eruption in the treatment of transverse root fractures. *J Am Dent Assoc* 1985; 111:270–272.

52. Biggerstaff RH, Sinks JH, Carazola JL: Orthodontic extrusion and biologic width realignment procedures: Methods for reclaiming nonrestorable teeth. *J Am Dent Assoc* 1986; 112:345–348.

53. Johnson GK, Sivers JE: Forced eruption in crown lengthening procedures. *J Prosthet Dent* 1986; 56: 424–427.

54. Molina DG, Miller CS: An esthetic extrusion device. *Gen Dent* 1987; 35:43–45.

55. Ross IF: Fracture susceptibility of endodontically treated teeth. *J Endod* 1980; 6:560–565.

56. Sorensen JA, Martinoff JT: Clinically significant factors in dowel design. *J Prosthet Dent* 1984; 52:28–35.

57. Goerig AC, Mueninghoff LA: Management of the endodontically treated tooth. Part I. Concept for restorative designs. *J Prosthet Dent* 1983; 49:340–345.

58. Shillingburg HT, Kessler JC: After the root canal—Principles of restoring endodontically treated teeth. *Okla Dent Assoc J* 1984; 74:19–24.

59. Halpern BG: Restoration of endodontically treated teeth—A conservative approach. *Dent Clin North Am* 1985; 29:293–303.

60. Lovdahl PE, Nicholls JI: Pin-retained amalgam cores vs. cast-gold dowel-cores. *J Prosthet Dent* 1977; 38:507–514.

61. Gelfand M, Goldman M, Sunderman EJ: Effect of complete veneer crowns on the compressive strength of endodontically treated teeth. *J Prosthet Dent* 1984; 52:635–638.

62. Nathanson D, Ashayeri N: New aspects of restoring the endodontically treated tooth. *Alpha Omegan* 1990; 83:76–80.

63. Standlee JP, Caputo AA, Collard EW, Pollack MH: Analysis of stress distribution by endodontic posts. *Oral Surg* 1972; 33:952–960.

64. Colley IT, Hampson EL, Lehman ML: Retention of post crowns: An assessment of the relative efficiency of posts in different shapes and sizes. *Br Dent J* 1968; 124:63–69.

65. Krupp JD, Caputo AA, Trabert KC, Standlee JP: Dowel retention with glass ionomer cement. *J Prosthet Dent* 1979; 41:163–166.

66. Johnson JK, Sakumura JS: Dowel form and tensile force. *J Prosthet Dent* 1978; 40:645–649.

67. Standlee JP, Caputo AA, Hanson EC: Retention of endodontic dowels: Effects of cement, dowel length, diameter and design. *J Prosthet Dent* 1978; 39:401–405.

68. Sorensen JA, Martinoff JT: Intracoronal reinforcement and coronal coverage: A study of endodontically treated teeth. *J Prosthet Dent* 1984; 51:780–784.

69. Frank AL: Protective coronal coverage of the pulpless tooth. *J Am Dent Assoc* 1959; 59:895–900.

70. Gutmann JL: The dentin-root complex: Anatomic and biologic considerations in restoring endodontically treated teeth. *J Prosthet Dent* 1992; 67:458–467.

71. Rud J, Omnell K-A: Root fractures due to corrosion—Diagnostic aspects. *Scand J Dent Res* 1970; 78:397–403.

72. Rosen H: Operative procedures on mutilated endodontically treated teeth. *J Prosthet Dent* 1961; 11:973–986.

73. Hoag EP, Dwyer TG: A comparative evaluation of three post and core techniques. *J Prosthet Dent* 1982; 47:177–181.

74. Sorensen JA, Engelman MJ: Ferrule design and fracture resistance of endodontically treated teeth. *J Prosthet Dent* 1990; 63:529–536.

75. Milot P, Stein RS: Root fracture in endodontically treated teeth related to post selection and crown design. *J Prosthet Dent* 1992; 68:428–435.

76. Kratochvil FJ: *Partial Removable Prosthodontics.* Philadelphia, WB Saunders Co, 1988, p 101.

77. Sorensen JA, Martinoff JT: Endodontically treated teeth as abutments. *J Prosthet Dent* 1985; 53:631–636.

78. Colman HL: Restoration of endodontically treated teeth. *Dent Clin North Am* 1979; 23:647–662.

79. Nayyar A, Walton RE, Leonard LA: An amalgam coronal-radicular dowel and core technique for endodontically treated posterior teeth. *J Prosthet Dent* 1980; 43:511–515.

80. Goerig AC, Mueninghoff LA: Management of the endodontically treated tooth. Part II. Technique. *J Prosthet Dent* 1983; 49:491–497.

81. Baum L: Dowel placement in the endodontically treated tooth. *J Conn State Dent Assoc* 1979;53:116–117.

82. Kovarik RE, Breeding LC, Caughman WF: Fatigue life of three core materials under simulated chewing conditions. *J Prosthet Dent* 1992; 68:584–590.

83. Christian GW, Button GL, Moon PC, England MC, Douglas HB: Post core restoration in endodontically treated posterior teeth. *J Endod* 1981; 7:182–185

84. Kern SB, von Fraunhofer JA, Mueninghoff LA: An in vitro comparison of two dowel and core techniques for endodontically treated molars. *J Prosthet Dent* 1984; 51:509–514.

85. Wirz J, Graber G, Widmer W: *Metallische Verankerungselemente in der Restaurativen Zahnmedizin.* Berlin, Quintessenz Verlag, 1987, pp 41, 51, 66, 105.

86. Standlee JP, Caputo AA, Holcomb J, Trabert KC: The retentive and stress-distributing properties of a threaded endodontic dowel. *J Prosthet Dent* 1980; 44:398–404.

87. Standlee JP, Caputo AA: The retentive and stress–distributing properties of split threaded endodontic dowels. *J Prosthet Dent* 1992; 68:436–442.

88. Fisher DW, Jeannet DJ, Kwan SK: An evaluation of methods for preparing teeth to receive retentiveposts [abstract 532]. *J Dent Res* 1982; 61:237.

89. Gegauff AG, Kerby RE, Rosenstiel SF: A comparative study of post preparation diameters and deviations using Parapost and Gates Glidden drills. *J Endod* 1988; 14:377–380.

90. Goldman M, DeVitre R, Tenca J: Cement distribution and bond strength in cemented posts. *J Dent Res* 1984; 63:1392–1395.

91. Christy JM, Pipko DS: Fabrication of dual-post veneer crown. *J Am Dent Assoc* 1967; 75:1419–1425.

92. Gerstein J, Burnell SC: Prefabricated precision dowels. *J Am Dent Assoc* 1964; 68:787–791.

93. Taylor AG: Dowel abutment crown. *Royal Canad Dent Corps Quart* 1963; 4:1–4.

94. Bartlett SO: Construction of detached core crowns for pulpless teeth in only two sittings. *J Am Dent Assoc* 1968; 77:843–845.

208

95. Dewhirst RB, Fisher DW, Shillingburg HT: Dowel-core fabrication. *J South Calif Dent Assoc* 1969; 37:444–449.

96. Shillingburg HT, Fisher DW, Dewhirst RB: Restoration of endodontically treated posterior teeth. *J Prosthet Dent* 1970; 24:401–409.

97. Baraban DJ: A simplified method for making posts and cores. *J Prosthet Dent* 1970; 24:287–297.

98. McMullen AF, Himel VT, Sarkar NK: An in vitro study of the effect endodontic access preparation has upon the retention of porcelain fused to metal crowns of maxillary central incisors. *J Endod* 1989; 15:154–156.

99. Shillingburg HT, Kessler JC: Restoration of crowned teeth after endodontic treatment. *Quintessence Int* 1982; 13:635–641.

100. Shillingburg HT, Jacobi R: Two-piece retrofit dowel-core: A case report. *Int J Periodont Rest Dent* 1987; 7:31–41.

Chapter 14

Preparations for Periodontally Weakened Teeth

Teeth that have been saved by periodontal therapy often need cast restorations. This may occur because of caries or previous damage, or the teeth may need to be splinted together to improve their stability. These teeth also may be needed as abutments for prostheses replacing missing teeth.

Preparation Finish Line

Restoration of a tooth around which there has been a loss of gingival height or other change in gingival architecture frequently requires modification of the tooth preparation. The type and location of the finish line may have a significant impact on the success of the restoration. An improperly designed preparation can unnecessarily damage the tooth and potentially compromise the longevity of the restoration and of the tooth itself. The proximity of the preparation finish line to the furcations can necessitate even further modification of the tooth preparation.

Location

The optimum location for the gingival finish line of a crown preparation is on enamel, away from the gingival sulcus. However, it is frequently necessary for the restoration margin to extend apically to cover an expanse of root surface that may have been affected by caries or erosion.

If an all-ceramic shoulder is used as the gingivofacial margin for a metal-ceramic crown, a 1.0-mm-wide shoulder will be required as the gingival finish line. This configuration is destructive under the best of circumstances when it is placed in the enamel of the clinical crown (Fig 14-1). Nevertheless, it is generally well-tolerated in mature teeth.

A shoulder is a poor choice when the margin must be placed on the root surface. The constricted, smaller diameter of the root will require that the axial reduction be extended into the tooth to a pulp-threatening depth to achieve the same 1.0-mm-wide shoulder (Fig 14-2). Aside from possible pulpal encroachment, this gross destruction of axial tooth structure weakens the natural structural durability of the tooth. Additionally, the shoulder has a greater potential for concentrating stresses that could ultimately lead to fracture of the tooth.

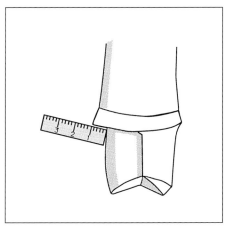

Fig 14-1 Preparation for a metal-ceramic crown on a maxillary premolar with a 1.0-mm shoulder in the usual position.

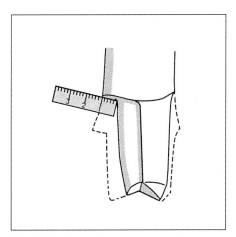

Fig 14-2 Preparation for a metal-ceramic crown on a maxillary premolar with a 1.0-mm shoulder apical to the CEJ. Notice the additional destruction of axial tooth structure required to produce the shoulder at this level.

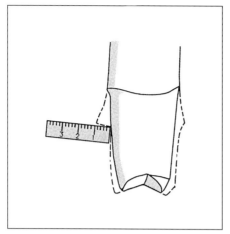

Fig 14-3 Preparation for a metal-ceramic crown on a maxillary premolar with a chamfer apical to the CEJ. The amount of axial reduction is similar to that required for a shoulder at the usual position.

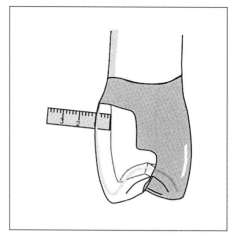

Fig 14-4 Wide gingival collar is used to blend the root contour with that required for a ceramic veneer of adequate thickness.

A chamfer finish line on the facial surface in this apical position will result in approximately the same depth of axial reduction as would a shoulder at the usual level (Fig 14-3). A metal-ceramic crown fabricated in such circumstances should have a wide metal gingival collar (Fig 14-4). Extension of the ceramic veneer to the gingival margin will create overcontouring or will require use of the more destructive shoulder.

Furcation Flutes

Sometimes the crown margins on a molar must extend far enough apically that the preparation finish line approaches the *furcation,* where the common root trunk divides into two or three roots (Fig 14-5). The designs of both the tooth preparations and the crowns for these teeth must be different from those customarily used. This is caused by the intersection of the preparation finish line with the vertical *flutes* or concavities in the common root trunk, extending from the actual furcation in the direction of the cementoenamel junction. When that occurs, the axial surface(s) of the tooth preparation occlusal to the inversion of the gingival finish line must also have vertical concavities or flutes[1] (Fig 14-6).

Examples can be seen in the mandibular furcation, which is frequently encountered by crown preparations that do not extend very far apically. The entrances to the facial and lingual furcations are 3 and 4 mm apical to the cementoenamel junction on mandibular first molars.[2] On the mesial, facial, and distal surfaces of maxillary first molars the furcation entrances are 3.6, 4.2, and 4.8 mm from the cementoenamel junction, respectively.[3] The flutes on a maxillary molar are seen less frequently, and their presence often is an indication of greater gingival recession and vertical bone loss.

The axial contours of crowns placed on teeth whose

furcation flutes are intercepted by preparation finish lines must likewise reflect the concavity rising from the furcation flute (Fig 14-7). The artificial crown should recreate the contours of the furcation flute and not follow the original crown contours.[4] The facial surface should be invaginated into a concavity above the bifurcation that extends occlusally until it meets the facial groove in the occlusal one-third of the facial surface.[5] The concavities usually merge with features originating on the occlusal surface. There must be no interruption in the vertical concavity rising at the margin of the restoration. Any horizontal ridge on the facial or lingual surface of the tooth that intersects with this concavity and blocks it will result in a plaque-retaining area (Fig 14-8).

There also will be concavities on the mesial and distal aspects of a maxillary molar arising from their respective furcations. They should be "softened" or blended into the surrounding axial surfaces of the crown. This will minimize the difficulty of cleaning those areas in the less accessible lingual embrasures of the posterior segments of the maxillary arch.

Root Resection

Root resection is a procedure in which the root is removed, irrespective of what is done with the crown.[1] The resection of a root also may be called a radectomy.[6] *Root amputation* is removal of a root without touching the crown.[1] A *hemisection* is a procedure in which the tooth is separated through the crown and the furcation,[1,7] producing two essentially equal-sized teeth. Although the widespread use of these procedures is fairly recent, similar procedures were described in the literature more than 100 years ago by Farrar,[8] Black,[9] and Tomes and Tomes.[10]

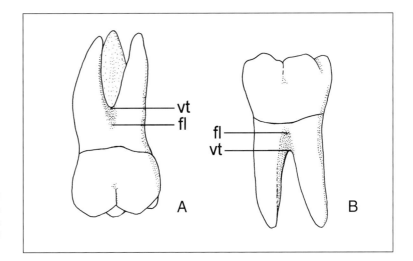

Fig 14-5 Facial furcations for a maxillary (A) and a mandibular (B) first molar. The portion of the furcation facing apically or toward the bone is the vault (vt), or roof. The vertical concavity on the common root trunk is the flute (fl).

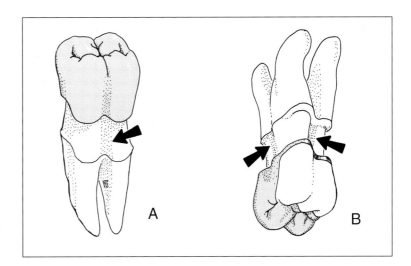

Fig 14-6 Vertical concavities in the axial walls of the tooth preparations *(arrows)* extend occlusally from the invaginations where the finish lines cross the furcation flutes on a mandibular (A) and a maxillary (B) molar.

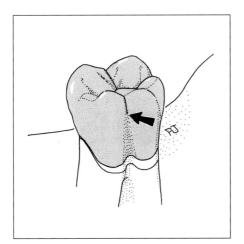

Fig 14-7 Anatomic facial groove of this mandibular first molar merges *(arrow)* with the vertical concavity extending from the furcation flute.

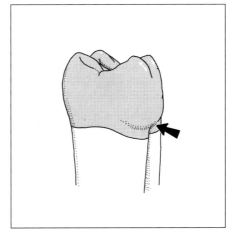

Fig 14-8 A horizontal ridge in the gingival third of the axial surface above the furcation flute will create a plaque-retaining area that is difficult to keep clean *(arrow)*.

Indications

One or more roots of a molar may be removed to eradicate areas of the tooth that create problems in the maintenance of good hygiene and plaque control. A root or roots can be eliminated because of an invasion or uncovering of the furcation by severe vertical bone loss.[7,11-13] The severe loss of bone or attachment around one root may also necessitate the removal of a root.[1,14-16] The concept of "periodontal strategic extraction" may simplify the periodontal treatment of an entire quadrant.[17] It also reduces the risk of extension of the lesion to the surviving roots of that tooth or to neighboring teeth.

In 58% of the maxillary and mandibular first molars examined by Bower,[18] furcation entrances were narrower than the width of the smallest curettes available. When the furcation entrance is that narrow, maintenance may be compromised by instrument inaccessibility, and resection may be the only way to create an area that can be adequately cleaned. Root removal can aid in reestablishing furcation control[15] by changing furcation anatomy to facilitate cleaning.[19]

Nevertheless, involvement of a furcation does not automatically require resection of a root. Hamp et al[20] reported a clinical study of 100 patients with 175 multirooted teeth afflicted with varying degrees of salvageable furcation involvement. About half were treated with root resection, while the others received scaling and root planing, furcation operations, or other procedures. Both groups retained all of their teeth during the 5-year period of the study. The actual percentages will vary among practitioners based on individual philosophies, patient acceptance, and a number of other factors.

Resection may be performed to salvage teeth with endodontic problems.[1,6,11-13,15,16] These encompass a wide variety of situations including perforations, irretrievable broken instruments, anatomic anomalies that would prevent successful instrumentation or obturation of a canal, and other nonspecific failures.

A tooth that has other sound roots can be saved by removing a root that has fractured,[11,13,16] or one afflicted with untreatable caries[14-16] that extends into it. Root resection is also done where roots of two adjacent teeth are in such close proximity that embrasure space is obliterated.[1,11,13,15] Resection of a root on one tooth may facilitate retention of both teeth. Indeed, the removal of a particular root may be accomplished as much to improve the prognosis of an adjacent tooth as that of the tooth being sectioned.

Contraindications

Fused roots,[11] or those that approximate other roots of the same tooth[15] are contraindicated for resections. If the furcation is too far apical, roots cannot be resected because there will be too little bone left to support the remaining roots.[11] The furcation must be in the coronal one-third to do a hemisection on a mandibular molar, and resections cannot be done on maxillary first premolars.[19]

If excessive alveolar support has been lost uniformly around all of the roots, nothing is gained by removing a root. The remaining roots will have no better support than the one removed. A root resection also may not be used if the root that is to be kept cannot be successfully treated endodontically.

Capacity of Resected Roots

Teeth that have been resected can be used as abutment teeth for fixed partial dentures, splints, or vertical stops for cantilever fixed partial dentures.[21] The retention of a strategic tooth by root resection may preclude the need for a removable partial denture.[22] Keep in mind, however, that their load-bearing ability has been lessened by their diminished attachment area. As the level of bone is lowered by periodontal disease, the surface area of periodontal attachment diminishes (Fig 14-9).

The mesial root of a mandibular first molar provides 37% of the attachment surface area and the distal provides 32%.[23] If the furcation is uncovered, 31% of the attachment area, which is imparted by the root trunk, has been lost. The mesiofacial, distofacial, and palatal roots of a maxillary first molar furnish 25%, 19%, and 24% of the attachment area, respectively.[24] The root trunk supplies 32% of the attachment for the tooth.

Removal of a corresponding root on a second molar will probably result in a similar percentage loss of support. However, the length of the root trunks of second molars tends to be both more variable and somewhat greater than that of first molars.[2] The total root surface areas of first and second molars differ by only 0.5% to 1.2%.[25]

Resection Technique

It is usually desirable to complete endodontic treatment before removing the root,[6,11,13-15,19] since a root canal will be transected during the surgery. However, often it is not possible to adequately evaluate the extent of furcation involvement until the flap has been reflected to permit a direct visual examination.[20] To avoid possible misunderstandings over the time, discomfort, and expense of a "needless" endodontic procedure on a tooth that cannot be saved because of the inability to separate the targeted root from the others, it is often necessary to do the resection first. The pulp should be protected by a provisional restoration, and endodontic therapy should be scheduled as soon as possible.

Begin the resection with a long, thin diamond to cut through the vault of the furcation.[15] Remove all traces of the resected root at the time of surgery. Do not leave any vestigial remnants of the furcation vault. They will act much as overhanging crown margins would, interfering

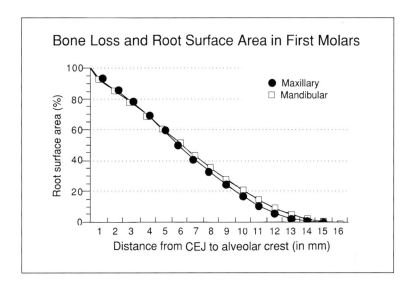

Fig 14-9 Relationship between vertical bone loss and the root surface area of maxillary[3] and mandibular[23] first molars.

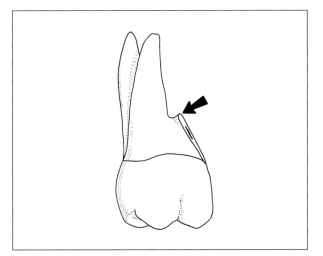

Fig 14-10 Any remnant of the resected root that is left *(arrow)* will impede plaque removal.

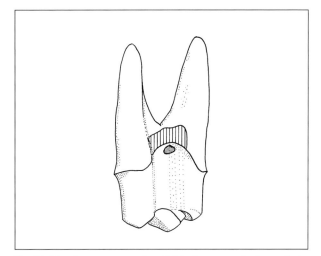

Fig 14-11 Crown preparation finish line extends beyond the pulp chamber *(small shaded area)*, but it need not encompass the entire root removal site *(cross-hatched area)*. Shown is a preparation on a maxillary molar with a resected distofacial root.

with plaque removal and increasing tissue inflammation (Fig 14-10).

If any ridges are discovered at the time the tooth is prepared for a crown, they should be smoothed over. An *intermediate bifurcational ridge* is present in 73% of mandibular first molars,[26] and there is a "bridge" of tooth structure connecting the distofacial and palatal roots of maxillary molars.[15] The finish line of the crown preparation should extend apically beyond the obturated pulp chamber (Fig 14-11). It is neither necessary nor desirable to extend the preparation finish line far enough apically to cover all areas of the root whose configuration has been altered by root removal.

If the root of a maxillary molar is being resected for periodontal reasons, there is usually enough coronal tooth structure so that the pulp chamber need only be filled with amalgam. A dowel is frequently not needed in this situation and might actually weaken a thin, isolated root rather than strengthen it.

If a dowel core is required because of coronal damage, a custom cast dowel core is preferable to a prefabricated dowel.[27] The minimal diameter of a periodontally weakened, root-resected segment does not permit a sufficient bulk of core material to remain around the dowel when the crown preparation is done.

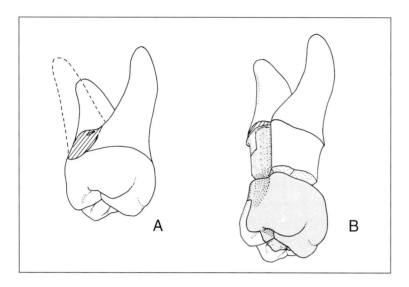

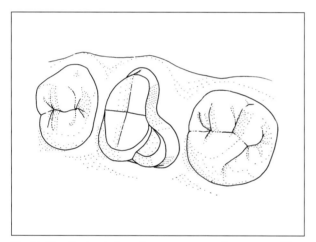

Fig 14-12 Proper contours for a distofacial root resection on a maxillary molar after the surrounding area has been smoothed (A). A metal-ceramic crown is fabricated for the preparation after a core is placed (B). The preparation does not cover all of the cut root surface.

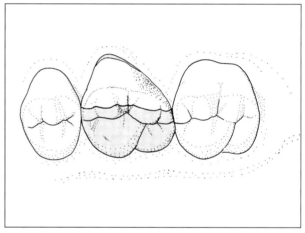

Fig 14-13 Occlusal view of a crown preparation on a maxillary first molar with no distofacial root.

Fig 14-14 Occlusal view of a metal-ceramic crown on a maxillary molar without a distofacial root.

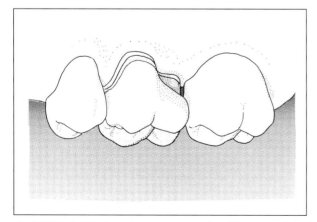

Fig 14-15 Facial view of a crown on a molar with a resected distofacial root. Note the pronounced concavity in the distogingival area.

Tooth Preparation and Crown Configuration

When a root has been removed from a tooth, both the tooth preparation and the contours of the crown will be different because of the altered tooth shape.

Maxillary Distofacial Root. The distal furcation of the maxillary first molar is susceptible to frequent periodontal involvement because of the proximity of the divergent distofacial root to the nearby second molar[2] and its inaccessibility to the patient. The distofacial root of a maxillary molar is the one that is most frequently removed[28] (Fig 14-12). Because the distofacial root is a relatively small one, the occlusal outline of the resulting preparation commonly resembles a lamb chop when viewed from the occlusal direction (Fig 14-13).

The completed restoration placed in this situation usually will not restore the complete occlusal outline of the

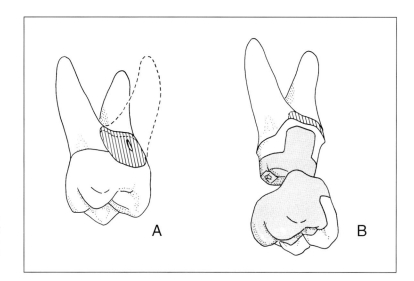

Fig 14-16 Mesiofacial root resection on a maxillary molar after the area surrounding the root attachment has been contoured (A). A metal-ceramic crown is used to restore the tooth after a core is placed (B).

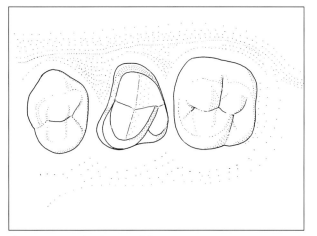

Fig 14-17 Occlusal view of the crown preparation on a maxillary molar with a resected mesiofacial root.

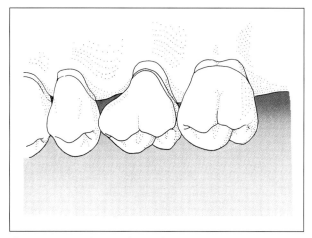

Fig 14-18 Facial view of a metal-ceramic crown on a maxillary molar whose mesiofacial root has been removed.

intact tooth. The distofacial embrasure is larger than usual, enabling the patient to keep the area clean (Fig 14-14). Making the distofacial cusp smaller generally does not create an esthetics problem, because the distofacial cusp is hidden by the mesiofacial cusp in normal tooth alignment.

The proximal contact is restored to its normal faciolingual size. In the finished restoration, it is important that the contours of the distofacial cusp apical to the contact area have a definite concave shape[15] (Fig 14-15). This insures that crown contours will be aligned with the root configuration in that critical area, preventing impingement on the gingiva.

Maxillary Mesiofacial Root. Loss of the mesiofacial root (Fig 14-16) represents a greater loss of support for the remaining tooth than does the loss of the distofacial root. The mesiofacial root accounts for 25% to 36% of the first molar root area, depending upon the amount of loss of bone around the root trunk.[23] If the mesiofacial root must be removed, the resulting occlusal outline tends to be more triangular in configuration because of the greater faciolingual dimension of the root that has been removed (Fig 14-17). Again, the finish line will extend apically past the pulp chamber, but it will not include all of the area where the mesiofacial root was removed. There will be a concavity gingivofacial to the proximal contact on the mesial surface of the crown (Fig 14-18).

Maxillary Palatal Root. In those situations where the palatal root has been removed from a maxillary molar, the palatal surface of the preparation will be flat, reflecting the general configuration of the remaining root stump (Fig 14-19). The tooth preparation will have an abbreviated faciolingual dimension. The central groove of the preparation is aligned with those of the occlusal surfaces

217

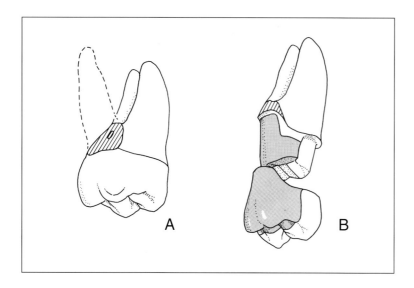

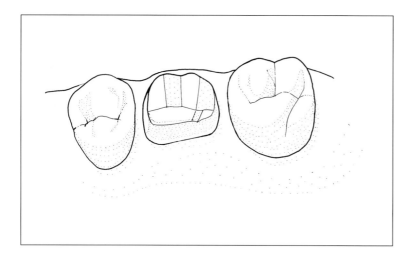

Fig 14-19 Area surrounding the root attachment of the palatal root of a maxillary molar after removal and smoothing (A). The tooth is restored with a metal-ceramic crown after it is built up with a core (B).

Fig 14-20 Occlusal view of a crown preparation on a maxillary molar with no palatal root.

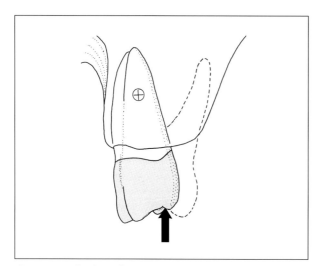

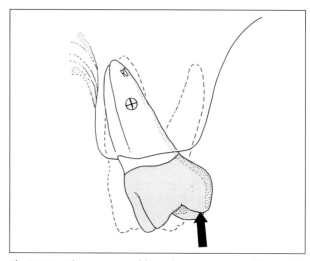

Fig 14-21 The lingual cusp on a crown made for a maxillary molar without a palatal root is very small.

Fig 14-22 The presence of lingual cusps on a maxillary molar deprived of the support of its palatal root would subject the tooth to torquing forces (arrow) that could tip the tooth lingually.

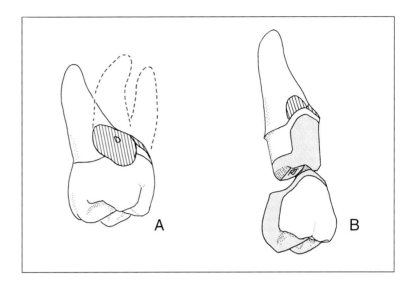

Fig 14-23 Correct contours for the attachment sites of the facial roots of a maxillary molar after resection and smoothing (A). A crown is placed over the preparation after core fabrication (B).

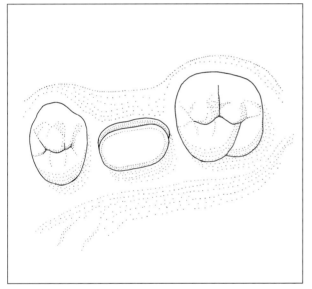

Fig 14-24 Occlusal view of a crown preparation on a palatal root reflects the cross-sectional shape of the root.

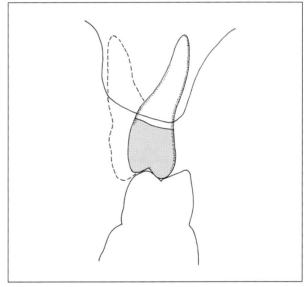

Fig 14-25 Occlusal contacts should occur on the lingual cusp tip. There should be minimal occlusion facial to the central groove of the crown.

of adjacent teeth (Fig 14-20). The facial cusps of the preparation will be near normal faciolingually. The lingual cusps will be quite small, possibly little more than a narrow ledge lingual to the central groove.

The preparation and resulting restoration usually will have a distinct concave flute on the facial surface arising from the facial bifurcation. Essentially there will be no lingual cusp[15] (Fig 14-21). The presence of lingual cusps would produce an area inaccessible to hygiene maintenance in the linguogingival segment of the crown. It would also create a severe torquing moment on the tooth, which could either tip the tooth lingually or fracture the tooth preparation under the crown (Fig 14-22).

Maxillary Facial Roots. When both of the maxillary facial roots are removed, only the palatal root remains (Fig 14-23). Preparation of the tooth overlying this root will result in either an oval or a circular configuration depending upon the shape of the root itself (Fig 14-24). The resulting crown should occlude with its mandibular counterpart in such a way that occlusal forces cannot be directed facially. This will place it in a near reverse occlusal or cross-bite relationship[15] (Fig 14-25).

Mandibular Hemisection. When separating the roots of mandibular molars, the possibilities are fewer since there are only two roots. Frequently one root is removed while the other remains. Saving the mesial segment

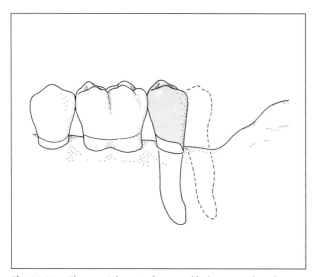

Fig 14-26 The mesial root of a mandibular second molar can effectively extend the occluding segment of the mandibular arch to serve as a stop for the opposing occlusion.

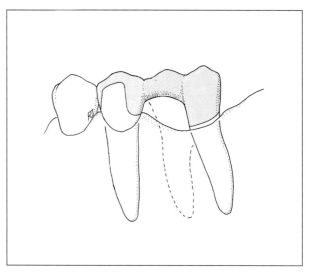

Fig 14-27 The distal root of a mandibular molar can serve as an abutment for a short-span prosthesis replacing the resected mesial root.

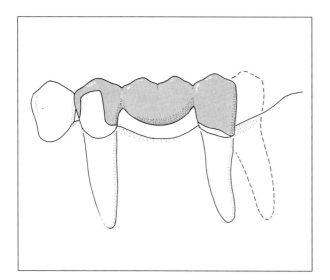

Fig 14-28 The mesial root of a mandibular second molar can be the abutment for a molar replacement fixed partial denture, but it offers less than one-third of the support of an unresected molar.

would be desirable if the molar in question were the last tooth in the arch (Fig 14-26) and the opposing teeth did not extend very far distal to the mandibular first molar. The distal root could be used as an abutment for a short-span fixed partial denture replacing the mesial root (Fig 14-27). Occasionally the one root may be used as the distal abutment for a longer-span fixed partial denture, replacing an entire molar (Fig 14-28). This must be viewed as a high-risk prosthesis, since the remaining distal root has slightly less than one-third of the alveolar support of the intact tooth with normal bone.[23]

If an effort is made to save both roots of the molar following the resection, the process is described as "bicuspidization."[16] If both roots are maintained, it is important that they be separated from each other to allow normal gingival embrasure spaces. Sometimes the roots are distinctly separate, angling out from the furcation and providing the separation naturally. However, if they are not naturally separated, some measure must be taken to accomplish it, or the crowns placed over those roots will have no embrasure space. The result will be a proximal contact that extends subgingivally to the marginal ridge.

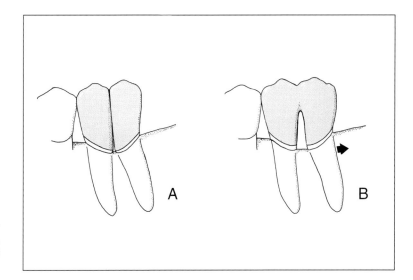

Fig 14-29 If the roots are not separated after resection, there will be no gingival embrasure (A). Orthodontic movement is one way of achieving separation (B).

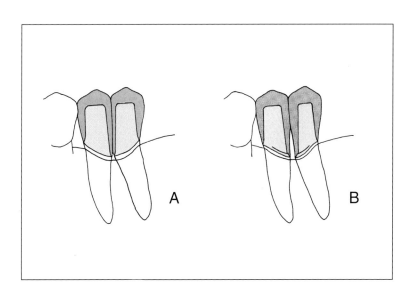

Fig 14-30 The contact that obliterates the gingival embrasures of restorations placed on a hemisected molar (A) can be alleviated in some cases by placing shoulders on the interradicular segments of the preparation that face each other across the former furcation (B).

The prognosis for teeth restored in such a manner is extremely poor. Separation may be accomplished by moving the roots apart orthodontically (Fig 14-29), or it may be accomplished with interradicular shoulders on the crown preparations on the separated roots[15] (Fig 14-30).

"Skyfurcation." Occasionally it may be desirable to separate the roots of a maxillary molar without removing a root. This is possible only if the roots are long, well-supported by bone, and distinctly separate. The roots are cut apart (Fig 14-31) and then rejoined by a "crown" that in reality is a very short interradicular splint with concave connectors from one root to the other. The occlusal configuration of the splint, or "crown," is pretty much that of an ordinary molar. This procedure, in effect, makes the furcation metal and moves it occlusally while separating the roots (Fig 14-32). This improves access to the furcation and protects a caries-prone area.[14,20]

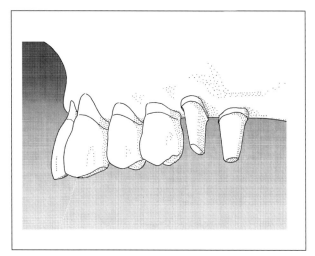

Fig 14-31 Roots of one tooth can be separated and prepared as individual teeth.

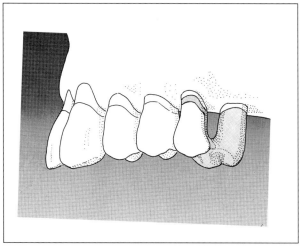

Fig 14-32 The crown placed over these resected roots reestablishes the furcation(s) in metal.

Success and Failure

Root resection does not guarantee success (Table 14-1). Ehrlich et al[29] reported an 87% success rate in furcation-involved teeth treated by root resection after 10 to 18 years. Ross and Thompson,[30] on the other hand, published a similar success rate (88%) for furcation-involved molars that were treated conservatively without root resection (Table 14-2). Hamp and associates[20] reported being able to maintain all 87 of the resected teeth in their study over a 5-year period, but they claimed equal success with 88 furcation-involved teeth that were kept intact over the same time period.

Langer et al[31] found that failures usually occurred 5 to 10 years after treatment, with 55% of the failures occurring in 5 to 7 years. The failure is more likely to be endodontic or restorative than periodontal in nature. This usually means that a root will fracture.

Mandibular roots are more likely to fail than maxillary roots. This probably is explained by the fact that resection of mandibular teeth always creates single-rooted segments. In the maxillary arch, a root resection will usually leave a tooth with two roots, providing it with additional support as well as stability.

Successful restoration of periodontally weakened teeth is aided by creating an occlusal scheme with canine-protected articulation, decreased vertical overlap, and flattened posterior cusps.[32]

Table 14-1 *Success Rates of Root Resection*

Years	Number of teeth	Percent success	Investigator
1–10	45	93	Bergenholtz[6]
5	87	100	Hamp et al[20]
1–7	34	97	Klavan[27]
10	100	62	Langer et al[31]
1–7	34	79	Erpenstein[12]
10–18	75	87	Ehrlich et al[29]
1–24	375	84	OVERALL

Table 14-2 *Success Rates of Nonresection Methods*

Years	Number of teeth	Percent success	Investigator
5–24	341	88	Ross and Thompson[30]
5	88	100	Hamp et al[20]
5–24	429	90	OVERALL

References

1. Appleton IE: Restoration of root-resected teeth. *J Prosthet Dent* 1980; 44:150–153.

2. Gher ME, Vernino AR: Root morphology–Clinical significance in pathogenesis and treatment of periodontal disease. *J Am Dent Assoc* 1980; 101:627–633.

3. Gher ME, Dunlap RW: Linear variation of the root surface area of the maxillary first molar. *J Periodontol* 1985; 56:39–43.

4. Yuodelis RA, Weaver JD, Sapkos S: Facial and lingual contours of artificial complete crown restorations and their effect on the periodontium. *J Prosthet Dent* 1973; 29:61–66.

5. Eissman HF, Radke RA, Noble WH: Physiologic design criteria for fixed dental restorations. *Dent Clin North Am* 1971; 15:543–568.

6. Bergenholtz A: Radectomy of multirooted teeth. *J Am Dent Assoc* 1972; 85:870–875.

7. Amen CR: Hemisection and root amputation. *J Periodontol* 1966; 4:197–204.

8. Farrar JN: Radical and heroic treatment of alveolar abcess by amputation of roots of teeth. *Dent Cosmos* 1884; 26:79–81.

9. Black GV. In Litch WF: *The American System of Dentistry,* vol 1. Philadelphia, Lea Brothers, 1886, p 997.

10. Tomes J, Tomes CS: *Dental Surgery,* ed 3. Philadelphia, P. Blakeston & Son, 1887, p 526.

11. Basaraba N: Root amputation and tooth hemisection. *Dent Clin North Am* 1969; 13:121–132.

12. Erpenstein H: 3-Year study of hemisectioned molars. *J Clin Periodontol* 1983; 10:1–10.

13. Marin C, Carnevale G, De Febo G, Fuzzi M: Restoration of endodontically treated teeth with interradicular lesions before root removal and/or root separation. *Int J Periodont Rest Dent* 1989; 9:43–57.

14. Rosen H, Gitnick PJ: Separation and splinting of the roots of multirooted teeth. *J Prosthet Dent* 1969; 21:34–38.

15. Abrams L, Trachtenberg DI: Hemisection—Technique and restoration. *Dent Clin North Am* 1974; 18:415–444.

16. Grant DA, Stern IB, Listgarten MA: *Periodontics,* ed 6. St Louis, CV Mosby Co, 1988, pp 921–949.

17. Amsterdam M, Rossman SR: Technique of hemisection of multirooted teeth. *Alpha Omegan* 1960; 53:4–15.

18. Bower RC: Furcation morphology relative to periodontal treatment—Furcation entrance architecture. *J Periodontol* 1979; 50:23–27.

19. Staffileno HJ: Surgical management of the furca invasion. *Dent Clin North Am* 1969; 13:103–119.

20. Hamp S-E, Nyman S, Lindhe J: Periodontal treatment of multirooted teeth. *J Clin Periodontol* 1975; 2:126–135.

21. Reinhardt RA, Sivers JE: Management of class III furcally involved abutments for fixed prosthodontic restorations. *J Prosthet Dent* 1988; 60:23–28.

22. Lloyd RS, Baer PN: Periodontal therapy by root resection. *J Prosthet Dent* 1960; 10:362–365.

23. Dunlap RW, Gher ME: Root surface measurements of the mandibular first molar. *J Periodontol* 1985; 56:39–43.

24. Hermann DW, Gher ME, Dunlap RM, Pelleu GB: The potential attachment area of the maxillary first molar. *J Periodontol* 1983; 54:431–434.

25. Jepsen A: Root surface measurement and a method for x-ray determination of root surface area. *Acta Odontol Scand* 1963; 21:35–46.

26. Everett FG, Jump EB, Holder TD, Williams GC: The intermediate bifurcational ridge: A study of the morphology of the bifurcation of the lower first molar. *J Dent Res* 1958; 37:162–169.

27. Klavan B: Clinical observations following root amputation in maxillary molar teeth. *J Periodontol* 1975; 46:1–5.

29. Ehrlich J, Hochman N, Yaffe A: Root resection and separation of multirooted teeth: A 10-year follow-up study. *Quintessence Int* 1989; 20:561–564.

30. Ross IF, Thompson RH: A long term study of root retention in the treatment of maxillary molars with furcation involvement. *J Periodontol* 1978; 49:238–244.

31. Langer B, Stein SD, Wagenberg B: An evaluation of root resections—A 10-year study. *J Periodontol* 1981; 52:719–722.

32. Kois JC, Spear FM: Periodontal prosthesis: Creating successful restorations. *J Am Dent Assoc* 1992; 123:108–113.

Provisional Restorations

It is important that the prepared tooth or teeth be protected and that the patient be kept comfortable while a cast restoration is being fabricated. By successful management of this phase of the treatment, the dentist can gain the patient's confidence and favorably influence the ultimate success of the final restoration. During the time between the preparation of the tooth and the placement of the final restoration, the tooth is protected by a *provisional restoration*. This type of restoration has also been known for many years as a *temporary restoration*. A good provisional restoration should satisfy the following requirements:

1. *Pulpal protection.* The restoration must be fabricated of a material that will prevent the conduction of temperature extremes. The margins should be adapted well enough to prevent leakage of saliva.
2. *Positional stability.* The tooth should not be allowed to extrude or drift in any way. Any such movement will require adjustments or a remake of the final restoration at the time of cementation.
3. *Occlusal function.* Being able to function occlusally on the provisional restoration will aid patient comfort, ward off tooth migration, and possibly prevent joint or neuromuscular imbalance.
4. *Easily cleaned.* The restoration must be made of a material and contour that will permit the patient to keep it clean during the time it is worn. If the gingival tissues remain healthy during the wearing of the provisional crown, there is less likelihood of a problem arising after cementation of the final restoration.
5. *Nonimpinging margins.* It is of utmost importance that the margins of a provisional restoration not impinge upon the gingival tissue.[1-4] The resulting inflammation could cause gingival proliferation, recession, or at the very least, hemorrhage during the impression or cementation. A damaging overhang can result from a preformed metal or resin provisional restoration that has not been contoured properly, while a custom resin provisional crown can produce a horizontal overhang if it is incorrectly trimmed. A restoration with drastically underextended margins also may result in a proliferation of gingival tissue.[5]
6. *Strength and retention.* The restoration must stand up to the forces to which it is subjected without breaking or coming off the tooth. Having to replace a provisional restoration is time-consuming and does not aid patient rapport. A broken provisional fixed partial denture can accelerate tooth movement. The restoration should also remain intact during removal so that it can be reused if necessary.
7. *Esthetics.* In some cases, the restoration must provide a good cosmetic result, particularly on anterior teeth and premolars.

Types of Provisional Restorations

There are numerous ways of providing protective coverage for teeth while permanent restorations are being fabricated. These range from zinc oxide–eugenol cement for small intracoronal inlay preparations, to provisional crowns and provisional fixed partial dentures.

Prefabricated vs Custom Restorations

Provisional restorations can be classified by whether they are prefabricated or custom made. Prefabricated forms include stock aluminum cylinders ("tin cans"), anatomic metal crown forms, clear celluloid shells, and tooth-colored polycarbonate crown forms. They can be used only for single-tooth restorations. Custom crowns and fixed partial dentures can be fabricated of several different kinds of resins by a variety of methods, direct or indirect.

Direct vs Indirect Techniques

Provisional restorations also can be classified by the method used for adapting the restoration to the teeth: the *direct technique* is done on the actual prepared teeth in the mouth, and the *indirect technique* is accomplished outside of the mouth on a cast made of quick-set plaster.

The direct technique is inviting to novices, because it eliminates the alginate impression and the plaster cast.

However, the direct reline is very technique-sensitive. In today's computer terminology, it is decidedly "user unfriendly." If the direct technique has any place in restorative dentistry, it is in the hands of experienced operators using a resin other than poly(methyl methacrylate).

The indirect technique is preferred over the direct technique for its accuracy.[6] To avoid locking into undercuts, a directly fabricated resin provisional restoration must be removed from the tooth before it has completely polymerized. Since poly(methyl methacrylate) shrinks approximately 8% when it polymerizes,[7] polymerization outside the mouth without a supporting form results in distortion and a less than optimal fit.[8,9] In a study of the marginal adaptation of provisional restorations, Crispin et al[10] showed that the marginal fit of poly(methyl methacrylate) provisional restorations could be improved nearly 70% by fabricating them indirectly.

The fit of provisional restorations made from almost all resins can be improved by using the indirect technique. For some materials, the improvement in fit obtained by using the indirect technique is as much or more than the improvement seen with poly(methyl methacrylate).[10] Monday and Blais[11] found better margins on poly(vinylethyl methacrylate) crowns made indirectly than those made either directly or by relining.

The indirect technique also is preferred for the protection that it provides the pulp,[6] particularly if poly(methyl methacrylate) is used. The placement of polymerizing poly(methyl methacrylate) on freshly cut dentin could lead to thermal irritation from the exothermic reaction or chemical irritation from the free monomer.[12,13] It has been reported that this produces an acute pulpal inflammation, as evidenced by an accumulation of neutrophilic leukocytes in the pulp horns.[14] This is another irritant added to a tooth that in most cases has already been subjected to caries, previous restorations, and high-speed cutting in the preparation of the tooth. It is an additional insult that should be avoided whenever possible. A further advantage of the indirect technique is that much of the work can be delegated to auxiliary personnel.

Resins for Provisional Restorations

There are several types of resins that can be used for making custom provisional restorations. Poly(methyl methacrylate) has been in use the longest. Poly(ethyl methacrylate), poly(vinylethyl methacrylate), bis-acryl composite resin, and visible light–cured (VLC) urethane dimethacrylate have come into common usage in recent years. Epimine resin, which for a decade also was used for this purpose, is no longer available. No one resin is superior in all respects,[15] and the restorative dentist must assess the advantages and disadvantages of each in selecting which to use (Table 15-1).

Techniques for Custom Provisional Restorations

The requirements for a good provisional restoration are most easily and completely met by a custom indirect restoration. There are a variety of techniques for making a mold to form the outer surface of a custom provisional restoration that provides the appearance of a tooth where needed, physiologic axial contours adjacent to the gingiva, occlusion with opposing teeth, proximal contact, and marginal fit. The inner surfaces will be shaped by a cast of the preparation(s).

Both elastomeric[1,2,8,16,18,22,23] and alginate[5,6,24] *overimpressions* have been used to shape the provisional restoration. An overimpression is made on the diagnostic cast, or in the mouth, before the tooth preparation is begun. An elastomeric impression provides excellent stability, but it is more expensive than alginate.

A *template* formed from clear thermoplastic resin also can be used for this purpose.[3,25-27] It is shaped on a diagnostic cast, using a vacuum forming machine or an impression tray filled with silicone putty. The template is filled with resin and applied to the prepared teeth or to a fast-setting plaster cast of the prepared teeth. Templates are very stable, and they can be adapted well enough to be used for checking preparation reduction or starting wax patterns.[27]

A thin *shell* crown or fixed partial denture can be made of autopolymerizing resin in an impression prior to the preparation appointment by alternately dripping monomer and gently blowing polymer with an atomizer.[28-30] The resulting form is relined after the tooth or teeth are prepared.[16,28] A second shell can be made from the same impression as a spare.[28] The shell also can be heat processed in a laboratory.[16]

Selected techniques are discussed in detail in the following pages. Although an overimpression is shown for making a provisional crown, and a clear resin template for a provisional fixed partial denture, they are interchangeable.

Overimpression-Fabricated Provisional Crown

The use of an alginate overimpression remains a popular technique, because it is always readily available in the dental operatory. It is easily adapted to intraoral use in the event that the proposed restoration of a tooth with amalgam is unexpectedly replanned as a cast restoration.

Table 15-1 *Characteristics of Resins Used for Provisional Restorations* [8,11,15–21]

Type	Brand	Manufacturer	Advantages	Disadvantages
Poly(methyl methacrylate)	*Alike* *Cr & Br Resin* *Duralay* *Jet*	GC America LD Caulk Reliance Dental Lang Dental	Good marginal fit[15] Good transverse strength[15] Good polishability[15] Durability[16]	High exothermic heat increase[17,18] Low abrasion resistance[15] Free monomer toxic to pulp[16] High volumetric shrinkage[16]
Poly(ethyl methacrylate)	*Snap*	Parkell Biomaterials	Good polishability[15] Minimal exothermic heat increase[17] Good stain resistance[15] Low shrinkage[8]	Surface hardness[15] Transverse strength[15] Durability[16] Fracture toughness[19]
Poly(vinylethyl methacrylate)	*Trim*	Harry Bosworth	Good polishability[15] Minimal exothermic heat increase[17] Good abrasion resistance[15] Good stain resistance[15] Flexibility[8]	Surface hardness[15] Transverse strength[15] Esthetics[8] Fracture toughness[19]
Bis-acryl composite	*Protemp II*	ESPE-Premier	Good marginal fit[15] Low exothermic heat increase[18] Good abrasion resistance[15] Good transverse strength[15] Low shrinkage[8]	Surface hardness[15] Less stain resistance[15] Limited shade selection[8] Limited polishability[8] Brittle[16]
VLC uerthane dimethacrylate	*Triad*	Dentsply York	High surface hardness[15] Good transverse strength[15] Good abrasion resistance[15] Controllable working time[20] Color stability[15]	Marginal fit[15] Less stain resistance[15] Limited shade selection[20] Expensive[11,21] Brittle

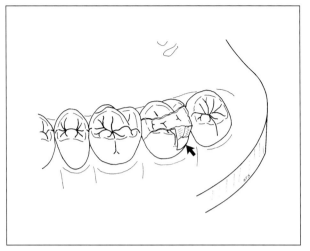

Fig 15-1 Defects, such as a missing cusp *(arrow),* should be filled in on the cast.

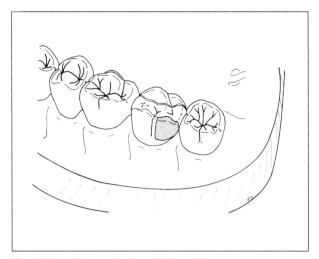

Fig 15-2 Utility wax is placed in the defect.

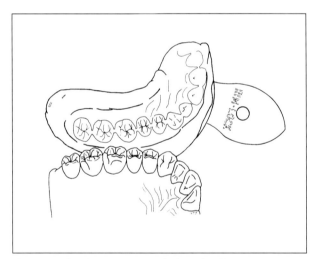

Fig 15-3 Overimpression is made from the diagnostic cast.

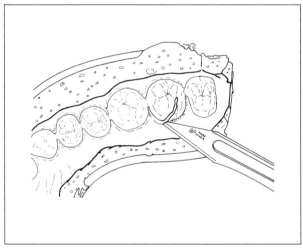

Fig 15-4 Thin edges in the gingival areas of the overimpression are cut away.

Overimpression Armamentarium

1. Diagnostic cast
2. Utility wax
3. No. 7 wax spatula
4. Quadrant impression trays (two, same side)
5. Alginate
6. Rubber bowl
7. Spatula
8. Quick-set plaster
9. Laboratory knife with no. 25 blade
10. Heavy-duty laboratory knife
11. Large camel-hair brush
12. Cement spatula
13. Dappen dish
14. Separating medium
15. Monomer and polymer
16. Medicine dropper
17. Heavy rubber band
18. Straight handpiece
19. Acrylic burs
20. Abrasive discs and Moore mandrel

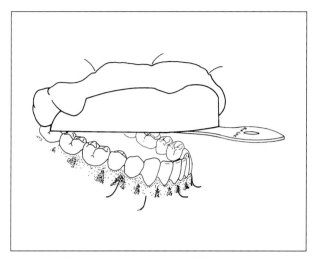

Fig 15-5 Alginate impression is made of the prepared tooth.

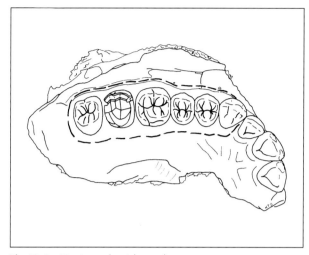

Fig 15-6 Untrimmed quick-set plaster cast.

The overimpression frequently is made in the patient's mouth while waiting for the anesthetic to take effect. However, if the tooth to be restored has any obvious defects, the overimpression should be made from the diagnostic cast (Fig 15-1). After any defects are filled and smoothed over with red utility wax, the diagnostic cast is immersed in a plaster bowl of water for 5 minutes (Fig 15-2). Wetting the cast in this manner will keep the alginate from adhering to it.

When the alginate has set, the overimpression is removed from the diagnostic cast and checked for completeness (Fig 15-3). A laboratory knife with a no. 25 blade is used to trim off all excess alginate. Thin flashes of impression material that replicate the gingival crevice are removed to insure that there will be no impediments to the complete seating of the cast into the overimpression later (Fig 15-4). The impression is wrapped in a wet paper towel and placed in a ziplock plastic bag for later use.

When the tooth preparation is completed, another quadrant impression is made in alginate (Fig 15-5). This impression is poured up with a thin mix of quick-setting plaster (Snow White Impression Plaster No. 2, Kerr Manufacturing Co, Romulus, MI) (Fig 15-6). Excess material should be trimmed off on a model trimmer when the plaster has set. The trimmed cast should have at least one tooth on either side of the prepared tooth, if possible. Areas of the cast that duplicate the soft tissues should be reduced as much as possible (Fig 15-7).

Check the occlusal surfaces and gingival crevices for any plaster nodules that will prevent complete seating. Then try the trimmed quick-set plaster cast in the overimpression to make sure that it will seat completely (Fig 15-8). Coat the prepared tooth and adjacent areas of the cast liberally with a "tin foil substitute" separating medi-

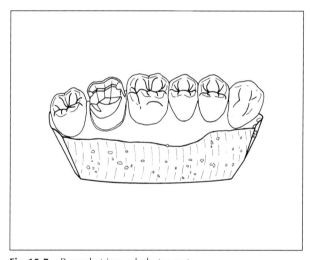

Fig 15-7 Properly trimmed plaster cast.

um (Alcote, LD Caulk Div, Dentsply International, Milford, DE) (Fig 15-9). Allow the material to dry before mixing the acrylic resin. Drying can be accelerated by the use of an air syringe.

Mix tooth-colored acrylic resin in a dappen dish with a cement spatula (Fig 15-10). Use 12 drops of monomer for each tooth being restored. Place the resin in the overimpression so that it completely fills the crown area of the tooth for which the provisional restoration is being made (Fig 15-11).

229

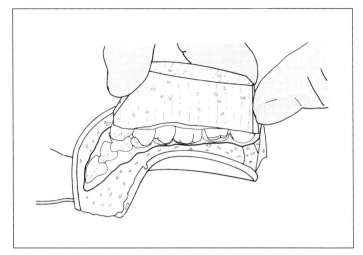

Fig 15-8 The cast is tried in the overimpression before proceeding.

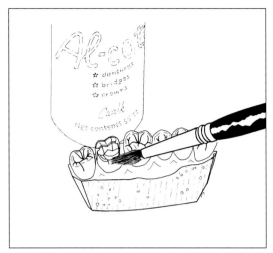

Fig 15-9 Separating medium is painted on the plaster cast.

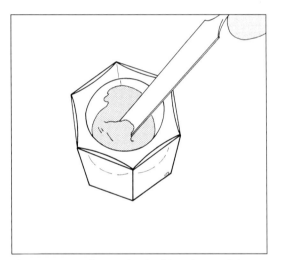

Fig 15-10 Acrylic resin is mixed in a dappen dish.

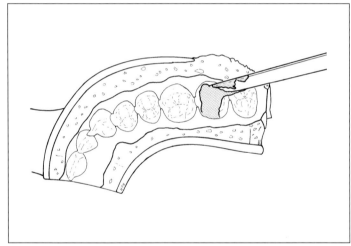

Fig 15-11 Resin is placed into the overimpression.

Seat the cast into the overimpression, making sure that the teeth on the cast are accurately aligned with the tooth impressions (Fig 15-12). The force used to seat the cast into the alginate impression is critical.[31] Excessive force can overseat the cast and uneven force can torque the cast, either of which will affect the restoration.

Once the cast has been firmly seated and the excess resin has been expressed, hold the cast in place with a large rubber band (Fig 15-13). It is important that the cast be oriented securely in an upright position so that the space between the cast and the impression that is filled with the resin forming the provisional restoration will not be distorted (Fig 15-14, A). If the cast is torqued to one side by the rubber band, the cast may be forced through the soft resin in some areas, resulting in a provi-

sional restoration that may be thin in those areas and thicker than desirable in others (Fig 15-14, B). If the cast is seated with too much force, or if the rubber band is wrapped around the assembly too many times, the cast may be forced through the resin occlusally, resulting in a provisional restoration with an occlusal surface that is too thin (Fig 15-14, C).

Place the overimpression–plaster cast assembly in a plaster bowl full of hot tap water for approximately 5 minutes, or into a pressure pot if one is available. Allowing a poly(methyl methacrylate) provisional restoration to polymerize in a pressure pot (Sure-Cure Pressure Unit, Howmedica Dental Div, Chicago, IL) under 20 psi will decrease porosity and increase the transverse strength of the restoration by 28%.[32]

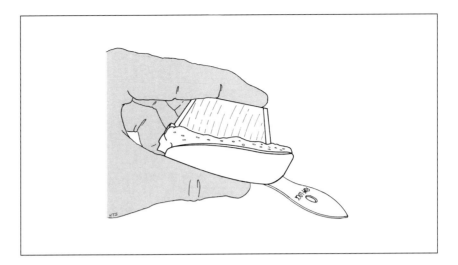

Fig 15-12 The cast is seated firmly in the overimpression.

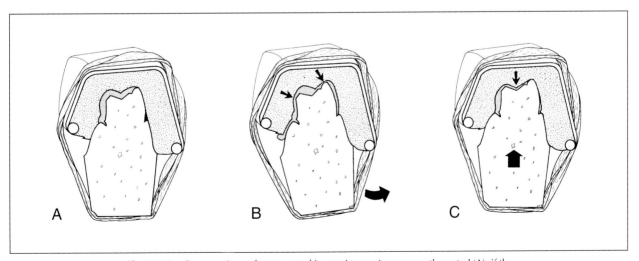

Fig 15-13 The cast is held in place with a rubber band.

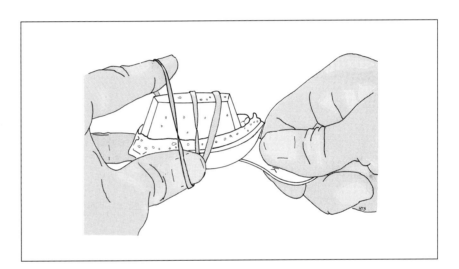

Fig 15-14 Cross sections of casts seated in overimpressions: correctly seated (A); if the cast is pushed to one side, the provisional restoration will be deficient (B); overseating of the cast will produce a provisional restoration with a thin occlusal surface (C).

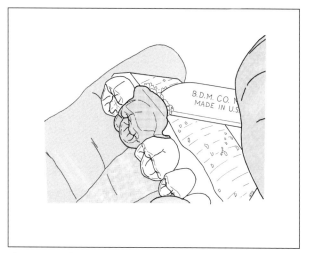

Fig 15-15 The cast can be broken to remove the provisional restoration.

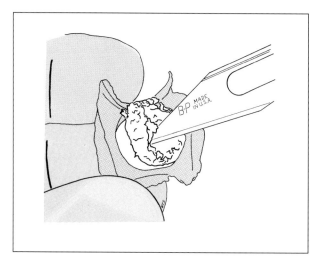

Fig 15-16 Any plaster remaining in the provisional restoration is removed.

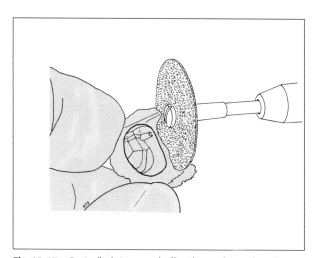

Fig 15-17 Resin flash is ground off with a carborundum disc.

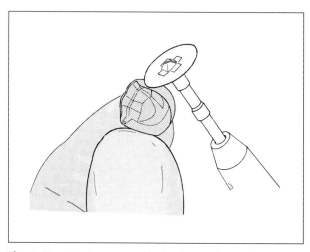

Fig 15-18 Margins are smoothed with a sandpaper disc.

When the resin has polymerized, remove the rubber band to disassemble the quick-set plaster cast from the overimpression. If the restoration is not easily removed from the cast, break the tooth off the plaster cast with a heavy-bladed laboratory knife (Fig 15-15). Use the sharp end of a thin-bladed knife or some other small, pointed instrument to remove any plaster that remains in the provisional restoration (Fig 15-16). Ease of removal is one of the advantages of using the weak, quick-set plaster.

Acrylic burs or coarse Moore discs are used to trim the excess resin from the provisional restoration (Fig 15-17). Before attempting to seat the restoration on the tooth, be sure to remove all resin extending beyond the preparation finish line into undercut areas. Smooth the axial surfaces near the margins of the restoration with a fine sandpaper disc (Fig 15-18).

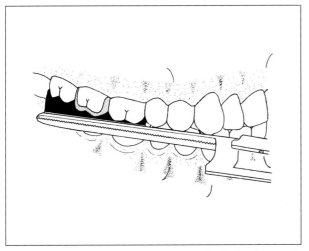

Fig 15-19 Occlusion on the restoration is checked in the mouth.

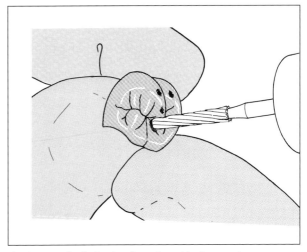

Fig 15-20 Occlusion is adjusted outside the mouth.

Cementation Armamentarium

1. Articulating paper
2. Miller forceps
3. Straight handpiece
4. High-speed handpiece
5. No. 171L FG bur
6. Muslin rag wheel
7. Pumice
8. Cement spatula
9. Paper pad
10. Zinc oxide–eugenol cement
11. Petrolatum
12. Explorer
13. Mouth mirror
14. Dental floss

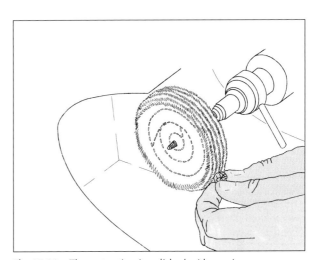

Fig 15-21 The restoration is polished with pumice.

Seat the provisional restoration on the tooth in the mouth. Check the occlusion with thin articulating paper (Fig 15-19). Remove the restoration from the tooth and adjust the occlusal prematurities with a nondentate bur (Fig 15-20). When the occlusion has been adjusted to make the patient comfortable, polish the restoration first with pumice and then polishing compound (Yellow Diamond Polishing Compound, Matchless Metal Polish Co, Chicago IL) on a muslin rag wheel (Fig 15-21). Besides making the provisional restoration easier to clean and more comfortable for the patient, polished materials are much less likely to discolor.[33]

To fit a provisional crown under an existing removable partial denture, undercontour the crown so it does not touch any rests or clasps on that tooth. Add resin to the outside of the crown, and while the resin is still soft, seat the crown on the tooth. To form the rest seat and guide planes on the crown, lubricate the partial denture with petrolatum and seat it over the provisional crown. Pump the partial denture up and down several times to insure

that it is not locked into any undercuts. Remove the crown from the tooth, smooth any rough areas, and polish the crown.

The restoration should be cemented with a temporary cement of moderate strength. After the zinc oxide–eugenol cement has been mixed to a thick, creamy consistency, an amount of petrolatum equal to 5% to 10% of the cement volume is incorporated to slightly reduce the strength of the cement (Fig 15-22). This will facilitate removal of the provisional restoration at a subsequent appointment. If the preparation is short or otherwise lacking in retention, the petrolatum should not be added.

It is not necessary to keep zinc oxide–eugenol cement dry while it is setting. In fact, moisture will accelerate the hardening. Coating the outside of the restoration with a thin film of petrolatum prior to cementation will aid in the

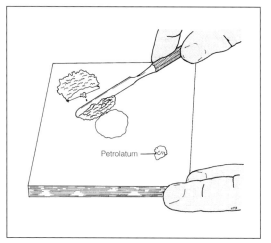

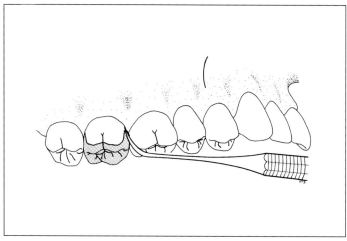

Fig 15-22 Zinc oxide–eugenol cement is often mixed with a small amount of petrolatum.

Fig 15-23 An explorer is used to remove cement from the gingival crevice.

removal of excess cement. After the cement has hardened, all excess must be removed from the gingival crevice. Use an explorer in accessible areas and dental floss interproximally (Fig 15-23).

Template-Fabricated Provisional Fixed Partial Denture

When a fixed partial denture is to be made for a patient, the provisional restoration should also be in the form of a fixed partial denture rather than individual crowns. In the anterior region it will provide a better cosmetic result. However, even in the posterior region, a provisional fixed partial denture will better stabilize the teeth and will afford the patient the opportunity to become accustomed to having a tooth in the edentulous space again.

Template Armamentarium

1. Diagnostic cast
2. Mor-Tight
3. No. 7 wax spatula
4. Denture tooth
5. Crown form
6. Vacuum forming machine
7. Coping material or temporary splint material
8. Quadrant impression trays
9. Silly Putty
10. Wire frame
11. Bunsen burner
12. Scissors
13. Laboratory knife with no. 25 blade
14. Heavy-duty laboratory knife
15. Large camel-hair brush
16. Cement spatula
17. Dappen dish
18. Separating medium
19. Monomer and polymer
20. Medicine dropper
21. Heavy rubber band
22. Straight handpiece
23. Acrylic burs
24. Abrasive discs and Moore mandrel

To make a template, place a metal crown form or a denture tooth in the edentulous space on the diagnostic cast (Fig 15-24). All of the embrasures should be filled with putty (Mor-Tight, TP Orthodontics, LaPorte, IN) to eliminate undercuts during adaptation of the resin template.

To facilitate removal of the template, a thin strand of putty can be placed around the periphery of the cast and on the lingual surface of the cast, apical to the teeth (Fig 15-25). Use a large acrylic bur to cut a hole through the middle of the cast (midpalatal or midlingual). Place a 5 x 5-inch sheet of 0.020-inch-thick resin (translucent Coping Material or transparent Temporary Splint Material, Buffalo Dental Manufacturing Co, Syosset, NY) in the frame of the vacuum forming machine (Sta-Vac, Buffalo Dental Manufacturing Co) with the shiny surface down (Fig 15-26). If temporary splint material is used, both sides will be shiny. Turn on the heating element of the machine and swing it into position over the plastic sheet.

As the resin sheet is heated to the proper temperature, it will droop or sag about 1.0 inch in the frame. If you are using coping material, it will lose its cloudy appearance and become completely clear (Fig 15-27). The cast should be in position in the center of the perforated stage of the vacuum forming machine. Turn on the vacuum.

Grasping the handles on the frame that holds the heated coping material, forcefully lower the frame over the perforated stage (Fig 15-28). Turn off the heating element and swing it off to the side. After approximately 30 seconds, turn off the vacuum and release the resin sheet from the holding frame. After removing the resin sheet from the frame, use a laboratory knife with a sharp no. 25 blade to cut through the resin over the Mor-Tight strand (Fig 15-29).

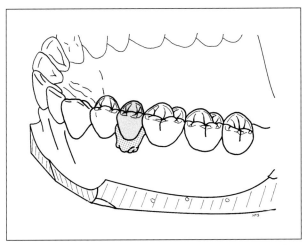

Fig 15-24 A crown form or a denture tooth is placed in the edentulous space on the diagnostic cast.

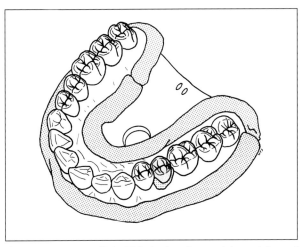

Fig 15-25 A rope of Mor-Tight is placed around the periphery of the cast.

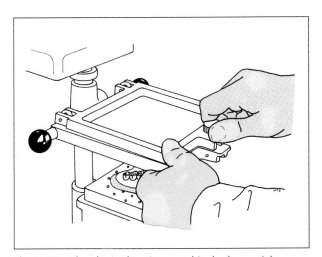

Fig 15-26 The plastic sheet is secured in the frame of the vacuum forming machine.

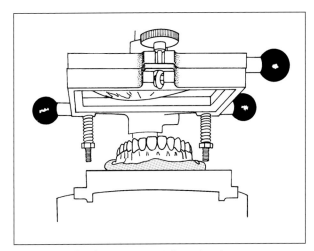

Fig 15-27 The plastic sags as it is heated to the proper temperature.

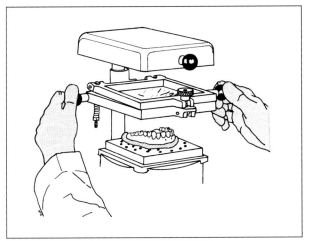

Fig 15-28 The frame is pulled down over the perforated stage of the vacuum forming machine.

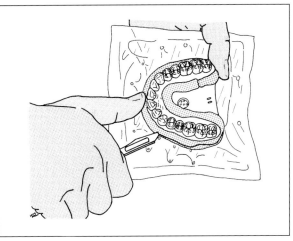

Fig 15-29 The plastic is cut to remove the template from the diagnostic cast.

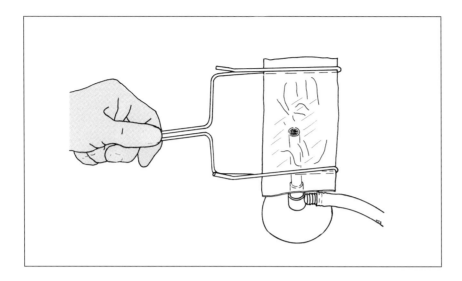

Fig 15-30 The plastic can be heated in a wire frame over a Bunsen burner.

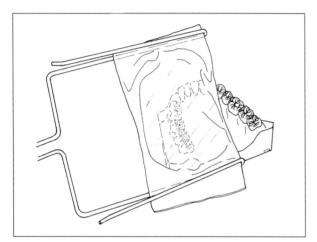

Fig 15-31 The plastic sheet is positioned over the diagnostic cast.

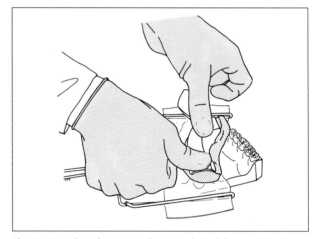

Fig 15-32 The plastic template is adapted by exerting heavy force on the impression tray of silicone putty.

If a vacuum forming machine is not available, it is still possible to fabricate a template for a provisional restoration. Fill a quadrant impression tray with a soft silicone putty available in most variety or toy stores (Silly Putty, Binney & Smith, Easton, PA). Cut a sheet of coping material in half and insert it, shiny side down, into a wire frame bent from a coat hanger. Heat the resin sheet over a Bunsen burner flame until it sags and becomes clear, which usually occurs in about 10 seconds (Fig 15-30).

Place the softened sheet over the cast (Fig 15-31). Forcefully seat the tray of silicone putty over the coping material (Fig 15-32). To accelerate cooling, blow compressed air on the plastic sheet and the impression tray. After about a minute, snap the tray off the cast (Fig 15-33). If the silicone putty sticks to the resin sheet, the putty can be easily removed by pulling it off in quick jerks. Rapid separation causes the silicone putty to exhibit brittleness that will result in easy removal. Replace the putty in its original container for later reuse. Separate the template from the diagnostic cast.

Trim the template, however it was fabricated, with a pair of scissors (Fig 15-34). It should extend at least one tooth on either side of the prepared teeth. Save those portions not needed for possible later use.

Upon completion of the preparations, make an alginate impression of them and pour it in fast-setting plaster. The plaster cast will include replicas of soft tissue and teeth that are not needed (Fig 15-35). Trim the cast so that it includes only one tooth on either side of the prepared teeth. Try on the template to verify its fit (Fig 15-36).

Coat the cast with Alcote separating medium and allow it to dry. Mix the acrylic resin in a dappen dish and place some on protected areas of the cast, such as interproximal spaces and in grooves and boxes (Fig 15-37). As the resin begins to lose its surface gloss and becomes slightly dull, fill the area for which the provisional fixed partial denture is being made (Fig 15-38). Place some extra bulk in the portion that will serve as the pontic.

Wrap rubber bands around the template and cast, being careful not to place them over the abutment prepa-

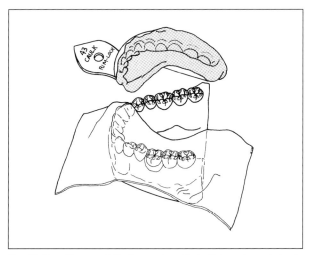

Fig 15-33 The tray full of putty is pulled off the adapted plastic template.

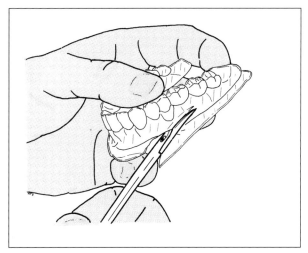

Fig 15-34 Excess is trimmed from the periphery of the template.

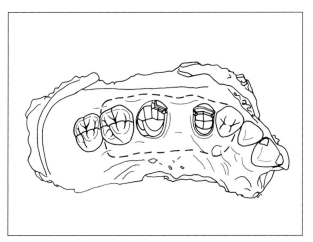

Fig 15-35 The quick-set plaster cast should be trimmed back to the dotted line.

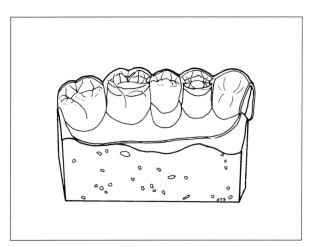

Fig 15-36 The template is tried on the cast to verify the fit.

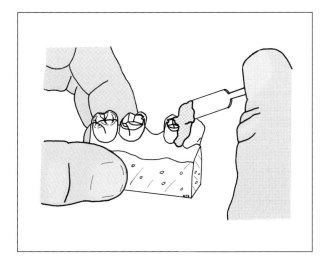

Fig 15-37 Some acrylic resin is placed in the interproximal areas of the cast.

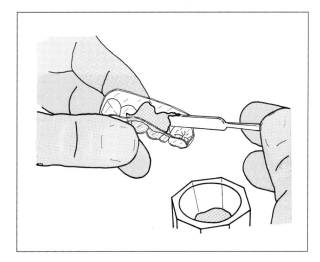

Fig 15-38 Resin is placed in the template.

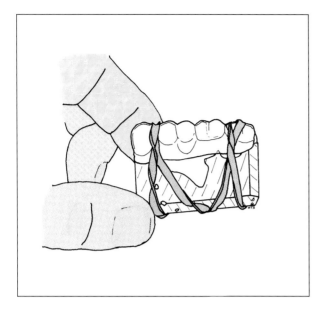

Fig 15-39 The template is held in position with rubber bands.

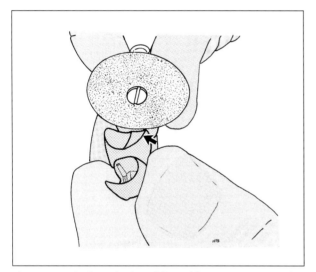

Fig 15-40 The lingual ridge of the saddle *(arrow)* is removed to open the lingual embrasure of the pontic.

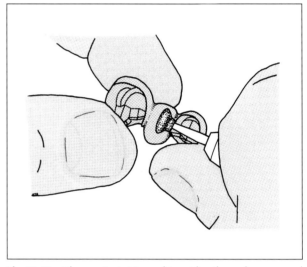

Fig 15-41 The pontic is trimmed to widen the embrasures and create cleanable contours.

rations, lest they cause the template to collapse in that area (Fig 15-39). Place the cast in a pressure pot if one is available. Otherwise, place it in warm (not hot) tap water to hasten polymerization. Hot water causes the monomer to boil, increasing porosity. Wait for about 5 minutes. Pry off the template and save it in case it is needed again. Before removing the provisional restoration from the cast, add resin to any voids or thin spots and place the cast back in warm water. Do not replace the template for this correction. Placing the unpolymerized resin back into water will prevent evaporation of monomer and the formation of a granulated, "frosted" surface.

Remove the fixed partial denture from the cast. Do not hesitate to break the cast if necessary. Trim off the excess acrylic resin. Use discs to trim the axial surfaces down to the margins. The pontic should be trimmed with discs and burs to open up the proximal embrasures (Fig 15-40). Remove the saddle configuration that was created by the crown form in the edentulous space (Fig 15-41). The pontic should have the same general shape that the pontic on the permanent prosthesis will have. This will insure that the patient will be comfortable and satisfied with the pontic form before the completed fixed partial denture is inserted.

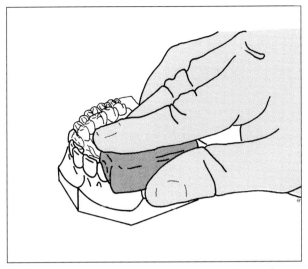

Fig 15-42 A silicone putty index is formed over the template on the diagnostic cast.

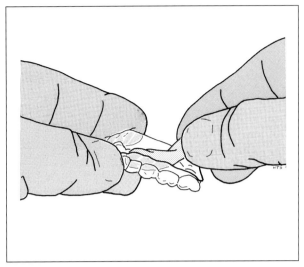

Fig 15-43 VLC resin is placed in the clear template.

Template-Fabricated VLC Provisional Restoration

A transparent template is essential to the use of a visible light–cured (VLC) resin (Triad, Dentsply International, York, PA), because the clear matrix allows the light access to the resin to initiate polymerization.

Template-VLC Armamentarium

1. Items in template armamentarium
2. Silicone impression putty
3. Triad resin
4. Model release agent (MRA)
5. Air barrier coating material (ABC)
6. Triad curing unit
7. Straight handpiece
8. Acrylic burs
9. Abrasive discs and Moore mandrel
10. Items in cementation armamentarium

Fabricate a template on the diagnostic cast. If the restoration is to be a fixed partial denture, set a metal crown form or denture tooth in Mor-Tight putty in the edentulous space. If a diagnostic wax-up has been made, soak the cast for 5 minutes and duplicate it with an alginate impression. Pour the impression in quick-set plaster.

Produce a template from a resin sheet on the vacuum forming machine. Trim the template and replace it on the cast. Mix a scoop of silicone impression putty with accelerator (Citricon, Kerr Manufacturing Co) and mold it around the template on the cast (Fig 15-42). This is needed to reinforce the unsupported template and prevent displacement by the highly viscous resin later.[20] Quick-set plaster also can be used to make this reinforcing

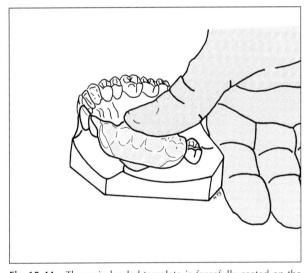

Fig 15-44 The resin-loaded template is forcefully seated on the quick-set plaster cast.

index. Set the template and the index aside until the teeth have been prepared.

Make an alginate impression of the prepared abutment teeth and pour a cast of quick-set plaster. Coat the cast with a layer of model release agent (MRA, Dentsply International), which is part of the resin system. Then place some of the Triad resin around the finish lines of the abutment preparations. Lay a strand of resin inside the clear template (Fig 15-43). "Enamel" resin can be placed in the incisal or occlusal portion of the template first to enhance esthetics.

Use firm pressure to seat the loaded template on the quick-set plaster cast of the prepared abutments (Fig 15-44). Compress the silicone putty index over the template

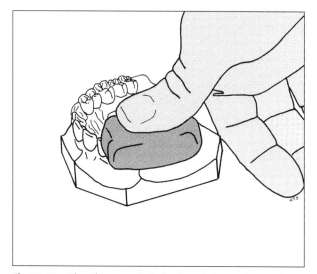

Fig 15-45   The silicone putty index is seated over the template.

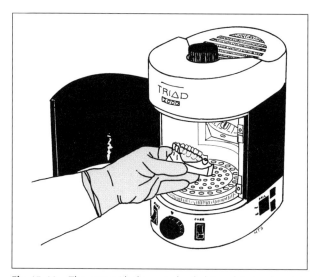

Fig 15-46   The cast with the resin-loaded template is placed in the light-polymerizing unit.

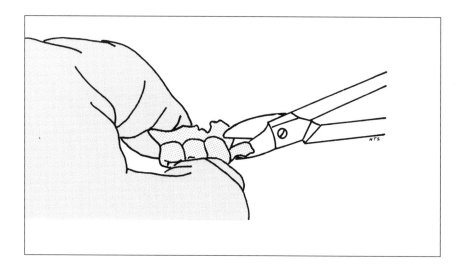

Fig 15-47   Excess resin is cut off with crown and bridge scissors.

to insure complete seating of the template and an even thickness of resin in the provisional restoration (Fig 15-45). In an alternative technique, the template can be seated into the silicone putty index before the resin is loaded into the template.[20] Remove the putty index from the cast, leaving the resin and template in position on the cast.

Place the cast in the Triad curing unit to polymerize the resin in the template for 4 minutes (Fig 15-46). Carefully remove the template and then the provisional restoration from the cast. Paint all surfaces of the restoration with air barrier coating material (ABC, Dentsply International). Place the provisional restoration back in the curing unit, tissue side up, for an additional 6 minutes. Retrieve the restoration from the curing unit and remove all of the ABC with a brush and water.

Trim as much excess material as possible with a pair of curved scissors (Fig 15-47). Finish trimming the axial surfaces to the margins with discs. Open the embrasures around the pontic with discs and burs. Be sure to remove the saddle form produced by the template. Polish the restoration with pumice and a high-shine polishing material (Yellow Diamond Polishing Compound, Matchless Metal Polish Co).

Another technique has been described in which the restoration is started in a template on the prepared teeth in the mouth.[21] Polymerization of the restoration is initiated by a 10-second application of a hand-held curing light. After the restoration is "frozen" in this manner, it is removed from the mouth and further exposed to the high-intensity curing light in the laboratory.

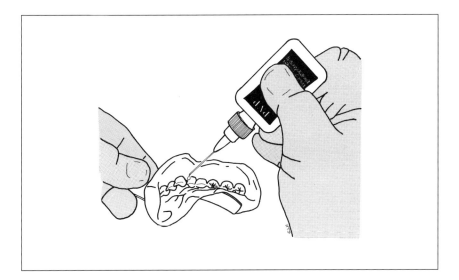

Fig 15-48 Monomer is applied to the overimpression with a needle-tipped liquid applicator.

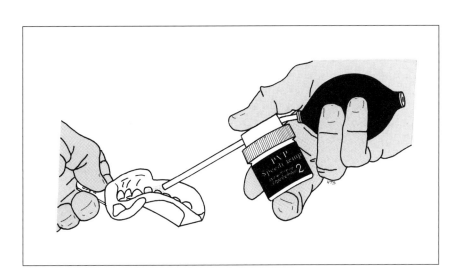

Fig 15-49 Enough polymer is applied to turn the surface of the impression dull.

Shell-Fabricated Provisional Restoration

A thin shell crown or fixed partial denture can be made from any of the acrylic resins, and then that shell can be relined indirectly on a quick-set plaster cast. It also can be relined directly in the mouth.[16,28,34,35] If the reline is done directly, a methacrylate other than poly(methyl) should be used. This technique can save chair time because the restoration is partially fabricated prior to the preparation appointment.

Care must be taken not to make the shell too thick. If too thick, the shell will not seat completely over the prepared teeth and it will need to be trimmed internally. This can be time-consuming and defeats any advantage gained by making it before the preparation appointment.

Shell Fabrication Armamentarium

1. Items in overimpression armamentarium
2. Items in cementation armamentarium
3. Liquid applicator
4. Powder blower

An overimpression is made from a diagnostic wax-up before the preparation appointment. Check it for completeness. Trim off thin flashes of impression material created by the gingival crevice to produce an extra bulk of resin near the margins. Use a plastic squeeze bottle with a fine tip (Liquid Applicator, Prairie Village Prosthetics, Prairie Village, KS) to deposit one drop of monomer on the facial and one drop on the lingual surface of the imprint of each tooth to be restored (Fig 15-48).[30] Keep

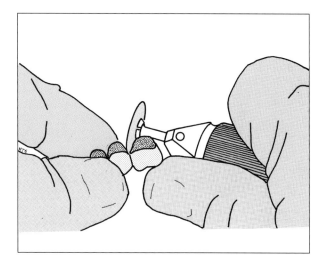

Fig 15-50 Gingival flash is removed and gingival embrasures are opened with a fine sandpaper disc.

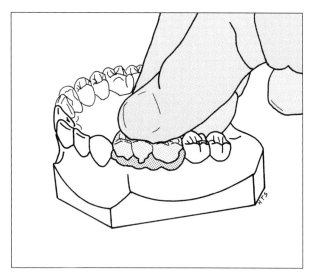

Fig 15-51 The resin-filled shell is seated on the prepared teeth on the cast.

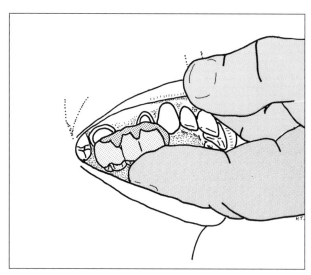

Fig 15-52 The resin-filled shell is seated on the prepared teeth in the mouth.

the monomer near the gingival portion of the impression to prevent excess from accumulating in the incisal or occlusal area. Extend the coverage by the resin to one tooth imprint on either side of the teeth being restored.[28]

With an insufflator (Powder Blower, Prairie Village Prosthetics), gently spray enough polymer onto the surface of the impression to absorb the monomer (Fig 15-49).[30] Repeat the process four times, inverting the impression frequently to allow the material to run down to the margins rather than puddling in the incisal or occlusal areas of the impression. Gently remove the shell from the impression after 4 minutes. Trim the flash from the gingival area and open the gingival embrasures with an abrasive disc (Fig 15-50).

When the teeth have been prepared, make a quadrant

alginate impression and pour it with a thin mix of quick-setting plaster. Trim off excess plaster on a model trimmer. Save one tooth on either side of the prepared tooth, if possible. Remove areas of the cast that duplicate soft tissues. Examine the cast for nodules that would prevent complete seating.

Try the shell gently on the cast to make sure it seats completely without binding. If it does bind, relieve the inner surfaces of the shells until the restoration seats completely and passively. Liberally coat the tooth preparations on the cast with separating medium and make sure it is dry before mixing the acrylic resin.

Monomer and polymer can be added directly to the shell and mixed there. The resin also can be mixed in a dappen dish and then transferred to the shell, complete-

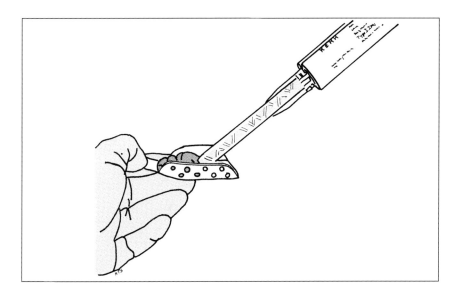

Fig 15-53 Impression material is loaded into a quadrant tray for the over-impression.

ly filling each tooth. Seat the shell onto the prepared teeth on the cast (Fig 15-51). Wrap a rubber band around the shell and cast, and place them in a plaster bowl full of hot tap water for approximately 5 minutes, preferably in a pressure pot. The use of a pressure pot will significantly increase the strength of the restoration.[32]

If the direct technique is employed, seat the shell on the prepared teeth in the mouth (Fig 15-52). When the resin becomes rubbery, elevate the restoration 2.0 mm and flush the teeth under it with water.[34] Pump the restoration up and down several times to eliminate undercuts. Then remove the restoration from the mouth and place it in warm water.

When the resin has polymerized, remove the rubber band and disassemble the shell from the plaster cast. If the restoration resists removal from the plaster cast, break the teeth off with a heavy-bladed laboratory knife. Use a small, pointed instrument to remove any plaster left in the provisional restoration. Trim excess resin from the provisional restoration with acrylic burs or coarse Moore discs. Smooth the axial surfaces of the restoration with a fine sandpaper disc, followed by pumice and polishing compound on a muslin rag wheel.

Overimpression-Fabricated Bis-acryl Composite Crown

Bis-acryl composite resin (Protemp II, ESPE-Premier, Norristown, PA) can be used to fabricate a provisional restoration on a quick-set plaster cast. Its polymerization produces very little heat, and it has minimal toxic effect on soft tissues and the pulp. It probably is as well suited as any resin for use in a direct technique, based on the study of materials by Wang et al.[15] Its use in making a direct provisional restoration is presented here, although it bears repeating that the direct technique is not a desirable one for novices.

Alginate makes a satisfactory overimpression, but this discussion will focus on the use of an elastomeric impression material, polyvinyl siloxane (Extrude Extra, Kerr Manufacturing Co), for the sake of presenting as many techniques as possible in this chapter. A heavy-bodied elastomeric material has the advantages of being very stable and difficult to distort. Its disadvantages include greater expense and extra time required for the impression material to polymerize.

Load a disposable aluminum sextant tray with impression material and make the overimpression while waiting for anesthesia (Fig 15-53). Trim the excess from the borders of the impression to facilitate accurate placement back in the mouth (Fig 15-54). Remove the webs of material between the imprints of individual teeth in the impression (Fig 15-55). These could interfere with complete reseating of the overimpression.

The margins of a provisional restoration may be thin or deficient because the overimpression was not seated straight, or because the thickness required for a resin restoration is greater than that needed for a metal restoration. To avoid this problem, use a no. 8 round bur to cut a trough in the gingival area of the facial and lingual surfaces of the tooth imprint(s) in which the restoration will be fabricated (Fig 15-56). This will produce a bead of material parallel with the margin of the resulting restoration (Fig 15-57). This insures adequate material in the margin, and the excess can be trimmed off during finishing.

After the tooth preparation has been completed, begin the provisional restoration. Check to be sure that the plastic catch is engaged in the vertical groove on the threaded plunger in the ratchet at the back end of the large blue syringe containing the Protemp II base material (Fig 15-58). To extrude one full measure of base paste onto a mixing pad, give the thumbscrew at the end of the threaded plunger one complete turn clockwise until it clicks (Fig 15-59). Check the simple ratchet on the

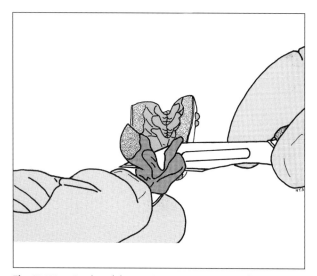

Fig 15-54 Border of the overimpression is trimmed.

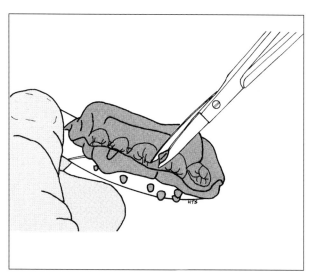

Fig 15-55 Impression material between the imprints of teeth is removed.

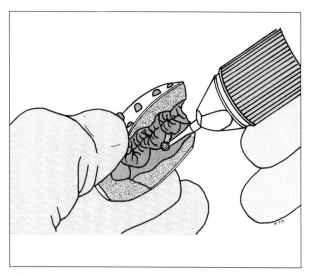

Fig 15-56 A gingival trough is cut with a no. 8 bur in the facial and lingual surfaces of the imprint of the tooth being restored.

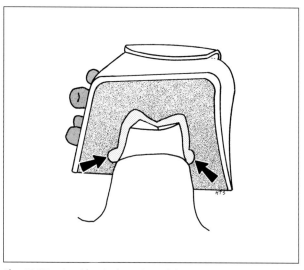

Fig 15-57 A midsagittal section of the overimpression and the provisional restoration shows a bulk of material *(arrows)* near the margins.

threaded center plunger of the smaller white, double-barreled catalyst paste syringe to see that it is in place (Fig 15-60). Express an equal amount of each of the two catalyst pastes onto the same pad by twisting the single threaded shaft one full revolution or "click" (Fig 15-61).

Mix the catalyst pastes and the base material with a cement spatula for approximately 30 seconds (Fig 15-62). Use the spatula to load the back end of a frosted plastic syringe (Fig 15-63). Place the resin in the overimpression with the syringe, as suggested by von Krammer[36] (Fig 15-64). Keep the syringe tip buried in resin and fill the cusp tip or incisal edge areas from the

bottom up to prevent voids in the completed provisional restoration. The use of an application syringe will frequently require a second unit of resin, but it greatly reduces the possibility of creating bothersome voids in the restoration.

Lubricate the prepared teeth with petrolatum and position the impression tray on them no later than 2 minutes from the start of mixing. Allow the resin to polymerize in the mouth for approximately 2 minutes. Check excess resin around the border of the tray for consistency. Do not rely on material left on the mixing pad as an indication of polymerization, because the reaction in the oral cavity at

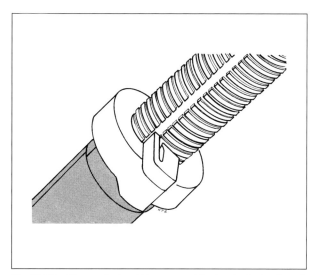

Fig 15-58 The catch should be engaged in the slot in the threaded plunger at the back of the base syringe.

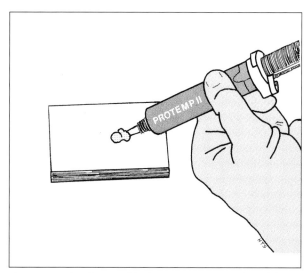

Fig 15-59 The plunger of the base syringe is rotated one full turn to produce one measure of base resin.

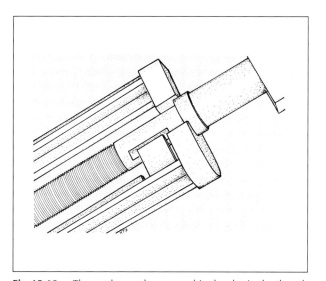

Fig 15-60 The catch must be engaged in the slot in the threaded middle plunger at the back of the catalyst syringe.

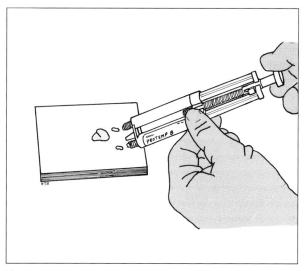

Fig 15-61 The threaded middle plunger of the catalyst syringe is rotated one click to produce enough catalyst to mix with one measure of base paste.

body temperature and 100% humidity will proceed more rapidly than on a mixing pad at room temperature. When the resin becomes elastic, it is ready for removal. That should occur no later than 6 minutes from the start of the mix.

Tease the restoration from the tooth (Fig 15-65) or from the impression (Fig 15-66). Remove as much excess as possible with scissors. Replace the provisional restoration on the tooth and ask the patient to close down on it several times. Then pump it several times to insure removability. Remove the restoration no later than 7 minutes from the start of mixing. Wipe off the air-inhibited,

unset resin with an alcohol sponge. If there are voids or other defects, they can be repaired by mixing another batch of resin and applying it to the affected area with an instrument. Repairs also can be effected by using VLC composite resins and a light.

Remove excess near the margins (including the intentional bead, if used) with fine abrasive discs. Place the restoration back on the tooth in the mouth. Test and adjust the occlusion if necessary. Polish the outer surfaces of the restoration with pumice and polishing compound. Seat the restoration with a temporary cement.

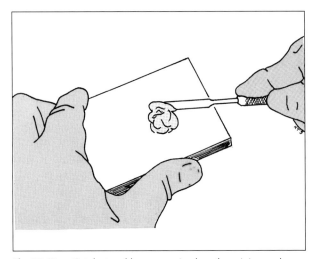

Fig 15-62 Catalyst and base are mixed on the mixing pad.

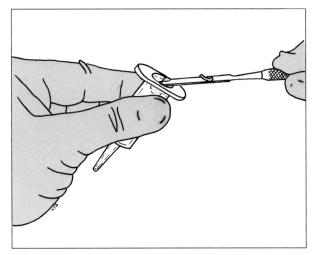

Fig 15-63 Syringe is loaded with mixed resin.

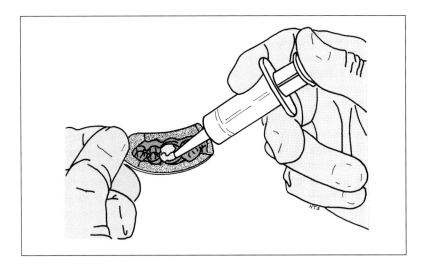

Fig 15-64 Mixed resin is expressed into the imprint of the tooth for which the provisional restoration is being fabricated.

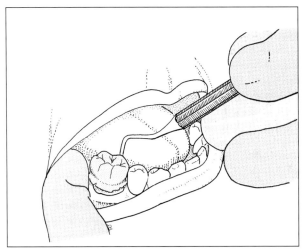

Fig 15-65 The rubbery provisional restoration is teased from the tooth.

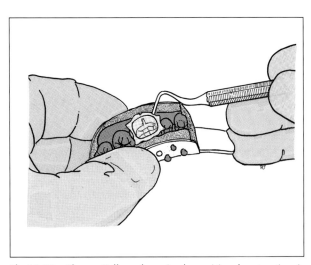

Fig 15-66 The partially polymerized provisional restoration is removed from the impression.

Techniques for Prefabricated Provisional Restorations

Clinical situations will arise in which it may not be possible or desirable to make a custom acrylic resin provisional crown. Prefabricated polycarbonate crowns are easily adapted to produce esthetic provisional crowns in an expeditious manner on prepared single anterior teeth in most patients.[37] A patient may present with an emergency situation in which a posterior tooth has fractured, and there is not time available for a definitive tooth preparation and a custom provisional crown. In those cases, a preformed anatomic metal crown form can be employed to protect the tooth and the patient made comfortable until sufficient time can be arranged for completing the treatment.

Anterior Polycarbonate Crown

A suitable provisional restoration can be made for single anterior teeth by the use of polycarbonate crowns. However, they frequently will require extensive alteration to correct morphologic discrepancies and improper contours.[31] If they are not carefully contoured, they will have horizontal overhangs that will be damaging to the gingiva.[5] To accomplish the recontouring that is required and to provide the necessary retention, the tooth-colored crown form must be relined with a resin. This can be accomplished with the greatest accuracy by doing the reline on a quick-set plaster cast of the prepared tooth.

Armamentarium

1. Anterior sectional impression tray (one only)
2. Alginate
3. Rubber bowl
4. Spatula
5. Quick-set plaster
6. Polycarbonate crown kit
7. Pencil
8. Straight handpiece
9. Acrylic bur
10. Coarse garnet disc on Moore mandrel
11. Burlew disc on mandrel
12. Large camel-hair brush
13. Cement spatula
14. Dappen dish
15. IPPA plastic instrument
16. Separating medium
17. Monomer and polymer
18. Medicine dropper
19. Muslin rag wheel
20. White polishing compound
21. Miller forceps
22. Articulating paper
23. Paper pad
24. Zinc oxide–eugenol cement
25. Petrolatum
26. Explorer
27. Mouth mirror
28. Dental floss

When the tooth preparation has been completed, make an alginate impression of the prepared tooth, using an anterior sextant tray (Fig 15-67). Apply alginate around the prepared tooth with the tip of the index finger. After the impression has been removed from the mouth, pour it up with a thin mix of fast-setting plaster (Kerr's Snow White Impression Plaster No. 2). Separate the cast from the impression as soon as a fingernail cannot score the cast (Fig 15-68).

Use the mold guide provided with the kit being utilized to determine the proper mesiodistal size for the crown form (Fig 15-69). Remove the corresponding size of crown from its compartment in the kit and place it on the prepared tooth on the cast or in the mouth. With a pencil, make a mark on the gingival portion of the labial surface (Fig 15-70). The distance from the pencil mark to the margin should equal the length discrepancy between the incisal edge of the crown form and the incisal edges of the adjacent teeth.

The excess gingival length is trimmed away with a large carborundum stone or an acrylic bur, using the pencil line as a reference mark (Fig 15-71). Try the shortened crown back onto the prepared tooth (Fig 15-72). If it is too tight interproximally, adjust it.

Paint the cast of the prepared tooth and the surrounding area with liberal amounts of a "tin foil substitute" separating medium (Alcote) (Fig 15-73). Accelerate the drying with an air syringe, and make sure that the cast is dry before starting to mix the resin.

Place four drops of monomer into a dappen dish and add tooth-colored polymer. While polycarbonate crowns are available in only one shade, it is possible to modify that shade somewhat by the shade of acrylic resin used to reline it. Fill the crown form with resin applied with an IPPA plastic instrument. When the acrylic resin just begins to lose its gloss, seat the crown form on the plaster cast, slowly expressing all the excess resin around the margins (Fig 15-74). Make sure that it is seated completely, and place it in a bowl of hot tap water to accelerate polymerization.

When the resin has polymerized completely, remove the provisional crown from the cast, breaking the cast if necessary. A coarse garnet disc on the straight handpiece is used to trim away the excess at the margins (Fig 15-75). In many cases this will mean that part of the original polycarbonate crown will be cut into and recontoured. Do not leave any sharp ledges or abrupt contour changes near the margin. If necessary, recontour the gingival half of the axial contours. Only in this way will it be possible to obtain a satisfactory provisional restoration by this technique.

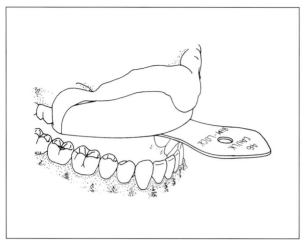

Fig 15-67 An anterior sectional tray is used to make an alginate impression of the prepared tooth.

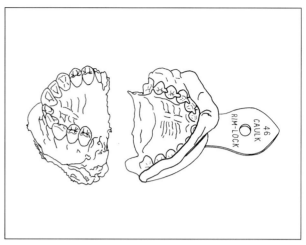

Fig 15-68 Quick-set plaster cast and the impression in which it was made.

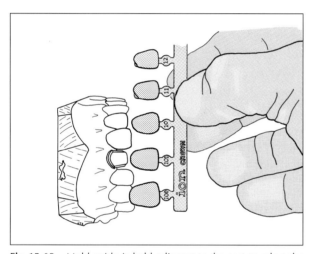

Fig 15-69 Mold guide is held adjacent to the cast to select the correct crown size.

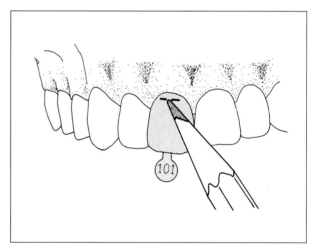

Fig 15-70 With the crown on the preparation, a mark is made at a distance from the labial margin that is equal to the amount by which the crown exceeds the height of adjacent teeth.

If the tooth is nonvital, or if a resin other than poly(methyl methacrylate) is used, the crown can be relined on the prepared tooth in the mouth. The preparation is coated with petrolatum, and the crown must be removed before the resin has polymerized to a stiffness that locks it into interproximal undercuts. Cut off as much of the rubbery excess as possible with a pair of curved scissors. Keep reseating and removing the crown until the relining resin has completely polymerized.

Place the crown on the prepared tooth in the mouth and check the occlusion with articulating paper (Fig 15-76). Adjust any high spots with a nondentate bur after removing the crown from the tooth. Smooth out the rough abraded areas in the lingual and incisal areas, as well as those surfaces recontoured near the margin, with a Burlew wheel in the straight handpiece (Fig 15-77).

Polish all surfaces of the provisional restoration with polishing compound (Yellow Diamond Polishing Compound, Matchless Metal Polish Co) on a muslin rag wheel (Fig 15-78). It is possible to return the crown to its original luster by this means. Coat the outer surface of the crown with petrolatum to prevent the cement from sticking to it. Cement the restoration with zinc oxide–eugenol cement. Make certain that all cement has been removed from the gingival crevice by using an explorer (Fig 15-79). Use dental floss interproximally to remove any cement left there.

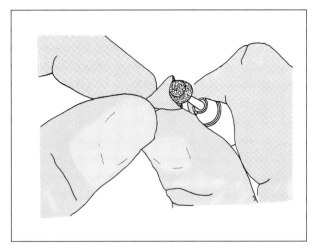

Fig 15-71 Excess gingival length that extends beyond the mark is cut off.

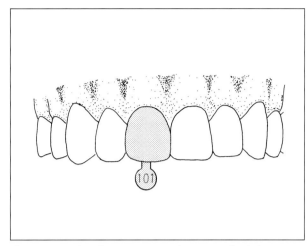

Fig 15-72 Polycarbonate crown after removal of the excess length. The tab is left on at this point to facilitate handling.

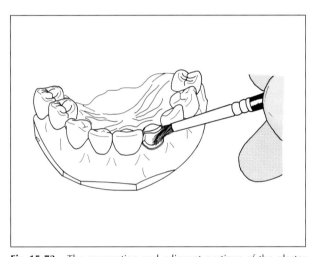

Fig 15-73 The preparation and adjacent portions of the plaster cast are painted with separating medium.

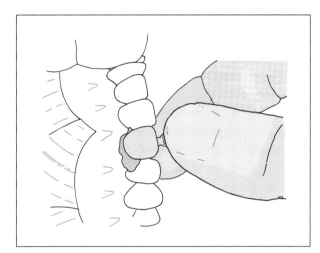

Fig 15-74 The crown filled with resin is placed onto the prepared tooth on the plaster cast.

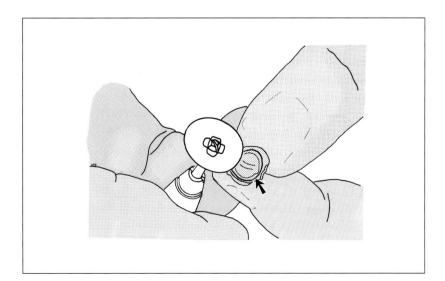

Fig 15-75 Gingival excess created by the expressed acrylic is trimmed back with a garnet disc until the margin coincides with the imprint of the finish line *(arrow)*.

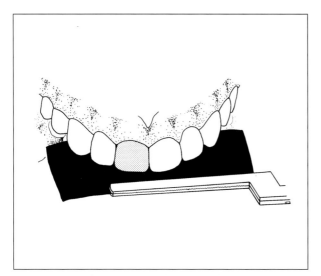

Fig 15-76 Occlusion is checked with articulating paper.

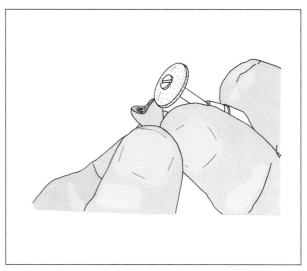

Fig 15-77 Axial surfaces near the margin are smoothed with a Burlew disc.

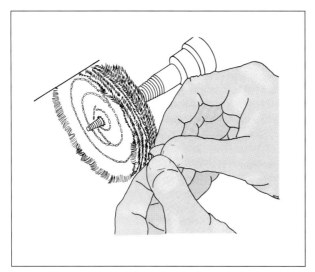

Fig 15-78 Axial surfaces are polished with white polishing compound on a muslin rag wheel.

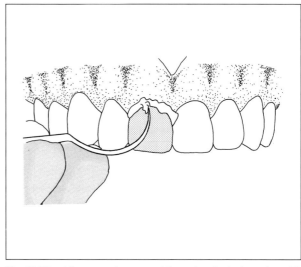

Fig 15-79 All cement is removed from the gingival crevice with an explorer.

Provisional Crown for an Endodontically Treated Tooth

It is often difficult to fabricate a provisional restoration for a tooth that has been prepared for a dowel core because there is so little intact supragingival tooth structure. This can be accommodated for in the use of a standard polycarbonate crown by placing a piece of paper clip or other stiff wire into the canal and placing the resin-filled crown down over that (Fig 15-80).[1,2,5]

Preformed Anatomic Metal Crown

Emergency cases involving fractured molars are one of the best indications for the use of preformed metal crowns. Zinc oxide and eugenol alone will not adhere to the tooth, and there is rarely enough time at the emergency appointment to fabricate a custom acrylic resin provisional crown. By using the preformed anatomic metal crown, it is possible to provide the patient with temporary coverage to protect the fractured tooth and prevent irritation of the tongue and mucosa.

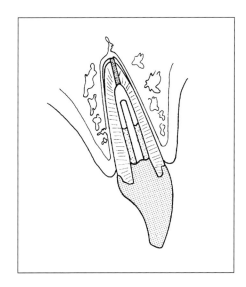

Fig 15-80 A pin is incorporated into a polycarbonate crown for use as a provisional restoration on a tooth prepared for a dowel core.

There are several systems available for this purpose, utilizing the same general principles. The procedure consists of:

1. Minimal tooth preparation
2. Measurement and selection of crown
3. Trimming and adaptation of gingival margin
4. Occlusal adjustment
5. Cementation

Armamentarium

1. High-speed handpiece
2. No. 170 bur
3. Measuring gauge
4. Crown forms
5. Stretching block
6. Crown and bridge scissors
7. Contouring pliers
8. Straight handpiece
9. Sandpaper disc on Moore mandrel
10. Articulating paper
11. Miller forceps
12. Cement spatula
13. Paper pad
14. Zinc oxide–eugenol cement
15. Petrolatum
16. LL 6-7 curved burnisher
17. Explorer
18. Mouth mirror
19. Dental floss

The maxillary molar with a lingual cusp fractured off is not an uncommon dental emergency (Fig 15-81). It is most easily protected on a short-term basis with a preformed metal crown (Iso-Form Temporary Crown, 3M Dental Products, St Paul, MN).

The tooth must be prepared minimally to create space for the restoration. The initial step is occlusal reduction, which follows the inclined planes of the occlusal surface (Fig 15-82). The depth will be 1.0 mm on the nonfunctional cusps and 1.5 mm on the functional cusps. A functional cusp bevel (on the lingual incline of the maxillary lingual cusp) is placed to a depth of 1.5 mm to complete the occlusal reduction (Fig 15-83).

Only enough proximal reduction is done to permit the seating of the crown. If an MOD amalgam restoration is present in the tooth, the proximal reduction is most easily accomplished by removing the amalgam in the boxes (Fig 15-84). The boxes are cut with a no. 170L or 171L bur. All caries is removed at this time. No effort is made to remove all of the existing restoration, nor to provide permanent bases or a completed preparation.

Each of the three measuring heads in the metal crown form kit has converging blades that measure a 1.0-mm range: 9 to 10 mm, 10 to 11 mm, and 11 to 12 mm (Fig 15-85). Hold the gauge in line with the contact points, resting it on the occlusal surfaces of the other teeth in the arch. Slide the blades until they wedge between the contacts of the teeth on either side of the preparation (Fig 15-86). The point at which the blades wedge indicates the dimension to be used for selection of the proper crown form.

The crown is tried on the tooth. If the gingival collar is too tight, the crown is placed on the appropriate post of the stretching block (Fig 15-87). There is a tapered post corresponding to each of the maxillary and mandibular molars, left and right. Flaring the margins is also required when there is a shoulder finish line. The crown is pushed

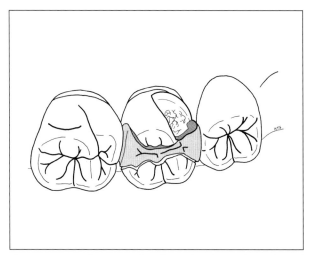

Fig 15-81 Maxillary second molar with a fractured distolingual cusp.

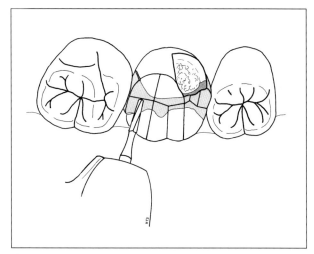

Fig 15-82 Occlusal clearance is obtained with a diamond or a no. 170 bur.

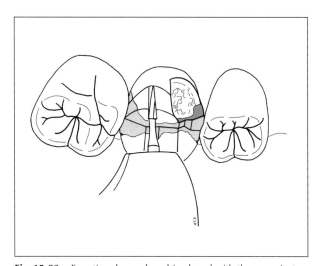

Fig 15-83 Functional cusp bevel is placed with the same instrument.

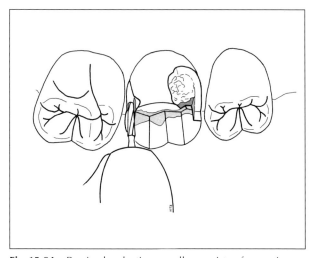

Fig 15-84 Proximal reduction usually consists of removing an existing amalgam restoration.

down on the post until an adequate amount of gingival flare is obtained.

The crown is placed on the tooth to evaluate its occlusogingival length. Compare the height of each marginal ridge of the crown with that of the adjacent tooth (Fig 15-88). Use crown and bridge scissors to remove an amount at the gingival margin equal to the marginal ridge height discrepancy (Fig 15-89). Festoon the margin to follow the contours of the gingival tissue.

Smooth rough spots and any irregularities in the gingival margin with a sandpaper disc (Fig 15-90). Use no. 114 contouring pliers to produce a slightly convex contour occlusal to the margins (Fig 15-91). The margin will be slightly constricted as a result.

Place the crown on the tooth and check the occlusion with articulating paper (Fig 15-92). Remove the crown and burnish areas on the occlusal surface that are in hyperocclusion. Open proximal contacts can be corrected by burnishing the proximal area from the inside of the crown.

Coat the outside of the crown with petrolatum to facilitate the removal of excess cement later. Mix zinc oxide and eugenol to a thick creamy consistency on a paper pad. Fill the crown with the cement and seat it on the prepared tooth with finger pressure (Fig 15-93).

Burnish the margins of the crown with an LL 6-7 curved burnisher before the cement hardens (Fig 15-94). Run dental floss through the proximal contacts to remove hardened cement from the interproximal areas (Fig 15-95). Use an explorer to remove all remaining subgingival cement (Fig 15-96). Make a final check of the margins to insure that they are not impinging on the gingiva.

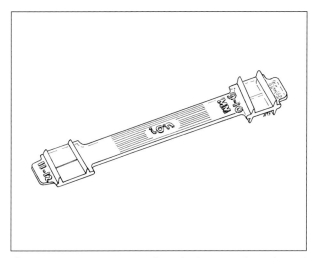

Fig 15-85 Measuring gauge for selecting a preformed metal crown.

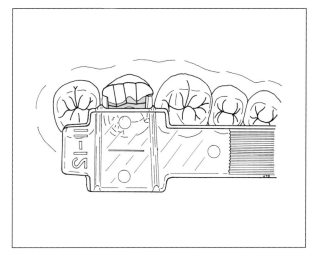

Fig 15-86 Mesiodistal measurement of the space is obtained.

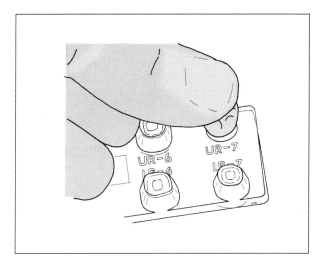

Fig 15-87 Gingival margins can be flared slightly on the stretching block.

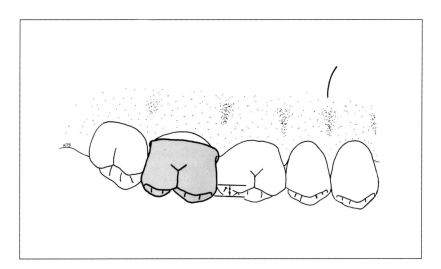

Fig 15-88 Marginal ridge height discrepancy between the restoration and the adjacent tooth is estimated.

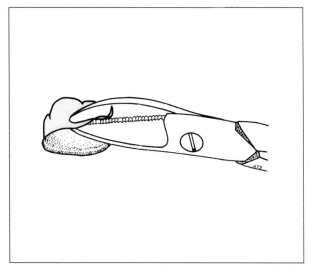

Fig 15-89   Estimated excess height is removed from the gingival margin.

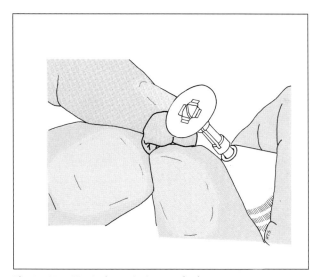

Fig 15-90   Gingival margin is smoothed.

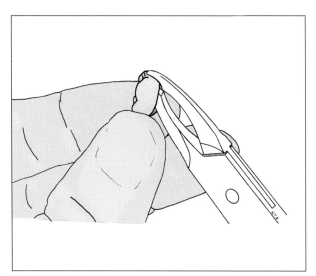

Fig 15-91   Axial surfaces are contoured with pliers.

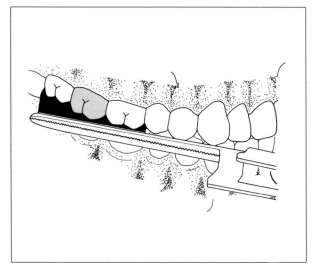

Fig 15-92   Occlusion is checked with articulating paper.

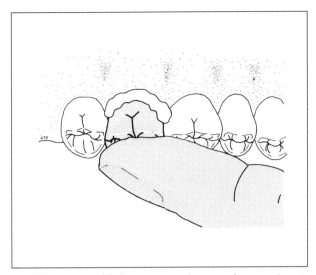

Fig 15-93 Crown filled with zinc oxide–eugenol cement is seated.

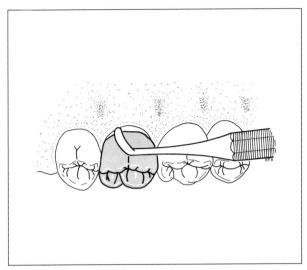

Fig 15-94 Margin is burnished.

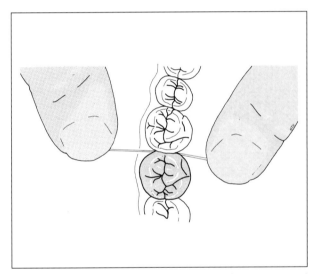

Fig 15-95 Excess cement is removed from the interproximal region with dental floss.

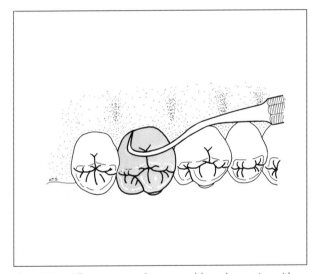

Fig 15-96 All cement must be removed from the crevice with an explorer.

References

1. Mumford JM, Ferguson HW: Temporary restorations and dressings. *Dent Pract Dent Rec* 1959; 9:121–124.

2. Segat L: Protection of prepared abutments between appointments in crown and bridge prosthodontics. *J Mich Dent Assoc* 1962; 44:32–35.

3. Knight RM: Temporary restorations in restorative dentistry. *J Tenn Dent Assoc* 1967; 47:346–349.

4. Rose HP: A simplified technique for temporary crowns. *Dent Dig* 1967; 73:449–450.

5. Behrend DA: Temporary protective restorations in crown and bridgework. *Aust Dent J* 1967; 12:411–416.

6. Fisher DW, Shillingburg HT, Dewhirst RB: Indirect temporary restorations. *J Am Dent Assoc* 1971; 82:160–163.

7. Phillips RW: *Skinner's Science of Dental Materials,* ed 9. Philadelphia, WB Saunders Co, 1991, p 193.

8. Lui JL, Setcos JC, Phillips RW: Temporary restorations: A review. *Oper Dent* 1986; 11:103–110.

9. Lockard MW, Wackerly J: Excellence in dentistry: Acrylic provisional crowns. *Dent Manage* 1987; 27:60–62.

10. Crispin BJ, Watson JF, Caputo AA: The marginal accuracy of treatment restorations: A comparative analysis. *J Prosthet Dent* 1980; 44:283–290.

11. Monday JJL, Blais D: Marginal adaptation of provisional acrylic resin crowns. *J Prosthet Dent* 1985; 54:194–197.

12. Grossman LI: Pulp reaction to the insertion of self-curing acrylic resin filling materials. *J Am Dent Assoc* 1953; 46:265–269.

13. Kramer IRH, McLean JW: Response of the human pulp to self-polymerizing acrylic restorations. *Br Dent J* 1952; 92:255–261, 281–297, 311–315.

14. Langeland K, Langeland L: Pulp reactions to crown preparation, impression, temporary crown fixation and permanent cementation. *J Prosthet Dent* 1965; 5:129–143.

15. Wang RL, Moore BK, Goodacre CJ, Swartz ML, Andres CJ: A comparison of resins for fabricating provisional fixed restorations. *Int J Prosthodont* 1989; 2:173–184.

16. Vahidi F: The provisional restoration. *Dent Clin North Am* 1987; 31:363–381.

17. Driscoll CF, Woolsey G, Ferguson WM: Comparison of exothermic release during polymerization of four materials used to fabricate interim restorations. *J Prosthet Dent* 1991; 65:504–506.

18. Moulding MB, Teplitsky PE: Intrapulpal temperature during direct fabrication of provisional restorations. *Int J Prosthodont* 1990; 3:299–304.

19. Gegauff AG, Pryor HG: Fracture toughness of provisional resins for fixed prosthodontics. *J Prosthet Dent* 1987; 58:23–29.

20. Haddix JE: A technique for visible light-cured provisional restorations. *J Prosthet Dent* 1988; 59:512–514.

21. Goldfogel M: Direct technique for the fabrication of a visible light-curing resin for provisional restorations. *Quintessence Int* 1990; 21:699–703.

22. Freese AS: Impressions for temporary acrylic resin jacket crowns. *J Prosthet Dent* 1957; 7:99–101.

23. Leary JM, Aquilino SA: A method to develop provisional restorations. *Quint Dent Technol* 1987; 11:191–192.

24. Leff A: An improved temporary acrylic fixed bridge. *J Prosthet Dent* 1953; 3:245–249.

25. Fiasconaro JE, Sherman H: Vacuum-formed prostheses. I. A temporary fixed bridge or splint. *J Am Dent Assoc* 1968; 76:74–78.

26. Sotera AJ: A direct technique for fabricating acrylic resin temporary crowns using the Omnivac. *J Prosthet Dent* 1973; 29:577–580.

27. Preston JD: *Ceramometal Restorations and Fixed Prosthodontic Esthetics.* Continuing education program presented by the University of Oklahoma College of Dentistry, Oklahoma City, OK, September 12, 1975.

28. Ferencz JL: Fabrication of provisional crowns and fixed partial dentures utilizing a "shell" technique. *N Y J Dent* 1981; 51:201–206.

29. Elledge DA, Hart JK, Schorr BL: A provisional restoration technique for laminate veneer preparations. *J Prosthet Dent* 1989; 62:139–142.

30. Elledge DA, Schorr BL: A provisional and new crown to fit into a clasp of an existing removable partial denture. *J Prosthet Dent* 1990; 63:541–544.

31. Fritts KW, Thayer KE: Fabrication of temporary crowns and fixed partial dentures. *J Prosthet Dent* 1973; 30:151–155.

32. Donovan TE, Hurst RG, Campagni WV: Physical properties of acrylic resin polymerized by four different techniques. *J Prosthet Dent* 1985; 54:522–524.

33. Crispin BJ, Caputo AA: Color stability of temporary restorative material. *J Prosthet Dent* 1979; 42:27–33.

34. Yuodelis RA, Faucher R: Provisional restorations: An integrated approach to periodontics and restorative dentistry. *Dent Clin North Am* 1980; 24:285–303.

35. Chiche GJ, Avila R: Fabrication of a preformed shell for a provisional fixed partial denture. *Quint Dent Technol* 1986; 10:579–581.

36. von Krammer R: An extrusion technique for handling autocuring acrylic resins. *J Prosthet Dent* 1988; 60:735–738.

37. Nayyar A, Edwards WS: Fabrication of a single anterior intermediate restoration. *J Prosthet Dent* 1978; 39:574–577.

Chapter 16

Fluid Control and Soft Tissue Management

Complete control of the environment of the operative site is essential during restorative dental procedures. For the patient's comfort and safety, and for the operator's access and clear visibility, saliva, as well as water introduced during instrumentation, must be removed from the mouth.

Control of the oral environment extends to the gingiva surrounding the teeth being restored. The gingiva must be displaced to make a complete impression and sometimes even to permit completion of the preparation and cementation of the restoration. Occasionally it is necessary to permanently alter the contours of the gingival tissues around the teeth or of the edentulous ridge to insure a better, longer-lasting result for the fixed restoration.

Fluid Control

The need for removal of fluids varies depending upon the task being performed. During the preparation of teeth, it is necessary to remove large volumes of water produced by a handpiece spray and to control the tongue to prevent accidental injury. When an impression is made or a restoration is cemented, there is a much smaller volume of fluid to be removed, but a much greater degree of dryness is required. Several types of attachments can be used with low-volume (saliva ejector) or high-volume vacuum outlets to remove fluids (Fig 16-1). Some combine the functions of fluid removal with isolation.

Rubber Dam

The rubber dam is the most effective of all isolation devices utilized in restorative dentistry. Its use is valuable in the removal of old restorations or excavation of caries when exposure of the pulp is a possibility. It also provides excellent isolation and access when a pin-retained amalgam or composite resin core is required before a cast restoration can be fabricated. Teeth with old or questionable endodontic treatments should be isolated in this

manner for dowel-core preparation, pattern fabrication, and cementation.

If the premise is accepted that the rubber dam is meant to be an instrument of convenience, it has only limited direct application in the area of cast restorations. It can be used during tooth preparation for inlays and onlays (if the occlusal reduction is done before the dam is placed), and it can be readily used for making impressions and cementing the same types of restorations. When used with elastomeric impression materials, the dam must be lubricated and the clamp must be removed or avoided. It should not be used with polyvinyl siloxane impression material, because the rubber dam will inhibit its polymerization.[1]

The occlusion must be adjusted on onlays before the actual cementation. Some would argue that the rubber dam can be used for preparation, impression, and cementation of all cast restorations. However, it is likely to produce more aggravation than assistance for the majority of dentists when its use is attempted with most full or partial veneer crowns.

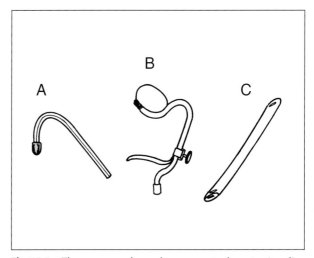

Fig 16-1 Three commonly used vacuum attachments: A, saliva ejector; B, Svedopter; C, vacuum tip.

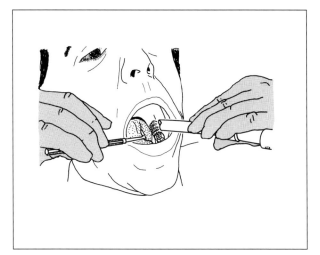

Fig 16-2 The vacuum tip can double as a cheek or tongue retractor.

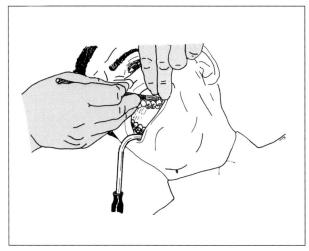

Fig 16-3 The saliva ejector can be used for evacuation when the maxillary arch is being treated.

High-Volume Vacuum

A high-volume suction tip is extremely useful during the preparation phase and is most effectively utilized with an assistant. When wielded by a knowledgeable assistant, it makes an excellent lip retractor while the operator uses a mirror to retract and protect the tongue (Fig 16-2). Its use is not practical during the impression or cementation phases.

Saliva Ejector

The simple saliva ejector can be utilized effectively in some situations by the lone dentist. It is most useful as an adjunct to high-volume evacuation, but it can be used alone for the maxillary arch. The saliva ejector is placed in the corner of the mouth opposite the quadrant being operated, and the patient's head is turned toward it (Fig 16-3). It can also be used very effectively on the maxillary arch for impressions and cementation simply by adding cotton rolls in the vestibule facial to the teeth being isolated. It can be used on the mandibular arch while a cotton roll holder positions cotton rolls facial and lingual to the teeth. Tongue control and fluid removal in this application may be less than ideal, however.

Svedopter

For isolation and evacuation of the mandibular teeth, the metal saliva ejector with attached tongue deflector is excellent. It can be used without cotton rolls during the preparation phase, with a mouth mirror as a lip retractor (Fig 16-4). By adding facial and lingual cotton rolls,

excellent tongue control and isolation is provided for impression making or cementation (Fig 16-5).

The Svedopter is most effective when it is used with the patient in a nearly upright position. In this position, water and other fluids collect on the floor of the mouth, where they are pulled off by the vacuum (Fig 16-6). If the patient is in a supine position, the throat and back of the mouth must fill with fluid before it reaches the level of the evacuation device.

Although this is an excellent device for the lone operator or one with only intermittent chairside assistance, it is not without its drawbacks. Access to the lingual surfaces of the mandibular teeth is limited. Because the device is made of metal, care must be exercised to avoid bruising the tender tissue in the floor of the mouth by overzealously cinching down the clamp that fits under the chin. The presence of mandibular tori usually precludes its use. Selection of an oversized reflector should be avoided, since it could cut into the palate above or trigger the gag reflex. The medium size seems to work best in most mouths.

For better positioning, the anterior part of the Svedopter should be placed in the incisor region, with the tubing under the patient's arm (Fig 16-7). This provides the security of having the tubing firmly under the patient's control. This is especially important if the saliva ejector tubing originates from a movable assistant's cart, a common design feature of many dental units today.

Antisialagogues

There are some patients for whom no mechanical device is effective in producing a dry enough field for impression making or cementation. For the patient who salivates excessively, some other measure may be nec-

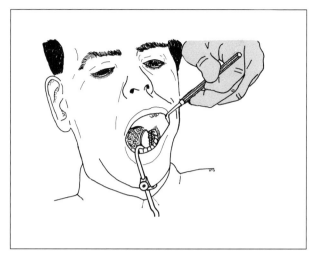

Fig 16-4 The Svedopter can be used on the mandibular arch during the preparation phase.

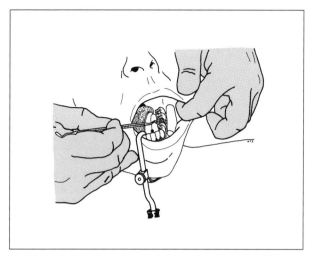

Fig 16-5 With cotton rolls, the Svedopter provides excellent isolation of a mandibular quadrant during the impression phase.

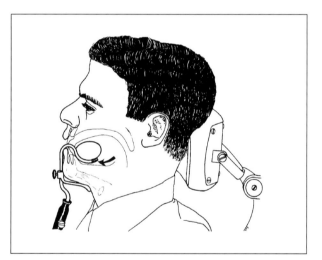

Fig 16-6 If the patient's head is upright, fluids collect on the floor of the mouth, where they are easily picked up by the Svedopter *(arrow).*

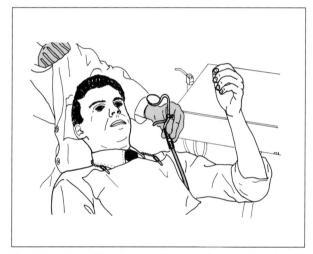

Fig 16-7 The tubing for the Svedopter is placed under the patient's arm to prevent any jerking on the attachment while it is in the mouth.

essary. Drugs can be used to control salivary flow. Methantheline bromide (Banthine) and propantheline bromide (Pro-Banthine), both manufactured by Schiapparelli Searle (Chicago, IL), have been used for this purpose.[2] They are gastrointestinal anticholinergics that act on the smooth muscles of the gastrointestinal, urinary, and biliary tracts, producing a dry mouth as a side effect.

Usually one 50-mg tablet of Banthine or 15-mg tablet of Pro-Banthine taken 1 hour before the appointment will provide the necessary control. If previous experience has shown this amount to be inadequate for a particular patient, the dosage can be doubled on subsequent appointments. The patient may experience drowsiness and blurred vision. Unfortunately, these substances also produce an unpleasant, bitter aftertaste.

Methantheline and propantheline are contraindicated in any patient with a history of hypersensitivity to the drugs, eye problems such as glaucoma, asthma, obstructive conditions of the gastrointestinal or urinary tracts, or congestive heart failure. They should not be used by lactating females. They may be potentiated by antihistamines, tranquilizers, and narcotic analgesics, and in the presence of corticosteroids they may increase ocular pressure.

Propantheline can be made tasteless by injecting 2.0 to 6.0 mg in solution intraorally. Onset of action occurs in 5 to 10 minutes, and the duration of a dry working environment is approximately 1.5 hours.[3] The drying effect can be prolonged after 1.5 hours by injecting an additional 2.0 to 3.0 mg of propantheline. Administration of larger doses at one time may result in bladder discomfort.

Another drug that has been shown to be effective as an antisialagogue is clonidine hydrochloride (Catapres, Boehringer Ingelheim Pharmaceuticals, Ridgefield, CT). Wilson et al[4] demonstrated that a 0.2-mg dose of this drug is as effective as 50 mg of Banthine in diminishing salivary flow. Clonidine hydrochloride is an antihypertensive agent, and it should be used cautiously in patients who are receiving other antihypertensive medication. Its principal side effect, besides a dry mouth, is drowsiness, which is not altogether undesirable in a patient undergoing a lengthy restorative dental appointment. The dose of 0.2 mg should be administered an hour before the appointment, and because of the sedative effect of the drug, someone should accompany the patient to do any driving.

Finish Line Exposure

It is essential that gingival tissue be healthy and free of inflammation before cast restorations are begun. To start tooth preparations in the face of untreated gingivitis makes the task more difficult and seriously compromises the chances for success. Because the marginal fit of a restoration is essential in preventing recurrent caries and gingival irritation, the finish line of the tooth preparation *must* be reproduced in the impression.

Obtaining a complete impression is complicated when some or all of the preparation finish line lies at or apical to the crest of the free gingiva. In these situations, the preparation finish line must be temporarily exposed to insure reproduction of the entire preparation. Control of fluids in the sulcus, particularly when a hydrophobic impression material is used, is also necessary, because liquids can cause an incomplete impression of the critical finish line area. These measures are accomplished by one or more of three techniques: mechanical, chemicomechanical, and surgical.[5] The surgical techniques can be further broken down into rotary curettage and electrosurgery.[6]

Mechanical

Physically displacing the gingiva was one of the first methods used for insuring adequate reproduction of the preparation finish line. A copper band or tube can serve as a means of carrying the impression material as well as a mechanism for displacing the gingiva to insure that the gingival finish line is captured in the impression.

One end of the tube is festooned, or trimmed, to follow the profile of the gingival finish line, which, in turn, often follows the contours of the free gingival margin (Fig 16-8). The tube is filled with modeling compound, and then it is seated carefully in place along the path of insertion of the tooth preparation (Fig 16-9). The technique has been utilized in restorative dentistry for many years.[7] It has been used with impression compound[7-10] and elastomeric materials.[11] Several types of die material can be used, depending on the material used for the impression. If the impression is made with an elastomeric material, the die can be formed of stone or electroplated metal[11]; if the impression is compound, the die can be made of amalgam[7,11] or electroplated metal.[8,9]

The use of copper bands can cause incisional injuries of gingival tissues,[12] but recession following their use is minimal, ranging from 0.1 mm in healthy adolescents[12] to 0.3 mm in a general clinic population.[13] Copper bands are especially useful for situations in which several teeth have been prepared. The likelihood of capturing all of the finish lines in one impression decreases as the number of prepared teeth increases. The use of a copper band could negate the necessity of remaking an entire full-arch impression just to capture one or two preparations.

A rubber dam also can accomplish the exposure of the finish line needed.[14] Generally it is used when a limited number of teeth in one quadrant are being restored and in situations in which preparations do not have to be extended very far subgingivally. It can be used with modified trays if the bow and wings of the clamp are blocked out. As mentioned previously, a rubber dam should not be used with polyvinyl siloxane impression material, because the rubber inhibits its polymerization.[1]

With the introduction of elastic impression materials, new means had to be used for displacing the gingiva. Plain cotton cord was used for sulcus enlargement,[15] physically pushing away the gingiva from the finish line. Unfortunately, its effectiveness is limited because the use of pressure alone often will not control sulcular hemorrhage. One group of investigators found that over half of the impressions preceded by the use of plain cotton cord had to be remade[16]; however, this may have been exaggerated by the fact that the cord was used dry.

Chemicomechanical (retraction cord)

By combining chemical action with pressure packing, enlargement of the gingival sulcus as well as control of fluids seeping from the walls of the gingival sulcus is more readily accomplished. Caustic chemicals such as sulfuric acid,[5] trichloracetic acid,[5,17] negatol (a 45% condensation product of meta cresol sulfonic acid and formaldehyde),[6] and zinc chloride[18] have been tried in the search for an effective chemical for gingival retraction, but their undesirable effects on the gingiva led to their abandonment.

Over the years, racemic epinephrine has emerged as the most popular chemical for gingival retraction. Surveys published in the 1980s document that cord impregnated with 8% racemic epinephrine is the most commonly used means of producing gingival retraction (Table 16-1).[19-21]

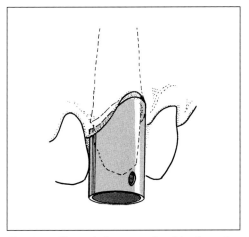

Fig 16-8 The end of a copper band is trimmed to follow the preparation finish line.

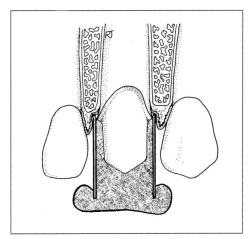

Fig 16-9 In a copper band impression, the band displaces the free gingiva.

Table 16-1 *Results of Surveys of Material Preferences for Gingival Retraction*

Investigators	Year published	Number of respondents	Epinephrine cord	Astringent cord	Electro- surgery	Misc or None
Shillingburg et al[19]	1980	3737	73%	24%	11%	7%
Donovan et al[20]	1985	495	79%	19%	5%	18%
Shaw and Krejci[21]	1986	814	55%	33%	2%	10%

The three criteria for a gingival retraction material are *(1)* effectiveness in gingival displacement and hemostasis, *(2)* absence of irreversible damage to the gingiva, and *(3)* paucity of untoward systemic effects.[20,22] Epinephrine produces hemostasis, and it causes local vasoconstriction, which in turn results in transitory gingival shrinkage. In research conducted on dogs, epinephrine produced slight tissue injury that healed in 6 days[23] to 10 days.[18] A study using human subjects showed that epinephrine cord did not produce significantly greater gingival inflammation than potassium aluminum sulfate or aluminum chloride.[24]

However, there is controversy surrounding the use of epinephrine for gingival retraction,[25] and its use is declining, particularly among dentists who have graduated since 1980.[21] Epinephrine causes an elevation of blood pressure and increased heart rate. Some investigators have found that the physiologic changes that occur when epinephrine-impregnated cord is placed in an intact gingival sulcus are minimal.[26-29] However, the heart rate increase and blood pressure elevation are more dramatic when the cord is applied to a severely lacerated gingival sulcus, or when cotton pellets soaked in epinephrine are applied.[29] The use of liquid, epinephrine-containing hemostatic agents is therefore not warranted in this situation; there are effective hemostatic agents without epinephrine available for such use.

For those patients with cardiovascular disease, hypertension, diabetes, hyperthyroidism, or a known hypersensitivity to epinephrine, a cord impregnated with some other agent *must* be substituted. Epinephrine also should not be used on patients taking Rauwolfia compounds, ganglionic blockers, or epinephrine-potentiating drugs.[30] Neither should patients taking monoamine oxidase inhibitors for depression receive epinephrine.[20]

Patients without the aforementioned contraindications can also exhibit "epinephrine syndrome" (tachycardia, rapid respiration, elevated blood pressure, anxiety, and postoperative depression).[6] The amount of epinephrine absorbed is highly variable, depending on the degree of exposure of the vascular bed,[31] as well as the time of contact and the amount of medication in the cord.[29,32] The amount of epinephrine lost (and presumed absorbed) from 2.5 cm of typical retraction cord during 5 to 15 minutes in the gingival sulcus is 71 µg.[33] This amount is slightly less than that obtained from receiving the injection of four carpules of local anesthetic containing a 1:100,000 concentration of epinephrine.[33] It also is approximately one-third the maximum dose of 0.2 mg (200 µg) for a healthy adult and nearly twice the recommended amount of 0.04 mg (40 µg) for a cardiac patient.[34]

Although the absorbed amounts reported by Kellam et al[33] are lower than estimates by some authors,[20] the patient nonetheless is receiving a large dose from the cord around one tooth. If cord is placed around more than one tooth, if more than one impression is made of a single tooth (not an uncommon occurrence in a teaching institution), and/or if an epinephrine-containing anesthetic is used, a patient could easily exceed the recommended maximum dosage of epinephrine.

Donovan and associates[20] report that only 3% of the dentists they surveyed recorded the patient's pulse, and fewer than 10% recorded blood pressures routinely. Given this, it is likely that few patients would receive even a rudimentary cardiovascular evaluation. The routine use of epinephrine in dentistry, even on healthy patients, has been questioned.[34]

Because epinephrine has been used successfully for nearly half a century, there is reluctance to abandon its use. However, the fact that many dentists manage without it proves that it is not indispensable. Its proper niche probably lies in utilization as an adjunct method in difficult situations where other agents have been ineffective. Even then it must be used only on healthy patients with no history of cardiovascular problems.

Aluminum chloride [$AlCl_3$], alum (aluminum potassium sulfate) [$AlK(SO_4)_2$], aluminum sulfate [$Al_2(SO_4)_3$], and ferric sulfate [$Fe_2(SO_4)_3$] are also used for gingival retraction[35] (Table 16-2). Investigators have compared several of these agents with epinephrine for displacement effectiveness, hemostasis, and tissue irritation.

No significant difference was found in sulcular width around teeth treated with alum- and epinephrine-impregnated cord before impressions (0.49 mm vs 0.51 mm, respectively).[36] In an in vivo study of 120 human teeth, Weir and Williams[37] found no significant difference between the hemorrhage control offered by cords impregnated with aluminum sulfate and those impregnated with epinephrine.

In a study conducted on dogs, Shaw et al[38] found no additional inflammation in gingival crevices in which dilute aluminum chloride (0.033%) was placed, but those receiving concentrated solutions (60%) demonstrated severe inflammation and necrosis. Another study on human subjects found no significant difference in gingival inflammation produced by alum-, aluminum chloride-, or epinephrine-impregnated cords.[24]

Over-the-counter drugs commonly used as nasal and ophthalmic decongestants show promise as gingival retraction agents.[36] Phenylephrine hydrochloride 0.25% (Neosynephrine, Winthrop Consumer Products Div, Sterling Drug, New York, NY) was found to be as effective as epinephrine and alum in widening the gingival sulcus, while oxymetazoline hydrochloride 0.05% (Afrin, Schering-Plough Health Care Products, Memphis, TN) and tetrahydrozoline hydrochloride 0.05% (Visine, Consumer Health Care Div, Pfizer, New York, NY) were 57% more effective.[36]

There is evidence to suggest that tissue hemorrhage can also be controlled indirectly by the adjunctive use of antimicrobial rinses. Sorensen et al[39] report lowered plaque, bleeding, and gingivitis indices with the administration of 0.12% chlorhexidine gluconate (Peridex, Proctor & Gamble, Cincinnati, OH) 2 weeks before tooth preparation, 3 weeks during provisional restorations, and 2 weeks after final restoration cementation.

Retraction Cord Armamentarium

1. Evacuator (saliva ejector, Svedopter)
2. Scissors
3. Cotton pliers
4. Mouth mirror
5. Explorer
6. Fischer Ultrapak Packer (small)
7. DE plastic filling instrument IPPA
8. Cotton rolls
9. Retraction cord
10. Hemodent liquid
11. Dappen dish
12. Cotton pellets
13. 2 x 2 gauze sponges

The operating area must be *dry*. An evacuating device is placed in the mouth, and the quadrant containing the prepared tooth is isolated with cotton rolls. The retraction cord is drawn from the dispenser bottle with sterile cotton pliers, and a piece approximately 5.0 cm (2.0 inches) long is cut off (Fig 16-10). If a twisted or wound cord is used, grasp the ends between the thumb and forefinger of each hand. Hold the cord taut and twist the ends to produce a tightly wound cord of small diameter (Fig 16-11). If a braided or woven cord is used, twisting is not necessary.

Be careful not to touch any of the cord other than the ends, which will be cut off later, with your gloved fingers. It has been postulated that handling the cord with latex gloves may indirectly inhibit polymerization of a polyvinyl siloxane impression.[40] If that happens, it will occur in that segment of the impression replicating the gingival crevice and the gingival finish line of the preparation.

The retraction cord should be moistened by dipping it in buffered 25% aluminum chloride solution (Hemodent, Premier Dental Products Co, Norristown, PA) in a dappen dish. Cords impregnated with either epinephrine or aluminum sulfate are twice as effective when saturated with aluminum chloride solution prior to insertion into the gingival crevice.[37] If there is slight hemorrhage in the gingival crevice, it can be controlled by the use of a hemostatic agent, such as Hemodent liquid (aluminum chloride). In any event, the cord must be slightly moist before it is removed from the sulcus.[41] Removing dry cord from the gingival crevice can cause injury to delicate epithelial lining that is not unlike the "cotton roll burn" produced

Table 16-2 *Principal Chemical in Brands of Gingival Retraction Cord*

Manufacturer	$AlCl_3$	$Al_2K(SO_4)_2$	$Al_2(SO_4)_3$	$Fe_2(SO_4)_3$	Epinephrine	Combination	None
Aseptico, Inc Kirkland, WA	—	Sulpak K-Alum Astringent R-24, 25, 26 (T)		—	Sulpak Epinephrine Vasoconstrictor R-34, 35, 36, (T)	Astringent Plus Vasoconstrictor R-44, 45–46 (T) (epinephrine + alum)	Sulpak Plain R-14, 15, 16 (T)
Belport Co, Inc Camarillo, CA	Gingi-Aid (T,W)	—	—	—	Gingi-Pak (T,W)	—	Gingi-Plain (T,W)
Miles Dental Prod South Bend, IN	—	—	Cutter Cord Aluminum Sulfate (W)	—	Cutter Cord Epinephrine (W)		—
Pascal Dental Mfg Bellevue, WA	—	—	Pascord (T) Siltrax A.S. (W)	—	Racord (T) Siltrax Epi (W)	Racord II (T,W) (epinephrine + zinc phenolsulfonate)	Retrax (T) Siltrax (W)
Premier Norristown, PA	Hemodent (T,W)	—	—	—	—		—
Sultan Dental Prod Englewood, NJ	—	Sulpak (T) Ultrax (W)	—	—	Sulpak (T) Ultrax (W) (4% epinephrine)	Sulpak (T) Ultrax (W) (4% epinephrine + alum)	—
Ultradent Salt Lake City, UT	—	—	—	Ultrapak & Astringedent (W)	—	—	Ultrapak (W)
Van R Oxnard, CA	GingiGel (W)	FlexiBraid (W) GingiYarn (T)	—	—	GingiYarn (T)	GingiBraid (W) FlexiBraid (W) GingiCord (T) (epinephrine + alum)	GingiBraid (W) GingiYarn (T)

T = twisted; W = woven (braided or knitted).

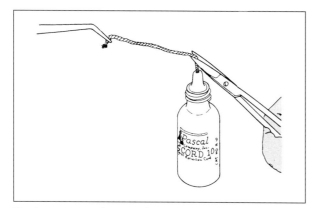

Fig 16-10 A 2-inch piece of retraction cord is cut off.

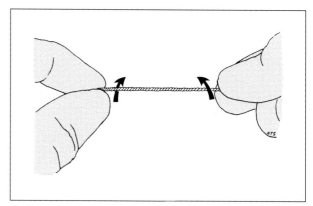

Fig 16-11 The cord is twisted to make it as tight and as small as possible.

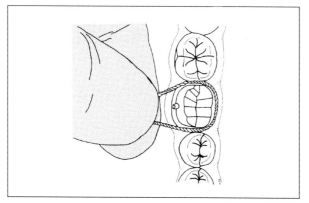

Fig 16-12 A loop of retraction cord is formed around the tooth and held tautly with the thumb and forefinger.

by prying an adhering cotton roll off the desiccated mucous membrane of the mouth.

Form the cord into a "U" and loop it around the prepared tooth (Fig 16-12). Hold the cord between the thumb and forefinger, and apply slight tension in an apical direction. Gently slip the cord between the tooth and the gingiva in the mesial interproximal area with a Fischer packing instrument or a DE plastic instrument IPPA (Fig 16-13, A). Cord placement is a finesse move, not a power play. Once the cord has been tucked in on the mesial, use the instrument to lightly secure it in the distal interproximal area (Fig 16-13, B).

Proceed to the lingual surface and begin working from the mesiolingual corner around to the distolingual corner. The tip of the instrument should be inclined slightly *toward* the area where the cord has already been placed; ie, the mesial (Fig 16-14, A). If the tip of the instrument is inclined away from the area in which the cord has been placed, the cord may be displaced and pulled out (Fig 16-14, B).

In some instances where there is a shallow sulcus or a finish line with drastically changing contours, it may be

necessary to hold the cord already placed in position with a Gregg 4-5 instrument held in the left hand. Placement of the cord can then proceed with the packing instrument held in the right hand (Fig 16-15). Gently press apically on the cord with the instrument, directing the tip *slightly* toward the tooth (Fig 16-16). Slide the cord gingivally along the preparation until the finish line is felt. Then push the cord into the crevice.

If the instrument is directed totally in an apical direction, the cord will rebound off the gingiva and roll out of the sulcus (Fig 16-17). If cord persists in rebounding from a particularly tight area of the sulcus, do not apply greater force. Instead, maintain gentle force for a longer time. If it still rebounds, change to a smaller or more pliable cord (ie, twisted rather than braided).

Continue on around to the mesial, firmly securing the cord where it was lightly tacked before. Cut off the length of cord protruding from the mesial sulcus as closely as possible to the interdental papilla (Fig 16-18). Continue packing the cord around the facial surface, overlapping the cord in the mesial interproximal area. The overlap must always occur in the proximal area, where the bulk of tissue will tolerate the extra bulk of cord. If the overlap occurs on the facial or lingual surface where the gingiva is tight, there will be a gap apical to the crossover, and the finish line in that area may not be replicated in the impression.

Pack all but the last 2.0 or 3.0 mm of cord (Fig 16-19). This tag is left protruding so that it can be grasped for easy removal. Tissue retraction should be done firmly but *gently,* so that the cord will rest at the finish line (Fig 16-20, A). Heavy-handed operators can traumatize the tissue, create gingival problems, and jeopardize the longevity of the restorations that they place. *Do not overpack!* (Fig 16-20, B).

Place a large bulk of gauze in the patient's mouth. This will make the patient more comfortable by having something to close on and, at the same time, it will keep the area dry (Fig 16-21). After 10 minutes, remove the cord slowly to avoid bleeding. Inject impression material only

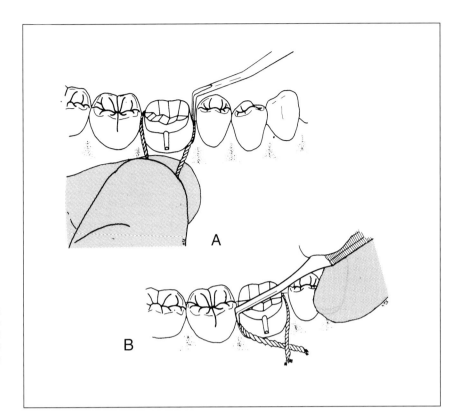

Fig 16-13 Placement of the retraction cord is begun by pushing it into the sulcus on the mesial surface of the tooth (A). It should also be tacked lightly into the distal crevice (B) to hold the cord in position while it is being placed.

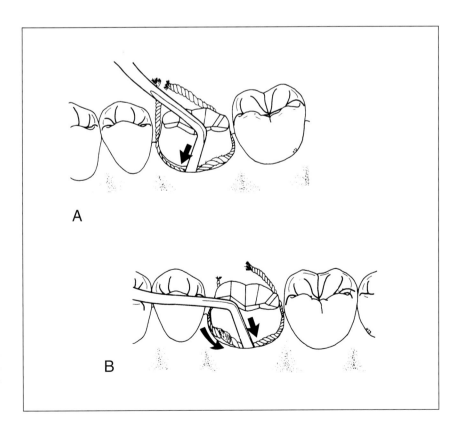

Fig 16-14 As the cord is being placed subgingivally, the instrument must be pushed slightly toward the area already tucked into place (A). If the force of the instrument is directed away from the area previously packed, the cord already packed will be pulled out (B).

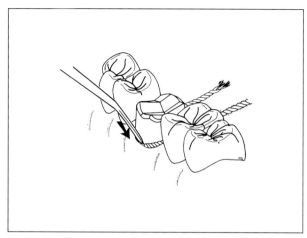

Fig 16-15   Occasionally it is necessary to hold the cord with one instrument while packing with the second.

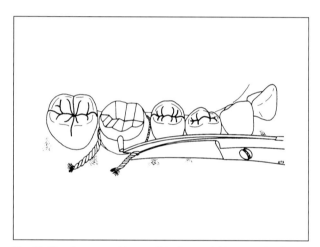

Fig 16-16   The instrument must be angled slightly toward the root to facilitate the subgingival placement of the cord.

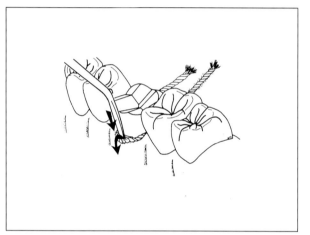

Fig 16-17   If the instrument is held parallel to the long axis of the tooth, the retraction cord will be pushed against the wall of the gingival crevice, and it will rebound.

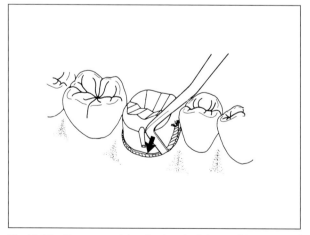

Fig 16-18   Excess cord is cut off in the mesial interproximal area.

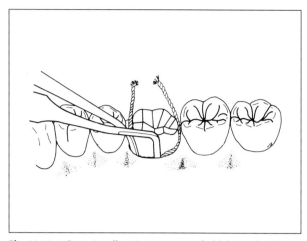

Fig 16-19   Placement of the distal end of the cord is continued until it overlaps the mesial. The force of the instrument must be directed toward the cord previously packed (to the distal in this case).

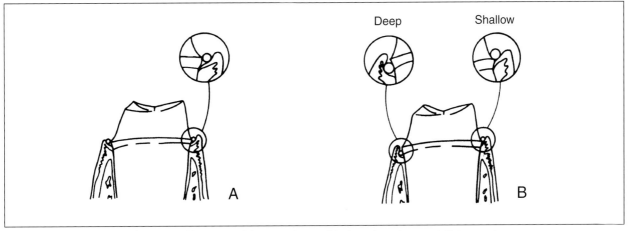

Fig 16-20 Placement of the retraction cord in the sulcus: A, correct; B, incorrect.

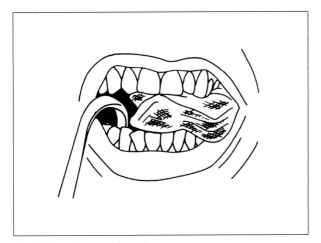

Fig 16-21 Gauze pack in place.

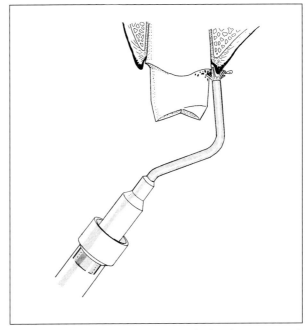

Fig 16-22 Ferric sulfate solution is applied to the gingiva with the tip of the special syringe.

if the sulcus remains clean and dry. It may be necessary to gently rinse away any coagulum, then lightly blow air on it. If active bleeding persists, abort the impression attempt. Electrocoagulation and ferric sulfate are sometimes effective in stopping persistent bleeding.

If ferric sulfate (Astingedent, Ultradent Products, Salt Lake City, UT) is used as the chemical, soak a plain knitted cord in it and place the cord in the gingival sulcus as just described. After 3 minutes, remove the cord. Load the 1.0-cc special syringe (Dento-Infusor) with the astringent chemical, and place a tip on the syringe. Use the fibrous syringe tip to rub or burnish cut sulcular tissue

until all bleeding stops (Fig 16-22). Using the tip in this manner will wipe off excess coagulum.

Keep the sulcus moist so that the coagulum will be easy to remove. Keep circling the preparation until bleeding has stopped completely. The solution usually will puddle in the sulcus when hemostasis is complete. Verify this by thoroughly rinsing the preparation with a water/air spray. The coagulum is black, and traces may linger in the sulcus for a few days.

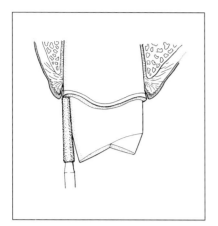

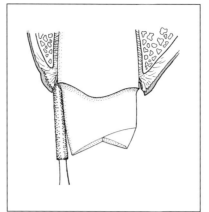

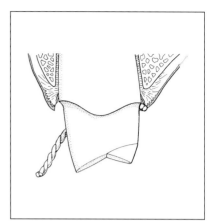

Fig 16-23 Prior to rotary curettage, a shoulder is formed at the level of the gingival crest.

Fig 16-24 A torpedo-tipped diamond simultaneously forms a chamfer finish line and removes the epithelial lining of the sulcus.

Fig 16-25 A cord is placed in the "troughed" sulcus for hemostasis.

Rotary Curettage

Rotary curettage is a "troughing" technique, the purpose of which is to produce limited removal of epithelial tissue in the sulcus while a chamfer finish line is being created in tooth structure.[42] The technique, which also has been called "gingettage,"[43,44] is used with the subgingival placement of restoration margins. It has been compared with periodontal curettage, but the rationale for its use is decidedly different.[42] Periodontal curettage is used to debride diseased tissue from the sulcus to allow re-epithelialization and healing.

The removal of epithelium from the sulcus by rotary curettage is accomplished with little detectable trauma to soft tissue, although there is a lessened tactile sense for the dentist.[45] Rotary curettage, however, must be done only on healthy, inflammation-free tissue[42,44] to avoid the tissue shrinkage that occurs when diseased tissue heals.[42]

The concept of using rotary curettage was described by Amsterdam in 1954.[45] The technique described here was developed by Hansing and subsequently enlarged upon by Ingraham.[44,48] Suitability of gingiva for the use of this method is determined by three factors: absence of bleeding upon probing, sulcus depth less than 3.0 mm, and presence of adequate keratinized gingiva.[44] The latter is determined by inserting a periodontal probe into the sulcus. If the segment of the probe in the sulcus cannot be seen, there is sufficient keratinized tissue to employ rotary curettage. Kamansky et al[47] found that thick palatal tissues responded better to the technique than did the thinner tissues on the facial aspect of maxillary anterior teeth.

In conjunction with axial reduction, a shoulder finish line is prepared at the level of the gingival crest with a flat-end tapered diamond (Fig 16-23). Then a torpedo-nosed diamond of 150 to 180 grit is used to extend the finish line apically, one-half to two-thirds the depth of the sulcus, converting the finish line to a chamfer (Fig 16-24).[42] A generous water spray is used while preparing the finish line and curetting the adjacent gingiva. Cord impregnated with aluminum chloride[42,47] or alum[43,44] is gently placed to control hemorrhage (Fig 16-25). The cord is removed after 4 to 8 minutes, and the sulcus is thoroughly irrigated with water. This technique is well suited for use with reversible hydrocolloid.[44]

Several studies have been done to compare both the efficacy and the wound healing of rotary curettage with those of conventional techniques. Kamansky and his associates reported less change in gingival height with rotary curettage than with lateral gingival displacement using retraction cord.[47] With curettage there was an apparent disruption of the apical sulcular and attachment epithelium, resulting in apical repositioning and an increase in sulcus depth. The changes were quite small, however, and they were not regarded as clinically significant.

Tupac and Neacy[43] found no significant histologic differences between retraction cord and rotary curettage. Ingraham et al[42] reported slight differences in healing among rotary curettage, pressure packing, and electrosurgery at different time intervals after the tooth preparation and impression. However, complete healing had occurred by 3 weeks with all techniques.

There is poor tactile sensation when using diamonds on sulcular walls, which can produce deepening of the sulcus.[47] The technique also has the potential for destruction of periodontium if used incorrectly,[44] making this a method that is probably best used only by experienced dentists.

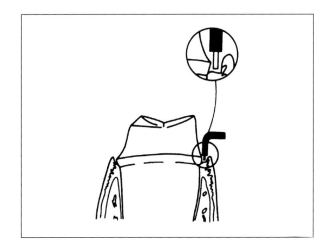

Fig 16-26 Electrosurgical electrode enlarges the gingival sulcus.

Electrosurgery

There are situations in which it may not be feasible or desirable to manage the gingiva with retraction cord alone. Even if the general condition of the gingiva in a mouth is healthy, areas of inflammation and granulation tissue may be encountered around a given tooth. This can be caused by overhangs on previous restorations or by the caries itself. It may have been necessary to place the finish line of the preparation so near the epithelial attachment that it is impossible to retract the gingiva sufficiently to get an adequate impression. In these cases, it may be necessary to use some means other than cord impregnated with chemicals to gain access and stop minor bleeding.

The use of electrosurgery has been recommended for enlargement of the gingival sulcus and control of hemorrhage to facilitate impression making (Fig 16-26).[48-50] Strictly speaking, electrosurgery cannot stop bleeding once it starts. If hemorrhage occurs, it first must be controlled with pressure and/or chemicals, and then the vessels can be sealed with a coagulating ball electrode.[51]

Electrosurgery has been described for the removal of irritated tissue that has proliferated over preparation finish lines,[52] and it is commonly used for that purpose. There has been concern expressed about the use of electrosurgery on inflamed tissue, based on an exaggerated response to an electrosurgical procedure.[53] Proximity to bone and lateral heat production may have been responsible for the response. Bone is very sensitive to heat.[54]

Electrosurgery is unquestionably capable of tissue damage. Most surgical instruments are dangerous if used improperly. Tremendous iatrogenic damage has been done over the years by the rotary handpiece, but no one has suggested that it not be used. Kalkwarf et al[55] reported that wounds created by a fully rectified, filtered current in the healthy gingiva of adult males demonstrated epithelial bridging at 48 hours and complete clinical healing at 72 hours. In a double-blind study on 27 patients, Aremband and Wade[56] detected no difference in healing in gingivectomies done by scalpel or electrosurgery. When variables are properly controlled in electrosurgery, untoward events in wound healing are rare.[57]

An electrosurgery unit is a high-frequency oscillator or radio transmitter that uses either a vacuum tube or a transistor to deliver a high-frequency electrical current of at least 1.0 MHz (one million cycles per second) (Fig 16-27). It generates heat in a way that is similar to a microwave oven heating food, or a diathermy machine producing heat in muscle tissue for physical therapy. Electrosurgery has been called surgical diathermy.[51]

Credit for being the direct progenitor of electrosurgery is generally given to d'Arsonval.[58,59] His experiments in 1891 demonstrated that electricity at high frequency will pass through a body without producing a shock (pain or muscle spasm), producing instead an increase in the internal temperature of the tissue. This discovery was used as the basis for the eventual development of electrosurgery.

Electrosurgery produces controlled tissue destruction to achieve a surgical result. Current flows from a small cutting electrode that produces a high current density and a rapid temperature rise at its point of contact with the tissue. The cells directly adjacent to the electrode are destroyed by this temperature increase. The current concentrates at points and sharp bends. Cutting electrodes are designed to take advantage of this property so they will have maximum effectiveness (Fig 16-28). The circuit is completed by contact between the patient and a ground electrode that will not generate heat in the tissue because its large surface area produces a low current density, even though the same amount of current passes through it.[60] The cutting electrode remains cold; this dif-

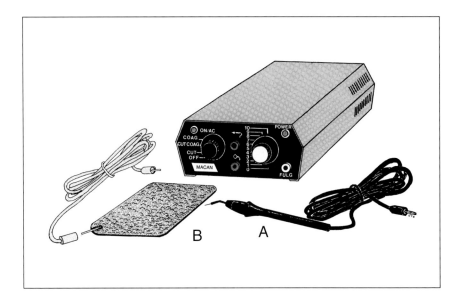

Fig 16-27 Typical electrosurgical unit with active electrode (A) and ground electrode (B).

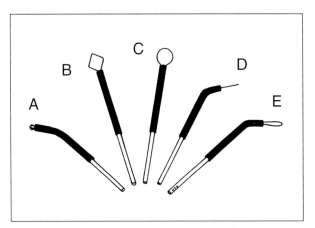

Fig 16-28 Five commonly used electrosurgical electrodes: A, coagulating; B, diamond loop; C, round loop; D, small straight; E, small loop.

fers from electrocautery, in which a hot electrode is applied to the tissue.

Types of Current. There are different forms of current that can be generated for electrosurgical use, depending on the type of machine (and circuitry) used or the setting on any given machine. These currents exhibit different wave forms when viewed on an oscilloscope. They are significant because each produces a different tissue response.

The *unrectified, damped* current is characterized by recurring peaks of power that rapidly diminish (Fig 16-29, A). It is the current produced by the old hyfurcator or spark gap generator, and it gives rise to intense dehydration and necrosis. It causes considerable coagulation, and healing is slow and painful. Sometimes referred to as the Oudin or Telsa current, it is not used routinely in dental electrosurgery today.

A *partially rectified, damped* (half-wave modulated) current produces a wave form with a damping in the second half of each cycle (Fig 16-29, B). There is lateral penetration of heat, with slow healing occurring in deep tissues. The damping effect produces good coagulation and hemostasis, but tissue destruction is considerable and healing is slow.

A better current for enlargement of the gingival sulcus is found in the *fully rectified* (full-wave modulated) current that produces a continuous flow of energy (Fig 16-29, C). Cutting characteristics are good and there is some hemostasis.

The *fully rectified, filtered* (filtered) is a continuous wave that produces excellent cutting (Fig 16-29, D). Healing of tissues cut by a continuous wave current will be better initially than tissues cut by a modulated wave. The continuous wave produces less injury to the tissue than does a modulated wave.[61] However, a controlled histologic study[62] found that after 2 weeks, healing of wounds produced by filtered current was not remarkably better than healing of wounds produced by nonfiltered full-wave modulated current.

Filtered current probably produces better healing in situations requiring an incision and healing by primary intention, because there is less coagulation of the tissues in the walls of the wound. This is not critical in those procedures done in conjunction with restorative dentistry, when either the inner wall of the gingival sulcus is removed, or modified gingivoplasty is accomplished by planing the surface of the tissue. In these cases, hemostasis is required, and moderate tissue coagulation is not only tolerated but desired.

Grounding. For the patient's safety, it is important that the circuit be completed by the use of the *ground elec-*

Electrosurgical Wave Forms

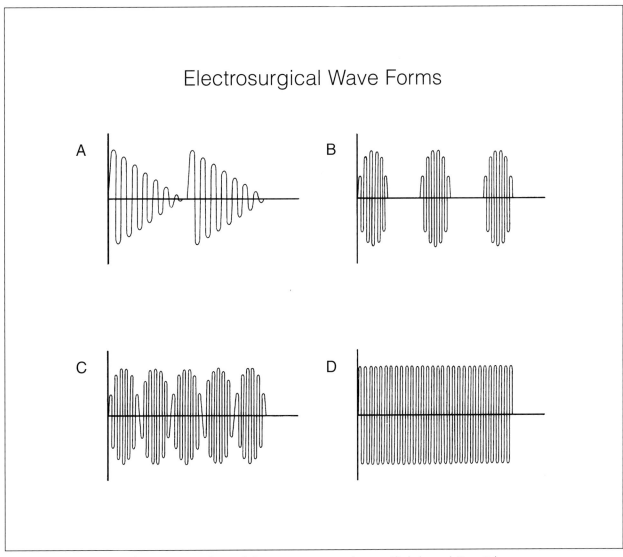

Fig 16-29 Four forms of electrosurgery current: A, unrectified, damped; B, partially rectified, damped (half-wave modulated); C, fully rectified (full-wave modulated); and D, fully rectified, filtered (filtered).

trode,[63] which is also known as a ground plate, indifferent plate, indifferent electrode, neutral electrode, dispersive electrode, passive electrode, or patient return (Fig 16-30). Some dentists, prompted by the unfortunate advertising of a few electrosurgical manufacturers, have chosen to dispense with the use of this vital piece of equipment. An electrosurgery unit will work without one, but it is neither as efficient nor as safe.

Grounding the chair is not an acceptable alternative. Current will be dissipated through the path of least resistance, and patient contact with a piece of equipment, including metal parts of the chair, could cause a burn.[64] It is acceptable, however, to permanently attach a metallic mesh grounding antenna to the chain *under* the uphol-

stery and insultated from all metal chain parts. This can do much to reduce patient anxiety.

The safe use of electrosurgery dictates that current flow be facilitated along the proper circuit from the generator to the active electrode, the patient, and back to the generator.[65] Because patient burns have been attributed to faulty grounding in many cases,[64,66,67] the *proper* grounding of a patient is considered to be the single most important safety factor when electrosurgery is used.[68]

Oringer[69] recommends that the ground be placed under the thigh rather than behind the back, as is often done. Contact with a small, bony protuberance, such as a vertebra or shoulder blade, could produce a high enough current density to cause a burn. The only pre-

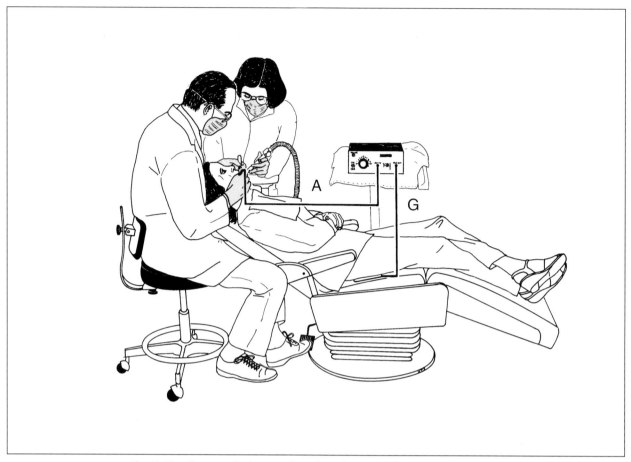

Fig 16-30 Electrosurgical current flows from the unit to the active (cutting) electrode (A) to the ground (G), and back to the unit.

caution to be observed in placing the ground under the legs is that the patient does not have keys in a pants pocket or is not wearing metal garters (the latter is unlikely in this day).

Contraindications. For reasons of safety, electrosurgery should *not* be used in some circumstances. It should not be employed on patients with cardiac pacemakers. The demand (synchronous) type of pacemaker, which is the most common, is designed to sense cardiac impulses (the R wave).[70] When bradycardia occurs because the heart does not emit an impulse, the pacemaker fires at an appropriate rate to keep the heart beating. External electromagnetic interference hinders the pacemaker's sensing function.[71] Incorrectly sensing the interference as an intrinsic myocardial impulse, the generator shuts down until the interference ceases, with consequences that could be quite serious for the patient. Electrosurgery will alter the normal function of a pacemaker,[72] and it presents a hazard to the patient who

wears one.[73] Shielding in recent pacemaker models diminishes the risks from extraneous electromagnetic interferences, but the use of electrosurgery is still contraindicated for those patients who wear pacemakers.[74]

Because it can produce sparks in use, electrosurgery should not be used in the presence of flammable agents. This does not present the risk in dentistry that it does in medicine, because flammable gases are not routinely employed as dental anesthetic agents. However, the use of topical anesthetics such as ethylchloride and other flammable aerosols should be avoided when electrosurgery is to be used.

Many fires in hospital operating rooms do not involve flammable anesthetics. Instead they occur when ordinary combustible materials are ignited in an oxygenated atmosphere that will support a fire.[63,65] There is a slight danger attached to the use of nitrous oxide with electrosurgery because of the enriched oxygen atmosphere that will be present in the oral cavity and nasopharynx.

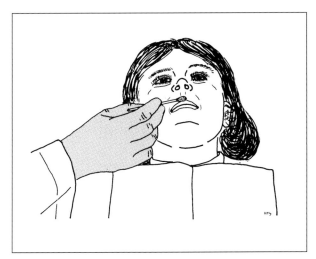

Fig 16-31   A small drop of a strongly scented oil is placed on the upper lip to help mask the unpleasant odor associated with electrosurgery.

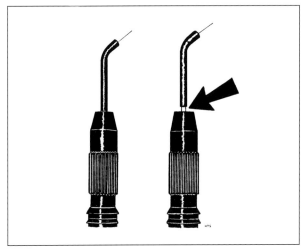

Fig 16-32   Electrodes must be completely seated in the hand-piece *(left).* If bare metal is left exposed anyplace but at the tip *(arrow),* the patient or the operator could be burned.

The number of reported cases involving flash fires caused by dental electrosurgery in the presence of nitrous oxide–oxygen analgesia is minimal. Oringer[75] describes two such occurrences. Given the right circumstances with an extremely dry mouth and an accumulation of oxygen, a small spark caused by the electrode touching a metallic restoration could conceivably set off a dry cotton packing. Therefore, whenever electrosurgery is used in the presence of nitrous oxide–oxygen analgesia, be sure that any cotton packing in the mouth is kept slightly moist,[63] if in fact it is not already that way from absorption of oral fluids.

Electrosurgery Armamentarium

1. Electrosurgery unit
2. Set of cutting electrodes
3. Cotton pliers
4. Mouth mirror
5. Fischer Ultrapak Packer
6. DE plastic filling instrument
7. High-volume vacuum with plastic tip
8. Wooden tongue depressor
9. Cotton rolls
10. Cotton-tipped applicator
11. Aromatic oil
12. Hydrogen peroxide
13. Dappen dish
14. Alcohol sponges (gauze, 4 x 4)
15. Retraction cord

Electrosurgery Technique

Before an electrosurgical procedure is done, verify that anesthesia is profound and reinforce it if necessary. With a cotton-tipped applicator, place a drop of a pleasant-smelling aromatic oil, such as peppermint, at the vermilion border of the upper lip (Fig 16-31). The odor from it will help to mask some of the unpleasant odor emanating from the mouth during electrosurgery.

Check the equipment to make sure all the connections are solid. Be especially certain that the cutting electrode is seated completely in the handpiece (Fig 16-32). If any uninsulated portion of it other than the cutting tip is exposed outside the handpiece chuck, it could produce an accidental burn on the patient's lip.

Proper use of electrosurgery requires that the cutting electrode be applied with very light pressure and quick, deft strokes. The pressure required has been described as the same needed to draw a line with an ink-dipped brush without bending the bristles (Fig 16-33). It is obvious that the electrode is being guided, and not pushed, through the tissue.

To prevent lateral penetration of heat into the tissues with subsequent injury, the electrode should move at a speed of no less than 7 mm per second.[54] If it is necessary to retrace the path of a previous cut, 8 to 10 seconds should be allowed to elapse before repeating the stroke.[54] This will minimize the buildup of lateral heat that could disrupt normal healing.

Initially set the power selector dial at the level recommended by the manufacturer and make adjustments as necessary. As the electrode passes through the tissue, it should do so smoothly without dragging or charring the tissue. If the tip drags and collects shreds of clinging tissue, the unit has been placed on a setting that is too low.

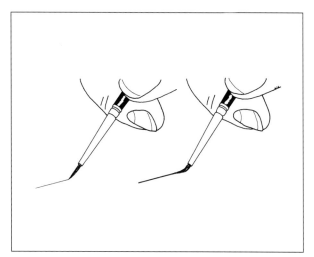

Fig 16-33 The cutting electrode should be used with the same light pressure used to draw a straight line with a brush without bending it *(left)*. The pressure exerted on the brush on the right would be excessive.

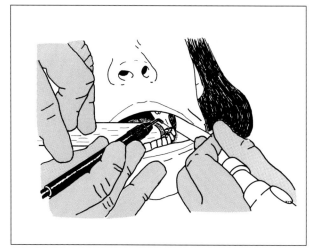

Fig 16-34 A plastic vacuum tip should be kept close to the surgical site and a wooden tongue blade used as a tongue retractor.

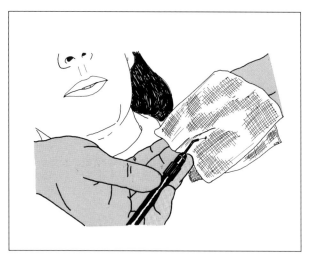

Fig 16-35 An alcohol sponge is used to wipe tissue debris from the cutting electrode.

On the other hand, if the tissue chars or discolors, or if there is sparking, the setting is too high. If an error must be made initially, it is better to have a setting that is slightly too high. Moist tissue will cut best. If it dries out, spray it lightly. Avoid collections of water, however, because that will increase resistance and decrease efficiency.

A high-volume vacuum tip should be kept immediately adjacent to the cutting electrode at all times to draw off the unpleasant odors that are generated (Fig 16-34). The tip must be plastic to prevent any burns that might be caused by accidental contact with the electrode. For the same reason, a wooden tongue depressor or plastic-handled mirror should be used rather than the metal-backed mouth mirror that would customarily be employed.

Stop frequently to clean any fragments of tissue from the electrode by wiping it with an alcohol-soaked 4 x 4 sponge (Fig 16-35). The electrode is completely safe as soon as the foot switch has been released. Proper technique with the cutting electrode can be summed up in three points:

1. Proper power setting
2. Quick passes with the electrode
3. Adequate time intervals between strokes

Gingival Sulcus Enlargement

Before any tissue is removed, it is important to assess the width of the band of attached gingiva. The electrosurgery tip is a surgical instrument; it cannot restore lost gingiva. If there is unattached alveolar mucosa too near the gingival crest, periodontal surgery, probably in the form of a gingival graft, must be employed to reinstate an adequate band of healthy, attached tissue.

To enlarge the gingival sulcus for impression making, a small, straight or J-shaped electrode is selected. It is used with the wire parallel with the long axis of the tooth so that tissue is removed from the inner wall of the sulcus.[50] If the electrode is maintained in this direction, the loss of gingival height will be about 0.1 mm.[48] Holding the electrode at an angle to the tooth, however, is likely to result in a loss of gingival height.

Around those teeth where the attached gingival tissue is thin and stretched tightly over the bone on the labial surface, there is a greater chance for a loss of gingival height. This is frequently true of maxillary anterior teeth, and particularly the canines, and is worth bearing in mind if the esthetic requirements are great and any gingival recession will be unacceptable.

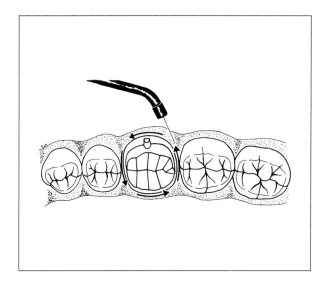

Fig 16-36 Passes to be made with the electrode can be practiced before turning on the power.

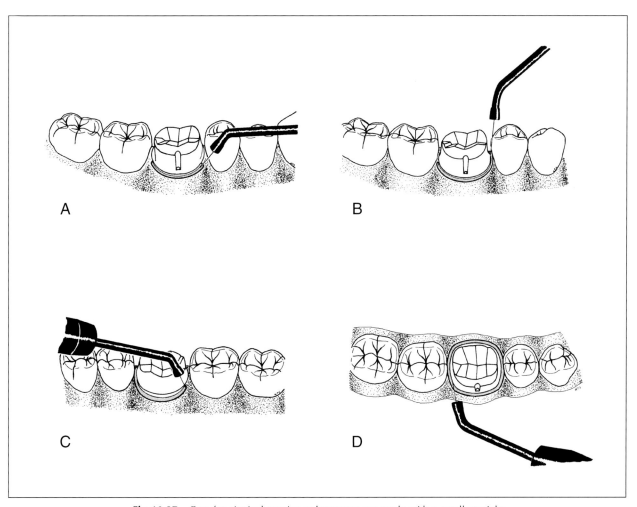

Fig 16-37 Cuts for gingival crevice enlargement are made with a small, straight electrode, without repeating any strokes until all others in the series have been made: A, facial; B, mesial; C, lingual; D, distal.

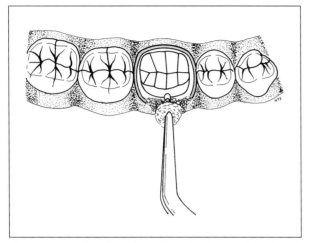

Fig 16-38 Debris from the enlarged sulcus is cleaned with hydrogen peroxide on a cotton pellet.

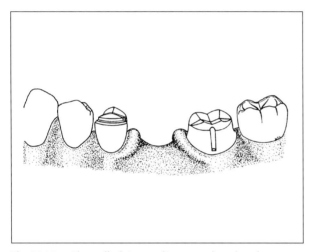

Fig 16-39 The cuff of tissue adjacent to the edentulous space interferes with a cleanable pontic and strong connectors.

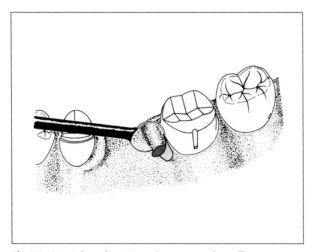

Fig 16-40 A large loop is used to remove the cuff.

With the electrosurgery unit off, the electrode is held over the tooth to be operated and the cutting strokes are traced over the tissue (Fig 16-36). Depress the foot switch before contacting the tissue, and then move the electrode through the first pass. A whole tooth should be encompassed in four separate motions: facial, mesial, lingual, and distal at a speed of no less than 7 mm per second (Fig 16-37, A to D).[54] If a second pass is necessary in any one area, wait 8 to 10 seconds before repeating that stroke.[54] This will minimize the production of lateral heat. Clean tissue debris off the electrode tip after each stroke. Use a cotton pellet dipped in hydrogen peroxide to clean debris from the sulcus (Fig 16-38). Better results are usually obtained if retraction cord is loosely packed in the enlarged sulcus before the impression is made.

Removal of an Edentulous Cuff

Frequently, the remnants of the interdental papilla adjacent to an edentulous space will form a roll or cuff that will make it difficult to fabricate a pontic with cleanable embrasures and strong connectors. Before a pontic is fabricated, an edentulous ridge should be examined carefully. If there are cuffs, they should be removed (Fig 16-39). Malone and Manning[49] found in a bilateral comparative study of gingivoplasties on 10 patients that there was no difference in healing between conventional surgery and electrosurgery. A large loop electrode is used for planing away the large roll of tissue (Fig 16-40). When this larger electrode is used, it requires a higher power setting of the unit.

Crown Lengthening

There are circumstances in which it may be desirable to have a longer clinical crown on a tooth than is present (Fig 16-41). If there is a sufficiently wide band of attached gingiva surrounding the tooth, this can be accomplished with a gingivectomy using a diamond electrode (Fig 16-42). It is frequently necessary to do a second series of cuts to produce a bevel around the first (Fig 16-43). This will produce a better tissue contour without hard-to-clean edges near the tooth (Fig 16-44). This "bevel" also must be done only on attached gingiva. When surgery leaves an extensive postoperative wound, as in this case, it is necessary to place a periodontal dressing, which should be changed in about 7 days.

The lengthened tooth that results from this surgery should afford better retention for any crown placed on it, with margin placement in an area of the tooth more accessible for cleaning. If the band of attached gingiva is too narrow, it must be made wider with a graft or an alternative restoration must be made for the tooth.

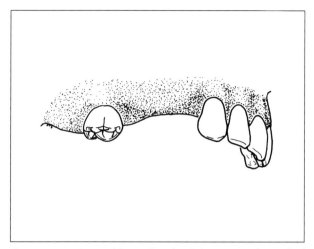

Fig 16-41 It is possible to "lengthen" the crown of a tooth if there is a wide band of attached gingiva.

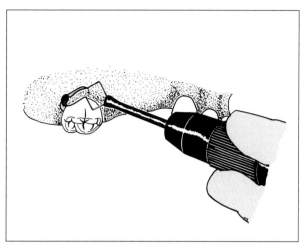

Fig 16-42 Gingivectomy is done with a loop electrode.

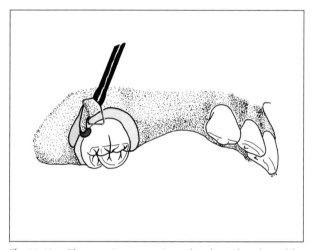

Fig 16-43 The same instrument is used to shape the edges of the previous cut to prevent a ledge of gingival tissue adjacent to the tooth.

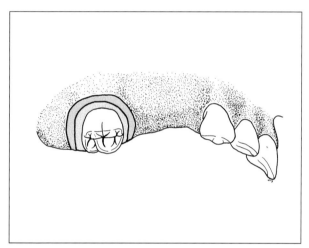

Fig 16-44 "Lengthened" tooth after completion of minor gingivectomy.

References

1. Noonan JE, Goldfogel MH, Lambert RL: Inhibited set of the surface of addition silicones in contact with rubber dam. *Oper Dent* 1985; 10:46–48.

2. *Accepted Dental Therapeutics,* ed 40. Chicago, American Dental Association, 1984, p 344–345.

3. Sapkos SW: The use of antisialagogues in periodontal and restorative dentistry. *Int J Periodont Rest Dent* 1984; 4(4):43–49.

4. Wilson EL, Whitsett LD, Whitsett TL: Effects of methantheline bromide and clonidine hydrochloride on salivary secretion. *J Prosthet Dent* 1984; 52:663–665.

5. Thompson MJ: Hydrocolloid—Its treatment and application in securing consistent accurate models for indirect inlays and fixed bridges. *Bull Okla Dent Assoc* 1949; 38:7–24.

6. Benson BW, Bomberg TJ, Hatch RA, Hoffman W: Tissue displacement methods in fixed prosthodontics. *J Prosthet Dent* 1986; 55:175–181.

7. Hovestad JF: *Practical Dental Porcelains.* St Louis, CV Mosby Co, 1924, p 34–36.

8. Miller IF: Fixed dental prosthesis. *J Prosthet Dent* 1958; 8:483–495.

9. Lucca JJ: The tube impression technique. *Dent Clin North Am* 1959; 3:113–123.

10. Ewing JE: Beautiful but glum—Porcelain jacket crowns. *J Prosthet Dent* 1954; 4:94–103.

11. Johnston JF, Mumford G, Dykema RW: *Modern Practice in Dental Ceramics.* Philadelphia, WB Saunders Co, 1967, p 84–94.

12. Ruel J, Schuessler PJ, Malament K, Mori D: Effect of retraction procedures on the periodontium in humans. *J Prosthet Dent* 1980; 44:508–515.

13. Coelho DH, Brisman AS: Gingival recession with modelling-plastic copper-band impressions. *J Prosthet Dent* 1974; 31:647–650.

14. Ingraham R, Bassett RW, Koser JR: *An Atlas of Cast Gold Procedures,* ed 2. Buena Park, CA, Uni-Tro College Press, 1969, p 47–48.

15. Thompson MJ: Exposing the cavity margin for hydrocolloid impressions. *J South Calif Dent Assoc* 1951; 19:17–24.

16. Pelzner RB, Kempler D, Stark MM, Lum LB, Nicholson RJ, Soelberg KB: Human blood pressure and pulse rate response to r-epinephrine retraction cord. *J Prosthet Dent* 1978; 39:287–292.

17. Sears AW: Hydrocolloid impression technique for inlays and fixed bridges. *Dent Dig* 1937; 43:230–234.

18. Harrison JD: Effect of retraction materials on the gingival sulcus epithelium. *J Prosthet Dent* 1961; 11:514–521.

19. Shillingburg HT, Hatch RA, Keenan MP, Hemphill MW: Impression materials and techniques used for cast restorations in eight states. *J Am Dent Assoc* 1980; 100:696–699.

20. Donovan TE, Gandara BK, Nemetz H: Review and survey of medicaments used with gingival retraction cords. *J Prosthet Dent* 1985; 53:525–531.

21. Shaw DH, Krejci RF: Gingival retraction preference of dentists in general practice. *Quintessence Int* 1986; 17:277–280.

22. Nemetz H, Donovan T, Landesman H: Exposing the gingival margin: A systematic approach for the control of hemorrhage. *J Prosthet Dent* 1984; 51:647–651.

23. Loe H, Silness J: Tissue reactions to string packs used in fixed restorations. *J Prosthet Dent* 1963; 13:318.

24. de Gennaro GG, Landesman HM, Calhoun JE, Martinoff JT: A comparison of gingival inflammation related to retraction cords. *J Prosthet Dent* 1982; 47:384–386.

25. Buchanan WT, Thayer KE: Systemic effects of epinephrine-impregnated retraction cord in fixed partial denture prosthodontics. *J Am Dent Assoc* 1982; 104:482–484.

26. Pogue WL, Harrison JD: Absorption of epinephrine during tissue retraction. *J Prosthet Dent* 1967; 18:242–247.

27. Houston JB, Appleby RC, DeCounter L, Callaghan N, Funk DC: Effect of epinephrine-impregnated retraction cord on the cardiovascular system. *J Prosthet Dent* 1970; 24:373–376.

28. Goldberg AT, Yoder JL, Thayer KE: Analysis of heart rate in dogs during retraction and impression procedures. *J Dent Res* 1971; 50:645–648.

29. Woychesin FF: An evaluation of the drugs used for gingival retraction. *J Prosthet Dent* 1964; 14:769–776.

30. Fisher DW: Conservative management of the gingival tissue for crowns. *Dent Clin North Am* 1976; 20:273–283.

31. Gogerty JH, Strand HA, Ogilvie AL, Dillie JM: Vasopressor effects of topical epinephrine in certain dental procedures. *Oral Surg Oral Med Oral Pathol* 1957; 10:614–622.

32. Forsyth RP, Stark MM, Nicholson RJ, Peng CT: Blood pressure responses to epinephrine- treated gingival retraction string in the rhesus monkey. *J Am Dent Assoc* 1969; 78:1315–1319.

33. Kellam SA, Smith JR, Scheffel SJ: Epinephrine absorption from commercial gingival retraction cords in clinical patients. *J Prosthet Dent* 1992; 68:761–765.

34. Malamed SF: *Handbook of Medical Emergencies in the Dental Office,* ed 3. St Louis, CV Mosby Co, 1987, p 288, 344–345.

35. Nemetz EH, Seibly W: The use of chemical agents in gingival retraction. *Gen Dent* 1990; 38:104–108.

36. Bowles WH, Tardy SJ, Vahadi A: Evaluation of new gingival retraction agents. *J Dent Res* 1991; 70:1447–1449.

37. Weir DJ, Williams BH: Clinical effectiveness of mechanical-chemical tissue displacement methods. *J Prosthet Dent* 1984; 51:326–329.

38. Shaw DH, Krejci RF, Cohen DM: Retraction cords with aluminum chloride: Effect on the gingiva. *Oper Dent* 1980; 5:138–141.

39. Sorensen JA, Doherty F, Flemmig T, Newman MG: Gingival enhancement in fixed prosthodontics: I. Clinical findings [abstract 2091]. *J Dent Res* 1988; 67:374.

40. de Camargo LM, Chee WWL, Donovan TE: Inhibition of polymerization of polyvinyl siloxanes by medicaments used on gingival retraction cords. *J Prosthet Dent* 1993; 70:114–117.

41. Anneroth G, Nordenram A: Reaction of the gingiva to the application of threads in the gingival pockets for taking impressions with elastic material. *Odontol Revy* 1969; 20:301–310.

42. Ingraham R, Sochat R, Hansing FJ: Rotary gingival curettage—A technique for tooth preparation and management of the gingival sulcus for impression taking. *Int J Periodont Rest Dent* 1981; 1(4):9–33.

43. Tupac RG, Neacy K: A comparison of cord gingival displacement with the gingitage technique. *J Prosthet Dent* 1981; 46:509–515.

44. Brady WF: Periodontal and restorative considerations in rotary curettage. *J Am Dent Assoc* 1982; 105:231–236.

45. Moskow BS: The response of the gingival sulcus to instrumentation. *J Periodontol* 1964; 35:112–126.

46. Ingraham R, Evens JK: I. Tissue management in cavity preparation. *Dent Dimen* 1975; 9:9–11, 32.

47. Kamansky FW, Tempel TR, Post AC: Gingival tissue response to rotary curettage. *J Prosthet Dent* 1984; 52:380–383.

48. Klug RG: Gingival tissue regeneration following electrical retraction. *J Prosthet Dent* 1966; 16:955–962.

49. Malone WF, Manning JL: Electrosurgery in restorative dentistry. *J Prosthet Dent* 1968; 20:417–425.

50. Podshadley AG, Lundeen HC: Electrosurgical procedures in crown and bridge restorations. *J Am Dent Assoc* 1968; 77:1321–1326.

51. Flocken JE: Electrosurgical management of soft tissues and restorative dentistry. *Dent Clin North Am* 1980; 24:247–269.

52. Patel MG: Electrosurgical management of hyperplastic tissue. *J Prosthet Dent* 1986; 56:145–147.

53. Ferreira PM, Fugazzotto PA, Parma-Benfenati S: Implications of the use of electrosurgical techniques in the presence of gingival inflammation. *Gen Dent* 1987; 35:17–21.

54. Kalkwarf KL, Krejci RF, Edison AR, Reinhardt RA: Lateral heat production secondary to electrosurgical incisions. *Oral Surg Oral Med Oral Pathol* 1983; 55:344–348.

55. Kalkwarf KL, Krejci RF, Wentz FM: Healing of electrosurgical incisions in gingiva: Early histologic observations in adult men. *J Prosthet Dent* 1981; 46:662–672.

56. Aremband D, Wade AB: A comparative wound healing study following gingivectomy by electrosurgery and knives. *J Periodont Res* 1973; 8:42–50.

57. Williams VD: Electrosurgery and wound healing: A review of the literature. *J Am Dent Assoc* 1984; 108:220–222.

58. Gonser DI: Theory of electrosurgical instrumentation. In Malone WF (ed): *Electrosurgery in Dentistry—Theory and Application in Clinical Practice.* Springfield, Charles C. Thomas Publishers, 1974, p 3.

59. Oringer M: *Electrosurgery in Dentistry,* ed 2. Philadelphia, WB Saunders Co, 1975, p 4.

60. Friedman J: The technical aspects of electrosurgery. *Oral Surg Oral Med Oral Pathol* 1973; 36:177–187.

61. Maness WL, Roeber FW, Clark RE, Cataldo E, Riis D, Haddad AW: Histologic evaluation of electrosurgery with varying frequency and waveform. *J Prosthet Dent* 1978; 40:304–308.

62. Sozio RB, Riley EJ, Shklar G: A histologic and electronic evaluation of electrosurgical currents: Nonfiltered full-wave modulated vs. filtered current. *J Prosthet Dent* 1975; 33:300–312.

63. Annex 2—The safe use of high frequency electricity in health care facilities. In *NFPA 99, Standard for Health Care Facilities.* Quincy, MA, National Fire Protection Association, 1993, pp 201–215.

64. Adams I: Potential hazards of an electro-surgical unit. *Hosp Admin Can* 1971; 13:37–38.

65. Neufeld GR: Principles and hazards of electrosurgery including laparoscopy. *Surg Gynecol Obstet* 1978; 147:705–710.

66. Battig GG: Electrosurgical burn injuries and their prevention. *AORN J* 1968; 8:48–54.

67. Becker CM, Malhotra IV, Hedley-Whyte J: The distribution of radiofrequency current and burns. *Anesthesiology* 1973; 38:106–122.

68. Billin AG: Patient safety and electrosurgery. *AORN J* 1971; 14:62–68.

69. Oringer M: *Electrosurgery in Dentistry,* ed 2. Philadelphia, WB Saunders Co, 1975, p 26.

70. Smyth NPD, Parsonnet V, Escher DJW, Furman S: The pacemaker patient and the electromagnetic environment. *JAMA* 1974; 227:1412.

71. Simon AB, Lindhe B, Bonnette GH, Schlentz RJ: The individual with a pacemaker in the dental environment. *J Am Dent Assoc* 1975; 91:1224–1229.

72. Walter C: Dental treatment of patients with cardiac pacemaker implants. *Quintessence Int* 1975; 8:57–58.

73. Rezai FR: Dental treatment of a patient with a cardiac pacemaker. *Oral Surg Oral Med Oral Pathol* 1977; 44:662–665.

74. Stamps JT, Muth ER: Reducing accidents and injuries in the dental environment. *Dent Clin North Am* 1978; 22:389–401.

75. Oringer M: *Electrosurgery in Dentistry,* ed 2. Philadelphia, WB Saunders Co, 1975, p 89.

Chapter 17

Impressions

An impression is an imprint or negative likeness. It is made by placing some soft, semi-fluid material in the mouth and allowing the material to set. Depending upon the material used, the set impression will be either hard or elastic. The impression materials most frequently used for cast restorations are elastic when removed from the mouth. From this negative form of the teeth and surrounding structures, a positive reproduction, or cast, is made.

The *indirect* technique for fabricating inlays, crowns, and fixed partial denture retainers has been a boon to the practice of dentistry. It allows most of the laboratory procedures involved in the fabrication of a restoration to be done away from the chair, substituting a gypsum cast for the actual tooth. If the restoration is to fit precisely, the cast on which it is made must be as nearly an exact duplicate of the prepared tooth in the mouth as possible. This means an accurate, undistorted impression of the prepared tooth must be made.

The impression must then be handled properly until it is poured up in a gypsum product. Impression making is an area of restorative dentistry where much abuse of materials occurs, and many an accurate impression has been distorted by improper handling or untoward delays between removal from the mouth and pouring.

An impression for a cast restoration should meet the following requirements:

1. It should be an exact duplication of the prepared tooth, including all of the preparation and enough uncut tooth surface beyond the preparation to allow the dentist and technician to be certain of the location and configuration of the finish line.
2. Other teeth and tissue adjacent to the prepared tooth must be accurately reproduced to permit proper articulation of the cast and contouring of the restoration.
3. It must be free of bubbles, especially in the area of the finish line and occlusal surfaces of the other teeth in the arch.

Comparison of Impression Materials

There are several types of impression materials that are accurate enough to be considered for cast restorations. The choice is based on personal preference, ease of manipulation, and, to some extent, economics. Accuracy is not a consideration in the choice among these materials because there are no clinically significant differences. The materials described here are reversible hydrocolloid, polysulfide, condensation silicone, polyvinyl siloxane, and polyether. The attributes of each are listed in Table 17-1, and costs of the different brands available are listed in Table 17-2.

Wettability

Each impression material has different handling characteristics. Finding the characteristics with which the dentist and auxiliaries can best work is an important consideration in choosing an impression material. Ease of pouring with gypsum products varies among the different impression materials. Impression materials can be classified as readily wettable by gypsum *(hydrophilic)* and resistant to wetting *(hydrophobic)*.

Irreversible hydrocolloid (alginate), reversible hydrocolloid, and polyether are hydrophilic and the easiest to pour. Polysulfide, polyvinyl siloxanes, and condensation-reaction silicones are the most hydrophobic, in ascending order, as indicated by their high contact angles (Fig 17-1).[1] The greater the contact angle, the greater the probability of air entrapment during pouring. Not only will the incidence of voids in the stone cast be greater,[2,3] but the voids will be larger.[3] Of at least equal clinical significance is the fact that materials exhibiting large contact angles are also more readily repelled by hemorrhage or other moisture in the gingival sulcus.

These findings certainly do not contraindicate the use of polyvinyl siloxanes, nor do they guarantee a good

Table 17-1 *Comparative Properties of Impression Materials*

Type	Type of tray	Setting time	Ease of removal	Finish line readability	Moisture tolerance	Pouring time	Tear strength	Pouring ease	Mixing ease	Odor/taste	Radi-opaque	Shelf life
Reversible hydrocolloid	Watercooled stock metal	5 min	Easy	Poor	Excellent	15 min	Weak	Good	None is needed, but conditioning is complicated	Good	No	24–48 months
Polysulfide rubber base	Custom	12–14 min	Moderate	Good	Acceptable	60 min	Good	Adequate	Moderate to difficult	Poor	Yes	18 months
Condensation silicone rubber base	Custom: two paste systems / Stock: Putty/reline	10 min	Easy	Good	Poor	60 min	Adequate	Poor to adequate	Easy	Good	No	12 months
Polyether rubber base	Custom: 4.0-mm spacer / Stock	5–6 min	Difficult	Good	Good	7 days	Adequate	Good	Moderate	Poor	No	24 months
Polyvinyl siloxane rubber base	Stock: single units / Custom: fixed partial denture / Stock: Putty/reline	6–8 min	Moderate to difficult	Good	Poor for standard "hydrophobic" brands; adequate for "hydrophilic" brands	7 days	Adequate	Poor for standard "hydrophobic" brands; adequate for "hydrophilic" brands	Easy for hand-mixed; very easy for cartridge systems	Good	No	24 months

Table 17-2 *Comparative Costs of Impression Materials*

| Type | Brand | Cost per milliliter (US $) | | |
		Tube	Cartridge	Putty
Reversible hydrocolloid	*Acculoid*	0.033	—	—
	Cartriloid	—	0.249	—
	Superbody	0.033	—	—
	Supersyringe	—	0.242	—
	Surgident	0.030	0.214	—
	Versatile	0.031	—	—
	Cohere	—	0.474	0.005*
	Duoloid	—	0.347	0.006*
Polysulfide rubber base	*Coe-flex*	0.102	—	—
	Neo-plex	0.127	—	—
	Omniflex	0.106	—	—
	Permalastic	0.126	—	—
	Super-Rubber	0.156	—	—
Condensation silicone rubber base	*Accoe*	0.292	—	0.103
	Citricon	0.195	—	0.079
	Cuttersil	0.143	—	0.056
	Elasticon	0.274	—	—
	Rapid	0.162	—	0.063
	Silene	0.182	—	0.063
Polyether rubber base	*Impregum–F*	0.177	—	—
	Permadyne	0.248	0.301	—
	Polyjel NF	0.153	—	—
Polyvinyl siloxane rubber base	*Baysilex*	0.148	0.249	—
	Cinch	0.093	0.150	0.150
	Correct	0.069	0.125	0.072
	Exaflex	0.192	—	0.086
	Examix	—	0.177	—
	Express	—	0.242	0.127
	Extrude	0.175	0.178	0.088
	Hydrosil	0.112	0.237	—
	Imprint	—	0.225	—
	Panasil	0.161	0.208	0.106
	Perfourm	0.171	0.229	0.097
	Permagum	0.352	0.246	0.200
	President	0.141	0.219	0.097
	Reflect	0.127	—	—
	Reprosil	0.116	0.198	0.124
	Supersil	0.224	0.260	0.181

*Irreversible hydrocolloid (alginate).

cast every time hydrocolloid is used. They require that caution be exercised in pouring an impression made of one of the materials whose surface is more difficult to wet. The use of a surfactant is also effective in reducing both the contact angle[1] and the number of voids trapped in the resulting cast.[3]

Viscosity

Viscosities for impression materials vary with the type of material. Light-bodied polysulfide and condensation silicone are the least viscous, and heavy-bodied polysulfide is the most viscous (Fig 17-2).[4] Viscosity will increase as time elapses after the start of mixing.[5] These materials exhibit lower viscosity when the shear rate (the speed at which a liquid flows under external forces) increases, which occurs when a material is expressed through a syringe.

This effect, called *shear thinning,* explains why a single-viscosity "monophasic" material can be placed in a tray, where "false body" (a higher apparent standing consistency) permits the material to stay in the tray without sagging or dripping, and yet the same material still can have sufficiently high fluidity (low viscosity) to be used in a syringe. A material that exhibits this property of becoming more fluid when the shear rate is increased by deforming or "disturbing" it (shaking, spatulating, or injecting through a syringe) is described as *thixotropic.*

The shear rate for injecting an impression material is 100 times as great as the shear rate for mixing the material.[4] The force required of the dentist is dependent on both the material and the syringe used. Forces as low as 2.6 lb for a condensation silicone/metal reusable syringe combination and as high as 112 lb for a polysulfide/large-diameter plastic disposable syringe combination have been reported.[6]

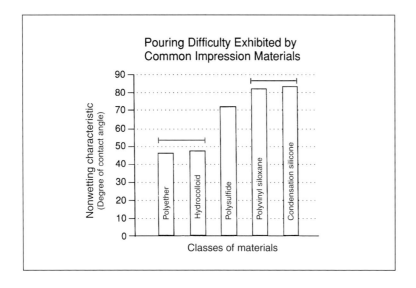

Fig 17-1 Degree of pouring difficulty for five types of impression materials as measured by the contact angle of gypsum on their surfaces. Adapted from data by McCormick et al.[1]

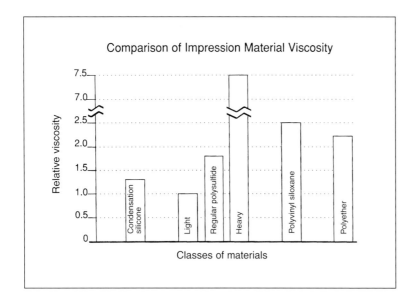

Fig 17-2 Comparison of the viscosity of five materials with light polysulfide 45 seconds after mixing. The viscosity of light polysulfide is arbitrarily assigned a value of 1.0, and the viscosities of the other materials are shown as a function of that. Based on data by Craig.[4]

Cost

While cost is not the primary factor in the selection of an impression material, it is one to be considered. A cost comparison of full-arch impressions made with commonly used impression materials is shown in Fig 17-3. The prices used for this comparison were the best available to private practitioners; they were found in fall 1993 catalogs from three US discount mail order dental supply dealers. Products not available from these companies were priced at the manufacturers' suggested retail prices. Bulk purchase or quantity discounts were used whenever they were available.

Although uniformly thin elastomeric impressions are more accurate,[7-9] only about one-third of surveyed dentists routinely employ custom trays.[10] Therefore, for this comparison, calculations were made for disposable stock plastic trays, stock metal trays, and custom resin trays. A volume of 33.3 mL was used for disposable trays, based on the mean volume of six sizes of spacer trays (GC America, Chicago, IL).[11] A volume of 38.4 mL was the mean for the 10 sizes of full-arch trays in the rimlock set (LD Caulk Div, Dentsply International, Milford, DE).[11]

The cost of a custom tray used here is that of the material only, assuming that office personnel make it. If a custom tray must be fabricated by a commercial laboratory, the expense would be prohibitive. Although hydrocolloid impressions were by far the least expensive, at an average cost of $2.10, this estimate made no provision for trays or for a conditioner, which is a very expensive piece of equipment.

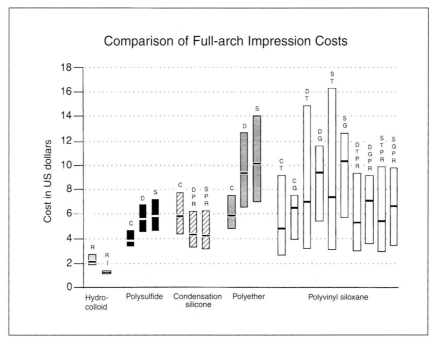

Fig 17-3 Comparison of the cost of full-arch impressions by type of tray and material. Each bar represents the range of impression cost, from least to most expensive, for that combination of material and tray. The horizontal line in each bar represents the average cost for that group. R = reversible, RI = reversible/irreversible, C = custom tray, D = disposable tray, S = stock tray, PR = putty/reline, T = tube-dispensed, G = gun/cartridge-dispensed. The volumes used for each type of impression tray are as follows: custom resin trays, 16.5 mL + 2.0 mL waste + 4.0 mL syringe; stock trays, 38.4 mL + 3.8 mL waste + 4.0 mL syringe; disposable trays, 33.3 mL + 3.3 mL waste + 4.0 mL syringe; putty reline (stock trays), 32 mL putty + 10 mL wash; putty reline (disposable trays), 27 mL putty + 10 mL wash; hydrocolloid impressions, 38.4 mL + cartridge + needle. Additional expenses include $0.43 for a disposable tray, $0.49 to $0.91 (depending on the brand) for a mixing tip for cartridge-dispensed polyvinyl siloxane, $1.15 for a custom tray, and $0.28 for a disposable hydrocolloid needle.

Of the elastomeric materials, polysulfide impressions in custom trays were the least expensive group, with a mean cost of $3.93, while cartridge-dispensed polyvinyl siloxanes in stock metal trays were the most expensive group, with an average cost of $10.27. Seventeen of the 21 groups studied had an average cost of less than $8.00. Of the 166 combinations of brand name, dispensing mode, and tray type, 73% were under $8.00 and 48% were under $6.00.

Reversible Hydrocolloid

Reversible (agar) hydrocolloid has seen extensive use as an impression material in the fabrication of cast gold restorations for more than 60 years.[12] Hydrocolloid was patented in 1925,[13] and it was introduced to the United States in the late 1920s.[14] Credit for its first use in the United States for fabricating cast restorations is given to J.D. Hart of Wewoka, Oklahoma, who began using it for that purpose in 1930.[14]

Reversible hydrocolloid is packaged as a semi-solid gel in polyethylene tubes. It is liquefied in a hydrocolloid conditioner by placing it in boiling water. As a liquid sol at this temperature, it is obviously too hot for intraoral use, so it is cooled in two stages: storage and tempering. In addition to lowering the temperature of the sol, tempering helps to increase the viscosity of the material in the tray so that it is more easily managed.

After the tray filled with tempered sol is placed in the mouth, cool tap water is circulated through the double-walled jacket of the tray to complete the gelation process. The material begins to gel near the cool tray first, spreading to the material adjacent to the oral tissues. Rapid cooling by excessively cold water can result in stress concentrations near the tray with possible distortion of the impression. The temperature should be 64°F to 70°F.[15] When the material is completely gelled, the impression is removed from the mouth and is ready to be poured. The cycle is thereby completed:

GEL	→	SOL	→	GEL
tube	→	conditioner	→	impression tray

Hydrocolloid is approximately 85% water, and the balance of this constituent is critical to the impression's accuracy. It can lose water by *syneresis* (water seeping from the surface), or by evaporation. It can also absorb water (if placed in contact with it) by *imbibition.* Numerous ways of storing impressions following removal from the mouth have been advocated: wet towels, humidors, water baths, and 2% potassium sulfate solution baths. The fact is that none is totally effective in preventing distortion; the impression begins distorting when it is removed from the mouth. The sooner it is poured, the less distortion there will be in the resulting cast.

The agar in hydrocolloid is a polysaccharide (a sulfuric ester of a linear polymer of galactose), which is obtained from seaweed.[15] Certain modifiers are added to improve the properties of the material. Sodium tetraborate increases the strength of the gel and the viscosity of the sol. The set of gypsum is retarded by contact with any gel, and the presence of borax tends to enhance this undesirable feature. The result could be a soft surface on the cast poured in the impression. Therefore, potassium sulfate is added to the hydrocolloid by the manufacturer to accelerate and harden the stone when it is poured into the impression. It also increases rupture strength and improves plastic deformation properties of the hydrocolloid.[16]

Reversible hydrocolloid impression materials have been strengthened considerably since their introduction,[17] and the process is ongoing. Some stones are more compatible with hydrocolloid impression material than others, reproducing surface detail more completely.[18] It is wise to check this feature before using a particular brand of stone with hydrocolloid. A bactericide such as thymol may be added to reduce bacterial growth. Plasticizers, fillers, flavoring agents, and pigments are added to the formula to constitute the final commercial product.

The ideal conditioner for preparing hydrocolloid for use has three baths (Fig 17-4):

1. *Liquefying bath.* Tubes of impression material and loaded syringes are boiled for 10 minutes in this bath (Fig 17-5). If the material is being reliquefied, it should be boiled for 12 minutes. To reach a boiling temperature of 212°F at higher altitudes, it is necessary to use propylene glycol in the boiling bath.
2. *Storage bath.* The tubes filled with liquefied material are moved to this bath, where they are stored at 150°F for a minimum of 10 minutes (Fig 17-6). Heavier-bodied materials may require storage at 152°F to 155°F.[15,17] Storage at higher altitudes also may require a higher storage temperature. The material can be stored for 5 days. If it has not been used by that time, it should be reliquefied by boiling it for 12 minutes.
3. *Tempering bath.* Loaded impression trays are tempered in this bath at 110°F to 115°F for 5 to 10 minutes immediately before placing them in the mouth. Heavier-bodied materials require less time, and a lower temperature requires less time. The tray should remain in the tempering bath for no less than 3 minutes.

The temperature in these three baths should be checked with a thermometer at regular intervals, since temperature variations can affect the viscosity and handling characteristics of the material. Water in the baths should be changed daily to minimize bacterial growth that occurs in many conditioners.[19] Iodophor disinfectant can be added to the water to further reduce the risk of cross-contamination.[19]

A technique combining reversible and irreversible hydrocolloid was described in 1951,[20] and a modified reversible hydrocolloid that could bond to alginate (irreversible hydrocolloid) was introduced in the late 1970s.[21] This system, also known as the *laminate technique,*[22] has the advantage of requiring less complicated (and less expensive) equipment for liquefaction and storage. The alginate in the tray, mixed with water at 70°F, cools the reversible hydrocolloid that has been injected around the prepared tooth, causing it to solidify. This eliminates the need for water-jacketed trays and tubing. The impression should be ready to remove from the mouth in 3 minutes, making it faster than other elastic materials. It is also less expensive.[23]

The principal disadvantage of combining reversible and irreversible hydrocolloids is the fast gelation time of the syringe material, which requires the impression to be handled very quickly.[24] There also have been problems with the syringe material separating from the alginate in the tray. Testing of the materials used has shown that some combinations of reversible hydrocolloid and alginate bond together better than others,[25] and that reversible/irreversible combination impressions have sufficient accuracy for clinical use.[21,24-26] Not surprisingly, bond strengths are greater between reversible and irreversible components made by the same manufacturer.[27] These combination systems are used by many dentists, but they have not supplanted the conventional reversible hydrocolloid impression materials.

Armamentarium

1. Hydrocolloid conditioning unit
2. Hydrocolloid in polyethylene tubes
3. Hydrocolloid in plastic cartridge
4. Nonaspirating anesthetic syringe
5. Water-cooled rim-lock sectional impression tray
6. Water-cooled rim-lock full-arch impression tray
7. Tacky stops
8. Tubing for trays

Impression Making With Hydrocolloid

Because only one accurate cast can be made from a hydrocolloid impression, two impressions are made: a sectional (quadrant) impression for making a die and a full-arch impression for the working cast. Be sure that the

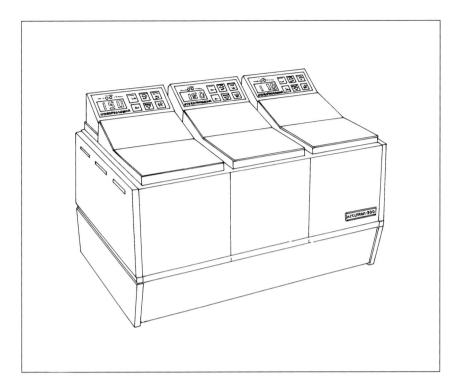

Fig 17-4 Hydrocolloid conditioner with three baths: liquefying *(left)*, storage *(center)*, and tempering *(right)*.

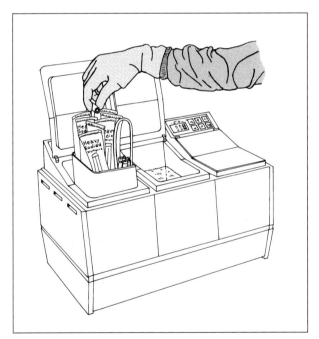

Fig 17-5 Tubes and cartridges of hydrocolloid are placed into the liquefying bath.

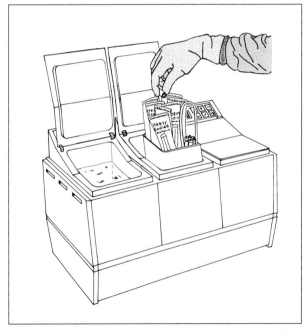

Fig 17-6 Tubes and cartridges are transferred from the liquefying bath to the storage bath.

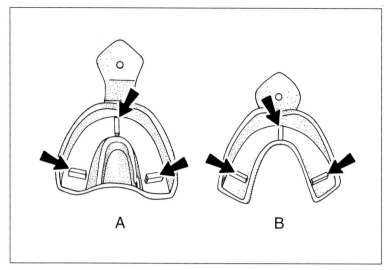

Fig 17-7 Rim-lock full-arch hydrocolloid impression trays, showing the optimal location of stops *(arrows)*. A, maxillary; B, mandibular.

patient has adequate anesthesia. If the impression is being made at a separate appointment subsequent to the preparation of the tooth, it is necessary to anesthetize the area again. Select the tray to be used and try it in the mouth to make certain that it fits.

Place adhesive plastic strips (Tacky Stops, Van R Dental Products, Los Angeles, CA) into the tray to keep the teeth from pushing all the way through to the tray when it is seated in the mouth. Position two of the stops, one on top of the other, at the rear of each side and in the front of the tray on full-arch trays (Fig 17-7). On quadrant trays, place stops at the front and rear. Make sure that the stops will contact unprepared teeth.

Isolate the quadrant containing the prepared tooth, insert the retraction cord, and place a large gauze pack in the mouth. Fill the impression tray with a tube taken from the storage bath and place the filled tray in the tempering bath (Fig 17-8). It should be allowed to temper for 10 minutes. Since tempering is a function of time as well as temperature, leaving the hydrocolloid in the tempering bath too long may bring it too near gelation and make it too stiff for making an impression. It is unacceptable to cool the material on the countertop at room temperature, as this is likely to cool only the surface layer.[13]

Screw a short, blunt 19-gauge needle onto the end of an anesthetic-type syringe that does not have a barb on the end of the plunger (Fig 17-9). Remove a plastic, anesthetic-type cartridge containing hydrocolloid from the storage bath (Fig 17-10). Insert it into the syringe (Fig 17-11) and express a small amount of material to make sure it is flowing freely.

Remove the 2 x 2 gauze squares from the patient's mouth. Blow a very light water/air mist on the prepared tooth before removing the retraction cord. The cord should be slightly moist, but not wet. Do not blow com-pressed air on the tooth after the retraction cord has been removed, since this may start hemorrhage in the sulcus.

Carefully remove the cord from the sulcus by grasping the free end in the mesial interproximal area with a pair of cotton pliers. Tease the cord out gently so that hemorrhage will not start (Fig 17-12). If an impression is being made of multiple preparations, remove the cord from the sulcus around each tooth, one at a time, immediately before the material is injected. Inject hydrocolloid from the syringe into the sulcus, starting in an interproximal area first (Fig 17-13). Hold the tip above the mouth of the crevice, taking care not to drag the tip along the gingiva. Proceed smoothly around the entire circumference of the preparation, pushing impression material before the tip.

An alternative way of applying the syringe material is called the *wet field technique*.[15] The prepared teeth are bathed in warm water, and syringe material is deposited in generous quantities only on the occlusal surfaces of the teeth. The relatively viscous tray material is counted on to force the lighter-bodied syringe material into the sulcus as the tray is seated. This technique should be used only on preparations that do not contain internal features, such as grooves, boxes, or isthmuses.

The assistant should remove the sectional tray from the tempering bath, wipe the surfaces of the hydrocolloid free of water, and connect the tray to the hoses. Give the syringe to the assistant in exchange for the tray. Seat the tray while the assistant connects the hoses to the unit. Hold the tray in place for 6 minutes while cool water flows through its tubes. Do not have the patient hold the hydrocolloid tray. It is too unstable, and a distorted impression could result.

While the sectional tray is setting in the patient's mouth, the assistant can fill the full-arch tray and place it in the

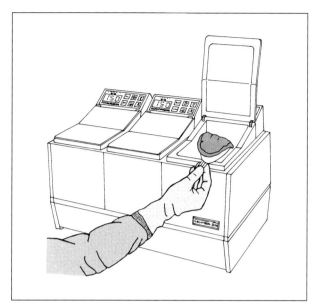

Fig 17-8 Tray filled with impression material is placed in the tempering bath.

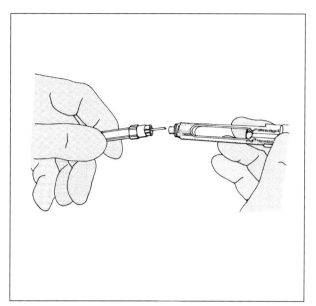

Fig 17-9 Blunt needle is attached to the impression syringe.

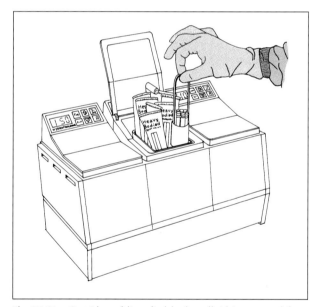

Fig 17-10 Cartridge of liquefied hydrocolloid is removed from the storage bath.

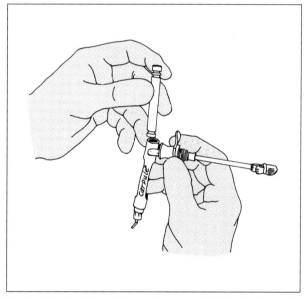

Fig 17-11 Cartridge of impression material is loaded into the syringe.

tempering bath. Remove the sectional impression with a quick motion, along the long axes of the teeth.[13] Check it for completeness, and wash it in cold tap water. Remove the excess moisture from the surface of the impression with air, but do not desiccate the material. Spray the impression or place it in an appropriate solution to disinfect it before pouring it.

Blow a very light water/air mist on the preparation and inject hydrocolloid around it again. It is usually not necessary to repack the sulcus with cord for the working cast impression. Place the full-arch tray and connect the tubes to the unit. Hold it in place for 6 minutes. Remove it with a snap. The impression of the opposing arch can be made with alginate (irreversible hydrocolloid).

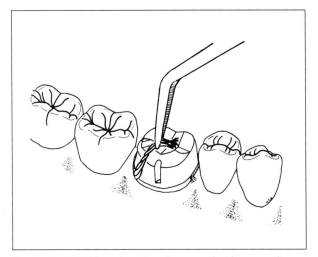

Fig 17-12 Cord from the sulcus is removed with cotton pliers.

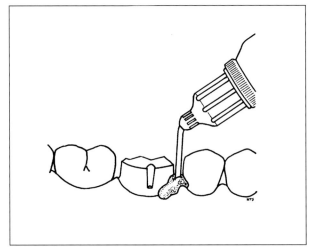

Fig 17-13 Hydrocolloid is injected into the sulcus.

Custom Resin Trays

Custom resin trays have been utilized in elastomeric impression techniques because these materials are more accurate in uniform, thin layers of 2 to 3 mm (Fig 17-14). Many authors advise against the use of stock trays because the uneven bulk of impression material is conducive to distortion.[7-9] However, it has been reported that the mean difference in material thickness between custom and stock trays is less than 1.0 mm, and that variations from uniform thickness exist in both custom and stock trays.[28]

Tray space seems to have no effect on the dimensional accuracy of monophasic polyvinyl siloxane impressions, except for the distance between fixed partial denture abutment preparations.[29] This distortion of interpreparation distance was first described by Gordon et al,[30] who reported that the interpreparation distance in casts made from polysulfide, polyvinyl siloxane, and polyether impressions was 45 to 100 μm greater when stock trays were used instead of custom acrylic resin or thermoplastic trays. They also reported 260-μm cross-arch discrepancies, which they attributed to stock tray flexibility.[30]

Smaller discrepancies have been reported for the length of dies poured in polyvinyl siloxane impressions in custom trays than those made from impressions in stock trays.[31] However, Bomberg et al[32] found no significant difference in the marginal fit of single-tooth restorations on casts made from polyvinyl siloxane impressions in stock and custom trays. Stock trays probably provide sufficient accuracy for single-tooth restorations, particularly if polyvinyl siloxane or polyether is used. However, if one-piece fixed partial dentures of three or more units are to be fabricated on the cast, the interpreparation and cross-arch discrepancies could have a significant impact on the fit of the restoration.

Efforts have been made to form a custom tray in the mouth by lining a stock tray with modeling compound. This is not a recommended technique because plasticizers in the elastomers attack and soften the compound.[33] The softened compound may allow some separation of the impression from the tray when it is removed from the mouth. The result could be distortion that would not be detected until the finished casting is tried in the mouth.

The custom tray must be rigid, and it should have stops on the occlusal surfaces of the teeth to orient the tray properly when it is seated in the mouth (Fig 17-15). The impression material must adhere firmly to the tray. This is achieved with a rubber adhesive packaged with the impression material. These adhesives are not interchangeable, so use only the type packaged with the brand of material being used. The adhesives used for polyether have the best tensile strength.[34,35] Condensation silicones exhibit the weakest tensile and peel bond strengths.[36] The strengths of some adhesives for polyvinyl siloxanes equal,[34,35] and others surpass, the strength of those used with polysulfide.[34,36,37]

The bonding strength of adhesives used with polyvinyl siloxanes can be improved nearly 50% by adding perforations to the tray, and approximately 140% by roughening the inner surface of an acrylic resin tray with 80-grit silicon carbide paper before adding the adhesive.[38] Polyvinyl siloxane putty does not adhere to its adhesive,[35,39] making good mechanical retention in the tray, such as perforations, mandatory when putty is used.

The composition of the tray also may have an effect on retention of the impression within the tray. The bonding of polyvinyl siloxane to trays made of a visible light–cured (VLC) urethane dimethacrylate resin (Triad Tray Material, Dentsply International, York, PA) seems to vary with the brand of impression material.[40-41] Dixon et al[41] reported the adhesion of Reprosil (LD Caulk Div, Dentsply International, Milford, DE) to VLC tray material to be about twice its retention to acrylic resin. However, Payne

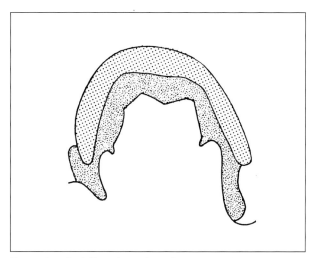

Fig 17-14 Faciolingual section of a custom impression tray, impression, and tooth preparation.

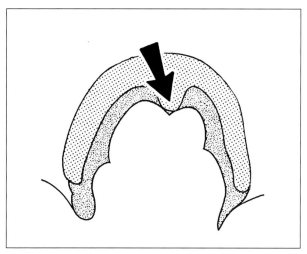

Fig 17-15 Faciolingual section of the stop *(arrow)* on a custom impression tray and impression.

and Pereira[40] found the bonding of Hydrosil (LD Caulk) to the same urethane dimethacrylate resin to be weak. The bond strength was nearly tripled by roughening the tray surface with a carbide bur.[40]

Polysulfide adhesive adheres at least as well to trays made of thermoplastic material (E-Z Tray, Oral Dynamics, Seattle, WA) as it does to acrylic resin, if the tray is formed over a foil-covered wax spacer.[37] Polysulfide and condensation silicones do not adhere as well to stock polystyrene trays as they do to custom acrylic resin trays, but polyether and polyvinyl siloxane adhere better to the former than to the latter.[35] Tjan and Whang[42] found no clinically significant differences in the accuracy of dies poured in polyvinyl siloxane impressions made in custom trays with adhesive only, perforations only, or both, on first pours. However, on second pours, impressions made in adhesive-coated trays were more accurate.

Tray Armamentarium

1. Diagnostic casts
2. Autopolymerizing acrylic resin (monomer and polymer)
3. Measuring vial for monomer
4. Measuring scoop for polymer
5. Waxed paper cup
6. Spatula
7. Baseplate wax
8. Aluminum foil
9. Laboratory knife with no. 25 blade
10. Bunsen burner
11. Matches
12. Arbor bands
13. Adhesive for impression material used

Tray Preparation

Heat a sheet of baseplate wax in a flame until it is softened. Fold it in half and place it on the diagnostic cast of the arch to be restored. Adapt it to the cast and trim any excess that extends more than 2 to 3 mm beyond the necks of the teeth. The wax will form a spacer for the impression material. A horseshoe-shaped form is used for both arches, with no palatal coverage on the maxillary arch.

Cut a 3 x 3-mm hole through the wax over posterior teeth on both sides of the arch and in the incisor area. The tray resin will touch the teeth in these areas, forming solid stops for the tray (Fig 17-16). On the side where the prepared tooth is situated, the stop should be distal to the preparation. There should be a protective layer between the wax and the tray resin to prevent the wax from impregnating the surface of the tray during the exothermic polymerization of the acrylic resin. A waxy layer on the inner surface of the tray will diminish bonding by the tray adhesive applied before placement of the impression material, resulting in distortion of the impression. Adapt a piece of aluminum foil over the wax and stone cast to provide separation.[43]

Mix the resin in the waxed paper cup, using one measure of powder and one vial of liquid. As soon as it is pliable and will not stick to your fingers, form it into a rod that is approximately the length of the dental arch (molar to molar, around the incisors). Flatten it out to form an oblong shape about 1 inch (2.5 cm) wide and 3/16 inches (5.0 mm) thick. Leave some extra bulk in the middle (Fig 17-17).

Place the acrylic resin on the arch and adapt it over the foil-covered wax. Mold it so that it just extends to the edge of the wax spacer under the foil. It should end at the distal surface of the last tooth on each side of the

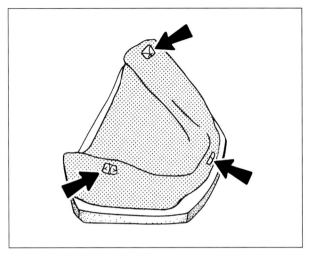

Fig 17-16 Cutouts for stops *(arrows)* in the spacer for fabrication of a custom impression tray.

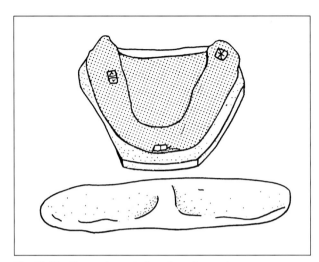

Fig 17-17 Tray resin ready for adaptation to the cast.

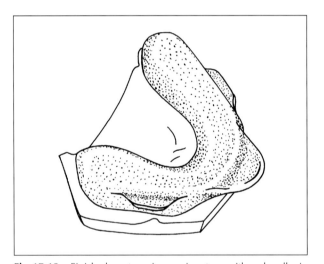

Fig 17-18 Finished custom impression tray with a handle in front and wings on the side to facilitate removal.

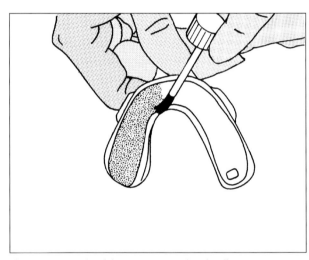

Fig 17-19 Inside of the tray is painted with adhesive.

arch. Make sure that the tray does not extend beyond the trimmed distal border of the cast in the retromolar area. The bulk left in the middle of the tray should be used to shape a horizontal handle in the middle and a narrow ledge or "wing" on either side of it (Fig 17-18). The wings can be used to get better leverage on the tray for removal from the mouth. Allow the resin to polymerize.

When the tray is hard, but still warm to the touch, remove it from the cast and peel out the aluminum foil and any wax adhering to it. Try the tray back on the cast to check for uniform clearance. Use an arbor band to cut back any areas that come too close to the cast, especially in the area of the prepared teeth. If any grinding must be done on the tray, smooth and polish those areas that will contact soft tissue before taking the tray to the

mouth. A rough, sharp border on the tray can lacerate the angles of the mouth when the tray is inserted.

The tray should be prepared at least 6 hours in advance. As the monomer undergoes polymerization, it shrinks. The dough could shrink as much as 8% before curing is completed.[44] Significant linear changes occur during the first 40 minutes of the fabrication of a tray, with some changes continuing to occur for up to 6 hours.[45] An acceptable result can be obtained with a tray that is at least 40 minutes old if the impression is poured quickly.[45] An acrylic resin tray can be stabilized against further shrinkage and distortion by boiling it.[46]

If the tray is made immediately before the impression is made, however, polymerization shrinkage and stress relaxation will be occurring while the impression is in the tray, resulting in distortion of that impression. Elastomeric impressions should not be stored in a moist environment, since an acrylic resin tray may imbibe water and distort.

Paint the inside of the tray with a thin, uniform coat of adhesive, using the one specified for the impression material being used (Fig 17-19). To achieve maximum adhesion of the impression material to the tray, allow it to dry for a minimum of 15 minutes.[43] If the adhesive has not been allowed to dry, the impression material may separate from the tray when it is removed from the mouth.

Polysulfide

Polysulfide is an elastomer that is also known as *mercaptan, thiokol,* or simply as *rubber base.* This latter term alone is incomplete and should be avoided. The material was developed as the matrix for solid-state fuels and oxidizers used in many space vehicles, including the boosters for the space shuttle program. The impression material is packaged in two tubes: a base and an accelerator. The base contains a liquid polysulfide polymer mixed with an inert filler. The accelerator, which is usually lead dioxide mixed with small amounts of sulfur and oil, acts as an oxidation initiator on terminal thiol groups on the polymer.

When these two pastes are mixed, the polymer chains are lengthened and crosslinked through the oxidized thiol groups. In clinical terms, this results first in an increased viscosity and finally in an elastic material. This polymerization is exothermic and is affected significantly by moisture and temperature.[47]

Polysulfide rubber base possesses much greater dimensional stability than does hydrocolloid. However, the polysulfide polymer does contract as curing occurs. Therefore, if maximum accuracy is to be obtained, a polysulfide impression should be poured within approximately 1 hour of removal from the mouth[48] or less.[49,50] Unpoured polysulfide impressions should never be sent to a laboratory.

Large undercut areas in the interproximal region should be blocked out in the mouth with soft wax. Otherwise, the impression may be "locked" in the mouth and be distorted by the excessive force that must be used to remove the tray from the mouth.

Because of the *hydrophobic* nature of this material, special care must be taken to insure that there is no moisture on the preparation when the impression is made. Thin layers of moisture on the surface can make the cast slightly larger, and moisture that becomes incorporated during the injecting process can cause folds, creases, and voids in the impression. This, in turn, will result in fins and assorted projections on the cast, rendering it useless. *Any* hemorrhage or fluid seepage in the sulcus will result in voids and bubbles that will obscure the finish line.

Polysulfide is unique among impression materials because it is radiopaque.[51] If a fragment becomes entrapped in the gingival sulcus or in a tissue space beyond an interrupted epithelial attachment, its exact location can be easily determined radiographically.[52] This property is the result of the presence of lead dioxide in the formula, which almost certainly contributes to its toxicity and tendency to irritate soft tissues when it becomes trapped.

Other impression materials can be made radiopaque by substituting radiopaque substances for the normal fillers used in making the impression material.[53] However, if the filler is not selected carefully, the altered composition may affect other properties of the impression material, such as setting or shelf life. At the present time, only one nonpolysulfide impression material, a polyvinyl siloxane (Blu-Mousse, Parkell, Farmingdale, NY), has been altered to make it radiopaque (personal communication, Dr Nelson Gendusa).

Impression Armamentarium

1. Polysulfide impression kit (regular base and accelerator)
2. Polysulfide impression kit (light base and accelerator)
3. Adhesive (butyl rubber cement)
4. Two disposable mixing pads
5. Two stiff spatulas
6. Syringe with disposable tip
7. Two 2 x 2-inch gauze sponges
8. Alcohol
9. Custom resin tray

Impression Making With Polysulfide

Be sure that the patient has adequate anesthesia. If the impression is being made at a separate appointment subsequent to the preparation of the tooth, it is necessary to anesthetize the area. Try the custom tray in the mouth to make sure it fits without impinging on the prepared tooth. Insert the retraction cord and place a large gauze pack in the mouth.

The following steps require an assistant. On one disposable mixing pad squeeze out 1.5 inches (4.0 cm) each of light (syringe) base and accelerator. On a second pad place 5.0-inch (12.5-cm) strips of regular (tray) base and accelerator. Pull the plunger from the injection syringe and set it aside. The tip and cap (if removable) should be on the barrel of the syringe.

The assistant should start mixing the tray material on one pad 30 seconds before the operator begins mixing the syringe material on the other. Pick up the dark accelerator on the spatula and incorporate it into the white base (Fig 17-20). Holding the spatula flat against the pad, mix with a back-and-forth motion, pressing hard against the pad. Change directions often to produce a smooth, homogenous mixture (Fig 17-21). Be careful not

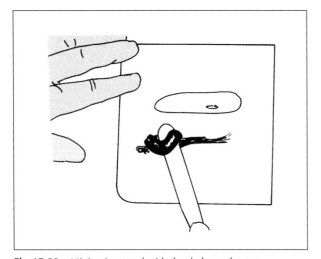

Fig 17-20 Mixing is started with the dark accelerator.

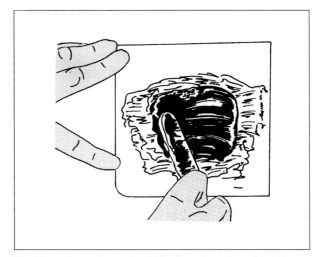

Fig 17-21 The mixture should be free of streaks and bubbles.

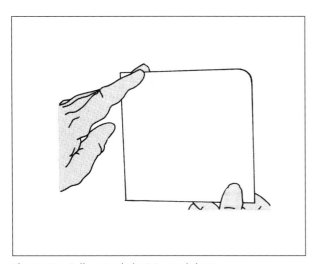

Fig 17-22 Fully extended mixing pad sheet.

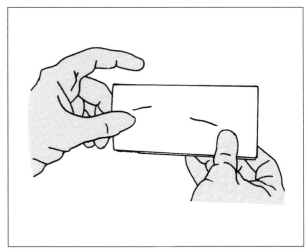

Fig 17-23 The sheet is folded in half.

to incorporate bubbles. Do not take more than 1 minute to mix it.

Fold a sheet previously removed from the mixing pad in half (Figs 17-22, 17-23) and then fold it to make a cone (Fig 17-24). Open it up and wipe the syringe material from the spatula onto the crease (Fig 17-25). Fold the cone over (Fig 17-26). Squeeze the syringe material from the cone into the back end of the syringe (Fig 17-27). Insert the plunger and express all the air from the syringe (Fig 17-28).

In a second method of loading the syringe, the back end of the syringe is brought in contact with the pad, and quick, closely spaced sweeps of the syringe will fill it, with a minimum of material spilled (Fig 17-29). In a third method, the syringe tip is removed and the front end of the syringe is buried in a collected mass of material on

the pad (Fig 17-30) or in a dappen dish. This technique unquestionably works, but the novice in a hurry can suck a lot of air into the syringe and make a mess in the process.

Remove the 2 x 2 gauze squares from the patient's mouth. Be sure that the retraction cord is slightly damp before removing it from the sulcus. Immediately inject polysulfide syringe material into the sulcus (Fig 17-31). Hold the tip just above the mouth of the crevice. Do not drag the tip along the gingiva. Proceed smoothly around the entire circumference of the preparation, pushing impression material ahead of the tip. Continue around the preparation until the entire tooth is covered.

Use an air syringe to direct a stream of air against the material (Fig 17-32) to spread it evenly over the surface of the preparation and drive it into small details such as

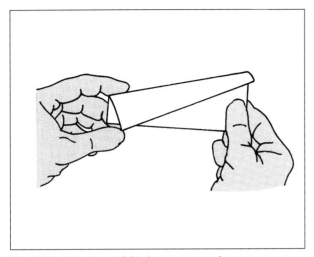

Fig 17-24   The sheet is folded once more to form a cone.

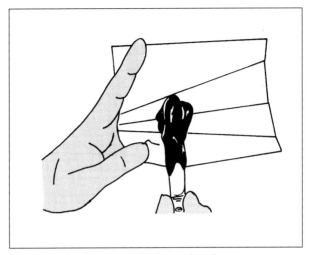

Fig 17-25   Impression material is wiped on the crease.

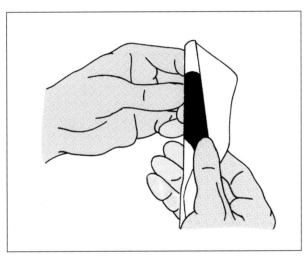

Fig 17-26   The paper is refolded to form the cone again.

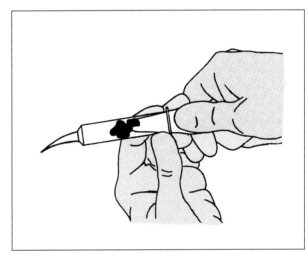

Fig 17-27   The cone is inserted into the syringe.

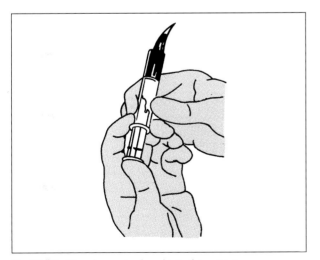

Fig 17-28   The plunger is placed into the syringe.

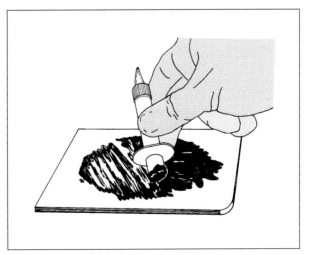

Fig 17-29   A syringe also can be loaded by scraping the back end across the mixing pad to scoop up material.

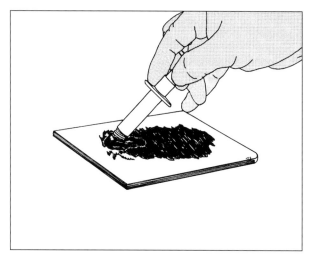

Fig 17-30 The syringe is loaded through the front end by aspirating the material.

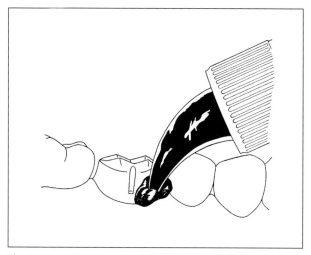

Fig 17-31 Impression material is injected into the sulcus.

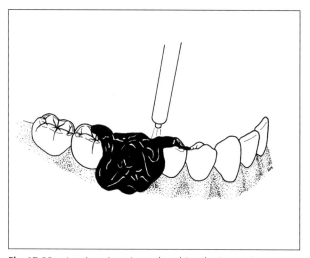

Fig 17-32 An air syringe is used to drive the impression material into the sulcus and preparation detail.

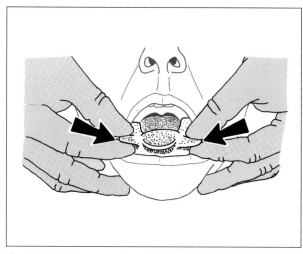

Fig 17-33 Wings on either side of the tray *(arrows)* are grasped to remove the impression from the mouth.

grooves and boxes.[54,55] Impression material is also forced more completely into the gingival crevice. Excessive pressure, prolonged air application, and use on patients with a thin band of attached gingiva should be avoided because of the possibility of producing interstitial emphysema. Seat the tray slowly until the stops hold the tray solidly in one position. The tray should be held with light pressure for 8 to 10 minutes without movement. The set of the material can be tested with a blunt instrument. When the material rebounds completely without leaving any trace, it has set.

After the material has polymerized, the impression is removed. The wings on the sides of the tray can be used for added leverage in this task (Fig 17-33). While it is customary to call for removing the tray suddenly or with a snap, it is more realistic to ask that the removal be as fast and in as straight a direction as possible. Only a silver-

back highland gorilla could remove a full-arch polysulfide impression with a snap. Rinse the impression to remove blood and saliva. Blow it dry and inspect it. An impression of the opposing arch can be made with alginate. Soak the impression in an appropriate disinfectant solution before pouring it.

Condensation Silicone

Condensation-reaction silicones are so named because of the nature of their polymerization reaction. They also could be called *organo-tin silicones,* which is a reference to their catalyst. The base paste is a liquid silicone polymer with terminal hydroxyl groups, mixed with inert fillers.

The reactor, a viscous liquid, consists of a crosslinking agent, ethyl silicate, with an organo-tin activator, tin octoate. When the two are mixed, the materials are crosslinked by a reaction between terminal hydroxyl groups on the polymer and ethyl orthosilicate.[56]

The condensation reaction occurs by the elimination of ethyl or methyl alcohol. The evaporation of this alcohol is believed to be responsible for shrinkage of the material and resultant poor dimensional stability.[57] Impressions made in silicone should be poured soon after removal from the mouth.[48,50] One of the problems in using condensation silicones has been its limited shelf life. This is caused by the instability of alkyl silicates in the presence of organo-tin compounds, which may result in oxidation of the tin.[47]

The technique for condensation silicone rubber base materials is similar in many ways to that for polysulfide. Two inches (5.0 cm) of base are mixed with two drops of accelerator to provide the material used in the syringe. Eight inches (20 cm) of base and eight drops of accelerator are used to form the quantity required to fill the average full-arch impression tray. Other aspects of the technique for the use of condensation silicone rubber base impressions are the same as those used for polysulfide impressions.

There are some condensation silicone impression materials that utilize a heavy-bodied "putty" relined with a thin "wash." These were developed to reduce the sizable dimensional change that begins to occur when a condensation silicone impression is not poured immediately. The putty has a silica filler content of 75%, which is more than double that in the wash.[58] As a result, there is a much lower dimensional change in the bulk of the impression. A preliminary impression is made with the highly filled, heavy-bodied putty in a stock tray. This will serve as a custom tray for a thin "wash" of a less highly filled, low-viscosity silicone.

The accuracy of the putty/reline has been found to be quite satisfactory,[59] with a minimal effect from a delayed pouring of up to 6 hours.[60] It does produce very slightly undersized dies.[60,61] The putty/reline condensation silicones have become much more popular with dentists than double-mix condensation silicones because they provide reasonable accuracy with delayed pouring and they do not require a custom tray.

Armamentarium

1. Silicone impression kit (putty, base, and accelerator)
2. Tray adhesive—poly(dimethyl) siloxane and ethyl silicate
3. Measuring scoop
4. Disposable mixing pad
5. Stiff spatula
6. Syringe with disposable tip
7. 2 x 2-inch gauze sponges
8. Stock trays (rim-lock or perforated)
9. Laboratory knife with no. 25 blade

Impression Making With Condensation Silicone

Before the preparation is begun, select a stock tray that fits the arch. Coat the inside of the tray with a thin, even coat of adhesive and allow it to dry (Fig 17-34). For a full-arch impression tray, place two scoops of putty (base) on the pad. Use one scoop for a sectional tray. Add six drops of accelerator for each scoop of base (Fig 17-35). Incorporate them on the pad with a spatula for a few seconds. Then transfer the material to the palm of the hand and knead it for 30 seconds. The material should be streak free.

Roll the base into a cigar shape and place it into a stock impression tray (Fig 17-36). Cover the base with a polyethylene spacer, and seat the tray in the mouth (Fig 17-37). Remove the tray from the mouth after the initial set has occurred (about 2 minutes). Peel off the spacer and remove any excess on the periphery of the tray with a sharp knife (Fig 17-38). Set the tray aside for use after the tooth has been prepared.

Be sure that the patient has adequate anesthesia. Isolate the quadrant containing the prepared tooth, place the retraction cord, and insert a large gauze pad in the mouth. The following steps require an assistant: Squeeze out 8 inches (20 cm) of the thin-wash silicone base onto the disposable mixing pad. Use 4 inches (10 cm) for a sectional tray. Add one drop of accelerator per inch of base. Mix with a spatula for 30 seconds; the mix should be free of streaks. Place about one-third of the wash material into the back end of the syringe. While you are inserting the plunger and expressing air, the assistant should place the rest of the material into the tray.

Remove the 2 x 2 gauze squares from the patient's mouth. Be sure that the retraction cord is slightly damp before removing it from the sulcus. If necessary, *gently* blow air on the prepared tooth to remove moisture from the tooth itself before the retraction cord is removed from the sulcus. If you blow compressed air on the tooth after the cord has been removed, hemorrhage may result.

Carefully remove the cord from the sulcus by grasping the free end in the interproximal region with cotton pliers. Tease the cord out *gently* so that hemorrhage will not start. Immediately inject syringe material into the sulcus. Hold the tip just above the mouth of the crevice. Do not drag the tip along the gingiva. Proceed smoothly around the entire circumference of the preparation, pushing impression material ahead of the tip. Do not skip any areas, but continue around the preparation until the entire tooth is covered. Give the syringe to the assistant in exchange for the loaded tray.

Seat the tray slowly until it is firmly in place. The tray should be held in place with no downward pressure for 6 minutes. Pressure exerted on the tray while the wash is polymerizing will produce stresses in the semi-rigid putty lining the impression tray. When the impression is removed from the mouth, the stresses will relax, resulting in deformation and distortion of the impression.

After the material has set, remove the impression as

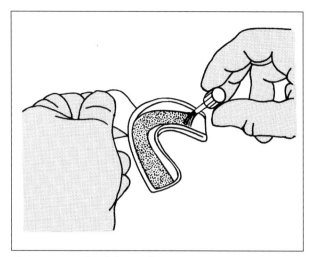

Fig 17-34 Inside of the stock impression tray is painted with adhesive.

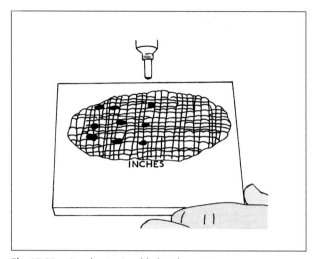

Fig 17-35 Accelerator is added to the putty.

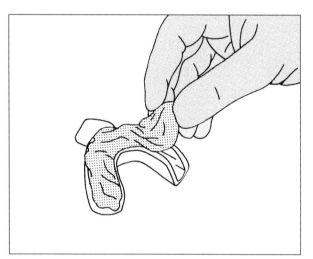

Fig 17-36 Putty is placed in the tray.

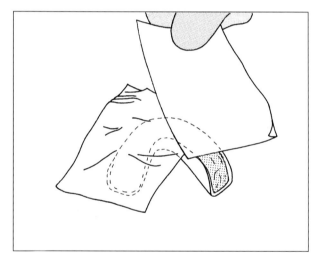

Fig 17-37 Spacers are placed over the tray.

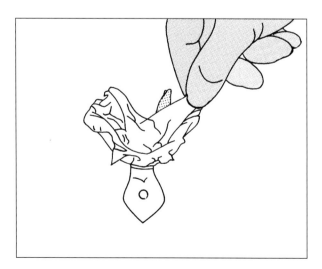

Fig 17-38 The spacers are removed from the tray.

quickly and as straightly as possible to prevent plastic deformation of the material. Rinse the impression to remove blood and saliva. Blow it dry and inspect it. Soak the impression in an appropriate disinfectant solution before pouring it. An impression of the opposing arch can be made with alginate.

Polyvinyl Siloxane

The dimensional stability of this group of impression materials is so much better than that of condensation silicone, and its reaction is so different that it deserves treatment as a separate variety of material. Polyvinyl siloxane silicone also is commonly called *addition silicone,* because of its setting reaction, sometimes *vinyl polysiloxane,* and even *vinyl silicone.*

The material usually is packaged as two pastes. One paste contains silicone with terminal silane hydrogen groups and an inert filler. The other paste is made up of a silicone with terminal vinyl groups, chloroplatinic acid catalyst, and a filler.[58] Upon mixing equal quantities of the two materials, there is an addition of silane hydrogen groups across vinyl double bonds with the formation of no by-products.[57] The result is an exceptionally stable material.[50,57,58]

Polyvinyl siloxane is least affected by pouring delays, or by second pours,[61] and it is still accurate, even when poured 1 week after removal from the mouth.[62] Early formulations of this material released hydrogen gas from the impression surface, resulting in voids in the surface of the setting stone cast.[63] If the impression was not poured within 15 minutes, then the best results were obtained by waiting 24 hours before pouring.[63] Modification of the formula by the addition of palladium to absorb the hydrogen has minimized this problem. Pouring should now be delayed for a short time, but it will be 15 to 30 minutes and not a day.

In its unaltered form, polyvinyl siloxane is hydrophobic.[1] Surfactants can be incorporated into the material to make it less hydrophobic and easier to pour. Casts poured in impressions made with altered "hydrophilic" polyvinyl siloxane exhibit 26% to 55% fewer trapped voids than casts poured in unaltered or conventional polyvinyl siloxane.[64] However, casts made in unaltered polyvinyl siloxane impressions whose surfaces have been treated with a surfactant at the time of pouring show a reduction in voids of 86%.[64]

Casts poured in "hydrophilic" polyvinyl siloxanes with intrinsic surfactants produce slightly less accurate casts with surfaces that are 14% to 33% softer than those poured in conventional polyvinyl siloxanes.[64] The incorporated surfactant makes electroplating more difficult, and it also makes the impression material more sensitive to the retardant action of sulfur.[47] Nonetheless, "hydrophilic" polyvinyl siloxanes will continue to be used because they are more convenient.

The two pastes can be packaged in separate tubes, or they can be placed in a twin-barreled cartridge. The cartridge is placed in a dispenser, or "gun," from which the contents of the two barrels are extruded through a mixing tip with multiple vanes or baffles that mix the two materials together. Mixing "guns" have become the most popular method of dispensing and mixing the material, eliminating the necessity of a spatula and a mixing pad.

Material dispensed and mixed in this manner costs more per milliliter, but reduced waste keeps the cost of the impression down.[65] It is certainly much cleaner. The system eliminates air entrapment, ensures consistently uniform ratios of catalyst and base, and prevents contamination.[66] Generally, automixed addition silicones exhibit fewer voids in an impression than do hand-mixed elastomers of the same type, although hand-mixing with some brands may produce fewer voids than automixing will with some other brands.[67]

Putty and light-bodied "wash" consistencies are made for this type of silicone also. The light-bodied syringe material is available either in separate tubes or in cartridges. If putty is used, it should not be dispensed or mixed while wearing latex gloves, because setting of the material may be impeded. The polymerization retardation probably results from sulfur derivatives in the latex.[68] The inhibition is not restricted to putty,[69] but the putty is more easily contaminated because it is hand-mixed.

The difficulty is not universal: Only some brands of impression material, in combination with some brands of gloves, cause retarded setting.[70] It also can result from contact with other latex items, such as a rubber dam.[71] This can even occur indirectly, when the impression material comes in contact with an object, such as a tooth, that has been touched by a glove, and not with the glove itself. This problem can be avoided by using vinyl gloves or overgloves during the handling of the impression material.[72]

Armamentarium

1. Dispenser
2. Cartridge (base and accelerator)
3. Mixing tip
4. Disposable mixing pad
5. Syringe with disposable tip
6. 2 x 2-inch gauze sponges
7. Custom impression tray
8. Tray adhesive

Impression Making With Polyvinyl Siloxane

Paint the custom tray with adhesive at least 15 minutes before the impression is to be made. If a tube-dispensed material is used in a double-mix technique, the assistant and operator start mixing material at about the same

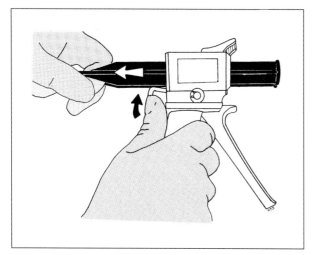

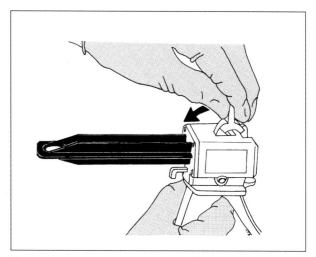

Fig 17-39 Release lever is pushed up with a thumb while the plunger is pulled back.

Fig 17-40 The retainer cap on top of the dispenser block is released.

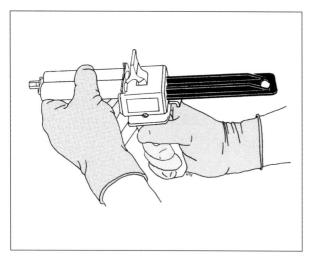

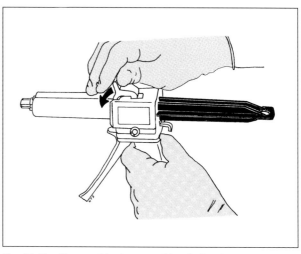

Fig 17-41 The cartridge flange is slid into the slots on the front of the dispenser.

Fig 17-42 The cartridge is secured by closing the retainer cap.

time. Mix with a spatula for about 45 seconds until all streaks are eliminated. Then load the syringe and tray.

If you are using a cartridge system, load a cartridge of light-bodied material into one dispenser and a cartridge of medium- or heavy-bodied material into another. It is still possible to use two cartridges even if you have access to only one dispenser. Prepare the dispenser, or gun, by pulling the ratcheted double plunger all the way back while pushing on the plunger release lever at the rear of the dispenser body (Fig 17-39). Lift up the retainer cap (a hinged locking device or removable locking plate) on the top of the dispenser, if there is one on your model (Fig 17-40). Slide the rear flange of the cartridge down into the slots on either side of the front of the dis-

penser until the cartridge is completely seated (Fig 17-41). Close the retainer cap (or replace it if it is removable) on the top of the dispenser, securing the cartridge flange to the dispenser (Fig 17-42).

Remove the cap from the end of the cartridge (Fig 17-43), and put the cap in a safe place where it will not be thrown out in the cleanup following the impression. Express a small quantity of impression material from the end of the cartridge before adding the mixing tip (Fig 17-44). This will insure that both barrels of the cartridge are clear and ready for use. Sometimes the end of the barrels become cross-contaminated, causing the formation of polymerized plugs in one or both sides of the nozzle. If this is not eliminated before adding the mixing tip and

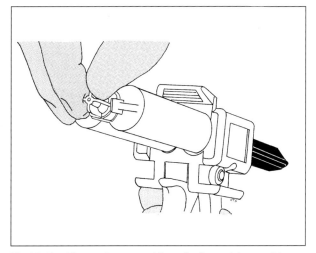

Fig 17-43   The cap is removed from the front of the cartridge.

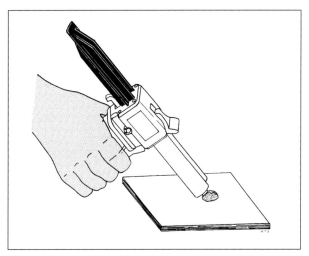

Fig 17-44   A small quantity of material is squeezed out to insure that the outlets are clear.

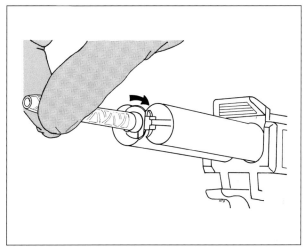

Fig 17-45   The mixing tip is attached to the end of the cartridge.

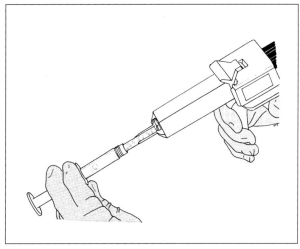

Fig 17-46   Material from the mixing tip is expressed into the syringe.

mixing the material, the dispenser will jam and the impression attempt will have to be aborted. Do not try to overpower a jammed dispenser by using more force on the trigger or handle. The end result could be a ruptured cartridge and a multicolored eruption of sticky impression material.

Place the mixing tip on the nozzle at the end of the cartridge of light-bodied material and rotate the mixing tip 90 degrees to lock it in place (Fig 17-45). Apply force to the handle of the dispenser until the mixing tip is filled with impression material. Insert the mixing tip into the front end of an impression syringe until it touches the face of the drawn-back plunger of the syringe (Fig 17-46). Express material into the syringe, slowly withdrawing the

mixing tip of the dispenser as you fill the syringe. Secure the clear tip on the syringe with the locking ring. Remove the gauze pack. Be sure that the retraction cord is slightly damp before removing it from the sulcus. Carefully remove the cord and inject the impression material, starting in one interproximal area and pushing the material ahead of the tip.

While the dentist applies the light-bodied material with a syringe, the assistant loads the tray with the medium- or heavy-bodied material (Fig 17-47). Exchange the syringe for the loaded tray and seat it firmly in the mouth. Hold it in place for 7 minutes from the start of mixing.

Remove the impression as quickly and straightly as possible to prevent distortion. Rinse, blow it dry, and

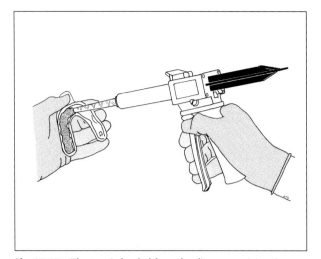

Fig 17-47   The tray is loaded from the dispenser mixing tip.

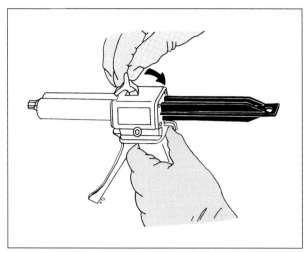

Fig 17-48   To remove the cartridge, the plunger is pulled back and the retainer cap or locking plate is opened.

inspect it. Place it in a disinfectant solution before pouring it. The impression of the opposing arch can be made with alginate. The mixing tip can be left on the cartridge as a cap. If it was contaminated, or if its bulk creates a storage problem, remove it from the cartridge and discard it. Replace the cap on the nozzle of the cartridge. Remove the locking plate from the top of the dispenser body (Fig 17-48). Remove the cartridge from the dispenser.

Polyether

Polyether is another type of elastomeric impression material that has become popular in the last 25 years. It is a copolymer of 1,2 epoxyethane and tetrahydrofuran that is reacted with an α, β unsaturated acid, such as crotonic acid, to produce esterification of the terminal hydroxyl groups.[73] The double bonds are reacted with ethylene amine to produce the final polymer. An aromatic sulfonate produces crosslinking by cationic polymerization. Polyether is packaged in two tubes using a much larger volume of base than accelerator (slightly less than 8:1).

The impression material exhibits accuracy on par with, or somewhat superior to, that of other elastomers. It has excellent dimensional stability even when pouring is delayed for prolonged periods of time.[48,50,74] It is accurate when poured 1 week after removal from the mouth.[62] Polyether has an affinity for water, making it hydrophilic. Impressions should not be stored in a humidor or moist environment. The material is stiff, and undercuts must be blocked out. Its resistance to tearing upon removal is roughly equal to that of silicone and less than that of polysulfide.[73] It is somewhat brittle.

Users of this impression material have experienced some problems with allergic reactions.[75,76] It was estimated that approximately 0.5% of those exposed to it exhibited a reaction to the aromatic sulfonate catalyst.[77] A material for provisional restorations that was capable of cross-sensitization has since been removed from the market, reducing potential sensitizing exposure to the allergen. When a patient experiences an allergic response to this material, however minor, polyether should not be used on that patient again.[78] This would be true with any material.

Armamentarium

1. Impression kit (base and accelerator)
2. Tray adhesive
3. Disposable mixing pad
4. Stiff spatula
5. Syringe with disposable tip
6. 2 x 2-inch gauze sponges
7. Custom resin tray

Impression Making With Polyether

Because of the accelerated setting time of this material, it is imperative that the operator be well organized and execute swiftly. Coat the custom tray with the adhesive supplied with the polyether. Express approximately 7.5 inches (19 cm) each of base and accelerator onto a disposable mixing pad. Mix with a spatula for about 1 minute until all streaks have been removed. Since contact with unmixed catalyst has been implicated in sensi-

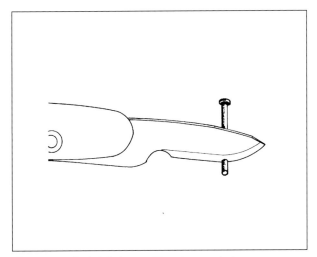

Fig 17-49 The bristle is cut with a sharp scalpel.

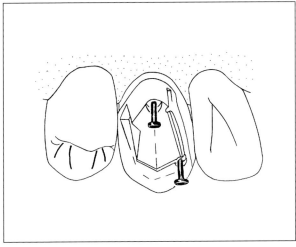

Fig 17-50 Bristles are used to duplicate the pin holes in the impression.

tization and allergic reactions, it is important that no unincorporated catalyst remain. Load the back end of the syringe. The material sets too fast and is too viscous to use a paper cone. The assistant should load the tray while the operator proceeds. Remove the gauze pack.

Be sure that the retraction cord is slightly damp before removing it from the sulcus. Carefully remove the cord from the sulcus and inject the impression material, quickly but carefully, starting in one interproximal area. Exchange the syringe for the loaded tray and seat the tray firmly in place in the mouth. Hold the tray in place for 4 minutes. Remove the impression. Rinse it and blow it dry. Inspect the impression and treat it with disinfectant. Because of polyether's tendency to absorb moisture, it is probably better to spray it than to soak it. The impression of the opposing arch can be made with alginate.

Polyether Urethane Dimethacrylate

This material (Genesis, LD Caulk Div, Dentsply, International, Milford, DE) appeared on the market briefly in the late 1980s. Although it was discontinued because of problems with surface polymerization, it is worthy of mention because it possessed some excellent features for an impression material. Hopefully it will reappear on the market at some future time. It is a polyether urethane dimethacrylate resin with a diketone initiator, an amine accelerator, and 40% to 60% silica filler.[79] It is used in a clear tray and is photoinitiated by 400- to 500-nm wavelength blue light, thus creating its most useful traits: a nearly unlimited working time coupled with a short setting time.

Impressions for Pin-Retained Restorations

To make an impression of a preparation for a pin-retained restoration, nylon bristles must be used to duplicate the pin holes. Impression materials will not fill the small-diameter holes being used. If a kit such as the V.I.P. (Coltene/Whaledent, Mahwah, NJ) is being utilized, use the nylon bristle supplied with a given diameter drill. It will be approximately 0.002 inch smaller in diameter than the drill. If it is necessary, shorten the bristle to prevent it from hitting the impression tray and being distorted. Cut it with a *sharp* scalpel (Fig 17-49). Do not use scissors, as they will bur the end of the bristle, making it difficult to remove from the pin hole.

Place a bristle in each of the pin holes (Fig 17-50). Proceed with the impression in the usual manner, making sure to inject *all* the way around the head of the bristle. Withdraw the impression in the line of draw of the preparation and pins. Pulling the impression off in another line may tear the bristle out.

Pour the impression in the usual way. When the stone has set, separate the impression and cast. The nylon bristle used to duplicate the pin hole will remain in the cast. Remove it by pulling it out with office pliers. If a second cast for a working cast is made, the pin hole will not be accurately reproduced. In this case, use a bur to create an oversized pin hole in the second cast so that the pin in the wax pattern will not touch stone when the pattern is transferred from the die to the working cast. Use of a working cast with a removable die eliminates the need for a second pour.

Lubricate the die with die lubricant and place a serrated iridioplatinum pin in the hole. Fabricate the wax pattern around the pin. Withdraw and invest the pattern in the usual way. Gold will be cast around the head of the pin. An alternative technique utilizes a nylon bristle of slightly smaller diameter than the pin hole in the cast. It is incorporated in the wax pattern and burns out in the oven.

There are often discrepancies at the bases of pins, caused by breakdown of investment in that area.[80] If this prevents seating of the casting in the mouth, countersink the orifice of the pin hole using a no. 2 or no. 4 round bur. Do not bur around the base of the pins, since this may weaken them. Prior to cementation, place a small wisp of cotton on a small reamer and coat the pin hole with Copalite. Then use a small reamer (reserved for this purpose) to apply cement to the pin hole. Rotate the reamer in a counterclockwise manner to carry the cement to the full depth of the pin hole. Apply cement to the pins themselves to insure they will be covered.

Disinfection of Impressions

Public as well as professional concern over *acquired immune deficiency syndrome* (AIDS) has forced a reevaluation of how the profession deals with blood-borne pathogens. These measures probably are as important, if not more so, for the prevention of the more prevalent hepatitis B (HBV) and the resurgent, drug-resistant strain of tuberculosis (MDR-TB). The dental impression certainly is one of the ways by which pathogens can leave the operatory and spread their risk abroad.

A detailed protocol is now required to insure that the previously overlooked impression is handled properly. The impression must be rendered harmless before being passed on to other people who will work with it, or with the gypsum cast made from it, outside the dental operatory. There are five types of chemical disinfectants that can be used for this purpose: chlorine compounds, combination synthetic phenolic compounds, glutaraldehydes, iodophors, and phenolic/alcohol combinations.[81]

A prolonged immersion in 2% glutaraldehyde or hypochlorite solution with 10,000 ppm available chlorine for 1 hour was recommended for disinfecting impressions in a 1973 World Health Organization report.[82] The recommendation of a 1-hour treatment has been reiterated on the rationale that all impressions are as potentially infectious as those coming from high-risk patients and should be treated accordingly.[83]

The most recent recommendations for the disinfection of impressions and casts published by the ADA Council on Dental Materials, Instruments, and Equipment; Council on Dental Practice; Council on Dental Therapeutics in 1988,[84] and amended in August 1991,[85] call for the immersion of polysulfide, condensation-reaction silicone, polyvinyl siloxane, polyether, and agar hydrocolloid in ADA-accepted disinfecting solutions that require immersion for no longer than 30 minutes.

An alternative technique, spraying, can be used on those materials most vulnerable to distortion.[85] This is done by rinsing the impression under running water; trimming excess impression material; spraying the entire impression, top and bottom (including the tray); and then sealing the impression tray in the bag for the time recommended for the disinfectant used.[81] The surface quality and dimensional stability of disinfected impressions have been the focus of numerous published reports.[86] Solutions requiring shorter immersion times should be selected for materials that are prone to distortion when immersed in water. Several investigators have found the surface detail and dimensional stability of alginate (irreversible) hydrocolloid impressions to be acceptable if immersed in sodium hypochlorite for 10 minutes.[87-89] Westerholm et al[90] found full-strength (5.25%) sodium hypochlorite to be the most effective disinfectant when sprayed on alginate. Similar treatment with some types of glutaraldehydes also produced acceptable results,[88,89,91] while others did not.[92,93]

There have been far fewer published studies of the effects of disinfectant solutions on agar (reversible) hydrocolloid. Those that have been done show that it is unaffected by a 10-minute immersion in 2% alkaline glutaraldehyde,[94] but immersion for 20 minutes or longer in the same solution will adversely affect dimensional stability[94-96] and surface detail.[95] Polyether, because of its hydrophilic properties, could present problems when immersed. However, it has been demonstrated to be dimensionally stable when immersed from 10 to 30 minutes in sodium hypochlorite,[92,93,97] glutaraldehyde,[91-93,97,98] iodophor,[91,93,97] and phenol solutions.[98,99]

Polysulfide has been demonstrated to have sufficient dimensional stability when immersed in sodium hypochlorite,[92,93,97,100,101] glutaraldehyde,[92,93,97,100,101] iodophor,[93,97,101] and phenol.[92,99,100,102] Sodium hypochlorite,[87,88] glutaraldehyde,[88,103] and phenol[88] can be used with conventional (condensation) silicones as long as immersion times do not exceed the recommended pouring times for the material.

Significantly fewer microorganisms are retained on the surface of polyvinyl siloxane impressions than on other materials, prior to disinfection.[104] Polyvinyl siloxanes generally display excellent tolerance to immersion in sodium hypochlorite,[87,88,92,97,98,100,101] glutaraldehyde,[92,97,98,100,101,103] iodophor,[93,97,101,103] and phenols.[88,92,99,100,102,103]

References

1. McCormick JT, Antony SJ, Dial ML, Duncanson MG, Shillingburg HT: Wettability of elastomeric impression materials: Effect of selected surfactants. *Int J Prosthodont* 1989; 2:413–420.

2. Lorren RA, Salter DJ, Fairhurst CW: The contact angles of die stone and impression materials. *J Prosthet Dent* 1976; 36:176–180.

3. Cullen DR, Sandrik JL: Wettability of elastomeric impression materials and voids in gypsum casts. *J Prosthet Dent* 1991; 66:261–265.

4. Craig RG: *Restorative Dental Materials,* ed 7. St Louis, CV Mosby Co, 1985, p 276.

5. Herfort TW, Gerberich WW, Macosko CW, Goodkind RJ: Viscosity of elastomeric impression materials. *J Prosthet Dent* 1977; 38:396–403.

6. Kishimoto M, Shillingburg HT, Duncanson MG: A comparison of six impression syringes. *J Prosthet Dent* 1980; 43:546–551.

7. Schnell RJ, Phillips RW: Dimensional stability of rubber base impressions and certain other factors affecting accuracy. *J Am Dent Assoc* 1958; 57:39–48.

8. Gilmore WH, Schnell RJ, Phillips RW: Factors influencing the accuracy of silicone impression material. *J Prosthet Dent* 1954; 4:94–103.

9. Eames WB, Sieweke JC, Wallace SW, Rogers LB: Elastomeric impression materials: Effect of bulk on accuracy. *J Prosthet Dent* 1979; 41:304–307.

10. Shillingburg HT, Hatch RA, Keenan MP, Hemphill MW: Impression materials and techniques used for cast restorations in eight states. *J Am Dent Assoc* 1980; 100:696–699.

11. Shillingburg HT, Brackett SE: Impression materials —A cost comparison. *J Okla Dent Assoc* 1984; 75:21–24.

12. Hart JD, Howard B: Hydrocolloids started here. *J Okla Dent Assoc* 1956; 45:10–12.

13. Engelman MA: Hydrocolloid: A reassessment for better dentistry. *N Y State Dent J* 1979; 45:383–388.

14. Hollenback GM: *Science and Technic of the Cast Restoration.* St Louis, CV Mosby Co, 1964, pp 86–87.

15. Phillips RW: *Science of Dental Materials,* ed 9. Philadelphia, WB Saunders Co, 1991, p 107–122.

16. Asgar K: Elastic impression materials. *Dent Clin North Am* 1971; 15:81–98.

17. Engelman MA, Kessler H, McEvoy R: New reversible hydrocolloid for recording the retracted gingival sulcus in fixed prosthodontics: Laboratory and clinical evaluation. *N Y J Dent* 1980; 50:251–263.

18. Eames WB, Rogers LB, Wallace SW, Suway NB: Compatibility of gypsum products with hydrocolloid impression materials. *Oper Dent* 1978; 3:108–112.

19. Powell GL, Fenn JP, Runnells R: Hydrocolloid conditioning units: A potential source of bacterial cross contamination. *J Prosthet Dent* 1987; 58:280–283.

20. Schwartz JR: The use of the hydrocolloids or alginates as impression materials for indirect or indirect-direct inlay construction procedure. *Dent Items of Interest* 1951; 73:379–389.

21. Appleby DC, Pameijer CH, Boffa J: The combined reversible hydrocolloid/irreversible hydrocolloid impression system. *J Prosthet Dent* 1980; 44:27–35.

22. Fusayama T, Kurosaki N, Node H, Nakamura M: A laminated hydrocolloid impression for indirect inlays. *J Prosthet Dent* 1982; 47:171–176.

23. Appleby DC, Cohen SR, Racowsky LP, Mingledorff EB: The combined reversible hydrocolloid/ irreversible hydrocolloid impression system: Clinical application. *J Prosthet Dent* 1981; 46:48–58.

24. Herring HW, Tames MA, Zardiackas LD: Comparison of the dimensional accuracy of a combined reversible/irreversible hydrocolloid impression system with other commonly used impression materials. *J Prosthet Dent*1984; 52:795–799.

25. Johnson GH, Craig RG: Accuracy and bond strength of combination agar/alginate hydrocolloid impression materials. *J Prosthet Dent* 1986; 55:1–6.

26. Linke BA, Nicholls JI, Faucher RR: Distortion analysis of stone casts made from impression materials. *J Prosthet Dent* 1985; 54:794–802.

27. Heisler WH, Tjan AHL: Accuracy and bond strength of reversible with irreversible hydrocolloid impression systems: A comparative study. *J Prosthet Dent* 1992; 68:578–584.

28. Bomberg TJ, Hatch RA, Hoffman W: Impression material thickness in stock and custom trays. *J Prosthet Dent* 1985; 54:170–172.

29. Tjan AHL, Nemetz H, Nguyen LTP, Contino R: Effect of tray space on the accuracy of monophasic polyvinylsiloxane impressions. *J Prosthet Dent* 1992; 68:19–28.

30. Gordon GE, Johnson GH, Drennon DG: The effect of tray selection on the accuracy of elastomeric impression materials. *J Prosthet Dent* 1990; 63:12–15.

31. Johnson GH, Craig RG: Accuracy of addition silicones as a function of technique. *J Prosthet Dent* 1986; 55:197–203.

32. Bomberg TJ, Goldfogel MH, Hoffman W, Bomberg SE, Flower B: Considerations for adhesion of impression materials to impression trays. *J Prosthet Dent* 1988; 60:681–684.

33. Phillips RW: *Skinner's Science of Dental Materials,* ed 7. Philadelphia, WB Saunders Co, 1973, p 148.

34. Nicholson JW, Porter KH, Dolan T: Strength of tray adhesives for elastomeric impression materials. *Oper Dent* 1985; 10:12–16.

35. Chai JY, Jameson LM, Moser JB, Hesby RA: Adhesive properties of several impression material systems: Part I. *J Prosthet Dent* 1991; 66:201–209.

36. Grant BE, Tjan AHL: Tensile and peel bond strengths of tray adhesives. *J Prosthet Dent* 1988; 59:165–168.

37. Hogans WR, Agar JR: The bond strength of elastomer tray adhesives to thermoplastic and acrylic resin tray materials. *J Prosthet Dent* 1992; 67:541–543.

38. Sulong MZAM, Setchell DJ: Properties of the tray adhesive of an addition polymerizing silicone to impression tray materials. *J Prosthet Dent* 1991; 66:743–747.

39. On making good impressions. *The Dental Advisor* 1984; 1(1):1–8.

40. Payne JA, Pereira BP: Bond strength of three nonaqueous elastomeric impression materials to a light-activated tray. *Int J Prosthodont* 1992; 5:55–58.

41. Dixon DL, Breeding LC, Bosser MJ, Nafso AJ: The effect of custom tray material type and surface treatment on the tensile bond strength of an impression material/adhesive system. *Int J Prosthodont* 1993; 6:303–306.

42. Tjan AHL, Whang SB: Comparing effects of tray treatment on the accuracy of dies. *J Prosthet Dent* 1987; 58:175–178.

43. Davis GB, Moser JB, Brinsden GI: The bonding properties of elastomer tray adhesives. *J Prosthet Dent* 1974; 31:647–650.

44. Phillips RW: *Science of Dental Materials,* ed 9. Philadelphia, WB Saunders Co, 1991, p 193.

305

45. Fehling AW, Hesby RA, Pelleu GB: Dimensional stability of autopolymerizing acrylic resin impression trays. *J Prosthet Dent* 1986; 55:592–597.

46. Pagliano RP, Scheid RC, Clowson RL, Dagefoerde RO, Zardiackas LD: Linear dimensional change of acrylic resins used in the fabrication of custom trays. *J Prosthet Dent* 1982; 47:279–283.

47. Phillips RW: *Science of Dental Materials,* ed 9. Philadelphia, WB Saunders Co, 1991, p 135–156.

48. Luebke RJ, Scandrett FR, Kerber PE: The effect of delayed and second pours on elastomeric impression material accuracy. *J Prosthet Dent* 1979; 41:517–521.

49. Hembree JH: Comparative accuracy of elastomer impression materials. *Tenn Dent J* 1974; 54:164–167

50. Eames WB, Wallace SW, Suway NB, Rogers LB: Accuracy and dimensional stability of elastomeric impression materials. *J Prosthet Dent* 1979; 42:159–162.

51. Shillingburg HT, Case JC, Duncanson MG, Kent WA: Radiopacity and color of elastomeric impression materials. *Quintessence Int* 1988; 19:541–548.

52. Kent WA, Shillingburg HT, Tow HD: Impression material foreign body: Report of a case. *Quintessence Int* 1988; 19:9–11.

53. Shillingburg HT, Wilkerson-Lyman SL, Duncanson MG: Radiopacity enhancement of an experimental vinyl polysiloxane impression material. *Quintessence Int* 1989; 20:657–663.

54. Harrop TJ, Middaugh DG: Forced air impression technique. *J Can Dent Assoc* 1967; 33:673–675.

55. Going RE: Accurate rubber base impressions. *J Prosthet Dent* 1968; 20:339–344.

56. Braden M, Elliott JC: Characterization of the setting process of silicone dental rubbers. *J Dent Res* 1966; 45:1016–1023.

57. McCabe JF, Wilson HJ: Addition curing silicone rubber impression materials. *Br Dent J* 1978; 145:17–20.

58. Craig RG: A review of properties of rubber impression materials. *J Mich Dent Assoc* 1977; 59:254–261.

59. Reisbick MH, Matyas J: The accuracy of highly filled elastomeric impression materials. *J Prosthet Dent* 1975; 33:67–72.

60. Tjan AHL, Whang SB, Tjan AH: Clinically oriented assessment of the accuracy of three putty-wash silicone impression techniques. *J Am Dent Assoc* 1984; 108:973–975.

61. Johnson GH, Craig RG: Accuracy of four types of rubber impression materials compared with time of pour and a repeat pour of models. *J Prosthet Dent* 1985; 53:484–490.

62. Tjan AHL, Whang SB, Tjan AH, Sarkissian R: Clinically oriented evaluation of the accuracy of commonly used impression materials. *J Prosthet Dent* 1986; 56:4–8.

63. Dhuru VB, Asgharnia MK, Mayer JC, Hassan K: Surface porosity of stone casts made from vinyl polysiloxane impression materials. *Oper Dent* 1986; 11:3–7.

64. Panichuttra R, Jones RM, Goodacre C, Munoz CA, Moore BK: Hydrophilic poly(vinyl siloxane) impression materials: Dimensional accuracy, wettability, and effect on gypsum hardness. *Int J Prosthodont* 1991; 4:240–248.

65. Crown and bridge impression materials. *The Dental Advisor* 1989; 6(2):1–8.

66. Keck SC: Automixing: A new concept in elastomeric impression material delivery systems. *J Prosthet Dent* 1985; 54:479–483.

67. Chong YH, Soh G, Lim KC, Teo CS: Porosities in five automixed addition silicone elastomers. *Oper Dent* 1991; 16:96–100.

68. Cook WD, Thomasz F: Rubber gloves and addition silicone materials. Current note no. 64. *Aust Dent J* 1986; 31:140.

69. Kahn RL, Donovan TE, Chee WWL: Interaction of gloves and rubber dam with poly(vinyl siloxane) impression material: A screening test. *Int J Prosthodont* 1989; 2:342–346.

70. Reitz CD, Clark NP: The setting of vinyl polysiloxane and condensation silicone putties when mixed with gloved hands. *J Am Dent Assoc* 1988; 116:371–375.

71. Noonan JE, Goldfogel MH, Lambert RL: Inhibited set of the surface of addition silicones in contact with rubber dam. *Oper Dent* 1985; 10:46–48.

72. Council on Dental Materials, Instruments, and Equipment: Retarding the setting of vinyl polysiloxane impressions. *J Am Dent Assoc* 1991; 122(8):114.

73. Braden M, Causton B, Clarke RL: A polyether impression rubber. *J Dent Res* 1971; 51:889–896.

74. Sawyer HF, Dilts WE, Aubrey ME, Neiman R: Accuracy of casts produced from three classes of elastomer impression materials. *J Am Dent Assoc* 1974; 89:644–648.

75. Nally FF, Storrs J: Hypersensitivity to a dental impression material: A case report. *Br Dent J* 1973; 134:244–246.

76. Duxbury AJ, Turner EP, Watts DC: Hypersensitivity to epimine containing dental materials. *Br Dent J* 1979; 147:331–333.

77. Van Groeningen G, Nater JP: Reactions to dental impression materials. *Contact Dermatitis* 1975; 1:373–376.

78. Blankenau RJ, Kelsey WP, Cavel WT: A possible allergic response to polyether impression material: A case report. *J Am Dent Assoc* 1984; 108:609–610.

79. Craig RG, Hare PH: Properties of a new polyether urethane dimethacrylate photoinitiated elastomeric impression material. *J Prosthet Dent* 1990; 63:16–20.

80. Schnepper HE, Baum L: Miniature parallel pins for retention of cast restorations. *J Prosthet Dent* 1961; 11:772–780.

81. Naylor WP: Infection control in fixed prosthodontics. *Dent Clin North Am* 1992; 36:809–831.

82. World Health Organization: *Technical Report Series 512, Viral Hepatitis.* New York, WHO, 1973.

83. Bergman B: Disinfection of prosthodontic impression materials: A literature review. *Int J Prosthodont* 1989; 2:537–542.

84. Council on Dental Materials, Instruments, and Equipment, Council on Dental Practice, Council on Dental Therapeutics: Infection control recommendations for the dental office and the dental laboratory. *J Am Dent Assoc* 1988; 116:241–248.

85. Council on Dental Materials, Instruments, and Equipment: Disinfection of impressions. *J Am Dent Assoc* 1991; 122(9):110.

86. Owen CP, Goolam R: Disinfection of impression materials to prevent viral cross contamination: A review and a protocol. *Int J Prosthodont* 1993; 6:480–494.

87. Minagi A, Fukushima K, Maeda N, Satomi K, Ohkawa S, Akagawa Y, et al: Disinfection method for impression materials: Freedom from fear of hepatitis B and acquired immunodeficiency syndrome. *J Prosthet Dent* 1986; 56:451–454.

88. Matyas J, Dao N, Caputo AA, Lucatorto FM: Effects of disinfectants on dimensional accuracy of impression materials. *J Prosthet Dent* 1990; 64:25–31.

89. Dellinger EL, Williams KJ, Setcos JC: Influence of immersion and spray disinfectants on alginate impressions [abstract 2045]. *J Dent Res* 1990; 69:364.

90. Westerholm HS, Bradley DV, Schwartz RS: Efficacy of various spray disinfectants on irreversible hydrocolloid impressions. *Int J Prosthodont* 1992; 5:47–54.

91. Johnson GH, Chellis KD, Gordon GE: Dimensional stability and detail reproduction of disinfected alginate and elastomeric impressions [abstract 2078]. *J Dent Res* 1990; 69:368.

92. Herrera SP, Merchant VA: Dimensional stability of dental impressions after immersion disinfection. *J Am Dent Assoc* 1986; 113:419–422.

93. Tullner JB, Commette JA, Moon PC: Linear dimensional changes in dental impressions after immersion in disinfectant solutions. *J Prosthet Dent* 1988; 60:725–728.

94. Minagi A, Yano N, Yoshida K, Tsuru HSE: Prevention of acquired immunodeficiency syndrome and hepatitis B. II: Disinfection method for hydrophilic impression materials. *J Prosthet Dent* 1987; 58:462–465.

95. Olsson S, Bergman B, Bergman M: Agar impression materials, dimensional stability and surface detail sharpness following treatment with disinfectant solutions. *Swed Dent J* 1987; 9:169–177.

96. Merchant VA, Radcliffe RM, Herrera SP, Stroster TG: Dimensional stability of reversible hydrocolloid impressions immersed in selected disinfection solutions. *J Am Dent Assoc* 1989; 119:533–535.

97. Langenwalter EM, Aquilino SA, Turner KA: The dimensional stability of elastomeric impression materials following disinfection. *J Prosthet Dent* 1990; 63:270–276.

98. Drennon DG, Johnson GH: The effect of immersion disinfection of elastomeric impressions on the surface detail reproduction of improved gypsum casts. *J Prosthet Dent* 1990; 63:233–241.

99. Drennon DG, Johnson GH, Powell GL: The accuracy and efficacy of disinfection by spray atomization on elastomeric impressions. *J Prosthet Dent* 1989; 62:468–475.

100. Merchant VA, McKneight MK, Cibirorowski CJ, Molinari JA: Preliminary investigation of a method for disinfection of dental impressions. *J Prosthet Dent* 1984; 54:877–879.

101. Merchant VA, Herrera SP, Dwan JJ: Marginal fit of cast gold MO inlays from disinfected elastomeric impressions. *J Prosthet Dent* 1987; 58:276–279.

102. Bergman M, Olsson S, Bergman B: Elastomeric impression materials. Dimensional stability and surface detail sharpness following treatment with disinfectant solutions. *Swed Dent J* 1980; 4:161–167.

103. Johnson GH, Drennon DG, Powell GL: Accuracy of elastomeric impressions disinfected by immersion. *J Am Dent Assoc* 1988; 116:525–530.

104. Jennings KJ, Samaranayake LP: The persistence of microorganisms on impression materials following disinfection. *Int J Prosthodont* 1991; 4:382–387.

Chapter 18

Working Casts and Dies

When good impressions have been made of the teeth prepared in the mouth, it is important that they be handled properly to insure that accurate and detailed casts will result. Obtaining good impressions requires the expenditure of time and effort by the operator, and it is a tedious procedure for the patient. A few simple steps should be followed in handling the casts to insure that costly and time-consuming remakes will not be required. The ease with which a restoration is fabricated, and the accuracy with which it will fit the mouth, are materially affected by the cast.

There are three requirements for good casts:

1. They must be bubble free, especially along the finish lines of the prepared teeth.
2. All portions of the cast must be distortion free.
3. The casts must be trimmed to insure access for carving wax pattern margins.

The *working cast* is the cast that is mounted on an articulator. To provide the most accurate articulation, it normally should represent the entire arch.[1] In the fabrication of the wax pattern, it is used to establish interproximal contacts, buccal and lingual contours, and occlusion with the opposing teeth. The *die* is a model of the individual prepared tooth on which the margins of the wax pattern are finished. There are two basic working cast and die systems: a working cast with a separate die and a working cast with a removable die.

Working Cast With a Separate Die

The working cast with a separate die is the simplest means of fabricating a working cast and die, since no procedures are required to create a die other than making a sectional cast and a full-arch cast. In addition to ease of fabrication, it also keeps the relationship between abutments fixed and immovable. This is a sure method of accurately orienting the preparation models to each other, which is considered an important step in minimizing casting adjustments.[2] Because the gingival tissue and other landmarks are intact, it is easier to obtain physiologically harmonious restoration contours when fabri-

cating the wax pattern (Yamada HN, personal communication, March 1972). One of the disadvantages encountered in the use of a working cast with a separate die is that the wax pattern must be transferred from one to the other. Inexperienced technicians are prone to do this more often than necessary, and in the process they destroy some of the internal adaptation of the wax pattern.

The working cast and the sectional cast for the die can be obtained from separate impressions or by pouring an elastomeric full-arch impression twice. If a double pour is utilized, the first cast is used for fabrication of the die.[3] This technique, unfortunately, can be used only with elastomeric impressions, since hydrocolloid is torn and distorted too much to be used for an accurate second pour.

Armamentarium

1. 500-cc Vac-U-Mixer and vacuum tubing
2. Vibrator
3. Water measure
4. Large and small spatulas
5. Die stone (Silky-Rock, Vel-Mix)
6. Humidor
7. Model trimmer
8. Straight handpiece and pear-shaped acrylic bur
9. Laboratory knife with no. 25 blade
10. Tanner carver
11. Colorbrite red pencil

Impression Pouring

The die and cast should have a hard enough surface to prevent surface abrasion when the wax pattern is fabricated. Therefore, one of the high-strength type IV (class II, "Densite") or high-strength, high-expansion type V stones should be used for fabricating the die.[4] An impression should be washed under cold running tap water, to remove mucous and saliva that may cover it, before disinfecting it in an appropriate solution.

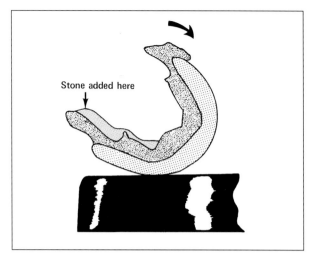

Fig 18-1 Stone is added to the impression in small increments above the preparation.

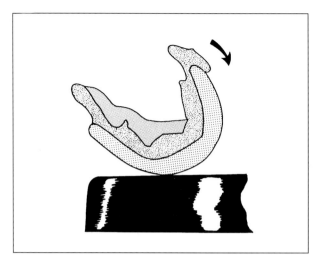

Fig 18-2 Tray is tilted to fill the preparation.

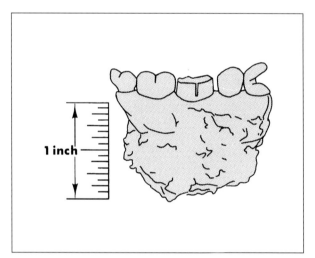

Fig 18-3 Stone is added to the impression so that the base of set stone will be 1 inch thick.

Place a measured amount of water in a plastic mixing bowl (Vac-U-Mixer, Whip Mix Corp, Louisville, KY) and add a measured amount of die stone to the water. Die impressions can be poured with 50 to 70 g of stone. It takes about 200 g for a full-arch impression. Follow the manufacturer's instructions for the correct water-powder ratio. This ratio can affect many of the properties of the set stone, including setting time, porosity, setting expansion, and the ultimate strength. It is important that the technique be standardized.

Mix water and stone by hand with the spatula until the powder is completely wet. Place the lid on the bowl, attach the vacuum tube to the plastic lid, and engage the drive nut on the top of the bowl in the larger drive chuck

of the power unit. Vacuum mix for 15 seconds. Disengage the drive nut from the drive chuck and vibrate the stone to the bottom of the bowl. Disconnect the vacuum tubing.

Remove excess moisture from elastomeric impressions. The wettability or pourability of an impression made of a hydrophobic impression material can be improved by using a surfactant on the impression.[5] Surfactants, applied by spraying, will reduce the number of voids trapped in the cast and increase the probability of obtaining a void-free cast.[6]

Excess moisture should also be blown from the surface of a hydrocolloid impression without actually desiccating it. The surface should be free of visible water, but it should still be shiny. If the surface of the hydrocolloid appears dull, it has been overdried and some distortion may occur. Use a small instrument to carry stone to the impression of the prepared tooth. Place a small amount of stone on the side of the impression above the preparation, and vibrate it until stone reaches the "bottom" (occlusal surface) of the preparation (Fig 18-1).

Tilt the impression so that stone flows slowly across the "bottom" of the preparation, displacing air as it moves (Fig 18-2). Add stone in small increments. If a large amount of stone is dropped into the preparation area, air will be trapped and a void will result in the cast. Continue adding stone in small increments from the original point so that the preparation will fill from the bottom up. After the preparation has been filled, pour stone into the tooth on either side of it in the impression. Build up the stone to a height of approximately 1.0 inch (2.5 cm) over the preparation to allow bulk for an adequate handle on the die (Fig 18-3).

To pour a full-arch impression, place the tray on the vibrator. Do not rest it on the impression material. Add small increments of stone to the distalmost area of one side of the impression. Slowly raise the distal end of the

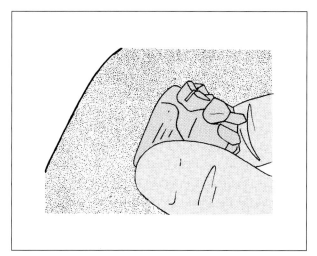

Fig 18-4 The die is first trimmed on a model trimmer.

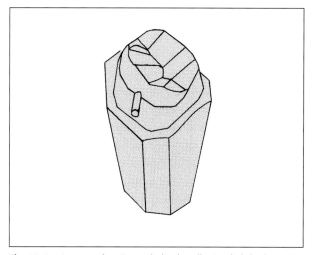

Fig 18-5 A properly trimmed die handle is slightly larger in diameter than the preparation.

impression so that stone will move mesially, flowing from tooth to tooth and filling each tooth imprint from the bottom. By tilting the impression tray in different directions, the flow of the stone can be controlled so that air will not be trapped. Add stone and vibrate until all the teeth in the arch are filled. If the impression being poured is of the mandibular arch, set the impression on the benchtop and fill in the open lingual space with a wet paper towel. This will enable a full base to be poured. Do not invert the impression before the initial set has occurred.[7] Allow the poured impression to set for at least 1 hour.[8] Do not separate the cast from the impression or begin preparing the dies until the hour has elapsed. If the impression is hydrocolloid, it should be placed in a humidor during this time.

Die Preparation

Carefully separate the poured cast from the impression. A material such as Super-Sep (Kerr Mfg Co, Glendora, CA) may be painted on the surface of the prepared teeth on the cast to guard against surface erosion or etching when the casts are trimmed. Liquid, prevulcanized latex has also been suggested for this purpose.[9] Wet the cast thoroughly before trimming excess stone from the working casts on the model trimmer. There should be no stone duplicating soft tissue in the peripheral area beyond the gingiva left on the cast.

Trim the cast from which the die is made on a model trimmer to remove all excess stone around the prepared tooth (Fig 18-4). Hold the cast by the base while cutting it down to form a handle on the die. If the die is held by the preparation portion while the handle is being trimmed, the die may be worn or chipped, resulting in an ill-fitting casting later.

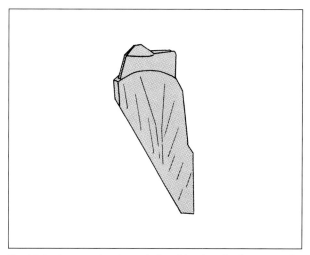

Fig 18-6 Improperly trimmed die with a handle that meets the preparation at an angle.

The handle of the die should be slightly larger in diameter than the preparation and octagonal in cross section (Fig 18-5). Its sides ought to be parallel or slightly tapered toward the base. The handle should parallel the long axis of the tooth. If the handle is made at an angle to the long axis of the tooth preparation, it will be more difficult to adapt the wax pattern margins (Fig 18-6). The handle should be approximately 1.0 inch (2.5 cm) long (Fig 18-7). If it is any shorter, it will be difficult to hold when the wax pattern is on it.

Use a pear-shaped acrylic bur to trim the die "apical" to the finish line of the preparation (Fig 18-8). Begin final trimming of the die with a sharp no. 25 blade (Fig 18-9). The area "apical" to the finish line should be smoothed

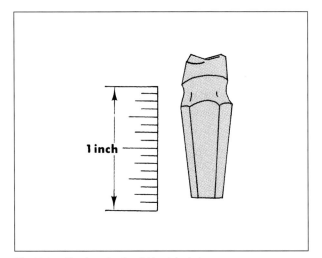

Fig 18-7 The handle should be 1 inch long.

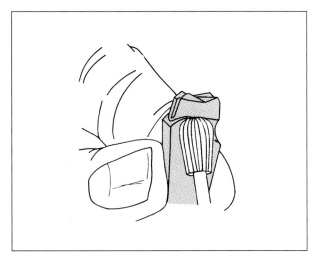

Fig 18-8 The die is trimmed with an acrylic bur.

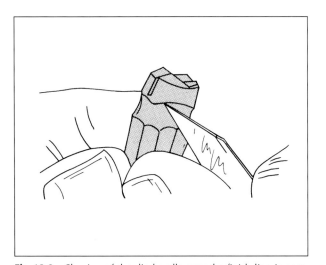

Fig 18-9 Shaping of the die handle near the finish line is completed with a scalpel.

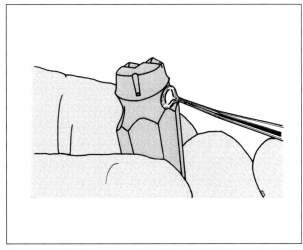

Fig 18-10 The die is smoothed below the finish line with the discoid end of a Tanner carver.

and made free of ridges with the discoid end of a Tanner carver (5T, Suter Dental Mfg Co, Chico, CA) (Fig 18-10). Irregularities in the stone will produce ripples in the wax when the margin finishing instrument rises and falls as it is guided over those rough spots in the stone. There also must be adequate access to rest a burnisher on this part of the stone die when the margins are finished (Fig 18-11).

The contour of the die "apical" to the finish line should approximate that of the root to facilitate good axial contours in the finished restoration (Fig 18-12). Sharply undercutting or "ditching" the die below the finish line is not advised and should not be required if there is an adequate finish line on the preparation. Because the instrument used for finishing the margins of the wax pattern will rest against this portion of the die, its angulation can be exaggerated by the undercut. This will result in a thick

gingival area on the restoration and an axial contour that is not conducive to good gingival health (Fig 18-13).

After the die has been trimmed, the finish line should be highlighted with a sharp Colorbrite red pencil[1] (Fig 18-14). This facilitates carving the margins of the wax pattern when wax obscures the preparation finish line. Do not use excessive pressure when marking the finish line, as it may be rounded over. A black, graphite pencil should not be used for this purpose. When used with the usual blue or green inlay waxes, a finish line outlined in black does not become more visible, but instead makes every wax pattern margin appear unsealed, or "open." In addition, the graphite, with its clay binder, may be carried into the investment on the pattern. Remnants of the clay binder could contaminate the margin of the casting.

Relief should be applied to the preparation area of the

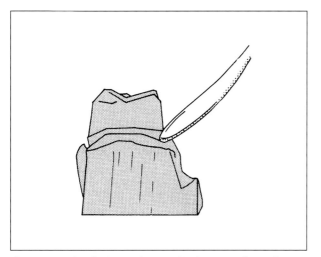

Fig 18-11 This die is too short, and it does not allow adequate access for margin finishing.

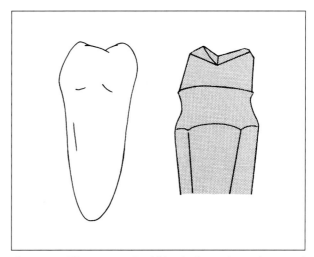

Fig 18-12 Die contours should be similar to those of a natural tooth.

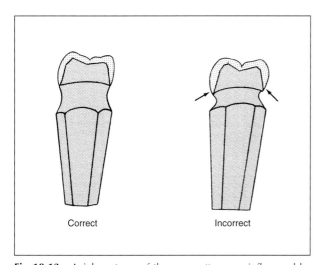

Correct   Incorrect

Fig 18-13 Axial contours of the wax pattern are influenced by die trimming.

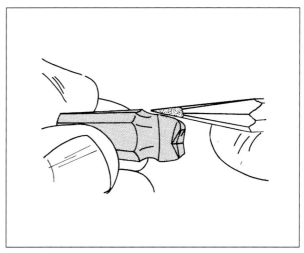

Fig 18-14 The preparation finish line on the die should be outlined with a red pencil.

die to provide space for cement.[10] Enamels and lacquers have been used for this purpose.[10,11] The thickness of the overall relief varies with the number of coats applied,[12] the brand used, and the care with which it is applied.[13] As a bottle of enamel or lacquer ages, the contents thickens due to evaporation.[12] Thinner must be added periodically. The number of coats will depend upon the material, but a relief of 20 to 40 μm is desired.[11,14] The tooth preparation on the die is painted to within 0.5 mm of the finish line (Fig 18-15).

A casting made on a relieved die will have space between it and the preparation when it is placed on the tooth in the mouth. When it is applied carefully, die relief material can be used on preparations with grooves and other internal features, although thicker relief agents tend to pool in the ends and corners of grooves.[13] Full veneer

crowns with grooves will seat more completely if a spacer is used, whether or not it is actually placed in the grooves.[15] A more detailed discussion can be found in Chapter 22.

A die hardening agent (cyanoacrylate or acrylic resin lacquer) can be applied to the finish line area of a die to prevent abrasion by waxing instruments during the fabrication of the wax pattern. However, the coating material should be used with care. It must have a low viscosity, and it must be applied lightly. The thickness of cyanoacrylates at the finish line can range from 1.0 to 25 μm, while acrylic lacquers can add 4.0 to 10 μm of thickness.[16] Unless the hardening agent is a thin one that is applied in a careful manner, it is possible to create an unacceptably thick relief over the finish line, which may produce an ill-fitting margin in the resultant casting.

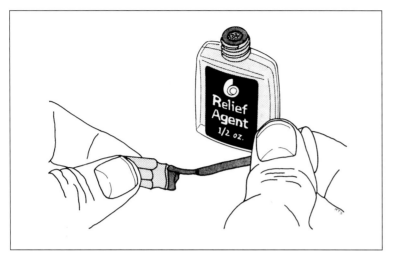

Fig 18-15   Die relief agent is painted on the preparation portion of the die.

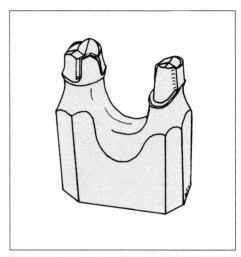

Fig 18-16   One-piece die for a fixed partial denture extending from second premolar to second molar.

When a one-piece casting without a solder joint is attempted in the fabrication of a fixed partial denture, a one-piece die will produce the most predictable result. The die for each preparation is left joined to the other by means of a common base (Fig 18-16). The edentulous ridge area is cut back to provide good access for visual examination and finishing of the margin.

Working Cast With a Removable Die

Dies that can be removed from the working cast have become very popular. They are convenient to use because wax patterns or copings need not be removed from their respective dies when they are transferred to the working cast. This is particularly important when making ceramic restorations, as the unfired material is quite fragile. A removable die eliminates discrepancies between a separate die and working cast that may be caused by impression distortion or deterioration between pours, or by a cast and die made from separate impressions that are not identical. A removable die also eliminates discrepancies that can occur when the die is coated with a relief agent and the working cast is not, or when they are coated with different thicknesses. The principal disadvantage of a removable die system is the risk of introducing an error in the pattern if the die does not reseat accurately in the working cast.

If a removable die system is used, it should satisfy these requirements[17]:

1. The dies must return to their exact original positions.
2. The dies must remain stable, even when inverted.
3. The cast containing the dies must be easy to mount on an articulator.

Several methods can be employed to allow the repositioning of a die in its working cast (Fig 18-17). Most of these devices can either be oriented in the impression before it is poured *(prepour technique)* or attached to the underside of a cast that has already been poured *(postpour technique)*. A tapered, flat-sided brass dowel pin can be used to orient the die of the prepared tooth into the working cast before pouring[1,18-20] or after.[21,22] Flat-sided, stainless steel dowel pins with attached positioning wires also can be prepositioned.[23,24] A different type of single dowel gains its stability from its curved shape (Outside Curve, Wimbledon Midwest, Midwest City, OK). The dowel tip protrudes from the side rather than the bottom of the base of the cast.

Single dowels are simple to use, but they do not provide as much antirotational resistance as double dowels (Twin Pin, Denerica Dental Corp, Northfield, IL, and J-Pin, National Keystone Products Co, Cherry Hill, NJ). Two separate dowels also can be cemented into parallel pin holes drilled in the underside of a cast, using a special drill press (Pindex, Coltene/Whaledent, Mahwah, NJ).

Preformed plastic trays use multiple horizontal die-contact tracks and vertical ribs to orient dies back into the cast.[25-27] They are especially useful for dies of teeth with dowel preparations that might be perforated by laboratory dowel pins protruding into the dowel space and for refractory dies onto which ceramic restorations will be fired.

Four systems are presented here:

1. Straight dowel pin
2. Curved dowel pin
3. Pindex system
4. Di-Lok tray

A fifth system, the Accutrac, is described in Chapter 24 in connection with the fabrication of veneers.

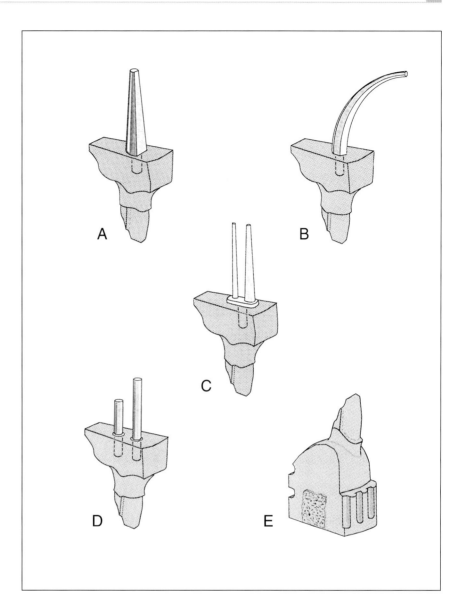

Fig 18-17 Types of antirotational devices used for removable dies: A, flat-sided single dowel; B, single curved dowel; C, double straight dowels with a common head; D, two separate parallel dowels; E, keyed plastic outer tray.

Straight Dowel Pin

This means of orienting dies has been in use for a number of years,[28] and most of the dowel systems are modifications of it. The brass dowel pin is one of the most accurate dowel types in terms of resisting horizontal displacement[26,29,30] and the second lowest in vertical deviation of four types of removable dies.[29] A dowel pin is positioned over each prepared tooth in the impression. The accurate placement of the dowels can be a problem: If the dowel pins are positioned inaccurately, they may impinge on the margins, weaken the die, or prevent the die from being easily removed from the cast.

Marking the desired location of the dowel on the periphery of the impression and then placing the dowel freehand after the stone has been poured can result in the dowel settling into the stone.[21] More consistently accurate placement can be effected by prepositioning

the dowel and stabilizing it in place before the stone is poured into the impression.[24]

There are devices made specifically for precise positioning of dowels before the pouring of an impression. One such device utilizes putty on a movable table to hold an impression in an exact, repeatable position, while pins are suspended above the impression from magnets on a larger immovable table.[31] Wire clips that can be stuck into the periphery of the impression can be purchased, or they can be fashioned from orthodontic wire.[32] The flat side of dowels also can be stabilized against the heads of horizontal straight pins protruding from putty along the periphery of the impression. A pin is positioned over the space above each tooth preparation.[33] Unfortunately, the dowels are guided by, but not attached to, the pins in this technique. It could work in the hands of an experienced technician, but it is not recommended for the novice.

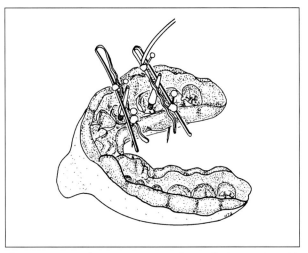

Fig 18-18 Dowel pins are positioned over the impression with bobby pins.

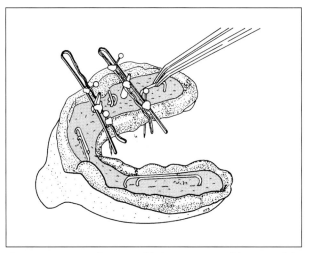

Fig 18-19 Paper clips are added to nonremovable parts of the unset first pour to provide retention for the second pour of stone.

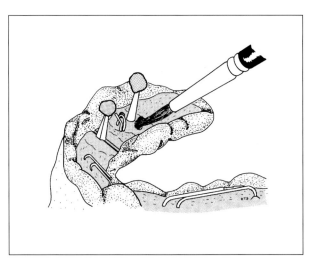

Fig 18-20 The stone around the dowel pins is lubricated.

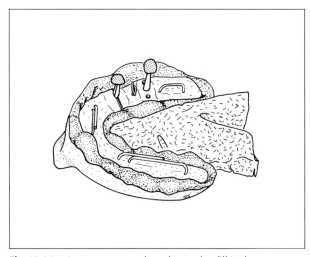

Fig 18-21 A wet paper towel can be used to fill in the open, center portion of the impression.

Dowel Pin System Armamentarium

1. 500-cc Vac-U-Mixer and vacuum tubing
2. Vibrator
3. Water measure
4. Large and small spatulas
5. Die stone (Silky-Rock, Vel-Mix)
6. Humidor
7. Dowel pins
8. Straight pins, bobby pins, and paper clips
9. Sticky wax and utility wax
10. Beavertail burnisher
11. Bunsen burner
12. Cotton pliers
13. Sable brush
14. Petrolatum
15. Model trimmer
16. Saw frame with blade
17. Laboratory knife with no. 25 blade
18. Straight handpiece and pear-shaped acrylic bur
19. Colorbrite red pencil

A number of items found in a dental laboratory are commonly used for orienting dowels: anesthetic needles, paper clips, bobby pins, and paper matches.[34] Place a dowel between the arms of a bobby pin, with the round side of the dowel in one of the corrugations and the flat side of the dowel against the flat arm of the bobby pin. Then position the bobby pin buccolingually across the impression so that the dowel pin will be centered directly over the preparation. Push a straight pin between the arms of the bobby pin and into the impression material

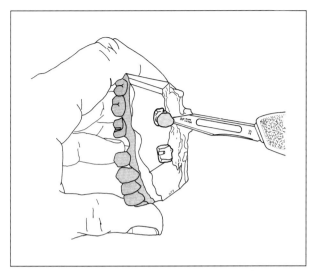

Fig 18-22 Wax at the ends of the dowel pins is located and removed.

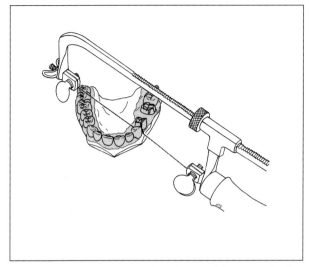

Fig 18-23 Dies are separated from the rest of the cast with a fine saw.

on both the buccal and the lingual surfaces of each tooth to have a dowel pin placed over it. Stabilize the dowel in the bobby pin, and the bobby pin itself against the straight pins with sticky wax (Fig 18-18).

Pour die stone into the impression, filling the impressions of the teeth and covering the knurled end of the dowel pin. The pin should parallel the long axis of the preparation, and it must not touch the impression. Paper clips or lock washers can be set into the stone before it sets, to provide retention for the base that will be added later (Fig 18-19). These retentive devices should be placed in other parts of the model that are not to be removed from the completed cast. It may facilitate removal of the die later if the teeth distal to the prepared tooth also are made removable by positioning a dowel pin over that segment of the cast.

When the stone has set, remove the straight pins and bobby pins from the impression. Place a small ball of soft utility wax on the tip of each dowel. A 1.0-inch (2.5-cm) length of plastic tubing with an inner diameter of approximately 0.5 inches also can be placed on the end of the dowel as an aid in locating the dowels after the base has been poured.[35] Cut a V-shaped buccolingual orientation groove or a round dimple on each die to aid in reseating the die completely and accurately during use. Then lubricate the stone around each dowel with a *thin* coat of petrolatum or commercially available separating medium to permit easy separation of the dies from the working cast later (Fig 18-20). Remove any excess lubricant.

Place a wet paper towel into the open lingual space. This will enable a complete base for the cast to be poured (Fig 18-21). When the base is poured, leave peaks and curls of stone projecting from the top of it to provide retention for the mounting plaster later. After the stone has set, remove the cast from the impression and trim the excess on a model trimmer. Use a sharp knife to uncover the spheres of utility wax and to remove them

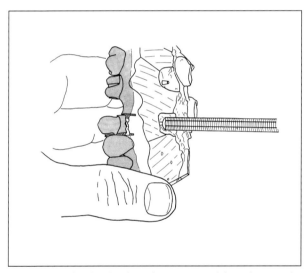

Fig 18-24 After the dies have been separated from the cast, the ends of the dowel pins are tapped to loosen the dies from the cast.

(Fig 18-22). Make certain that all wax is removed and that no stone chips are left around the apex of the dowel pin. Allow the stone to harden for 24 hours.

When the stone is hard and dry, use a saw frame with a thin blade to cut through the layer of die stone (Fig 18-23). There should be a cut on the mesial and distal side of each die, and the cuts should taper toward each other slightly from occlusal to gingival. Gently tap on the end of the dowel with an instrument handle to loosen the die (Fig 18-24). Take the die from the cast and trim away excess stone gingival to the finish line (Fig 18-25). Complete the trimming of the die with a no. 25 blade in the laboratory knife and then mark the finish line with the red pencil.

Repeat the procedure for each die on the cast. Check

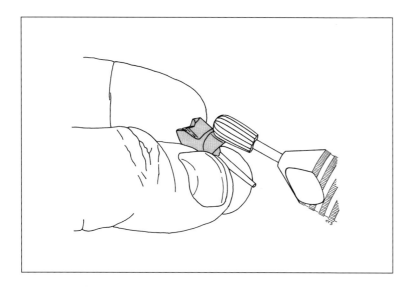

Fig 18-25 Base of the die is trimmed with an acrylic bur.

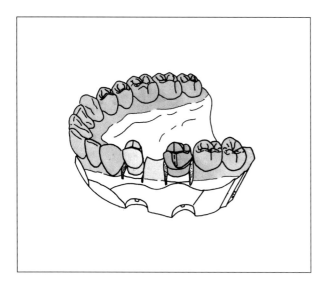

Fig 18-26 Dies are reseated into the cast.

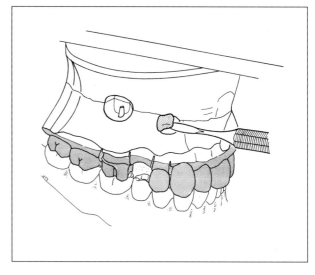

Fig 18-27 After the casts have been mounted, wax is removed from the ends of the dowel pins.

the surfaces of the working cast and tapered dowel hole to make absolutely certain that they are free of any particles or debris. The successful use of any removable die technique is contingent upon keeping the dies and cast free of stone chips, wax shavings, or any other debris. The failure of dies to reseat completely is probably caused by debris in the keyways,[29] and the resultant wax patterns will be inaccurate. Reseat the dies to make certain that they will seat completely and will be stable (Fig 18-26).

Place utility wax back into the wells around the tips of the dowels to protect them from plaster contamination. Soak the cast in water and mount it on the articulator using mounting stone. When the stone has set, remove the wax covering the tips of the dowels (Fig 18-27). Again make certain that no chips of stone or wax are left in the wells. This type of dowel also can be cemented into holes drilled into the flat underside of a cast that has already been poured.[22]

Curved Dowel Pin

Curved dowels can be incorporated into a working cast by fixing the dowels to the impression before it is poured, or by cementing the dowels into holes drilled in a previ-

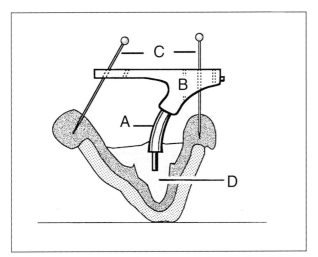

Fig 18-28 Cross section of an impression showing the relation of a curved dowel (A), positioning bar (B), straight pins (C), and first pour of die stone (D) to the impression.

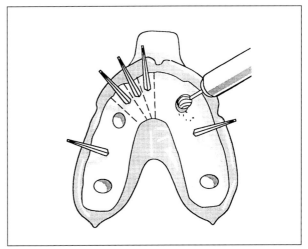

Fig 18-29 Depressions are made about 2.0 mm deep on either side of the dowels in the two large segments of the cast that will carry the unprepared teeth. The broken lines indicate where the cast will be sectioned later.

ously poured cast. To install pins before pouring the impression, use finger pressure to insert a curved dowel, tip first, into the large opening in a positioning bar. With that bar oriented faciolingually, hold the assembly so that the head of the dowel extends 1.0 to 2.0 mm into the impression of the prepared tooth. The tail of the dowel normally points facially. However, if a tooth is in linguoversion, reverse the direction of the dowel for easier removal.

Insert a straight pin through one of the three holes in the facial aspect of the bar and into the facial flange of the impression. Place another pin through one of the holes in the lingual aspect of the bar and into the lingual portion of the impression (Fig 18-28). The dowel should not touch the impression, and its head should approximately parallel the long axis of the tooth. Repeat this procedure for all prepared teeth and any pontic areas. If the restoration is a fixed partial denture, a dowel must also be placed near the center of each segment of unprepared teeth. This will allow removal of these segments of the stone cast to provide better access to the gingival margins of the retainer wax patterns.

Vibrate a mix of die stone into the impression until it covers the heads of the dowels and 1.0 to 2.0 mm of the thicker hexagonal bodies of the dowels. This will fill the impression to a level approximately 4.0 mm above the gingival finish lines. After the die stone has hardened, carefully extract the two straight pins and slide the positioning bar off each dowel. To assist in orienting each large segment of unprepared teeth in the cast, cut a 2.0-mm-deep hole on either side of each dowel with a large acrylic bur (Fig 18-29).

Paint the stone with petrolatum so that it will later separate from the base of the cast (Fig 18-30). Also apply a *thin* coat of petrolatum to the exposed parts of the dowels. Box the impression with wax, allowing the tails of the

dowels to extend slightly through the heat-softened wax (Fig 18-31). Fill the boxed impression with yellow dental stone. The dowels should be covered by at least 2.0 mm of stone, except for the tips that are embedded in the boxing wax.

After the stone has hardened, remove the boxing wax and make vertical saw cuts on either side of each die, being careful not to damage the preparation finish lines (Fig 18-32). The cuts must extend completely through the die stone to the underlying base. Separate each segment from the working cast by pressing or tapping on the protruding tail of the curved dowel with a knife handle (Fig 18-33).

To place the dowels after the cast has been made, pour the impression with die stone to form a horseshoe-shaped working cast. Trim the bottom of the cast flat on a model trimmer to a level no more than 10 mm from the necks of the teeth (Fig 18-34). Thin casts require less sawing, and short dies are more stable than longer ones. Drill a 5.0-mm-deep hole in the bottom of the cast directly under the center of each prepared tooth, pontic area, and segment containing unprepared teeth (Fig 18-35). These holes can be made with a 2.0-mm-diameter (no. 47 or 0.0785-inch) drill in a handpiece or with a drill press (Pindex system, Coltene/Whaledent, Mahwah, NJ). If a removable segment will be larger than the width of two teeth, the stone on each side of the dowel hole should be keyed to a depth of about 2 mm with a large acrylic bur (Fig 18-36).

Try a curved dowel into each hole to make sure the head will seat completely. Clean the hole with a drill if necessary. Cement dowels into the holes one at a time, placing a drop of cyanoacrylate cement into each hole (Fig 18-37). Seat the heads completely (Fig 18-38), with the tails of the dowels pointing facially (Fig 18-39).

After the cement has hardened, brush a *thin* layer of

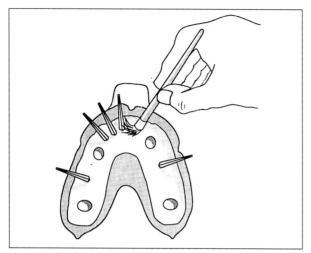

Fig 18-30 Thin coat of petrolatum is applied to the stone and dowels.

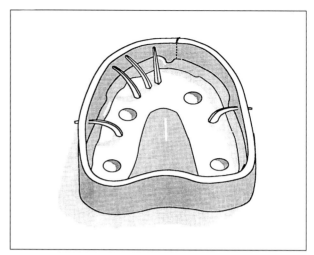

Fig 18-31 Boxing wax is placed around the impression, with the tips of the dowels sticking through.

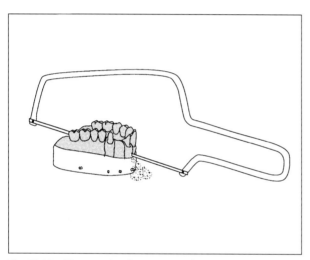

Fig 18-32 The completed cast is sawed.

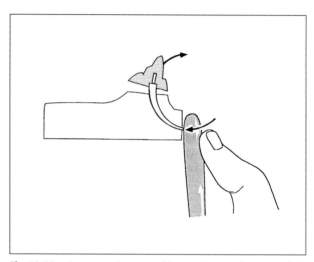

Fig 18-33 A segment is removed by pressing on the exposed tip of its curved dowel.

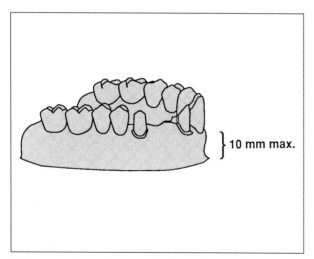

10 mm max.

Fig 18-34 The working cast is trimmed to receive cemented dowels.

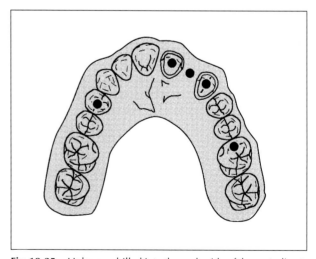

Fig 18-35 Holes are drilled into the underside of the cast, directly under the indicated locations.

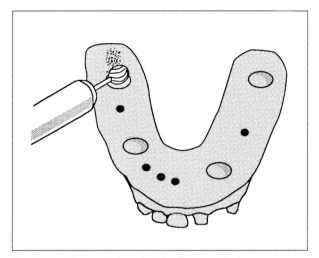

Fig 18-36 The cast is keyed with a large acrylic bur.

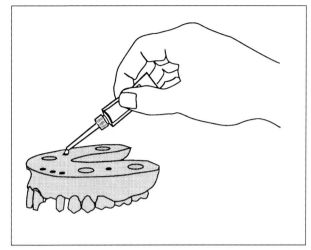

Fig 18-37 A drop of cyanoacrylate cement is placed into each of the drilled holes.

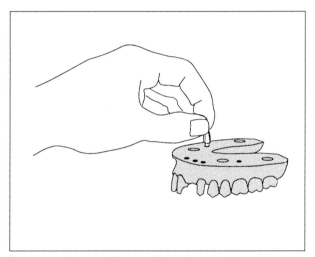

Fig 18-38 The head of a curved dowel is seated into the cement-lined hole.

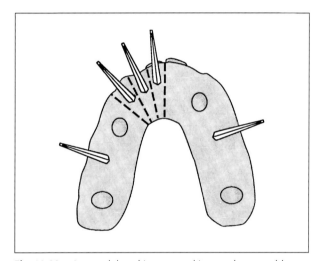

Fig 18-39 A curved dowel is cemented into each removable part of the working cast. Broken lines indicate where the segments will be separated by saw cuts after the base is poured.

petrolatum onto the flattened surface of the cast and the exposed portions of the dowels. Box the cast, pour a base, and separate the dies as described previously.

Pindex System

In the Pindex system (Coltene/Whaledent, Mahwah, NJ), a reverse drill press is used to create a master cast with dies that can be removed and replaced repeatedly with great precision (Fig 18-40). The impression is poured without positioning and attaching dowel pins beforehand. The machine accurately drills parallel holes from the underside of a trimmed cast.

Pour the impression in the usual manner, adding approximately 20 mm of stone beyond the edge of the tray (Fig 18-41). This should allow enough stone to trim

the cast to a desired thickness later without having to add more die stone. If stone is added to the base, the additional stone may separate from the underside of the dies when the pins are placed or when the dies are removed for trimming.

Allow the cast to set for 60 minutes, remove it from the impression, and repour the impression for a backup cast. Thoroughly wet the cast prior to trimming to prevent the accumulation of sludge on the prepared teeth. Use a model trimmer to flatten the heels of the cast. Then trim the bottom of the cast, resting the heels on the table of the trimmer (Fig 18-42). The cast should be trimmed until all rough, irregular, and undercut areas are removed from its underside. It should sit perfectly flat on a tabletop, and its thickness from base to preparation finish line must be a minimum of 15 mm (Fig 18-43). If the bottom of the cast is flat, it insures that the pin holes drilled into it will be parallel.[36]

Use the model trimmer to remove the excess stone on

321

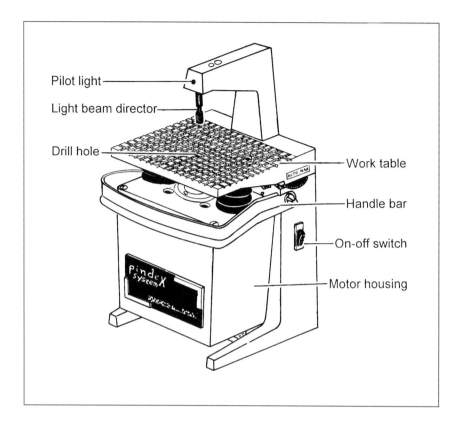

Pilot light

Light beam director

Drill hole

Work table

Handle bar

On-off switch

Motor housing

Fig 18-40 Parts of the Pindex machine.

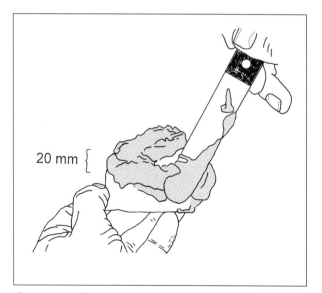

20 mm

Fig 18-41 Sufficient stone to allow for trimming is added.

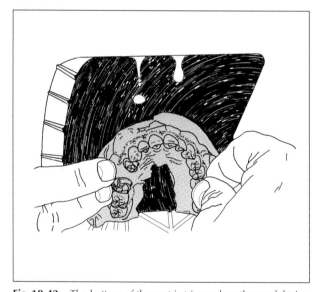

Fig 18-42 The bottom of the cast is trimmed on the model trimmer.

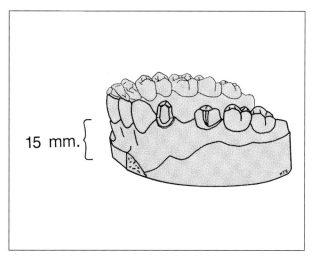

Fig 18-43   The cast should be 15 mm thick, exclusive of the teeth.

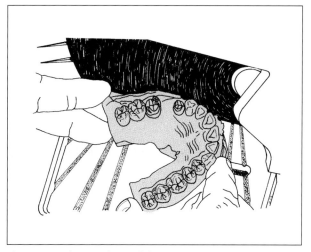

Fig 18-44   The periphery of the cast is trimmed on the model trimmer.

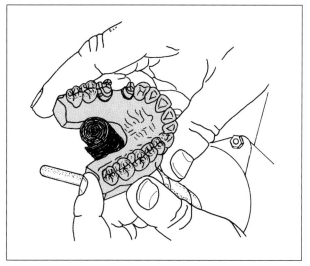

Fig 18-45   The palate/tongue area is trimmed with an arbor band.

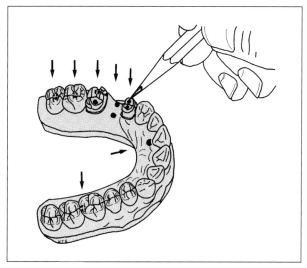

Fig 18-46   Location of the pin holes is marked with a pencil.

the periphery of the cast (Fig 18-44). Wash the cast to remove any debris that was deposited on it during grinding. Remove any excess stone in the palate/tongue area with an arbor band on a lathe (Fig 18-45). The lingual border of the cast should taper slightly toward the base to facilitate removal of the dies from the cast later. The faciolingual width of the cast should be approximately 20 mm. Use a pencil to mark the desired location of the pins on the occlusal surfaces of the teeth or preparations. There should be two pins for each die, two for each pontic (edentulous) area, and two pins in each terminal segment containing unprepared teeth (Fig 18-46).

Use the switch on the side of the machine to turn it on. A red pilot light will indicate that it is running. Place the prepared cast on the worktable and align the first pencil

mark with the illuminated dot from the light beam director (Fig 18-47). Using both hands, exert firm downward pressure on the cast with the thumbs.

Grasp the handle bar with the remaining fingers (Fig 18-48). This enables the operator to stabilize the cast as the drill assembly moves upward, cutting the pin holes. Raise the handle bar with slow, even pressure, timing the cycle to take 3 to 5 seconds. When the proper depth has been reached, the red pilot light will go off, indicating that the hole is finished. Do not force the bar any farther. Using the above technique, complete the drilling of all the pin holes. For best results, the cast should be slightly damp to prevent dust formation and excessive chipping around the pin holes. However, "damp" does not mean dripping wet.

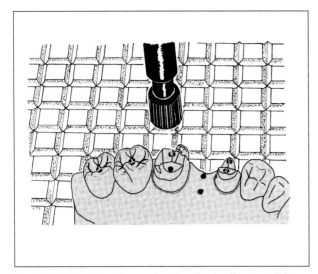

Fig 18-47 Pencil marks are placed under the illuminated dot.

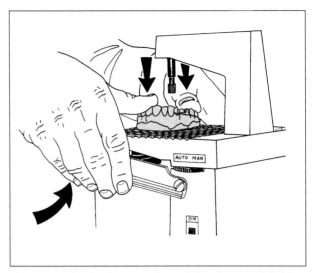

Fig 18-48 The thumbs are used to stabilize the cast while lifting the handle bar with the fingers.

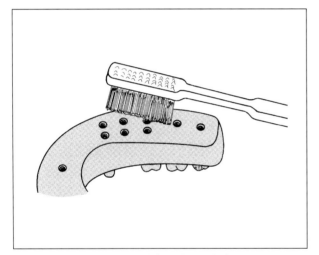

Fig 18-49 Debris is removed from the pin holes.

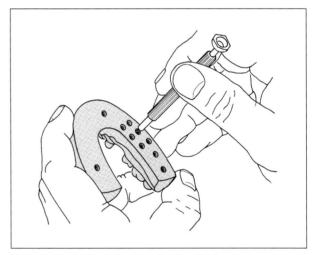

Fig 18-50 The pin holes are refined with a hand reamer.

Use compressed air and a toothbrush to remove debris from the pin holes (Fig 18-49). Use a hand reamer to remove any residual debris from the pin holes (Fig 18-50). Prior to cementation, try in the pins to insure complete seating. The collar of the pin should be flush with the base of the cast to avoid creating an undercut. The few minutes required for a precementation try-in can prevent the cast from being ruined during cementation.

Any commercially available cyanoacrylate cement can be used to lute the pins in their holes. The cast must be thoroughly dry. Apply a small amount of cement to the end of each pin (Fig 18-51). Excess cement in a closely fitting pin hole may create enough hydraulic pressure to prevent complete seating. Pin placement will be facilitated by placing the short pins in the lingual/palatal holes first (Fig 18-52). Placing the long pins in the facial holes makes the ends of the dowel pins more accessible for easy die removal after the casts are mounted.

When the cement has dried, place the sleeves over the pins with the flat sides of their bases facing each other (Fig 18-53). Place the white sleeves on the long pins and the gray sleeves on the short pins. Apply a *thin* coat of petrolatum to the bottom of the cast as a separating agent (Fig 18-54). Wipe off all excess with a cotton roll, a finger tip, or a dry cotton-tipped applicator. Visible excess lubricant left on the cast will create a space between the cast and its base, which could cause seating errors when the dies are repositioned after separation from the cast.

Place a small amount of molten wax in the ends of the short sleeves to prevent the sleeve from filling with stone when the secondary base is added (Fig 18-55). Run a strip of utility wax along the ends of the long pins to facilitate removal of the dies later (Fig 18-56). Place a small ball of wax on the ends of isolated pins on the contralateral side of the cast.

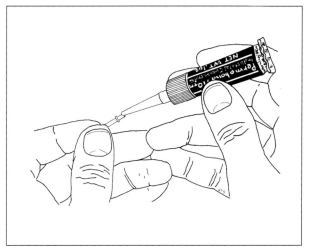

Fig 18-51 Cyanoacrylate cement is placed on the pins prior to cementing the pin tips.

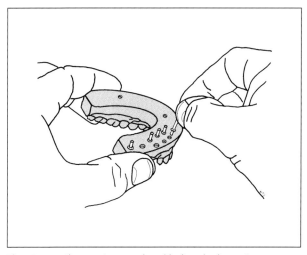

Fig 18-52 Shorter pins are placed before the long pins.

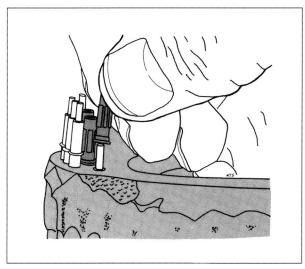

Fig 18-53 White sleeves are placed on the long pins and gray sleeves on the short pins.

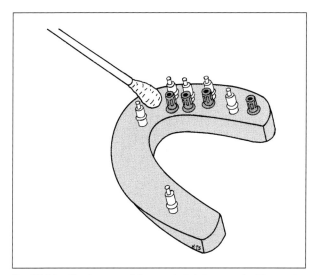

Fig 18-54 The bottom of the cast is lightly coated with petrolatum.

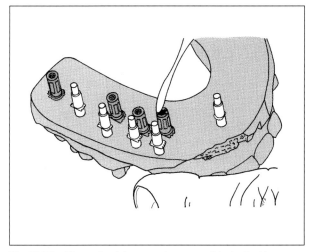

Fig 18-55 The ends of the gray sleeves are blocked with wax.

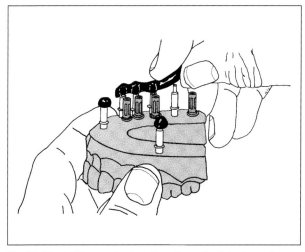

Fig 18-56 Utility wax is placed on the ends of the long pins.

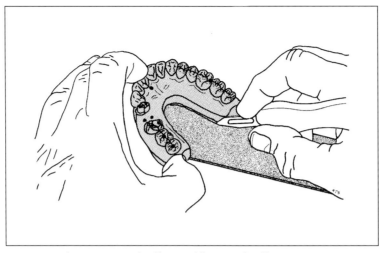

Fig 18-57   A palatal/tongue filler is made of boxing wax.

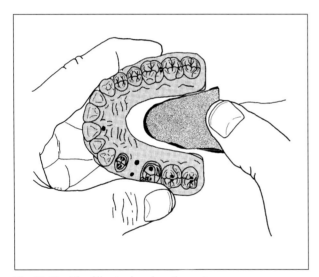

Fig 18-58   The filler is placed on the cast.

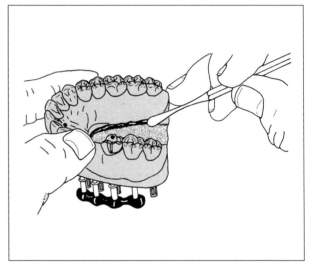

Fig 18-59   The filler is seated to the cast.

Two methods can be used to add the base to the cast. The first is the conventional method of boxing a cast. Using the cast as a template, cut a palate/ tongue filler from a strip of boxing wax (Fig 18-57). Place the U-shaped piece of wax in the appropriate area (Fig 18-58) and secure it to the die-stone cast with a hot no. 7 wax spatula (Fig 18-59).

Adapt a strip of boxing wax around the periphery of the cast and seal it with a hot instrument (Fig 18-60). The utility wax should be closely adapted to keep stone from leaking into the gingival crevices and axial surfaces of the teeth. Pour the base in type III stone (Microstone, Whip Mix Corp, Louisville, KY). Beginning in the area of the pins, add small increments of stone until they completely cover the pins (Fig 18-61).

The second technique utilizes specially designed base formers that are available in both full-arch and quadrant molds. The depth of the mold is identical to the length of the long pins. Once again, Microstone is utilized for the base. Using a vibrator, fill the base former with stone (Fig 18-62). Add a small amount of stone to the bottom of the cast in the area of the pins, carefully vibrating it between the pins (Fig 18-63).

Invert the cast and seat it slowly in the base former until the wax on the ends of the pins contacts the bottom of the mold (Fig 18-64). Be careful not to bury the cast in the stone. Remove excess as it wells up around the periphery of the cast. The base should set for a minimum of 30 minutes. After removal of the wax or the base former, wet the cast and then trim it on a model trimmer. The periphery of the cast should be trimmed until the junction of the die stone and the base stone is smooth and distinct.

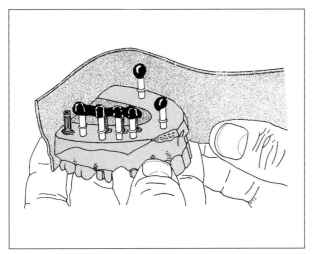

Fig 18-60 Boxing wax is applied around the cast.

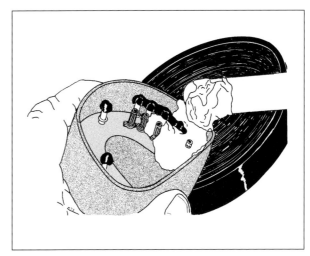

Fig 18-61 The base is poured in Microstone.

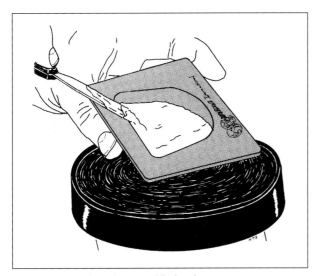

Fig 18-62 The base former is filled with Microstone.

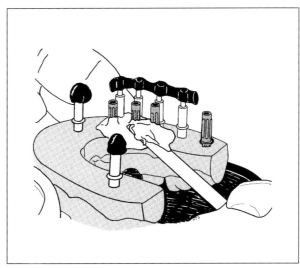

Fig 18-63 Stone is vibrated around the bases of the pins.

Allow the cast to dry before attempting to section and trim the dies. The pinned cast can be removed from the base in one piece, which permits sectioning of the cast into dies from the underside. This is particularly desirable in cases in which there is limited interdental space and therefore the possibility of damage to the finish lines.[37] For a routine three-unit fixed partial denture, the dies usually can be sectioned from the occlusal aspect. Because the finish lines are visible in this approach, the novice usually finds it less intimidating.

With either method of sectioning the dies, the first step is to remove the utility wax placed on the ends of the long pins (Fig 18-65). Next mark the desired location of the saw cuts on the facial and lingual aspects of the cast with pencil lines (Fig 18-66). To remove the cast in one piece, use the handle of an instrument to lightly tap all of the exposed pins (Fig 18-67). Continue the tapping until the pinned cast is loosened from the base. Remove the cast and extend the pencil lines onto the underside of the cast to indicate the location of the desired saw cuts.

Use a saw to section the dies from the underside (Fig 18-68). The saw cut should end approximately 1 to 2 mm short of the finish line with the final separation accomplished by squeezing the two parts gently together. In this manner, the parts can be broken cleanly without damage to the finish lines.

To section the dies from the occlusal aspect, the operator must initiate the saw cut slowly, carefully avoiding the finish line of the preparation (Fig 18-69). To prevent scoring of the contralateral teeth, the first saw cut should be made mesial to the section containing the prepared teeth. The uninvolved section or quadrant is removed.

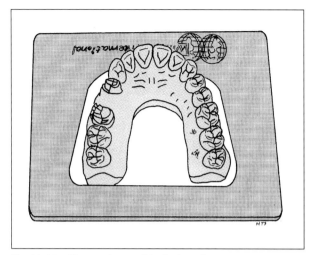

Fig 18-64   The cast is seated in the base former.

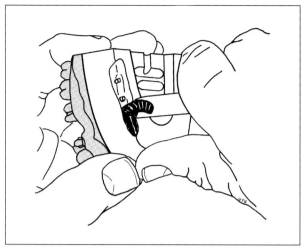

Fig 18-65   Wax over the long pins is removed.

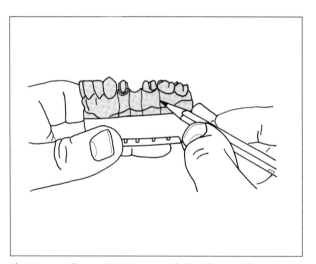

Fig 18-66   The saw cuts are premarked with a pencil.

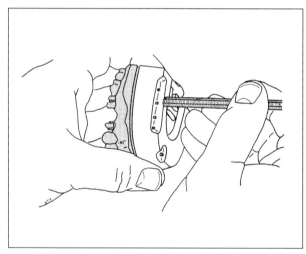

Fig 18-67   The cast is removed by tapping the pins with an instrument handle.

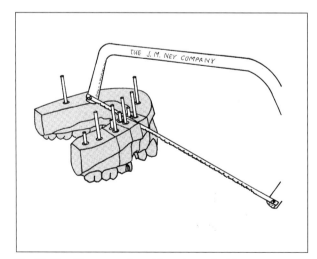

Fig 18-68   Dies are sectioned from the underside.

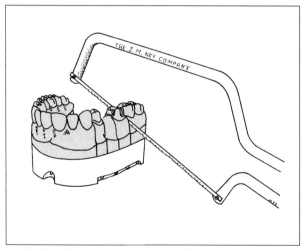

Fig 18-69   Dies may also be sectioned from the occlusal aspect of the cast.

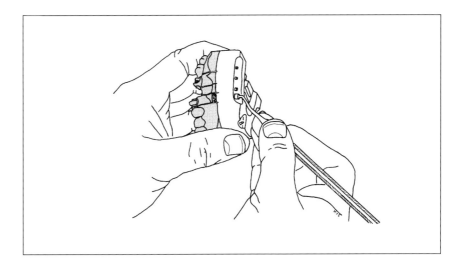

Fig 18-70 A large condenser can also be used to loosen the dies.

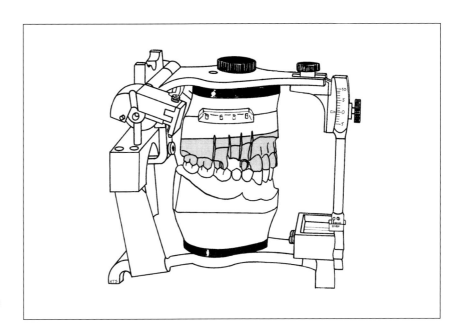

Fig 18-71 The completed cast on the articulator.

This allows ready access and freedom of movement when the dies are sectioned. The saw cut must be carried all the way through the stone before attempting to remove the die.

To remove a single die, a large amalgam condenser or the handle of an instrument is used to push on the end of the exposed pin until the die is loosened from the base (Fig 18-70). To allow easy removal of the dies during the subsequent laboratory procedures, the saw cuts should be parallel or taper slightly in toward the pins. If the base of the die is wider than the preparation, the die will be locked in and much of the efficiency of a removable die system will be lost.

After the dies are sectioned, trim them in the conventional manner. Mark the finish lines with a red pencil.

Apply die hardener and die spacer according to the manufacturer's instructions. Before mounting the cast on the articulator, evaluate the height of the base. If the height of the base is too great, it will prevent closure of the articulator. Check this before mixing the mounting stone. If the base needs to be reduced, remove the pinned sections of the cast before grinding the base on a model trimmer.

Reassemble the two sections and place a small amount of utility wax on the ends of the die pins. This will prevent the mounting stone from blocking access to the pins. Once the mounting stone has set, remove the wax on the pins. The cast is ready for fabrication of the wax pattern (Fig 18-71).

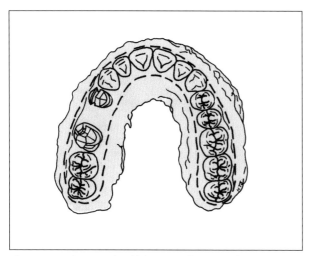

Fig 18-72 The cast should be poured in a U shape, with no stone in the center.

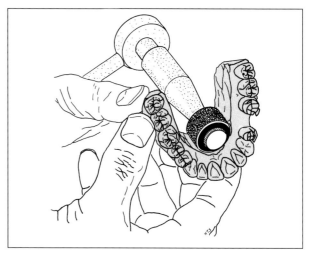

Fig 18-73 The lingual side of the cast base is trimmed with an arbor band.

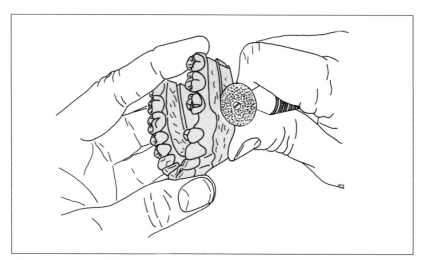

Fig 18-74 Horizontal grooves are cut in the base to give it retention.

Di-Lok Tray

A snap-apart plastic tray with internal orienting grooves and notches also can be used to reassemble the working cast and die. In two studies it was found to have the least vertical error.[29,38] Like all removable die systems, great care must be taken to keep it clean so that the parts will fit together with the greatest possible accuracy. Before using the tray for any given case, examine the mounting of the diagnostic casts on the articulator to determine whether there is space for the bulky tray. When the casts must be mounted near the upper member of the articulator, or near the hinge axis, some alternate technique must be employed.

Di-Lok Tray Armamentarium

1. 500-cc Vac-U-Mixer and vacuum tubing
2. Vibrator
3. Water measure
4. Large and small spatulas
5. Die stone (Silky-Rock, Vel-Mix)
6. Humidor
7. Di-Lok tray
8. Model trimmer
9. Arbor band on dental lathe
10. Straight handpiece, separating disc on mandrel, pear-shaped acrylic bur
11. Saw frame with thin blade
12. Colorbrite red pencil

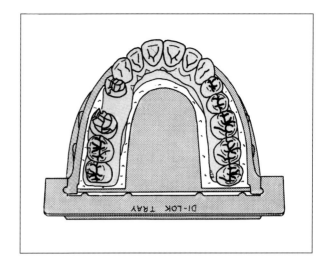

Fig 18-75 The cast is placed into stone in the tray.

Pour the entire full-arch impression with die stone. Keep the stone restricted to the U-shaped arch, building it up to a height of approximately 1.0 inch (2.5 cm). There should be no stone in the open lingual area and as little as possible on the vestibular roll of the impression. When the stone has set for 1 hour, separate it from the impression. The U-shaped cast, with an open lingual area, must be trimmed so that it will fit into a Di-Lok tray (Fig 18-72).

Trim the outer, or buccal, side of the cast on a model trimmer, tapering it toward the base. Allow the cast to dry out thoroughly and then trim the inner, or lingual, side of the cast on an arbor band on a dental lathe (Fig 18-73). Try the cast into the Di-Lok tray to make sure that it will fit. Score the base of the cast with a separating disc in a straight handpiece (Fig 18-74). Place one or two horizontal grooves on the inner and outer aspects of the cast to provide undercuts for holding the cast in stone in the tray.

Soak the base of the cast in water for about 5 minutes. Mix stone and vibrate it into the tray until the tray is approximately three-quarters full. Seat the cast into the tray, jiggling it slightly as it settles to eliminate bubbles. The cervical lines of the teeth should be about 4 mm above the edge of the tray when the cast has been seated. Wipe off the excess stone that has been expressed along the edge of the cast and over the shoulder of the tray. The working cast is now invested in a layer of stone within the tray (Fig 18-75). Allow the stone to set until it is hard and dry.

To complete the dies, the cast must be removed from the tray. Disassemble the tray by lifting the back up, and then slide the buccal segment forward (Fig 18-76). The cast can be most easily loosened by rapping sharply on the front of the base of the tray with the handle of a laboratory knife (Fig 18-77). After the cast has been slightly displaced, slide it forward and remove it from the tray base.

With a saw frame and a thin saw blade, cut between the prepared tooth and the adjacent tooth (Fig 18-78). The saw cut should start in the interdental papilla area and extend downward on a very slight taper. The die will be slightly wider mesiodistally at its base than at the gingival finish line of the prepared tooth.

The occlusal saw cut should extend approximately three-quarters of the way through the stone base. Use finger pressure to break the die and attached teeth from the cast (Fig 18-79). In the same manner, separate the die from the portion of the cast attached to it. This small area of stone that remains in intimate contact with adjacent segments, along with the vertical ribs in the tray, is responsible for the accurate relationship of the die(s) to the cast.[36] Repeat the process for every prepared tooth on the cast.

Remove excess stone gingival to the finish line with a pear-shaped acrylic bur (Fig 18-80). Finish trimming and blending the concave area adjacent to the finish line with a laboratory knife with a no. 25 blade. Mark the finish line itself with a red pencil to assist in locating it when making the wax pattern.

Check the tray for any thin stone flash that remains from embedding the cast in stone. Remove all stone particles from the tray by brushing it thoroughly with a stiff toothbrush. Blow it dry with compressed air. When the tray is completely clean, reassemble the dies and other parts of the cast in the tray. Slide the buccal facing onto the base of the tray from the front. Place the back down over the lugs on the buccal facing, locking the tray together (Fig 18-81). To attach the Di-Lok tray to the articulator, place the cast into a facebow or in occlusion with a previously mounted diagnostic cast if it is available. Put mounting stone on the articulator ring and on the bottom of the tray, which has undercut rails on it. When the stone has set, the articulated cast in the Di-Lok tray is ready for the fabrication of the wax pattern (Fig 18-82).

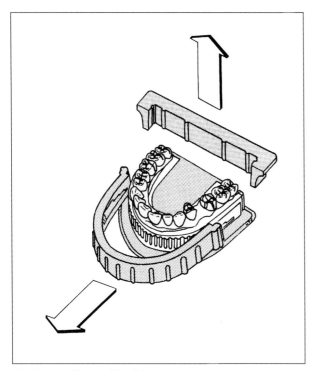

Fig 18-76 Disassembly of the cast.

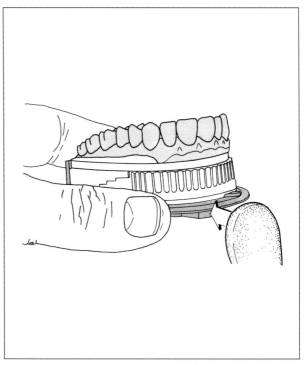

Fig 18-77 The cast is jarred loose from the tray base by tapping on the front of the base.

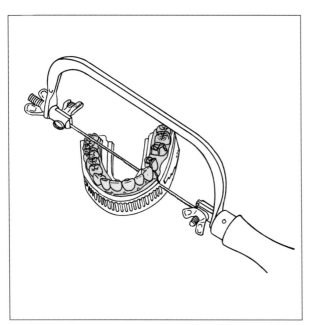

Fig 18-78 A saw cut is made on each side of the prepared tooth.

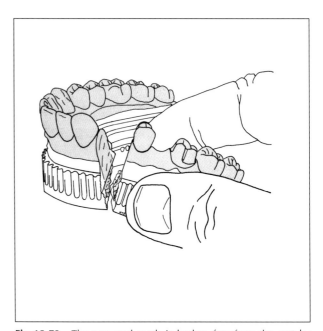

Fig 18-79 The prepared tooth is broken free from the cast by hand. Do *not* pry them apart.

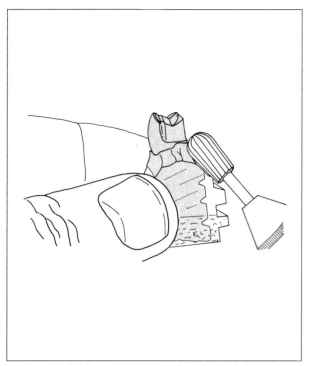

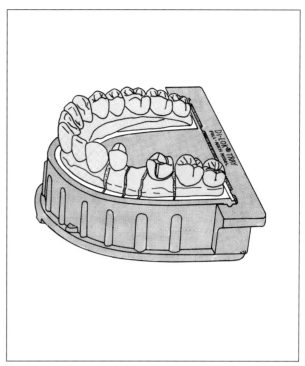

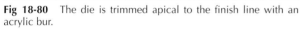

Fig 18-80   The die is trimmed apical to the finish line with an acrylic bur.

Fig 18-81   The cast and die(s) are reassembled in the tray.

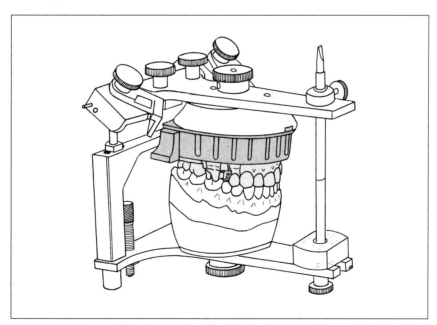

Fig 18-82   The cast and tray mounted on the articulator.

References

1. Rudd KD, Strunk RR, Morrow RM: Removable dies for crowns, inlays and fixed partial dentures. *J Prosthet Dent* 1970; 23:337–347.

2. Saunders M: The orientation of dies in restorative dentistry. *Br Dent J* 1964; 117:133–138.

3. Thompson MJ: A standardized indirect technic for reversible hydrocolloid. *J Am Dent Assoc* 1953; 46:1–18.

4. Phillips RW: *Skinner's Science of Dental Materials,* ed 9. Philadelphia, WB Saunders Co, 1991, p 86.

5. McCormick JT, Antony SJ, Dial ML, Duncanson MG, Shillingburg HT: Wettability of elastomeric impression materials: Effect of selected surfactants. *Int J Prosthodont* 1989; 2:413–420.

6. Cullen DR, Mikesell JW, Sandrik JL: Wettability of elastomeric impression materials and voids in gypsum casts. *J Prosthet Dent* 1991; 66:261–265.

7. Rudd KD, Morrow RM, Bange AA: Accurate casts. *J Prosthet Dent* 1969; 21:545–554.

8. Phillips RW, Ito BY: Factors affecting the surface of stone dies poured in hydrocolloid impressions. *J Prosthet Dent* 1952; 2:390–400.

9. Wiskott A: Laboratory procedures and clinical implications in the making of casts. *Quintessence Int* 1987; 18:181–192.

10. Fusayama T, Ide K, Hosada H: Relief of resistance of cement of full cast crowns. *J Prosthet Dent* 1964; 14:95–106.

11. Eames WB, O'Neal SJ, Monteiro J, Roan JD, Cohen KS: Techniques to improve the seating of castings. *J Am Dent Assoc* 1978; 96:432–437.

12. Gardner FM, Vermilyea SG: The variability of die-spacer film thickness. *Gen Dent* 1985; 33:502–503.

13. Donovan T, Wright W, Campagni WV: Use of paint-on die spacers in preparations with grooves. *J Prosthet Dent* 1984; 52:384–388.

14. Campagni WV, Preston JD, Reisbick MH: Measurement of paint-on die spacers used for casting relief. *J Prosthet Dent* 1982; 47:606–611.

15. Campagni WV, Wright W, Martinoff JT: Effect of die spacer on the seating of complete cast gold crowns with grooves. *J Prosthet Dent* 1986; 55:324–328.

16. Campagni WV, Prince J, Defreese C: Measurement of coating agents used for surface protection of stone dies. *J Prosthet Dent* 1986; 55:470–474.

17. Cowell TA, Moore J: New technic for sectional model production for inlay and bridgework. *J Am Dent Assoc* 1965; 71:1387–1390.

18. Kimball HD: Hydrocolloid in restorative operative dentistry—Technique and principles. *Dent Digest* 1949; 55:64–71.

19. Mann AW: A critical appraisal of the hydrocolloid technique: Its advantages and disadvantages. *J Prosthet Dent* 1951; 1:733–749.

20. Dilts WE, Podshadley AG, Ellison E, Neiman R: Accuracy of a removable die-dowel pin technique. *J Dent Res* 1971; 50:1249–1252.

21. Carl W, Garlapo DA, Brown MH: Modified impression procedure and removable die preparation. *Quintessence Int* 1974; 5:39–44.

22. Smith CD, Nayyar A, Koth DL: Fabrication of removable stone dies using cemented dowel pins. *J Prosthet Dent* 1979; 41:579–581.

23. Reed GM: New concept in precision dowels. *J Am Dent Assoc* 1968; 76:321–324.

24. Stern AJ, Vernon HM: Development of a new tool in restorative dentistry. *J Prosthet Dent* 1969; 21:536–544.

25. Benfield JW, Lyons GV: Precision dies from elastic impressions. *J Prosthet Dent* 1962; 12:737–752.

26. Covo LM, Ziebert GJ, Balthazar Y, Christensen LV: Accuracy and comparative stability of three removable die systems. *J Prosthet Dent* 1988; 59:314–318.

27. Richardson DW, Sanchez RA, Baker PS, Haug SP: Positional accuracy of four die tray systems. *J Prosthet Dent* 1991; 66:39–45.

28. Hohlt FA, Phillips RW: Evaluation of various methods employed for constructing working dies from hydrocolloid impressions. *J Prosthet Dent* 1956; 6:87–93.

29. Dilts WE, Podshadley AG, Sawyer HF, Neiman R: Accuracy of four removable die techniques. *J Am Dent Assoc* 1971; 83:1081–1085.

30. Myers M, Hembree JH: Relative accuracy of four removable die systems. *J Prosthet Dent* 1982; 48:163–165.

31. Troendle KB, Troendle GR, Cavozos E: Positioning dowel pins for removable dies. *J Prosthet Dent* 1981; 46:575–578.

32. George TA, Holmes JR: The dowelklip: A device for dowel pin placement. *J Prosthet Dent* 1985; 53:276–278.

33. Robinson FB, Block B: Dowel pin positioning technique for fixed partial denture working casts. *J Prosthet Dent* 1981; 46:215–216.

34. Balshi TJ, Mingledorff EB: Matches, clips, needles, or pins. *J Prosthet Dent* 1975; 34:467–472.

35. Stone TE, Welker WA: A method for locating dowel pins in artificial stone casts. *J Prosthet Dent* 1980; 44:345–346.

36. Miranda FJ, Dilts WE, Duncanson MG, Collard EW: Comparative stability of two removable die systems. *J Prosthet Dent* 1976; 36:326–333.

37. Netti CA, Yard RA, Withrow G, Nagy WW: Saw modification for underside die cutting. *J Prosthet Dent* 1990; 64:621–624.

38. Hembree JH, Brown T: Relative accuracy of several removable die systems. *J Acad Gen Dent* 1974; 22:31–33.

Chapter 19

Wax Patterns

The wax pattern is the precursor of the finished cast restoration that will be placed on the prepared tooth. Inasmuch as the wax pattern will be duplicated exactly through the investing and casting technique, the final restoration can be no better than its wax pattern; ie, errors and oversights in the wax pattern will only be perpetuated in the casting. A few extra minutes spent on the wax pattern can often save hours that might be spent correcting the casting.

There are two accepted ways of fabricating a wax pattern:

1. The *direct* technique, in which the pattern is waxed on the prepared tooth in the mouth
2. The *indirect* technique, in which the pattern is waxed on a stone cast made from an accurate impression of the prepared tooth

The indirect technique offers the advantage of allowing most of the procedure to be done away from the chair. It affords an opportunity for visualization of the restoration and ready access to waxing the margins. Because it allows a technician to fabricate the pattern, the indirect technique has become the most popular means of fabricating cast restorations.

The selection of the wax used in fabricating a wax pattern is important. Type I waxes are formulated for making intraoral wax patterns. Type II waxes, made for the fabrication of wax patterns extraorally, have a slightly lower melting point. Therefore, when an indirect wax pattern is made, the wax used should meet ADA specification no. 4, type II. The wax should be of some color, such as blue, green, or red, that will contrast with and be easily distinguishable from the stone die. There are several requirements of a good inlay wax[1]:

1. It must flow readily when heated, without chipping, flaking, or losing its smoothness.
2. When cooled, it must be rigid.
3. It must be capable of being carved precisely, without chipping, distorting, or smearing.

Stresses occur in the inlay wax as a result of the heating and manipulation of the wax during fabrication of the pattern. Wax, a thermoplastic material, "relaxes" as these stresses are released. The result is distortion, which is exhibited as a poor fit. To minimize this distortion, patterns should never be left off the die, and they should be invested as soon as possible after fabrication.

Wax Pattern Fabrication

Armamentarium

1. PKT (Thomas) waxing instruments (no. 1, no. 2, no. 3, no. 4, and no. 5)
2. Beavertail burnisher
3. No. 7 wax spatula
4. Sable brush
5. No. 2 pencil
6. Laboratory knife with no. 25 blade
7. Cotton pliers
8. Bunsen burner
9. Inlay casting wax
10. Zinc stearate powder
11. Die lubricant

Coping Fabrication

The first step in making a wax pattern is the fabrication of a thin coping, or thimble, on the die. The coping is usually made of wax, but heated resin sheets also can be used for this purpose. Vacuum-adapted polystyrene[2] and pressure-formed polypropylene[3] have been used to make metal-ceramic crown patterns. This type of coping also can be used with partial veneer crowns[4] and even pin-retained castings.[5] If the coping is made on a separate die, it then will be transferred to the articulated working cast, where it will serve as the foundation for the axial contours and occlusal morphology to be added there. If it is formed on a removable die, the die is replaced in the master cast.

To prevent the wax from sticking to the die stone, coat the die thoroughly with die lubricant and allow it to soak in for several minutes (Fig 19-1). If the surface of the die appears dry after this period of time, repeat the application. Remove any excess lubricant with a gentle stream of compressed air.

Flow wax over the surface of the preparation on the die, using quick strokes of a hot no. 7 wax spatula (Fig 19-2). Overlap and remelt the margins of wax already

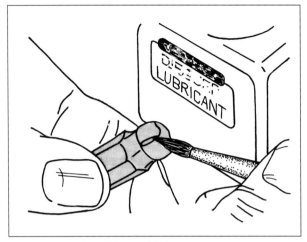

Fig 19-1 The die is lubricated before waxing.

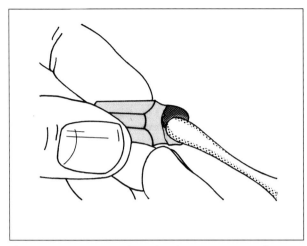

Fig 19-2 Wax coping is formed with a no. 7 wax spatula.

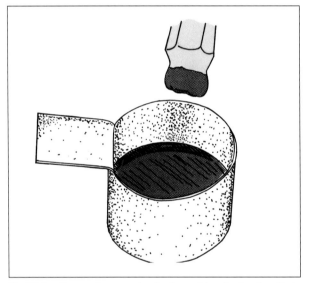

Fig 19-3 The coping can also be formed by dipping the die in molten wax.

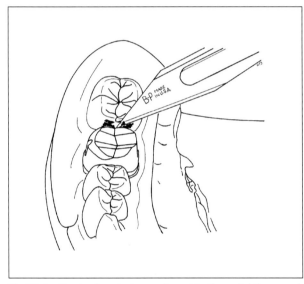

Fig 19-4 Proximal contacts on adjacent teeth are *lightly* scraped.

placed on the die. If small amounts of wax are placed on the die without remelting the edges of the previously applied wax, or if wax is applied with an instrument that is not hot enough, flow lines, or voids, will be produced on the internal surface of the wax pattern. Dipping the die into a small metal container filled with molten wax is yet another method that can be used for developing a uniform, thin initial coping of wax on the die (Fig 19-3).

To insure that the finished restoration will have adequate proximal contact with the teeth adjacent to it, the wax pattern should be *slightly* oversized mesiodistally. This will provide enough bulk in the contact areas to allow casting, finishing, and polishing without creating an open contact in the finished restoration. The best way of

achieving this is to remove a small amount of stone from the proximal surfaces of the teeth on the cast on either side of the prepared tooth. To control the amount of stone removed from the proximal surfaces of the cast, blacken them with a no. 2 pencil. Then use a laboratory knife with a sharp no. 25 blade to scrape off the graphite (Fig 19-4).

If using a separate die, lubricate the working cast and place the wax coping on it. It may be necessary to remove the wax 1.0 mm from the marginal periphery of the pattern to insure that it will seat all the way on the working cast. Stone also may be removed from the area of the cast that reproduces gingiva adjacent to the finish line of the prepared tooth.

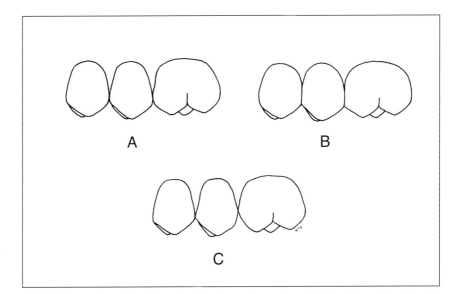

Fig 19-5 Occlusogingival dimension of proximal contacts: A, correct; B, too large; C, too small.

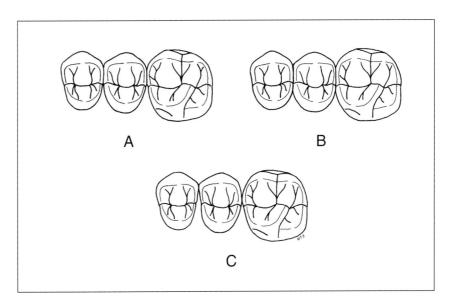

Fig 19-6 Faciolingual dimension of proximal contacts: A, correct; B, too broad; C, too narrow.

Axial Contours

The proximal contacts and the facial and lingual axial contours of the wax pattern should be established at this time. The proximal contacts of posterior teeth are located in the occlusal third of the crowns, except for the contacts between the maxillary first and second molars, which are located in the middle third.[6] The contact must be more than just a point occlusogingivally, but it must not extend far enough cervically to encroach on the gingival embrasure (Fig 19-5). The axial surface of the crown cervical to the proximal contact should be flat or slightly concave. There can be no encroachment upon the interdental papilla.[7,8] A flat contour may be the optimum shape because it is easiest to floss.[9] Overcontouring of the proximal surfaces apical to the contacts by making these areas convex will produce severe inflammation of the gingiva.[10]

The proximal contacts are located slightly to the facial aspect of the middle of the posterior teeth, except for the contacts between maxillary first and second molars, which are generally centered faciolingually.[6] As a result, the lingual embrasures are slightly larger than the facial embrasures. Contacts that are too narrow allow fibrous foods to wedge between the teeth, and contacts that are excessively wide faciolingually do not adequately deflect food from the gingival tissue (Fig 19-6).

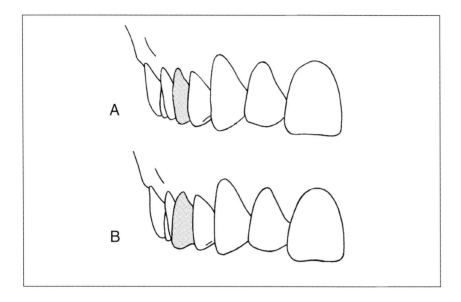

Fig 19-7 Facial contours of a restoration should be in harmony with those of adjacent teeth: A, correct; B, incorrect.

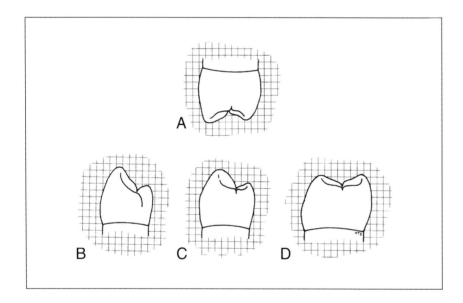

Fig 19-8 Height of contour on the facial surface of all posterior teeth extends horizontally 0.5 mm beyond the plane of the root. On the lingual surface of maxillary teeth (A) and mandibular first premolars (B), the height of contour also extends 0.5 mm, but it increases to 0.75 mm on mandibular second premolars (C) and 1.0 mm on mandibular molars (D).

The corresponding surfaces of the adjacent teeth make an excellent guide for judging the contours of the facial and lingual surfaces of the wax pattern. If these teeth are in a position that is nearly normal, and if they have not been subjected to poorly contoured axial restorations, the facial and lingual contours of the wax pattern should be harmonious with them (Fig 19-7).

The height of contour on the facial surface of posterior teeth usually occurs in the cervical third. It also occurs in the cervical third on the lingual surface of maxillary premolar and molars; but on mandibular teeth, it occurs in the middle third. The facial contours of both maxillary and mandibular posterior teeth extend approximately 0.5 mm beyond the outline of the root at the cementoenamel junction (Fig 19-8). The amount of lingual prominence differs between maxillary and mandibular teeth. It is 0.5 mm on maxillary teeth and mandibular first premolars, about 0.75 mm on mandibular second premolars, and nearly 1.0 mm on mandibular molars.[11]

Emergence Profile

The part of the axial contour that extends from the base of the gingival sulcus past the free margin of the gingiva has been described as the *emergence profile* by Stein and Kuwata[12] (Fig 19-9). The emergence profile extends to the height of contour, producing a straight profile in the

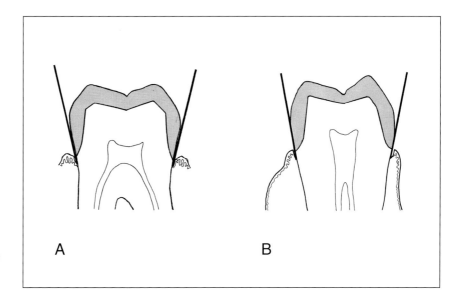

Fig 19-9 Emergence profile of the proximal surfaces (A) and of the facial and lingual contours (B).

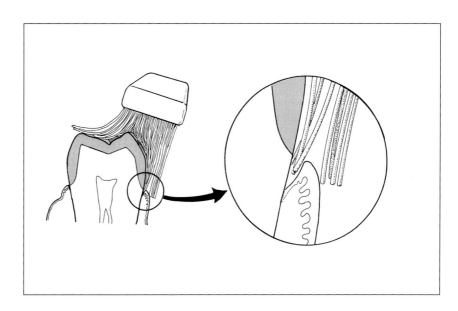

Fig 19-10 A straight emergence profile allows toothbrush bristles to reach into the gingival sulcus.

gingival third of the axial surface. The apparent curvature of an axial surface usually breaks down into a series of intersecting straight lines when it is examined closely. This has been confirmed by photographic analysis of several hundred natural teeth.[13] Production of a straight profile should be a treatment objective in restoring a tooth,[14,15] because it facilitates access for oral hygiene measures (Fig 19-10). The straight profile is easily evaluated with a periodontal probe.

The most common error relating to axial contour is the creation of a bulge or excessive convexity (Fig 19-11). Parkinson[16] reported that metal-ceramic crowns had a mean faciolingual width of 0.71 mm greater than that of unrestored contralateral teeth serving as controls. Full

gold crowns were 0.36 mm wider. Facial and lingual contours of teeth have been described in some detail.[11,17] Through the years, undue importance probably has been attributed to a "protective" role of the axial contour in the cervical region. As a result, both dentists and dental technicians frequently create a bulge where there should be none, as well as place it apically in the cervical region. Overcontoured restorations with large convexities promote the accumulation of food debris and plaque, and gingival inflammation is encouraged rather than prevented.[10,18-25]

There does not seem to be any justification for a "protective bulge." The small amount of facial bulge that exists in primary and adolescent human teeth and the

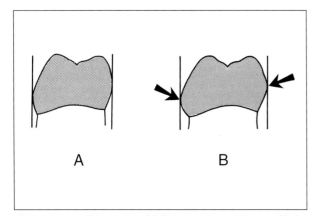

Fig 19-11 Axial contours of full veneer crowns on mandibular molars: A, correct; B, overcontoured.

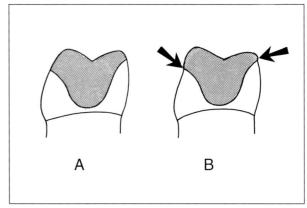

Fig 19-12 Restoration contours should blend smoothly with the contours of surrounding tooth structure: A, correct; B, incorrect.

dentitions of other species lies subgingivally without any apparent trauma to the gingiva from lack of "protection." Peg lateral incisors also lack cervical bulges, but they exhibit no deleterious gingival effects.[21] In addition, many clinicians have observed the phenomenon of prepared teeth that have gone without provisional restorations for a considerable amount of time with no gingival overgrowth or inflammation.

Experimental data indicate that while overcontouring produces gingival inflammation, undercontouring does not. In a study on dogs, Perel[26] found that overcontouring produced inflammatory and hyperplastic changes in 4 weeks, while undercontouring produced no significant changes. This was subsequently verified in human subjects by Sackett and Guildenhuys,[23] who found that the gingiva around nearly two-thirds of overcontoured restorations showed degradation, inflammation, and alteration of morphology 6 to 7 weeks after restoration placement. Because of its destructive potential, overcontouring should be avoided. It is better to undercontour than to overcontour.[24,26,27]

If the restoration is an onlay or a partial veneer crown, the areas in which it meets the axial surface of the tooth should be blended into smooth, continuous contours (Fig 19-12). Bulges, depressions, and other discrepancies should be eliminated in the wax pattern before proceeding to investing and casting.

Occlusal Morphology

Waxing of the occlusal surface is deferred until the axial surfaces are essentially complete. Since the occlusal scheme for the restoration is established in the wax pattern, no discussion of wax patterns would be complete without mention of occlusal theory and the effects of articulation on the occlusal surface of the wax pattern.

During centric closure in the normal dentition, the lingual cusps of the maxillary posterior teeth and the buccal cusps of the mandibular posterior teeth make contact with the occlusal fossae or the marginal ridges of the opposing teeth. They grind food like a mortar during mastication and are called *functional cusps*. On the other hand, the buccal cusps of the maxillary molars and the lingual cusps of the mandibular molars do not contact the opposing teeth. These cusps act like the rim of a pestle to prevent food from overflowing, and they protect the buccal mucosa and the tongue by keeping them away from the functional cusps. Since these cusps do not make direct contact with opposing teeth, they are called *nonfunctional cusps*.

The occlusal scheme can be classified by the location of the occlusal contact made by the functional cusp on the opposing tooth in centric relation (Table 19-1). There are two types: *cusp-fossa* (Fig 19-13, A) and *cusp–marginal ridge* (Fig 19-13, B). The locations of the occlusal contacts in each type are listed in Tables 19-2 and 19-3.

Cusp–Marginal Ridge Arrangement

The cusp–marginal ridge relation is the type of occlusal scheme in which the functional cusp contacts the opposing occlusal surfaces on the marginal ridges of the opposing pair of teeth, or in a fossa (Fig 19-14). Therefore, a cusp–marginal ridge occlusion is basically a one-tooth-to-two-teeth arrangement. Since the majority of adults exhibit the cusp–marginal ridge type of occlusion, it is an occlusal pattern widely utilized in daily practice.

The waxing technique used for cusp–marginal ridge occlusion was originally devised by E.V. Payne and was the first wax-added technique for functional waxing.[28] The same technique, modified by the use of color-coded waxes, has become a widely used method for teaching functional waxing.[29]

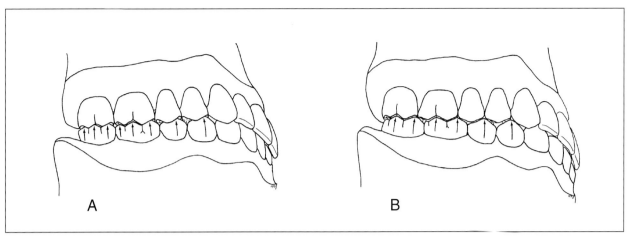

Fig 19-13 Cusp alignment for a cusp-fossa occlusion (A) and a cusp-marginal ridge occlusion (B).

Table 19-1 *Classification of Occlusal Arrangements*

	Cusp-fossa	Cusp–marginal ridge
Location of occlusal contact on opposing teeth	Occlusal fossae only	Marginal ridges and occlusal fossae
Relation with opposing tooth (teeth)	Tooth-to-tooth	Tooth–to–two teeth
Advantages	Occlusal forces are directed parallel with the long axis of the tooth; these forces are near the center of the tooth, placing very little lateral stress on the tooth	This is the most natural type of occlusion and is found in 95% of all adults; it can be used for single restorations
Disadvantages	Since this type of occlusion is rarely found in natural teeth, it usually can be used only when restoring several contacting teeth and the teeth opposing them	Food impaction and the displacement of teeth may arise if the functional cusps wedge into a lingual embrasure
Application	Full mouth reconstruction	Most cast restorations done in daily practice

Table 19-2 *Mandibular Cusp Placement*

Mandibular buccal cusps	Maxillary occlusal surfaces	
	Cusp–marginal ridge	Cusp-fossa
First premolar	Mesial marginal ridge of the first premolar	Mesial fossa of the first premolar
Second premolar	Distal marginal ridge of the first premolar and mesial marginal ridge of the second premolar	Mesial fossa of the second premolar
Mesiobuccal cusp of the first molar	Distal marginal ridge of the second premolar and mesial marginal ridge of the first molar	Mesial fossa of the first molar
Distobuccal cusp of the first molar	Central fossa of the first molar	Central fossa of the first molar
Distal cusp of the first molar	Usually nonfunctional	Distal fossa of the first molar
Mesiobuccal cusp of the second molar	Distal marginal ridge of the first molar and the mesial marginal ridge of the second molar	Mesial fossa of the second molar
Distobuccal cusp of the second molar	Central fossa of the second molar	Central fossa of the second molar
Distal cusp of the second molar	Usually not present	Usually nonfunctional

Table 19-3 *Maxillary Cusp Placement*

Maxillary lingual cusps	Mandibular occlusal surfaces	
	Cusp–marginal ridge	Cusp-fossa
First premolar	Distal fossa of the first premolar	Distal fossa of the first premolar
Second premolar	Distal fossa of the second premolar	Distal fossa of the second premolar
Mesiolingual cusp of the first molar	Central fossa of the first molar	Central fossa of the first molar
Distolingual cusp of the first molar	Distal marginal ridge of the first molar and mesial marginal ridge of second molar	Distal fossa of the first molar
Mesiolingual cusp of the second molar	Central fossa of the second molar	Central fossa of the second molar
Distolingual cusp of the second molar	Distal marginal ridge of the second molar	Distal fossa of the second molar

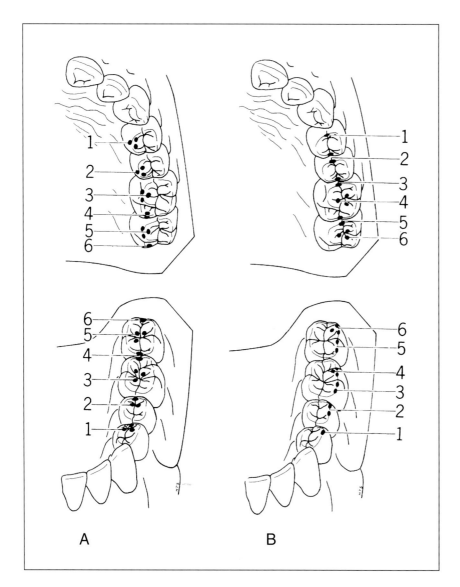

Fig 19-14 Cusp placement and occlusal contacts for a cusp–marginal ridge occlusion: A, contacts of maxillary lingual cusps on mandibular teeth; B, contacts of mandibular buccal cusps on maxillary teeth. The cusps and the matching areas of contact on the opposing teeth are numbered sequentially from anterior (1) to posterior (6).

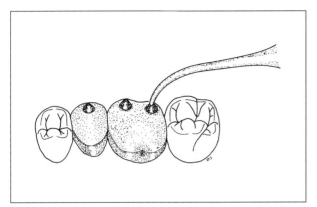

Fig 19-15   Cones for buccal cusps: PKT no 1.

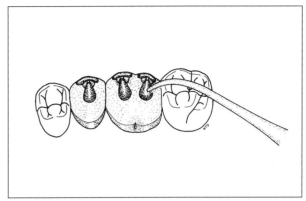

Fig 19-16   Buccal ridges and triangular ridges: PKT no. 1.

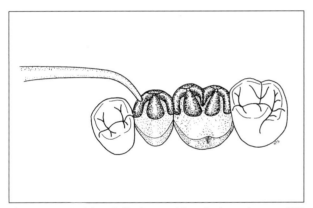

Fig 19-17   Mesial and distal cusp ridges for buccal cusps: PKT no. 1.

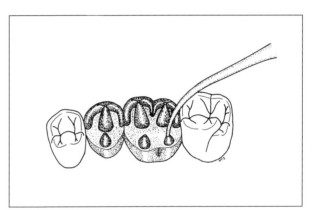

Fig 19-18   Cones for lingual cusps: PKT no. 1.

Cusp–Marginal Ridge for Maxillary Teeth

When making a maxillary wax pattern, place cones for the buccal cusps with a PKT no. 1 instrument. They should be placed as far buccally as possible (Fig 19-15). The length of a maxillary buccal cusp is determined by moving the articulator into a protrusive and a working lateral excursion. The tip should be shortened so that it *barely* misses the opposing mandibular cusp tip, if a canine-protected occlusion is being developed. If the cusp tips of the wax pattern are longer than the cusps of adjacent natural teeth, shorten the cones on the pattern.

Form the buccal ridges of the buccal cusps by adding wax to the buccal aspect of the buccal cones (Fig 19-16). These ridges, when viewed in profile from the mesial, give the buccal surface its proper overall contour. Add the triangular ridges with a PKT no. 1 instrument. Each triangular ridge extends from the central groove of the tooth to the cusp tip. These ridges are called triangular

because they are much wider at their base than at the cusp tip. They should be convex to allow for occlusal contact points. Check for occlusal contacts on the triangular ridges. Dust the occlusal surface with zinc stearate. Then close the articulator and move it through excursions. Remove unwanted contacts and trim those that are too large.

Form mesial and distal cusp ridges on each cone with the PKT no. 1. These ridges should form inclines away from the cusp tip (Fig 19-17). Place the articulator into lateral and protrusive excursions to check the mesial and distal ridges. The inclines of these ridges should mirror the inclines of the mesial and distal cusp ridges of the opposing teeth. The inclines of the cusp ridges on the maxillary wax pattern should not touch the opposing teeth.

Position the cones for the lingual (functional) cusps (Fig 19-18). Each cone should be located mesiodistally so that it will be in line with the opposing fossa or mar-

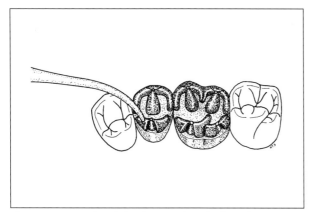

Fig 19-19   Mesial and distal cusp ridges for lingual cusps: PKT no. 1.

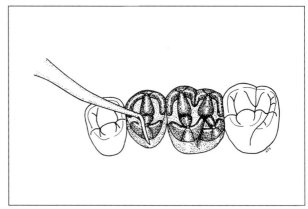

Fig 19-20   Lingual ridges and triangular ridges: PKT no. 1 and no. 4.

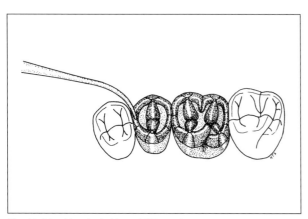

Fig 19-21   Marginal ridges: PKT no. 1.

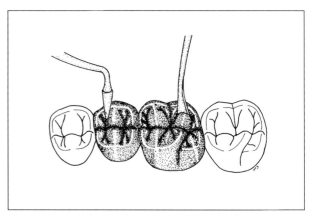

Fig 19-22   Supplemental anatomy: PKT no. 3 and no. 5.

ginal ridge with which it should occlude. The cones for a maxillary premolar are usually located slightly mesial to the mesiodistal center of the tooth. The mesiolingual cones for molars are centered between the two buccal cusps. Each mesiolingual cusp should be located so that it will fall opposite the buccolingual center of the opposing tooth. Dust the cone with zinc stearate and close the articulator to check its height. Contacts should occur on the sides of the cone near the tip, but not actually on the tip itself.

Add the mesial and distal ridges to the lingual cusps with the PKT no. 1 (Fig 19-19). The addition of these ridges completes the lingual perimeters of the occlusal table. The cusp ridges diminish in height from the cusp tip to the marginal ridges. Dust the pattern with zinc stearate and check the occlusal contacts.

Add lingual ridges to the cusps to complete the lingual axial contour (Fig 19-20). Smooth them with a PKT no. 4. Also add triangular ridges to the cusps at this time. The triangular ridges should be convex to form contact points with opposing cusps.

Form marginal ridges by uniting the mesial and distal ridges of the buccal cusps with the mesial and distal ridges of the lingual cusps (Fig 19-21). The height is determined by the height of the cusp tips of the opposing teeth.

Supplemental anatomy is formed by the junction between triangular ridges and adjacent cusp or marginal ridges (Fig 19-22). Use the PKT no. 5 to refine the ridges, and smooth the grooves with a PKT no. 3. Do *not* carve the grooves with these instruments.

Cusp–Marginal Ridge for Mandibular Teeth

The buccal cusps of mandibular premolars are approximately one-third the mesiodistal width of the teeth. They are placed at the junction of the buccal one-third and the lingual two-thirds of the mandibular tooth (Fig 19-23). This positioning will place them near the buccolingual middle of the opposing teeth. They are placed mesiodistally so they will be in line with the opposing fossae or

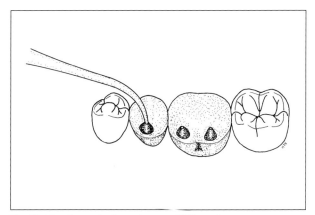

Fig 19-23   Cones for buccal cusps: PKT no. 1.

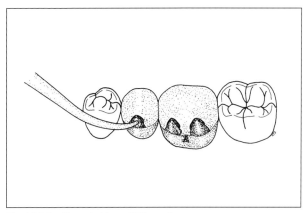

Fig 19-24   Buccal ridges: PKT no. 1.

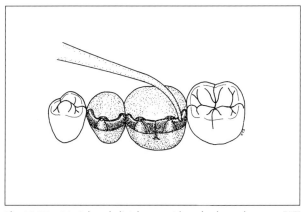

Fig 19-25   Mesial and distal cusp ridges for buccal cusps: PKT no. 1.

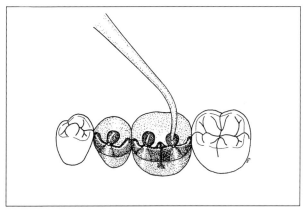

Fig 19-26   Triangular ridges: PKT no. 1.

marginal ridges with which they should occlude. The length of the mandibular buccal cusp is determined by contact in the fossa or on the marginal ridges of the maxillary teeth. Dust the cone with zinc stearate and close the articulator to adjust its height.

Place buccal ridges on the buccal cusps by applying wax from the tip of the cone to its base with a PKT no. 1 (Fig 19-24). This will produce the outline of the final contour of the buccal surface. Dust the pattern and check it in centric and lateral excursions to make sure that it is not overcontoured. Be careful not to melt the tips of the cones at this time.

Add mesial and distal ridges to the buccal cusps, and complete the buccal contour by blending these ridges into the buccal surface (Fig 19-25). Check the inclines of these new ridges for compatibility by moving the articulator through excursions.

Add triangular ridges to the buccal cusps with a PKT no. 1 (Fig 19-26). The base of these ridges should form the central groove of the occlusal surface. The ridges are convex to insure contact points with opposing teeth.

Next position the cones for the lingual (nonfunctional) cusps. They should be placed as far lingually as possible (Fig 19-27). To prevent working-side interferences on molars, place the cones as far apart mesiodistally as possible. On premolars position them mesially or distally to avoid any working-side interference. The lingual cusps should be shorter than the buccal cusps. In natural teeth, the lingual cusp is 3.3 mm shorter than the buccal cusp on the mandibular first premolar and 2.0 mm shorter than the buccal cusp on the mandibular second premolar.[30]

After all the mandibular lingual cusps have been placed, view them from the lingual as the articulator is moved through a working-side excursion. This insures that the lingual cusps will function opposite a maxillary embrasure or groove without interference.

Add lingual ridges to the lingual cusps to form the outline of the lingual contour. Then add broad-based, convex triangular ridges with a PKT no. 1 (Fig 19-28). They will converge *slightly* toward the central fossa. The contacts formed by each opposing cusp should form a *tripod* configuration.

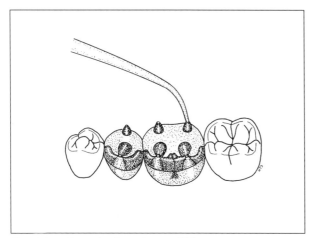

Fig 19-27 Cones for lingual cusps: PKT no. 1.

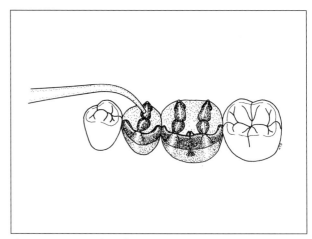

Fig 19-28 Triangular ridges: PKT no. 1.

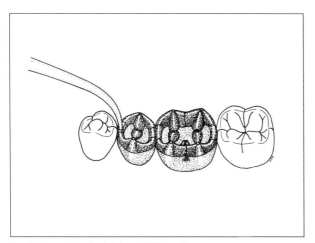

Fig 19-29 Marginal ridges: PKT no. 1.

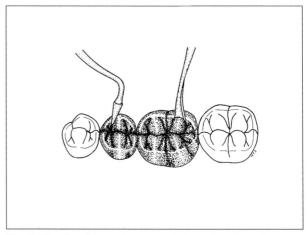

Fig 19-30 Supplemental anatomy: PKT no. 3 and no. 5.

Form marginal ridges by joining the buccal and lingual cusp ridges (Fig 19-29). The form of the mesial marginal ridges on mandibular premolars and first molars is determined arbitrarily, since they are not ordinarily in occlusion.[29] Smooth all grooves and fossae with the PKT no. 3 (Fig 19-30). Round and finish the ridges with the PKT no. 5.

Cusp-Fossa Arrangement

The cusp-fossa relation is an occlusal pattern in which each functional cusp is nestled into the occlusal fossa of the opposing tooth (Fig 19-31). It is a tooth-to-tooth arrangement. Although considered to be an ideal occlusal pattern, it is rarely found in its pure form in natural teeth.

Each centric cusp should make contact with the occlusal fossa of the opposing tooth at three points. The contact points are on the mesial and distal incline and the inner facing incline of the cusp, producing a tripod contact. Since the cusp tip itself never comes in contact with the opposing tooth, the cusp tip can be maintained for a long time with a minimum of wear.

The mandibular functional cusps arise opposite the middle (buccolingually) of the maxillary tooth. Similarly, the maxillary functional cusps are positioned halfway between the mandibular buccal and lingual cusp tips. Therefore, occlusal forces are transmitted along the long axes of the teeth.

The functional cusps of the maxillary posterior teeth become *slightly* shorter as they progress distally. Nonfunctional cusps are made slightly shorter than func-

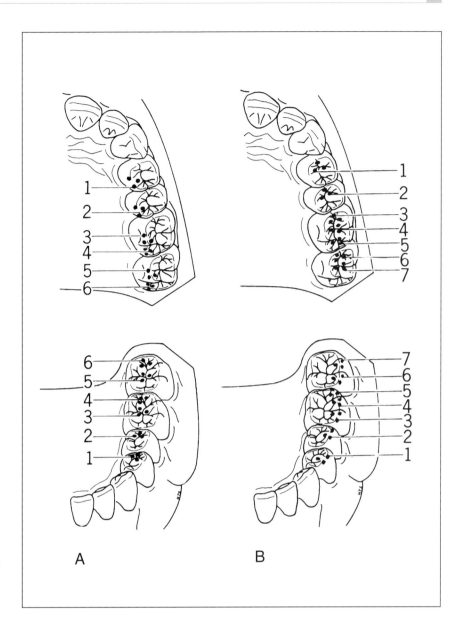

Fig 19-31 Cusp placement and occlusal contacts for a cusp-fossa occlusion: A, contacts of maxillary lingual cusps on mandibular teeth; B, contacts of mandibular cusps on maxillary teeth. The cusps and the matching areas of contact on the opposing teeth are numbered sequentially from anterior (1) to posterior (6 or 7).

tional cusps to insure clearance in excursive movements. The nonfunctional cusps also become slightly shorter from anterior to posterior. The resulting anteroposterior curvature of the occlusal plane is called the *curve of Spee*. Presence of this feature in a reconstructed mouth helps to prevent protrusive interferences. The left-right curvature resulting from the nonfunctional cusps being shorter than the functional cusps is the *curve of Wilson*. Its presence prevents interferences in lateral excursions.

The technique used for producing wax patterns with an exclusively cusp-fossa occlusion was developed by P.K. Thomas.[31] The method, as described in the following pages, will develop a cusp-fossa relationship. It is important to keep in mind, however, that the same technique, utilizing the same sequence of morphologic develop-

ment, can be used with excellent results for developing a cusp–marginal ridge occlusal relationship. When the cusp–marginal ridge arrangement is the desired end result, cusp placement is altered slightly.

The development of a cusp-fossa occlusion is best accomplished by waxing two opposing quadrants simultaneously. Therefore, this description will present the waxing of maxillary and mandibular occlusal surfaces in a concurrent stepwise progression. Locate the functional cusps first. The mandibular buccal cusps will nestle in the fossae of the opposing maxillary teeth. To accomplish this, place the cones for mandibular buccal cusps with a PKT no. 1 (Fig 19-32). They should be located approximately one-third the distance from the buccal to the lingual surface. Position them mesiodistally to fall into the appropriate fossae (see Table 19-2).

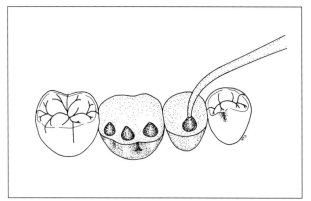

Fig 19-32   Cones for mandibular buccal cusps: PKT no. 1.

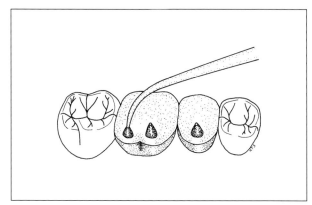

Fig 19-33   Cones for maxillary lingual cusps: PKT no. 1.

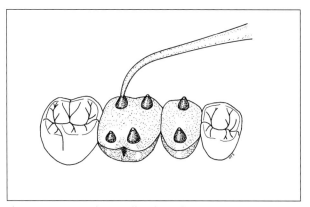

Fig 19-34   Cones for maxillary buccal cusps: PKT no. 1.

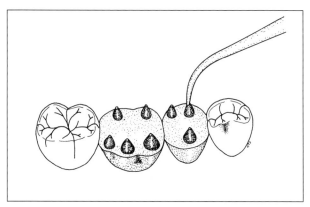

Fig 19-35   Cones for mandibular lingual cusps: PKT no. 1.

Then place the cones for the maxillary lingual cusps (Fig 19-33). Position them buccolingually so they will be over the middle of the opposing mandibular tooth. The mesiolingual cusp cones on the maxillary molars should be located as far distally as possible. The distolingual cones should have no contacts with opposing teeth.

Next place the nonfunctional cusps. The maxillary buccal cusp cones and the mandibular lingual cusp cones should be formed slightly shorter than the functional cusp cones (Fig 19-34). However, esthetic considerations should be given to the lengths of the buccal cusp cones of the maxillary premolars. Place the mandibular lingual cusps as far lingually and, on molars, as far from each other as possible (Fig 19-35). They are also shorter than the buccal cusps.

When nonworking movements are induced, the mesiolingual cusp cone of the maxillary molars should pass between the distal and the distobuccal cones of the mandibular teeth. During lateral excursions to the working side, the buccal cones of the maxillary premolars will pass distal to the buccal cones of the mandibular premolars.

Add the marginal ridges and cusp ridges (both mesial and distal) next, starting on the mesial of the maxillary

teeth, with a PKT no. 1 (Fig 19-36). The highest points on the occlusal surfaces are the tips of the cusp cones. The marginal ridges should never be higher than the cusps. Form the mandibular cusp and marginal ridges in a like manner, starting from the distal aspect (Fig 19-37). The cusp tips and the edges of the marginal ridges should be as sharp as possible. The buccolingual dimension of each occlusal table formed by the ridges should be approximately 55% of the overall buccolingual dimension of the respective tooth.

Dust the occlusal surfaces with zinc stearate and close the casts together on the articulator. The marginal ridges of opposing arches should be in close contact in the intercuspal position. Care must be taken to avoid leaving spaces between the maxillary and mandibular teeth. Place the side being waxed into both working and nonworking lateral excursions to remove any interferences.

During the working movement, the buccal cusp of each maxillary premolar passes distal to the buccal cusp of its counterpart in the mandibular arch. Therefore, it may be necessary to place a small depression in the distal incline of the buccal cusp of the mandibular premolar to allow the buccal cusp of the maxillary tooth to pass

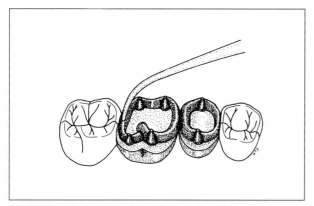

Fig 19-36 Maxillary marginal ridges and cusp ridges: PKT no. 1.

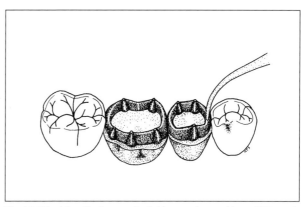

Fig 19-37 Mandibular marginal ridges and cusp ridges: PKT no. 1.

through easily without interference (Fig 19-38). This depression has been referred to as the "Thomas notch."

In a working excursion, the mesiobuccal cusp of a maxillary molar will pass through the buccal groove, distal to the mesiobuccal cusp of the mandibular molar. At the same time, the distobuccal cusp of the maxillary molar will pass through the distobuccal groove distal to the distobuccal cusp of the mandibular molar. The lingual cusps of the mandibular molars must be short enough so they will not collide with the cusps of the maxillary molars during the working movement.

Wax in the maxillary lingual ridges to provide the silhouette of the final contour of the lingual surface (Fig 19-39). Form the buccal cusp ridges on the mandibular buccal cusps in a similar manner (Fig 19-40). Use the PKT no. 1 to fill in any voids or discrepancies between the crest of the cusp ridges and the facial and lingual axial contours of the maxillary teeth. Smooth the contours with a PKT no. 4 (Fig 19-41). Repeat the process on the mandibular teeth (Fig 19-42). This completes the "fish's mouth," so named because of the appearance of the cusp and marginal ridges at this point.

Build up the triangular ridges for each of the cusps of the maxillary teeth with the PKT no. 1 (Fig 19-43). The bases of these ridges will form the central groove of the occlusal surface. The bases should be broader than the apex (at the cusp tip), and the ridges should be convex to provide contact points with the opposing cusps. Repeat the process for the mandibular cusps (Fig 19-44). Check the occlusion in the intercuspal position and the excursions as well.

Eliminate all voids remaining on the occlusal surface of the maxillary teeth (Fig 19-45). Place wax with a PKT no. 2. Supplemental anatomy is formed by the junction between the triangular ridge and the adjacent cusp or marginal ridges. Use the PKT no. 5 to refine the ridges. Follow the same procedure on the mandibular teeth (Fig 19-46). Developmental and supplemental grooves are formed in a combination of "U" and "V" shapes in cross section. Smooth the grooves with a PKT no. 3. Do *not* carve them with this instrument.

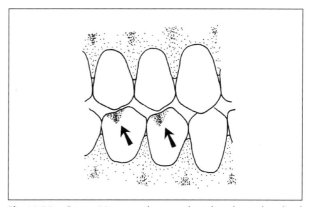

Fig 19-38 Concavities may have to be placed on the distal inclines of the buccal cusps of mandibular premolars *(arrows)* to accommodate the free passage of the buccal cusps of the maxillary premolars in a working-side excursion.

Dust the wax patterns with zinc stearate and check the occlusal contacts in the intercuspal and excursive positions. Tripod contacts should be formed about the cusp tips and in the fossae.

In nonworking movement, the mesiolingual cusp of a maxillary molar passes through the area distal to the distobuccal cusp of the mandibular molar (Fig 19-47). Therefore, a notch or groove should be formed on the distal incline of the distobuccal cusp. As a result, in a cusp-fossa occlusion, all mandibular molars are formed with three cusps.

At the same time, the distobuccal cusp of the mandibular molar moves in a mesiolingual direction across the buccal incline of the mesiolingual cusp of the maxillary molar (Fig 19-48). This may produce a nonworking interference. To prevent such an interference, it is often necessary to place a groove on the mesiolingual cusp of the maxillary molar. This groove, often referred to as "Stuart's groove," begins in the central fossa and is directed mesiolingually. It provides an escapeway for the mandibular distobuccal cusp in a nonworking movement.

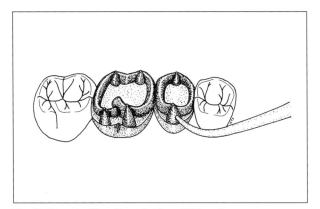

Fig 19-39   Maxillary lingual ridges: PKT no. 1.

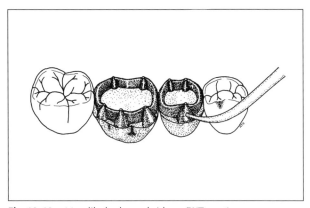

Fig 19-40   Mandibular buccal ridges: PKT no. 1.

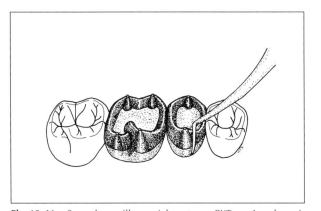

Fig 19-41   Smooth maxillary axial contours: PKT no. 1 and no. 4.

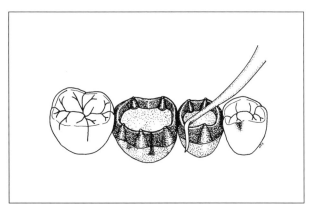

Fig 19-42   Smooth mandibular axial contours: PKT no. 1 and no. 4.

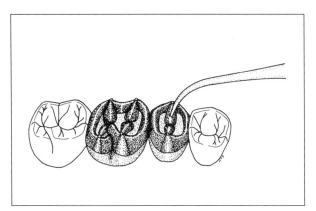

Fig 19-43   Maxillary triangular ridges: PKT no. 1.

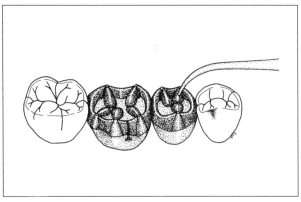

Fig 19-44   Mandibular triangular ridges: PKT no. 1.

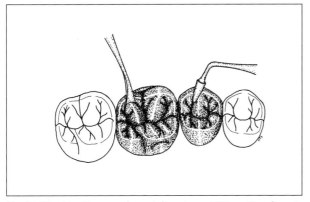 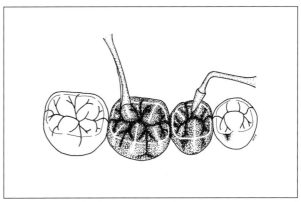

Fig 19-45 Maxillary supplemental anatomy: PKT no. 3 and no. 5.

Fig 19-46 Mandibular supplemental anatomy: PKT no. 3 and no. 5.

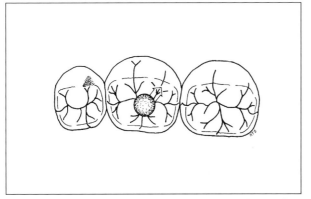 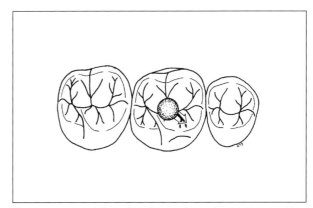

Fig 19-47 Path followed by the mesiolingual cusp of a maxillary molar on the occlusal surface of a mandibular molar during a nonworking excursion.

Fig 19-48 Path followed by the distobuccal cusp of a mandibular molar on the occlusal surface of a maxillary molar during a nonworking excursion.

Margin Finishing

Remove the pattern from the working cast and place it back on the freshly lubricated die. Make certain that the red line on the die finish line is still distinct. Smooth any roughness on the axial surfaces with a slightly warm beavertail burnisher. Remelt the entire marginal periphery with a hot PKT no. 1, making sure that the wax is melted through to the die (Fig 19-49).

This will result in a depression or "trough" 1 to 2 mm wide and·extending along the entire length of the marginal periphery of the wax pattern (Fig 19-50). Eliminate the depression by adding wax with a hot beavertail burnisher (Fig 19-51).

Carve the excess wax almost to the margin with a PKT no. 4 (Fig 19-52). Finish "carving" the margin with a warm beavertail burnisher (Fig 19-53). The instrument and the way in which it is used results in a combination of melting, burnishing, and carving of the margins.

The reader may, in time, develop a technique with specific instruments that differs from those above. One principle is of paramount importance: *Do not approach the finish line on the die with a sharp instrument.* Any sharp instrument that can remove die material as the wax margins are carved will produce a casting that will not fit the prepared tooth.

The margin is a critically important area of any wax pattern. While a good margin may not insure the success of a casting, a poor one can almost guarantee its failure.

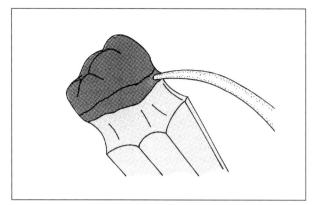

Fig 19-49   Margin is remelted with a PKT no. 1.

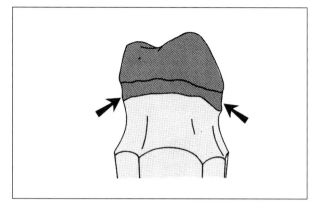

Fig 19-50   A depression *(arrows)* remains near the margin.

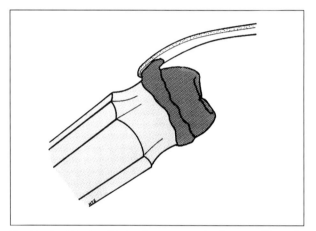

Fig 19-51   Wax is added to the margin with a beavertail burnisher.

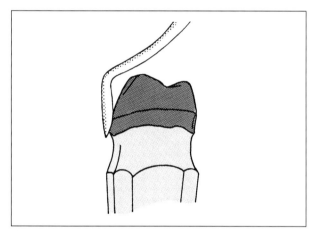

Fig 19-52   Excess wax is removed with a PKT no. 4.

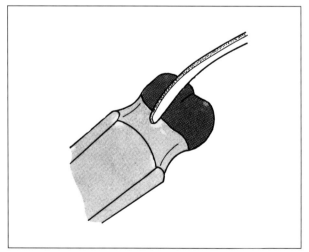

Fig 19-53   Margins are finished with a beavertail burnisher.

Check the margin carefully for the following discrepancies:

1. *Overwaxed margins.* Areas in which wax has been carried past the finish line may break off when a pattern is withdrawn from the die, resulting in a short, or "shy" margin. If the overwaxed area does not break during withdrawal of the pattern, it may spring back. When cast in metal, this area will no longer bend as it once did in wax, and the casting may be prevented from seating all the way on the tooth.
2. *Short margins.* A margin that is not waxed all the way to the red finish line will not provide an adequate seal for the finished restoration.
3. *Ripples.* Any roughness in the wax near the margin will be duplicated in the casting. If allowed to remain on the finished, cemented restoration, these rough areas will serve as a collecting point for plaque and may lead to irritation and inflammation of the adjacent

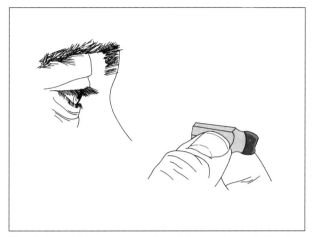

Fig 19-54 Finished margin is viewed from an "apical" direction.

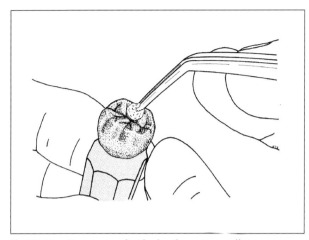

Fig 19-55 Grooves are finished with a cotton pellet.

gingival tissues. Do not count on being able to remove these irregularities once the casting has been made, since their elimination at that time frequently entails an undesirable change in contour.

4. *Thick margins.* A thick, rounded margin will result in poor sealing of the restoration and poor axial contours that will ultimately cause periodontal problems. The margin of a wax pattern must come to a fine edge.

5. *Open margins.* The open margin is a gremlin that haunts the wax pattern. It can be the result of any of the previously mentioned problems. Attention to detail is essential to produce closed margins. The wax pattern margins must be burnished and melted, as well as cut, to insure close adaptation of the wax to the die in the marginal area.

Carefully inspect the margin by turning the die so that the margin can be viewed from a gingival direction (Fig 19-54). This is one of the great advantages of the indirect technique. A properly trimmed die will aid in this inspection, just as it facilitated access to the margin during the marginal adaptation phase.

To finish the occlusal grooves, hold a very small cotton pellet in cotton pliers and dip it in the die lubricant. Run the pellet carefully through the grooves with the cotton pliers (Fig 19-55). Exercise caution so that the occlusal contacts so painstakingly developed in the waxing phase will not be destroyed.

To finish the axial surface use a cotton roll, one end of which has been dipped in die lubricant (Fig 19-56). Rub this end across the surfaces to be smoothed. Buff the dry end of the roll across the wet wax until a smooth surface is obtained. Do not employ excessive or prolonged buffing action near the margins; they will be destroyed in the process. Remove all lubricant from the pattern when polishing is completed. Any lubricant left on the pattern when it is invested can cause surface roughness in the casting.

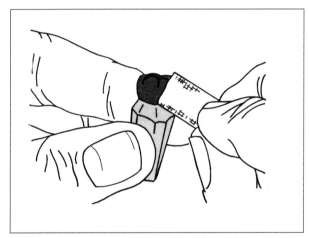

Fig 19-56 Axial surfaces are smoothed with a cotton roll dipped in die lubricant.

Depressions cannot be polished away. They can be removed only by removing the material around the depression, resulting in a change in contour. Depressions are better removed by filling them with wax and then smoothing them.

The purpose of finishing is to provide a smooth surface for casting. Tricks employed to polish the surface only serve to highlight the irregularities they seek to cover. Concentrate on a truly smooth surface—not a highly polished, irregular one. With a good investing and casting technique, the casting should be quite smooth and will require a minimum of finishing.

Wax is softer than metal. Anything that can be done in wax, as opposed to doing it later in metal, should be. In wax, anything can be done in a fraction of the time, with less effort, and with better results.

References

1. Phillips RW: *Skinner's Science of Dental Materials,* ed 9. Philadelphia, WB Saunders Co, 1991, p 387.

2. Weiss PA: New design parameters: Utilizing the properties of nickel-chromium superalloys. *Dent Clin North Am* 1977; 21:769–785.

3. El-Sherif MH, Shillingburg HT, Smith KS: A plastic shell technique for fabricating porcelain-fused-to-metal coping patterns. *Quint Dent Technol* 1987; 11:383–388.

4. Dumais MH: Use of polypropylene copings to simplify the waxing procedure for mesio-occlusodistal and partial veneer crowns. *Quintessence Int* 1990; 21:897–902.

5. Dumais MH: Using polypropylene copings to simplify the laboratory phase of making pin-retained castings. *QDT Yearbook* 1988; 12:135–139.

6. Burch JG, Miller JB: Evaluating crown contours of a wax pattern. *J Prosthet Dent* 1973; 30:454–458.

7. Skurow HM, Lytle JD: The interproximal embrasure: Wax pattern. *Dent Clin North Am* 1971; 15:641–647.

8. Tjan AHL, Freed H, Miller GD: Current controversies in axial contour design. *J Prosthet Dent* 1980; 44:536–540.

9. Burch JG: Ten rules for developing crown contours in restorations. *Dent Clin North Am* 1971; 15:611–618.

10. Morris ML: Artificial crown contours and gingival health. *J Prosthet Dent* 1962; 12:1146–1156.

11. Jordan RE, Abrams L: *Kraus' Dental Anatomy and Occlusion,* ed 2. St Louis, Mosby-Year Book, 1992, p 265.

12. Stein RS, Kuwata M: A dentist and a dental technologist analyze current ceramo-metal procedures. *Dent Clin North Am* 1977; 21:729–749.

13. Croll BM: Emergence profiles in natural tooth contour. Part I: Photographic observations. *J Prosthet Dent* 1989; 62:4–10.

14. Koidis PT, Burch JG, Melfi RC: Clinical crown contours: Contemporary view. *J Am Dent Assoc* 1987; 114:792–795.

15. Croll BM: Emergence profiles in natural tooth contour. Part II: Clinical considerations. *J Prosthet Dent* 1990; 63:374–379.

16. Parkinson CF: Excessive crown contours facilitate endemic plaque niches. *J Prosthet Dent* 1976; 35:424–429.

17. Ash MM: *Wheeler's Dental Anatomy, Physiology and Occlusion,* ed 7. Philadelphia, WB Saunders Co, 1993, p 119.

18. Herlands RE, Lucca JJ, Morris ML: Forms, contours, and extensions of full coverage restorations in occlusal reconstruction. *Dent Clin North Am* 1962; 6:147–162.

19. Hazen SP, Osborne JW: Relationship of operative dentistry to periodontal health. *Dent Clin North Am* 1967; 11:245–254.

20. Perel ML: Periodontal considerations of crown contours. *J Prosthet Dent* 1971; 26:627–630.

21. Yuodelis RA, Weaver JD, Sapkos S: Facial and lingual contours of artificial complete crown restorations and their effects on the periodontium. *J Prosthet Dent* 1973; 29:61–66.

22. Ehrlich J, Hochman N: Alterations on crown contour—Effect on gingival health in man. *J Prosthet Dent* 1980; 44:523–525.

23. Sackett BP, Gildenhuys RR: The effect of axial crown overcontour on adolescents. *J Periodontol* 1976; 47:320–323.

24. Jameson LM, Malone FP: Crown contours and gingival response. *J Prosthet Dent* 1982; 47:620–624.

25. Sorensen JA: A rationale for comparison of plaque-retaining properties of crown systems. *J Prosthet Dent* 1989; 62:264–269.

26. Perel ML: Axial crown contours. *J Prosthet Dent* 1971; 25:642–649.

27. Wagman SS: The role of coronal contour in gingival health. *J Prosthet Dent* 1977; 37:280–287.

28. Huffman RW: Occlusal morphology, in Guichet NF: *Procedures for Occlusal Treatment—A Teaching Atlas.* Anaheim, CA, Denar Corp, 1969, p 98.

29. Lundeen HC: *Introduction to Occlusal Anatomy.* Lexington, MA, Lexington Books, 1969.

30. Shillingburg HT, Kaplan MJ, Grace CS: Tooth dimensions—A comparative study. *J South Calif Dent Assoc* 1972; 40:830–839.

31. Thomas PK: *Syllabus on Full Mouth Waxing Technique for Rehabilitation.* San Diego, Instant Printing Services, 1967.

Chapter 20

The Functionally Generated Path Technique

The functionally generated path technique utilizes a different approach to achieve occlusal harmony between the restoration and the other teeth in the mouth. Rather than employing an articulator to simulate the movement of the mandible, this technique uses a tracing made in the mouth to capture the pathways traveled by the opposing cusps in mandibular function. In this situation, the articulator is reduced to the role of a simple hinge.

The functionally generated path technique is presented here as an alternative method for fabricating single-tooth restorations. It relies on recording in a simple, yet precise, manner the pathways traveled by the cusps in the border movements of the mandible. Wax is adapted over the occlusal surface of the prepared tooth. The patient occludes the teeth in an intercuspal position and moves the mandible through all excursions. By this process, the tips of the opposing cusps act as recording styli that carve, in three dimensions in wax, a record of the border movements in all mandibular positions.[1] Stone is brushed and poured onto the wax record in the mouth to produce a functional core. The stone core is then utilized in the fabrication of posterior tooth restorations.

This method was first described by Meyer as a means of obtaining the "functional occlusal path" for bridges fabricated by a direct/indirect technique[2] and for dentures.[3] At one time it was identified quite strongly with bilateral balanced occlusion, but it is also possible to use the technique to obtain a unilateral balanced occlusion or a mutually protected occlusion.

The technique does have the advantage of permitting simple, inexpensive instrumentation for single-tooth restorations. This constitutes an appropriate use for the straight line articulator.[4,5] It demands a minimum of chair time, especially during the try-in and cementation phase.[6] Finally, it is a relatively easy technique to learn.

The technique was adapted for use in complete occlusal rehabilitation by Mann and Pankey.[7-10] Based on a spherical theory of occlusion, calipers are used to locate a center of rotation. From this center, the mandibular diagnostic cast is reduced to bring the occlusal surfaces of the mandibular teeth into harmony with the surfaces of the theoretical sphere, with a uniform amount of reduction (1.6 mm). Buccal and lingual preparation plane guides are made on the diagnostic cast to permit duplication of the reduction in the mouth.

After the mandibular teeth in the mouth have been reduced and subsequently restored to an ideal plane, a functionally generated recording of the mandibular cusp paths is made. It is used to produce a stone functional core or index against which the maxillary restorations are fabricated. In this manner, the mandibular and maxillary teeth are restored separately. This stepwise approach to occlusal rehabilitation offers a definite financial advantage to the patient. The treatment, and therefore the cost to the patient, can be spread out over a longer period of time.

A prerequisite for the use of this technique for the restoration of a single tooth is the presence of an optimal occlusion. The technique perpetuates existing occlusion, good or bad. Correct anterior guidance must be present and there must be an absence of posterior interferences when the restoration is made. If there are any interferences, they will guide the mandible and help perpetuate the occlusal discrepancy. There can be no missing or broken down opposing teeth. Badly rotated, carious, or poorly restored teeth will not provide the occlusal pathways needed for shaping the occlusal surface.

Functional Core and Wax Pattern Fabrication

Armamentarium for Functional Tracing

1. Petrolatum
2. Cotton-tipped applicator
3. Cavity varnish
4. Tacky wax
5. PKT waxing instruments
6. Bunsen burner
7. Die lubricant
8. Mounting stone
9. Spatula
10. Plaster bowl
11. Sable brush
12. Functional index tray
13. Laboratory knife with no. 25 blade
14. Custom impression tray
15. Impression material (base and accelerator)

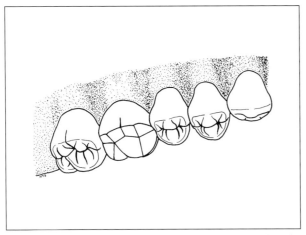

Fig 20-1 The tooth is ready for the functional tracing when the occlusal reduction is completed.

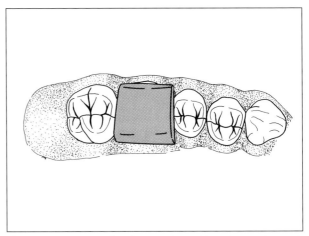

Fig 20-2 A square of tacky wax is positioned over the tooth being prepared.

16. Mixing pad
17. Syringe
18. Bite registration frame
19. Bite registration paste
20. Die stone
21. Di-Lok tray
22. Twin-Stage Occluder

Fabrication of Functional Core

Equilibrate the occlusion to eliminate all posterior interferences. Evaluate and note working-side tooth contacts to determine whether they form a mutually protected (canine guidance) or unilaterally balanced (group function) occlusion. This is essential to assist in determining the type of occlusal scheme to be produced in the final restoration.

The technique to be described is primarily for use in fabricating restorations on maxillary teeth. It can be used for restorations on mandibular teeth, but only if the occlusal contours of the maxillary teeth have been perfected first.[11]

Begin the preparation for the cast restoration by doing the occlusal reduction (Fig 20-1). Before proceeding on, however, the functional tracing should be made. The larger occlusal table that is present before axial reduction will afford greater stability to the wax tracing.

Apply petrolatum with a cotton-tipped applicator to the occlusal surfaces of the opposing quadrant. Apply cavity varnish (Copalite, Teledyne Getz, Elk Grove Village, IL) to the occlusal surface of the prepared tooth to help the wax to adhere more securely. Cut a piece of wax

(Synthetic Tacky Wax, Harry J Bosworth Co, Skokie, IL) in a square slightly larger than the occlusal surface of the tooth being restored. Attach the square of wax to a PKT no. 2 waxing instrument and soften it over a Bunsen burner flame. While the varnish on the occlusal surface is still sticky and the wax is soft, tack the wax to the tooth being restored (Fig 20-2).

Guide the patient into a retruded closure in centric relation (Fig 20-3). Then guide the patient through all excursions, moving first into working (Fig 20-4). From a working excursion, guide the patient back to centric relation and then into a nonworking movement (Fig 20-5). Have the patient return again to centric relation and then into protrusive (Fig 20-6). The patient should be guided through combination movements as well: working protrusive and nonworking protrusive. Finally, the patient should just "mill around" to ensure adequate clearance for the opposing cusps in function.

Have the patient open. Remove any excess tacky wax that has been displaced onto the occlusal surfaces of adjacent teeth. Examine the wax to see that it is still firmly attached to the prepared tooth. Stability of the tracing is extremely important; any movement of the tracing will result in an inaccurate core. Numerous solutions have been offered for this problem, ranging from cast bases to intraoral bandages.[12] The tacky wax should remain in position over the single prepared tooth without any other devices, but it is best to check it frequently. If it has been jarred loose, repeat the process. The patient should repeat all excursions and combinations of mandibular movements. Then inspect the surface of the wax to make sure that there are no voids.

A tray of some sort should be used to hold the stone in place in the mouth to make the functional core. Tongue

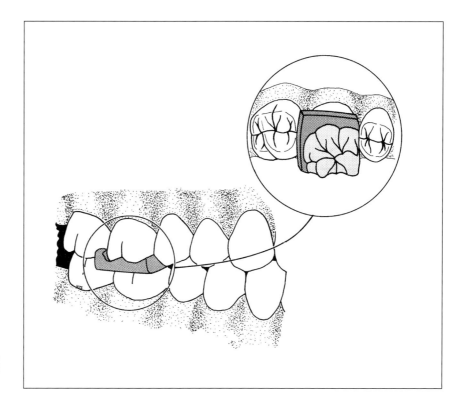

Fig 20-3 The tracing is begun by having the patient close in the retruded position.

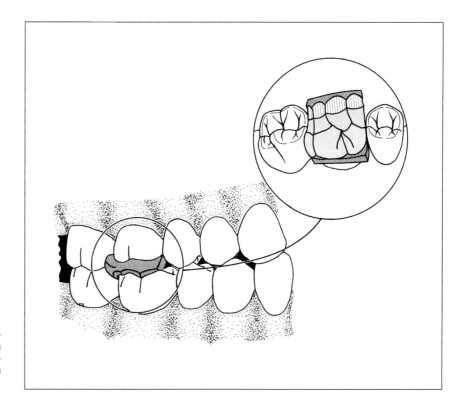

Fig 20-4 Paths of the cusps in working excursion are recorded. The area and direction of these excursive movements are demonstrated by fine lines in the inset.

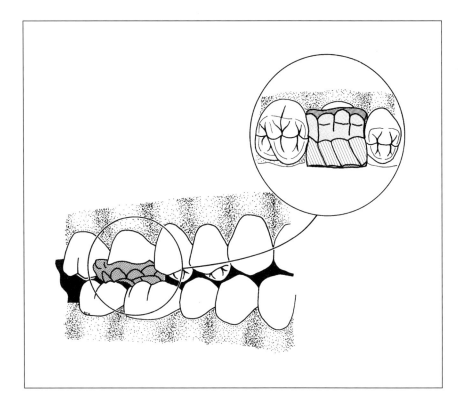

Fig 20-5 Paths of the cusps in the nonworking excursion are recorded next.

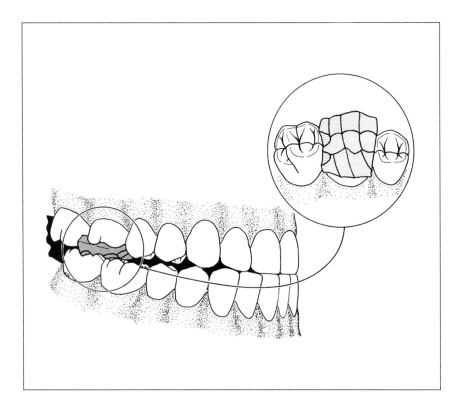

Fig 20-6 Protrusive paths are recorded last.

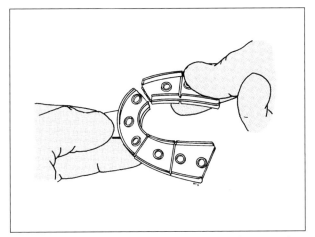

Fig 20-7 Unneeded portion of the functional index tray is broken off.

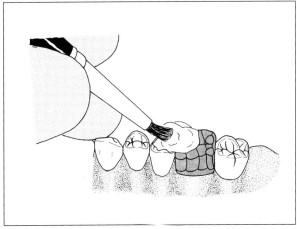

Fig 20-8 The functional core is begun by brushing mounting stone on the functional tracing.

blades and denture tooth cards can be employed for this purpose, but a functional index tray (Index Tray, Crown Enterprises, Oklahoma City, OK) offers definite advantages. It is curved to fit the arch, and it has undercuts to hold the stone in position. The tray should extend to include the anterior teeth for added stability. Break off the unneeded portion and discard it (Fig 20-7).

Paint the wax with a die lubricant (Microfilm, Kerr Manufacturing Co, Romulus, MI) to reduce surface tension and insure a smooth, complete functional core. Make a creamy mix of mounting stone and paint it on the surface of the functional wax tracing with a sable brush (Fig 20-8). Be especially careful not to incorporate any voids between the wax and the stone. Load the functional index tray with a layer of mounting stone 6.0 mm (0.25 inch) thick. Position it on the occlusal surfaces of the quadrant so that it covers at least one tooth on each side of the prepared tooth.

If the prepared tooth is the most distal tooth in the arch, the index should cover the three teeth mesial to the preparation. Carefully support the tray full of stone without any movement until it is set (Fig 20-9). Keep some of the unused stone on the spatula to use as an indicator for setting of the stone in the mouth. The procedure is very similar to that of making a plaster index for soldering.

When the stone has set, remove it and carefully examine its occlusal surface. It should be free of any bubbles or voids in the part that was formed by the tracings on the tacky wax. This stone replica of the movements of the cusp tips is called the *functional core*. It is also referred to as the *functional index* or the *counter die*.

Trim the surface of the core with a sharp laboratory knife (Fig 20-10). The indentations in the core produced by the occlusal surfaces of the teeth should be no more

than 3.0 mm deep. The rest of the tooth preparation should be completed at this time. Make an impression of the quadrant containing the prepared tooth, using a custom acrylic tray made previously (Fig 20-11).

It is possible to fabricate a restoration using only the functional core for an opposing model. It is very helpful, however, to have an anatomic cast against which you can occlude the wax pattern. This is especially helpful for the novice waxer who might have trouble recognizing various anatomic features on the functional core.

Obtain an occlusal registration at the intercuspal position using bite registration paste in a bite registration frame. Have the patient rehearse closing completely into a position of maximum intercuspation with nothing in the mouth. Try in the tray to make sure that the brace across its posterior end will not interfere with the closure of the most distal molars. Cover both sides of the gauze on the frame with a layer of zinc oxide–eugenol paste approximately 1 mm deep. Instruct the patient to close completely into the paste in the manner previously rehearsed. Steady the frame by holding onto the small handle projecting from the front end of it (Fig 20-12).

Allow the material to set for several minutes. Check the border with an instrument to see that it has set completely. Ask the patient to "snap open." Remove the frame and inspect the imprint of the mandibular teeth, which is actually a shallow impression in zinc oxide–eugenol paste, for completeness (Fig 20-13). Insert the temporary restoration and dismiss the patient.

Disinfect the functional core and the elastomeric impression. Pour the impression with die stone, forming a base approximately 20 mm (0.75 inch) thick. When the stone has set, remove the cast from the impression. Carefully position the functional core on the quadrant

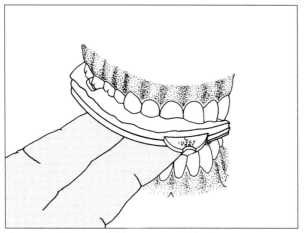

Fig 20-9   The tray is held in position while the stone sets.

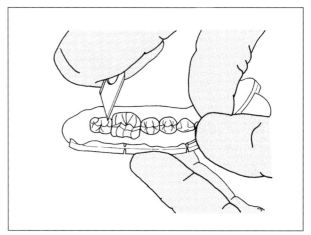

Fig 20-10   Excess mounting stone is trimmed from the functional core.

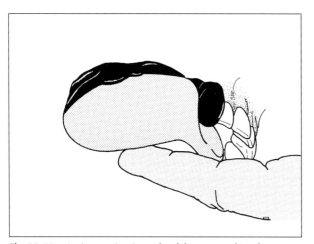

Fig 20-11   An impression is made of the prepared tooth.

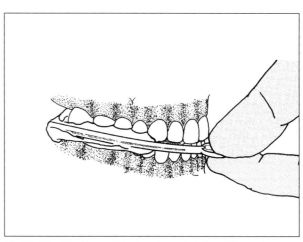

Fig 20-12   The bite registration frame is held while the bite registration paste sets.

cast of the prepared tooth. It should fit exactly. If there is any discrepancy or crack, however small, between the cast and the stone functional core, there will be an occlusal error in the restoration.

Attach a quadrant die tray (Di-Lok, Di-Equi Dental Products, Wappingers Falls, NY) with mounting stone to the lower member of an articulator with two upper members (Twin-Stage Occluder, Teledyne Hanau, Buffalo, NY). Trim the base of the cast containing the prepared tooth so the cast will fit into the die tray. The finish line of the tooth preparation should be about 0.25 inch above the top edge of the die tray.

Score the sides of the base of the cast with horizontal cuts to aid retention in the die tray. Soak the cast in water for a few minutes, keeping the teeth dry. Vibrate a mix of stone into the tray so that it is approximately two-thirds full. Insert the base of the cast into the stone, vibrating it

gently by hand to seat the cast completely (Fig 20-14). Be careful not to get any stone on the prepared tooth. Allow any excess stone to run over the sides of the Di-Lok tray. Carefully wipe away the excess and set the articulator aside to allow the stone in the tray to set.

Pour the remaining stone into the imprints of the mandibular teeth in the disinfected zinc oxide–eugenol bite registration. Place a small portion of wet stone on a paper towel and squeeze out the excess moisture to increase the body and stiffness of the stone. Create a base approximately 0.5 inch thick on the occlusal registration. Leave undercuts on the base for later attachment to the articulator.

Once again place the functional core on the cast in the die tray and confirm that it still fits accurately. Attach it to the cast with sticky wax. Move the incisal guide pin in or out of one of the upper members of the Twin-Stage

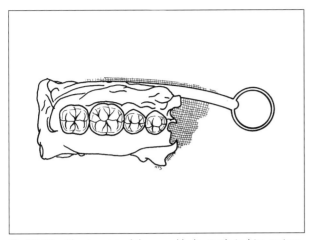

Fig 20-13 The imprint of the mandibular teeth in bite registration paste will be used to form the anatomic cast and to mount it.

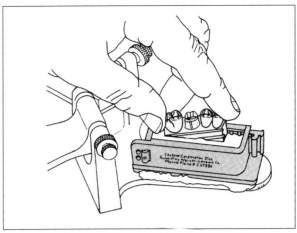

Fig 20-14 The cast is placed in wet stone in the Di-Lok tray.

Occluder until the upper member of the articulator clears the top of the functional core by 0.5 inch. Firmly tighten the set screw on the incisal guide pin. Check and tighten the locknut on the axis of each of the two upper members of the instrument. There must be absolutely *no* lateral play in the instrument; if there is, the occlusal surface of the wax pattern will be in error. Attach the functional core to that upper member of the articulator with mounting stone.

When the stone has set, open the articulator and remove all sticky wax from the teeth on the cast in the die tray. On the maxillary side of the zinc oxide–eugenol bite registration, trim away any small fins that fit into occlusal embrasures between the teeth. Carefully fit the zinc oxide–eugenol bite registration on the cast of the maxillary teeth in the Di-Lok tray. Make sure that it seats completely without any rocking or wobbling. Attach the registration to the teeth in the die tray with sticky wax. If the handle of the bite registration frame interferes with closure of the articulator, cut off the handle.

Adjust the incisal guide pin up or down on the other upper member of the Twin-Stage Occluder so the upper member of the articulator will clear the top of the anatomic cast by about 0.5 inch. Attach the anatomic cast to the upper member with mounting stone.

Remove the cast from the Di-Lok tray. Saw about halfway through the base from the occlusal surface on both the mesial and distal sides of the prepared tooth. Make facial and lingual cuts that are continuations of the occlusal cuts. Break the sections apart to isolate the die, then trim the die apical to the finish line. (Refer to Chapter 18 for a more complete description of the technique.) Mark the contact areas of the approximating teeth with a sharp no. 2 lead pencil. Lightly scrape the pencil marks with a laboratory knife to check for adequate bulk of material in the proximal contact areas of the finished casting. Reassemble the die and sections of the quadrant cast in the die tray.

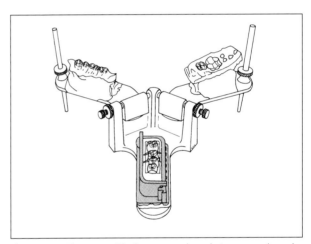

Fig 20-15 The cast with the prepared tooth is mounted on the lower member of the Twin-Stage Occluder. The anatomic cast is seen on the upper left member and the functional core on the upper right member.

The mounting is ready for the fabrication of the wax pattern. Mount the cast with the prepared tooth in the die tray on the lower member of the articulator (even if it is a maxillary cast). Mount the functional core on one of the upper members of the articulator and mount the anatomic cast on the other (Fig 20-15). The Verticulator (JF Jelenko, Armonk, NY) is another instrument that is made for use with the functionally generated path technique. It is extremely rigid and provides a precise alignment of cast and functional core. It also utilizes a second upper member (removable, not hinged) that can be employed with the anatomic cast. A plane line hinge articulator can be used for this purpose, but it does not permit the use of an anatomic cast.

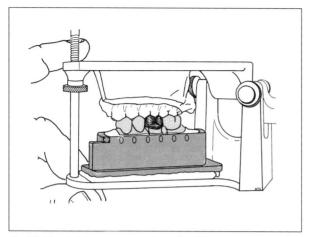

Fig 20-16 Axial contours and proximal contacts are checked before proceeding to the occlusal surface.

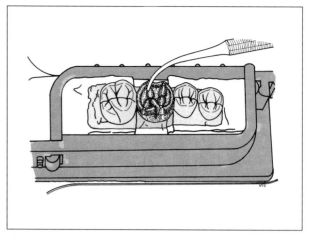

Fig 20-17 The wax-added technique is used to form the occlusal morphology.

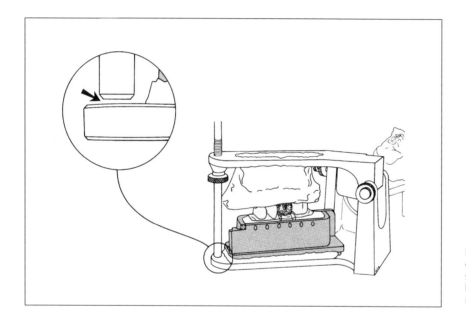

Fig 20-18 With the functional core closed against the wax pattern, there should be no discrepancy *(arrow)* between the guide pin and the lower member of the articulator.

Wax Pattern Armamentarium

1. Twin-Stage Occluder
2. Laboratory knife with no. 25 blade
3. Bunsen burner
4. Sable brush
5. No. 7 wax spatula
6. PKT (Thomas) waxing instruments (no. 1, no. 2, no. 3, no. 4, and no. 5)
7. Beavertail burnisher
8. Cotton pliers
9. Die lubricant
10. Inlay wax
11. White shoe polish
12. Cotton pellets
13. Cotton roll

Wax Pattern Fabrication

Remove the die from the Di-Lok tray and lubricate the preparation thoroughly with die lubricant. Allow it to soak in for several minutes and reapply if all of it is absorbed. Flow wax over the surface of the preparation on the die, using quick, overlapping strokes of a hot no. 7 wax spatula. Each time more wax is added, remelt that portion already on the die. Form the facial and lingual axial contours and the proximal contacts of the wax pattern at this time (Fig 20-16). Be especially careful to avoid overcontouring of the axial surfaces.

Initially, the occlusal portion of the wax pattern should be waxed against the anatomic cast to aid in visualizing cusp location more effectively. The wax-added technique can be used to position the cones for the cusp tips.

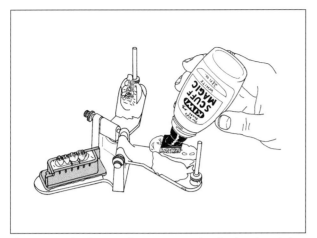

Fig 20-19 The functional core is painted with white liquid shoe polish.

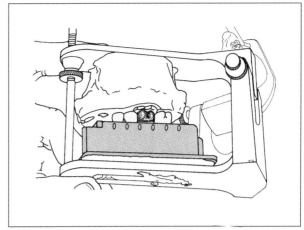

Fig 20-20 To mark the wax pattern, the freshly painted functional core is closed against it.

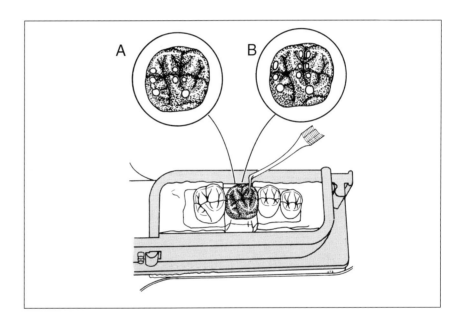

Fig 20-21 Occlusal contacts on the wax pattern for mutually protected occlusion, A, and unilaterally balanced occlusion, B.

Marginal ridges and cusp ridges complete the outline of the occlusal table, and then they are blended into the axial contours. Triangular ridges are placed next (Fig 20-17).

The occlusal portion of the pattern can be completed by waxing against the functional core. Make certain that the incisal guide pin is in contact with the base of the articulator when the wax pattern is completed (Fig 20-18). If this simple precaution is overlooked, the occlusal surface can be well formed but in an unacceptable superocclusion.

Paint white liquid shoe polish on the functional core (Fig 20-19). Close the articulator so the functional core is brought in contact with the occlusal surface of the wax pattern (Fig 20-20). The shoe polish will leave white marks on the occlusal surface of the wax pattern corresponding to the contacts in function. Carve off any areas

in white that are not part of the desired centric or excursive contact pattern.

If the restoration is to be in a mutually protected relationship (ie, with a canine lift), there should be no contact other than the centric contacts on the lingual incline of the buccal cusp (Fig 20-21, A). If, on the other hand, the restoration is to be fabricated to a group function, the lingual incline of the buccal cusp should maintain continuous contact with the functional core (Fig 20-21, B). In no case should the nonworking inclines (the buccal slopes of the maxillary lingual cusps) have any contact with the functional core.

Once the occlusal contact design has been established, finish the wax pattern by adding supplemental grooves and sluiceways. Blend in any roughness on the axial surfaces with a warm beavertail burnisher. Remelt

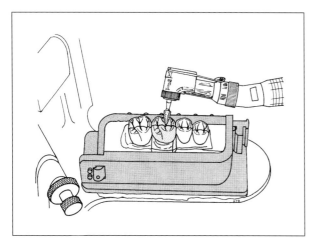

Fig 20-22 The restoration is adjusted to fit against the functional core.

the entire marginal periphery with a hot PKT no. 1, taking care to melt the wax all the way through to the die. Eliminate the resulting trough-like depression along the margin by adding wax with a hot beavertail burnisher. Carve away the bulk excess with a PKT no. 4 and finish the margins with a warm beavertail burnisher.

Attach a sprue to the wax pattern, invest it, burn it out, and cast the restoration. After the casting has been cleaned and pickled, remove the sprue and blend the contour of the sprue attachment area into the surrounding contours of the restoration. Try the casting back on the die and check to see that it is completely seated.

Close the functional core against the casting and check the incisal guide pin to see if it is again in contact with the articulator base. If it is slightly out of contact, as

is frequently the case, place no. 10 silk typewriter ribbon across the casting and close the functional core against it to mark the restoration. Carefully adjust the casting with a green stone until the pin is once again in contact with the articulator base (Fig 20-22). If the technique has been followed carefully to this point, adjustment should be minimal.

This functionally generated path technique is simple and can produce excellent results. Because of its simplicity, it is sometimes the object of derision by dentists who do not use it. Simplicity should not be confused with inaccuracy. The technique is capable of producing very accurate results, but it demands care and meticulous attention to detail.

There are variations of the technique that can be used to achieve the same result. An interocclusal record can be used to form the functional core.[13] After the functional wax tracing has been made, an acrylic rather than a stone index is formed. It is attached to the teeth opposing the prepared tooth, and when the interocclusal impression is made of the opposing quadrants, the index is recorded opposite the prepared tooth. When the two casts are mounted and removed from the impression, the cast bearing the prepared tooth is articulated against a functional core.

The functionally generated path effect can also be achieved in selected instances by rubbing two full-arch casts together.[11] Since any limitation of movement will result in interferences, casts must be mounted on an articulating device that permits total freedom in all directions. Light, flexible spring articulators accomplish this best. Any pronounced anterior guidance must be removed from the casts to prevent the cusp incline of the restoration from being overcontoured to match the anterior guidance.

References

1. Zimmerman EM: Modifications of functionally generated path procedures. *J Prosthet Dent* 1966; 16:1119–1126.

2. Meyer FS: Cast bridgework in functional occlusion. *J Am Dent Assoc* 1933; 20:1015–1030.

3. Meyer FS: A new simple and accurate technique for obtaining balanced and functional occlusion. *J Am Dent Assoc* 1934; 21:195–203.

4. Meyer FS: Can the plane line articulator meet all the demands of balanced and functional occlusion in all restorative work? *J Colo Dent Assoc* 1938; 17:6–16.

5. Meyer FS: The generated path technique in reconstruction dentistry. Part II. Fixed partial dentures. *J Prosthet Dent* 1959; 9:432–440.

6. Benfield JW: Advantages of functional bite technic in reducing chair time. *N Y J Dent* 1962; 32:296–297.

7. Mann AW, Pankey LD: Oral rehabilitation. Part I. Use of the P-M instrument in treatment planning and in restoring the lower posterior teeth. *J Prosthet Dent* 1960; 10:135–150.

8. Pankey LD, Mann AW: Oral rehabilitation. Part II. Reconstruction of the upper teeth using a functionally generated path technique. *J Prosthet Dent* 1960; 10:151–162.

9. Mann AW, Pankey LD: Oral rehabilitation utilizing the Pankey-Mann instrument and a functional bite technique. *Dent Clin North Am* 1959; 3:215–230.

10. Mann AW, Pankey LD: The Pankey-Mann philosophy of occlusal rehabilitation. *Dent Clin North Am* 1963; 7:621–636.

11. Dawson PE: *Evaluation, Diagnosis and Treatment of Occlusal Problems,* ed 2. St Louis, CV Mosby Co, 1989, pp 410–433.

12. King RC: Stabilizing functional chew-in wax records. *J Prosthet Dent* 1971; 26:601–603.

13. Getz EH: Functional "check-bite impressions" for fixed prosthodontics. *J Prosthet Dent* 1971; 26:146–153.

Chapter 21

Investing and Casting

Arriving at a completed casting after fabrication of a wax pattern involves three steps: *(1) investing*—surrounding the wax pattern with a material that can accurately duplicate its shape and anatomic features, *(2) burnout*—removal of the wax pattern so that a mold is created into which the molten alloy can be placed, and *(3) casting*—introducing the molten alloy into the previously prepared mold. The apparent simplicity of the above steps may belie their importance in obtaining accurately fitting castings. Few experiences in dentistry are more frustrating than having finished a casting that will not fit and therefore cannot be used in the patient's mouth.

Dental Casting Alloys

A brief review of the alloys used for casting restorations should aid in an understanding of the laboratory procedures employed to obtain well-fitting castings. Many different classification systems have been devised for the alloys used in dentistry, based on either noble metal content (noble, seminoble, base), cost (precious, semiprecious, nonprecious), or physical properties (types I to IV).

Alloys of the *noble metals* (gold, platinum, and palladium) with additional silver, copper, and zinc have been used for cast restorations since the introduction of the lost wax technique to dentistry around the turn of the century. There is evidence that Philbrook first described the lost wax method in 1897.[1] However, Taggart is generally credited with introducing the technique to the profession in 1906,[1-3] because he seemed to appreciate the significance of the idea, and he expended considerable time and effort in developing it.[1]

The most widely used alloy for cast all-metal restorations contains approximately 75% gold and is therefore designated as 18-karat gold, which means that it is 18/24 pure. The noble metals impart tarnish resistance and ductility to dental alloys, silver lightens the color and adds ductility, copper increases the hardness and strength, and zinc reduces oxidation.[4]

The noble alloys are sometimes referred to as "precious" metals, but the terms are not synonymous. The term "precious" alludes to the cost of the metal, while "noble" refers to its chemical behavior.[5] The elements gold and platinum happen to be both noble and precious. Palladium is noble, but is much less expensive. At times silver has gained enough in value to approach the classification of "precious," but it tarnishes and is *not* a noble metal.

The ADA and Identalloy Classification System for Noble Dental Alloy[6] has been adopted for the purpose of filing claims with third-party payers. This classification is as follows:

- *High-noble alloys* have a noble metal content of 60% or greater. At least 40% of the alloy must be gold.
- *Noble alloys* must be at least 25% noble metal.
- *Predominantly base alloys* have a noble metal content of less than 25%.

Often the major constituents of an alloy will be used to describe it (eg, gold-palladium, silver-palladium, nickel-chromium).

From 1934 to 1968, the US government maintained the price of gold at $35 an ounce. Since this price control has ended, the price of gold has risen on the world market, creating increasing pressure to use alloys that cost less. *Semiprecious* (seminoble, economy) alloys meet this requirement. They include the silver-palladium alloys and all alloys that contain more than 10% and less than 75% gold.[7]

The mechanical properties and handling characteristics of semiprecious alloys are much like those of standard gold alloys. However, greater corrosion is associated with lower noble metal content. Many of the alloys with lower gold content can be used with the same investments and with similar casting techniques as alloys with higher gold content. Silver-palladium alloys melt at slightly above 2,000°F (1,090°C), and therefore can only be melted with gas-oxygen torches or electric induction casting machines.

A steep rise in the cost of the noble metals and silver in 1973–1974 led to a widespread interest in *base metal alloys,* which are also referred to as nonprecious or non-noble. A logical transition was the adaptation of materials similar to those already in common usage for the fabrication of removable partial denture frameworks. These alloys possess desirable properties such as low cost, increased strength and hardness, higher fusion temperature, and less distortion during porcelain firing. They have been promoted for use in all-metal crowns, metal-ceramic crowns, long-span fixed partial dentures, and resin-bonded fixed partial dentures. There are several formulae utilizing nickel, chromium, and cobalt, with nickel-chromium alloys being the most popular. In the absence of noble metals, these alloys achieve their tarnish resistance in the mouth by formation of a surface monolayer of chromium oxide.[8]

Disadvantages of nickel-chromium alloys include possible excessive oxide formation, difficulty in finishing and polishing, and questionable biocompatibility. Beryllium is a common component of such alloys, added to limit oxide formation and improve castability. It has been identified as a potential carcinogen[9] and poses a potential hazard to laboratory personnel who might inhale beryllium or beryllium compounds as dust if appropriate precautions are not observed.[10] Beryllium concentration at the surface of the casting is far out of proportion to the percentage of beryllium in the rest of the casting, and the beryllium and nickel each potentiate the dissolution of the other in an acidic solution.[11] Occlusal wear as well as dissolution can be a factor in the release of nickel and beryllium in an artificial oral environment.[12] The extent of ingestion of the dissolved beryllium is unknown, but it is thought to be cumulative.[11] Its long-term effects, if any, are not known.

Nickel is capable of eliciting an allergic response from sensitive individuals. It produces more cases of allergic dermatitis than do all other metals combined.[13] Approximately 4.5% of the general population demonstrate a sensitivity to nickel, with a reaction being 10 times more likely to occur in women than in men.[14] Therefore, the use of nickel-chromium restorations is definitely contraindicated for patients with a known sensitivity to nickel. However, a retrospective study of 915 cast restorations in 335 patients found no higher rate of adverse responses of the mucosa around cemented base-metal restorations than around restorations made of gold alloys.[15]

An argument can be made for caution in adopting newer low-cost alloys. Even if no actual harm comes to the patients, there is always the danger that the news media will seize upon isolated reports of health hazards as they did recently with amalgam in the US and palladium-copper alloys in Europe.[16] The prospect of frightened patients demanding removal of previously placed restorations should make dentists think long and hard about utilizing untried alloys. At today's prices the cost of the alloy in a crown, even if it has a high noble metal content, constitutes a relatively minor part of the fee to the patient.

Base metal alloys also present a challenge to both dentists and dental technicians because of the many ways in which they differ from gold alloys in physical properties, handling characteristics, and fabrication techniques. Because of the presence of high-fusing elements, these alloys have a much higher melting temperature (2,300 to 2,600°F, or 1,260 to 1,430°C).[17] This necessitates the use of a multiorifice gas-oxygen torch and phosphate-bonded investment with a high-heat burnout (1,500 to 1,700°F, or 815 to 930°C).[18] It has been reported that more consistent castings can be obtained through the use of induction casting, which requires the use of expensive equipment.[19] The yield strength for nickel-chromium alloys can be as low as 260 MPa (37,700 psi), but the majority of them are above 517 MPa (75,000 psi) and many exceed 690 MPa (100,000 psi). This is much higher than the 207 to 275 MPa (30,000 to 40,000 psi) yield strength of Firmilay, a type III gold. The percent of elongation is also high, with many alloys exceeding 25.[17] However, the ability to manipulate the alloy is limited by the great force required to effect deformation (as evidenced by the high yield strength).

Titanium and its alloys have attracted great interest in recent years as an alternative to gold. Titanium's great biocompatibility has been proven through its widespread use as an implant material. Although chemically active, and therefore non-noble, it rapidly forms a thin, inert oxide layer when exposed to air. Among its other advantages are low cost, low thermal conductivity, and capability of bonding to resin cements[20] and to porcelain.[21] Its principal drawback is the difficulty in making castings. Pure titanium melts at 3,035°F (1,668°C) and reacts readily with conventional investments and oxygen. Therefore, it must be cast and soldered with special equipment in an oxygen-free environment. New alloys of titanium with nickel that can be cast by more conventional methods are being developed. These are reported to release very little ionic nickel and bond well to porcelain.[21] New methods of forming titanium crowns and copings by CAD/CAM (computer-aided design/computer-aided milling) technology avoid the problems of casting altogether.[22]

For many years, dental alloys were classified by the ADA according to *physical properties* and noble metal content as either type I, II, III, or IV. The ANSI/ADA specification no. 5 for dental casting alloys was revised in 1988, dropping reference to composition because of the successful use of a great number of new alloys with little or no noble metal content.[23] Yield strength and elongation are still specified for the four types, but now an alloy's composition, hardness, and melting range are only required to be within a certain percentage of that stated by the manufacturer.

The specification calls for type III alloys to have a yield strength between 200 and 340 MPa, and an elongation of at least 12% in the annealed state. The percent of elongation is a measurement of ductility and determines how much margins can be closed by burnishing. An alloy with a lower "type" number (eg, type I) will be softer, more burnishable (higher percent elongation), and weaker (lower yield strength) than an alloy with a higher "type" number (eg, type IV). Type I alloys are recommended for small inlays; type II for larger inlays and onlays; type III for onlays, crowns, and short-span fixed partial dentures; and type IV for thin veneer crowns, long-span fixed partial dentures, and removable partial dentures.

Independent of the just-mentioned classifications, special alloys are required for veneering with porcelain. They vary widely in their composition, and they also may be classified as either high-noble, seminoble, or base metal alloys. They share the unique requirements of having a fusion temperature 300 to 500°F (165 to 280°C) higher than that of porcelain, a coefficient of thermal expansion near that of porcelain, and the ability to form an oxide layer that will provide a strong bond to porcelain. They all tend to have a higher yield strength and lower percent elongation than type III gold.[17]

The ultimate choice of an alloy will depend on a variety of factors, including cost, rigidity, castability, ease of finishing and polishing, corrosion resistance, compatibility with specific brands of porcelain, and the personal preferences of both the dentist and the technician fabricating the restoration.

Investment Materials

An investment must fulfill three important requirements:

1. It must reproduce precisely the detailed form of the wax pattern.
2. It must provide sufficient strength to withstand the heat of burnout and the actual casting of the molten metal.
3. It must expand sufficiently to compensate for the solidification shrinkage of the alloy.

Shrinkage Compensation

Of great importance in the investing of wax patterns is the fact that the molten alloys used for dental restorations shrink upon solidification: gold alloys by approximately 1.5%[24] and nickel-chromium alloys by as much as 2.4%.[8] If the mold is not made correspondingly larger than the original wax pattern, the resultant casting will be that much smaller. For inlays and cast dowel cores, which are intracoronal and intraradicular, respectively, a slight net shrinkage is acceptable. However, if the restoration is a crown, which is extracoronal, net shrinkage may prevent it from seating completely on the tooth preparation. For crowns, therefore, it is necessary to compensate for the solidification shrinkage of the specific alloy used by expanding the mold enough to at least equal the shrinkage.

There are four mechanisms that can play a role in producing an expanded mold: *(1)* setting expansion of the investment, *(2)* hygroscopic expansion, *(3)* wax pattern expansion, and *(4)* thermal expansion.

Setting Expansion. Setting expansion of the investment occurs as a result of normal crystal growth. The expansion probably is enhanced by silica particles in the investment interfering with the forming crystalline structure of the gypsum, causing it to expand outward.[25] This type of expansion, in air, normally is about 0.4%, but expansion is partially restricted by the metal investment ring.

Hygroscopic Expansion. Hygroscopic expansion may be employed to augment normal expansion. The investment is allowed to set in the presence of water, producing additional expansion.[26,27] Hollenback[28] reported that maximum expansion could be achieved by immersing an investment-filled ring in a 100°F (38°C) water bath. This often has been interpreted as being due to hygroscopic expansion of the investment. It has been theorized that the water in which the investment is immersed replaces the water used by the hydration process. This maintains the space between the growing crystals, allowing them to continue expanding outward, rather than restricting them.[27]

Hygroscopic expansion ranges from 1.2% to 2.2%.[25] More controlled amounts of hygroscopic expansion may be achieved by adding a measured amount of water to the setting investment.[29] Hygroscopic expansion does occur in an unrestricted trough or an expandable investment ring.[26,27] However, in a lined, rigid, metal ring, the expansion attributed to hygroscopic expansion is more likely due to expansion of the wax pattern caused by the elevated temperature of the water in which the pattern has been immersed.[30]

Wax Pattern Expansion. Expansion of the wax pattern while the investment is still fluid occurs when the wax is warmed above the temperature at which it was formed. The heat may come from the chemical reaction of the investment or from a warm water bath in which the ring is immersed. Invested wax patterns allowed to set under water at room temperature actually exhibit slightly less expansion than do those that set in air at the same temperature, whereas invested patterns that set at 100°F without immersion in water expand just as much as those that set under water at the same temperature.[30]

The *low-temperature burnout technique* employs a combination of wax pattern expansion and thermal expansion of the mold. After the investment-filled ring is removed from a 100°F (38°C) water bath, the ring is heated to only 900°F (482°C) before casting to produce the additional expansion needed.

Thermal Expansion. Thermal expansion of the investment occurs when the investment is heated in the burnout oven. Heating of the mold also serves to eliminate the wax pattern and to prevent the alloy from solidifying before it completely fills the mold. The *high-temperature burnout technique* relies primarily on thermal expansion of the mold. The investment around the wax pattern is allowed to harden in air at room temperature, and then it is heated to approximately 1,200° F (650°C). At this temperature, the investment and metal ring expand enough to compensate for the shrinkage of the gold alloy.

Regardless of which technique is employed, a precise routine for investing, burning out, and casting must be adhered to in order to achieve consistent results.

Two kinds of investments are in common usage for the fabrication of cast restorations: those bonded with *gypsum* are used for alloys that fuse below 1,975°F (1,080°C), and those bonded with *phosphate* are used for higher-fusing alloys. The two types of investment are incompatible with each other, so mixing bowls used for one should not be used with the other. The manufacturer's instructions for a particular brand should be followed.

Gypsum-Bonded Investments

The gypsum-bonded investments are used with types I, II, and III gold alloys. These investments are themselves classified as type I for use with the high-temperature technique, or type II for the low-temperature technique. After setting, both types of investment are composites containing a matrix of gypsum with silica as a refractory filler, and certain chemical modifiers. The gypsum matrix, α-calcium sulfate hemihydrate, comprises 30% to 35% of the investment and acts as a binder. The refractory material, either quartz or cristobalite, makes up 60% to 65% of the investment and provides the thermal expansion for the investment.[31]

The rigid metal ring in which setting takes place must be lined with a compressible material to allow setting expansion to occur in a radial direction. Expansion can be controlled to some extent by varying the thickness of the liner.[32] Thermal expansion is achieved in the burnout oven through the normal expansion that occurs upon heating the silica (quartz and cristobalite), as well as through phase changes that occur in the material.

Investing Armamentarium

1. 200-cc Vac-U-Spat bowl and lid
2. Vacuum tubing
3. Vac-U-Vestor (Whip Mix Corp, Louisville, KY)
4. Rubber crucible former
5. Casting ring (32-mm diameter)
6. Plastic water measure
7. Spatula
8. PKT (Thomas) waxing instruments (no. 1 and no. 4)
9. Cotton pliers
10. Bunsen burner
11. Matches
12. Sticky wax
13. Sprue formers (hollow plastic)
14. One package (50 g) of investment
15. Four-inch (10 cm) strip of cellulose ring liner

Sprue Former Attachment

The *sprue former* is a small-diameter pin or tube made of wax, plastic, or metal. A 10-gauge (2.6-mm diameter) sprue former can be used on most patterns, while the 12-gauge (2.0-mm diameter) is used on small premolar patterns. One end of the sprue former is attached to the wax pattern and the other end to the crucible former (a conical rubber base). After the investment has hardened, the crucible former is removed from the ring, leaving a funnel-shaped entrance to the mold. The channel left by the sprue former following burnout is the sprue, an inlet for the gold that will be forced into the mold. A sprue former as large as possible should be used on each pattern.[28] If the sprue is too thin or too long, the gold may solidify in the sprue before it does in the larger cavity formed by the wax pattern. If this happens, molten gold cannot be drawn from the reservoir ("button") as the casting solidifies, and *shrink-spot porosity* will occur in the bulkiest part of the casting.

The sprue former should be attached to the wax pattern at its point of greatest bulk, avoiding centric occlusal contacts if possible. It is attached at an angle to allow the incoming gold to flow freely to all portions of the mold (Fig 21-1). If the sprue is directed at a right angle to a flat wall of the mold, a "hot spot" may be created at that point. This will keep the alloy adjacent to it molten after the rest of the casting has solidified, causing *suck-back porosity*.[25] Uneven expansion of the mold and entrapment of air bubbles in the occlusal fossae may also result from this position of the sprue.

Select a hollow plastic sprue former and place it inside the crucible former and casting ring for measurement. The sprue former should be just long enough so that the highest point on the wax pattern will be 6.0 mm from the end of the ring. If the pattern is too close to the end of the ring, the molten alloy may blast through the investment during casting; if it is too far, gases may not escape rapidly enough to permit complete filling of the mold with alloy. Remove the sprue former from the crucible former and shorten it with a sharp knife if necessary.

If the hole in the crucible former is too large to firmly grasp the sprue former, fill the hole with soft wax. With a PKT no. 1 instrument, drop a small bead of sticky wax onto the proposed site of attachment on the pattern. Place the sprue former into the molten bead of sticky wax. If the wax is hot enough, a small amount will be drawn into the lumen of the sprue by capillary action. This creates a strong union between sprue former and pattern, provided there is no movement as the wax hardens.

Melt in the sticky wax around the sprue former–wax pattern junction with the PKT no. 1 instrument to provide a smooth conduit for the molten alloy (Fig 21-2). Do not expose the wax pattern to prolonged heat during this procedure. Avoid overbulking the sprue former attachment because this will increase the risk of shrink-spot porosity and also make removal of the sprue from the casting more difficult. The sprue former also should not be constricted at its attachment to the wax pattern. The

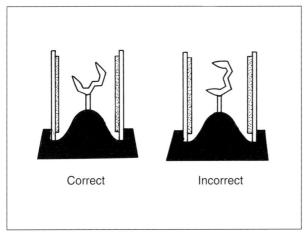

Fig 21-1 Sprue placement on the wax pattern and orientation of the pattern in the ring.

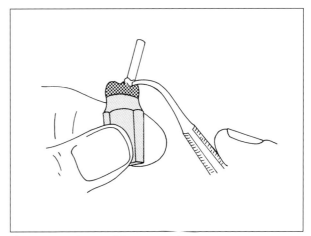

Fig 21-2 Attachment of the sprue to the wax pattern.

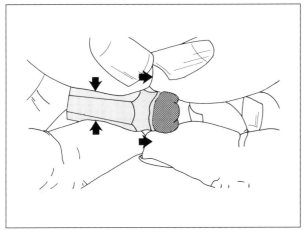

Fig 21-3 Wax pattern is removed from the die by indirect finger pressure.

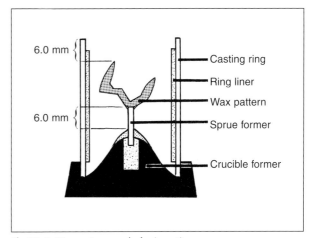

Fig 21-4 Wax pattern ready for investing.

best castability and least porosity is produced by a sprue former–wax pattern junction that is either straight or slightly flared.[33]

During the time period between removal of the wax pattern from the die and hardening of the investment, deformation will occur as stresses in the wax are released. To minimize this time, all the armamentarium must be at hand, the ring liner should be in place, and the water should be measured out before the pattern is removed. To remove the wax pattern from the die, lightly grasp it on the proximal surfaces with the thumb and forefinger of the left hand, being careful not to exert any pressure on the sprue former. Hold the die between the thumb and forefinger of the right hand and gently squeeze them together. This squeezing action by the right hand will exert gentle pressure against the tips of the fingers of the left hand and will usually lift the pattern from the die (Fig 21-3). If gentle pressure will not lift the pattern, place a small piece of rubber dam over the pattern to prevent slippage by the fingers. Do not exert a direct pulling action with the left

hand. Except in the situation described below, do not remove a pattern by the sprue former.

Difficulty can be encountered in removing an inlay pattern from the die, since there is usually insufficient bulk to draw the pattern without exerting distorting force on the sprue former. In this situation, the sprue should parallel the path of insertion of the restoration to prevent torquing of the pattern with attendant distortion of its margins. A small loop of gold zephyr wire with turned-up ends can be heated and embedded into the occlusal surface of the wax pattern and used as a handle for removal with cotton pliers.

To produce uniform expansion, surround the pattern on all sides with investment that is as uniform in thickness as possible. The closer to the center of the ring that the pattern is placed, the greater will be the expansion.[34,35] With pliers, push the sprue former down into the soft wax in the top of the crucible former until the top of the pattern is 6.0 mm below the end of the ring (Fig 21-4). To provide adequate bulk of gold during solidification, the sprue itself should be no longer than 6.0 mm (it can be shorter). To correct any discrepancy in length, add soft wax onto the sprue former, thus lengthening the crucible former and shortening the exposed sprue former. Smooth the wax around the base of the sprue former.

Investing Procedure

For a single crown or onlay, use a metal casting ring with an outside diameter of 32 mm. Place a resilient liner on the inside of the ring to provide a buffer of pliable material against which the investment can expand to enlarge the mold. If there is no room for expansion outward, the expansion forces will be exerted inward toward the mold, resulting in distortion of the casting. The layer of soft material between the investment and the wall of the ring also permits easier removal of the investment and casting from the ring later.

An alternative method uses a split plastic casting ring that offers no resistance to the setting expansion. The plastic ring is removed before the invested pattern is placed into the oven. This technique allows easier escape of gas from the mold during casting, but the mold is more vulnerable to cracking.

For many years, asbestos was used to line casting rings, but it has been removed from the market because of concern over its carcinogenic properties.[36] Ceramic paper (Kaoliner, Dentsply/York Div, York PA) and cellulose paper (Ring Liner Non-Asbestos Cellulose, Whip Mix Corp, Louisville, KY) are now used as substitutes for asbestos. It has been pointed out, however, that the ceramic material contains fibers in the size range likely to produce lung tumors in rats, and therefore may be no less hazardous than asbestos.[37,38]

The ceramic material does not readily absorb water except under vacuum.[39] The cellulose material, on the other hand, does absorb water, and in doing so becomes thicker and more compressible.[40] Cellulose liners burn out before the casting is made, allowing unrestricted thermal expansion and easy escape of gases from the mold during casting. However, this deprives the investment of support by the ring, and may result in cracking of the investment and fins on the casting. The manufacturers recommend that approximately 3.0 mm of ring at each end be left unlined so that the investment will be partially supported by direct contact with the ring after the liner has burned out.

Place a dry strip of cellulose liner approximately 9.5 cm long into a 32-mm-diameter casting ring, carefully adapting the strip to the walls of the ring with no overlap. The liner should be 3.0 mm short of both ends of the ring. This will allow supporting contact of the investment with the ring after the cellulose liner has burned out. It is also theorized that this restriction near the open end will provide for more uniform expansion.[41] Dip the ring into water to wet the liner, then gently shake off the excess. Theoretically, the water in the liner adds a degree of

hygroscopic expansion to the setting expansion, but it also reduces the powder-water ratio, which in turn will reduce the thermal expansion of the investment.

As a result, the net expansion with a dry liner will be slightly greater than with a wet liner.[42] However, because the effect of a dry liner depends on its volume relative to that of the investment, which varies with the diameter of the ring, a damp liner is preferred for the sake of consistency. Do not compress the wet liner against the ring because its cushioning effect will be reduced. Rotate the ring firmly onto the crucible former, being careful to avoid snapping movements or contact of the wax pattern with the ring.

Air bubbles in the investing material adjacent to the wax pattern will result in nodules on the casting. The incidence of visible nodules on the internal surface of full gold crowns with five commonly employed methods of investing was reported by Johnson.[43] Vacuum mixing produced the best results with open or vacuum pouring, allowing the investment to set under pressure or in open atmosphere. Hand-mixing with an open pour produced nearly three times as many nodules, while open pouring and allowing the invested pattern to set under vacuum produced 10 times as many nodules. The same study reported that painting the wax pattern with a surface-tension–reducing agent produced mixed results. This agent produced castings with 12% fewer nodules with the open pour technique, but 22% more nodules with the vacuum pour technique.

In another study, only 17% of the castings produced by open investing were bubble free, while 95% of those done in molds made by vacuum investing were free of bubbles.[44] Experienced technicians probably can obtain smooth castings with either vacuum pouring or open pouring.[45] Although the open pour technique is more popular with experienced technicians because of the unimpeded view of the pattern as it is covered with investment, it is easier for the novice to obtain good results with vacuum pouring.

The procedure for investing a pattern for a single-tooth restoration to be cast in type II or III gold with the *vacuum mix, vacuum pour technique* is as follows: Place the assembled ring and crucible former into the hole at the top of the Vac-U-Spat investor (Fig 21-5). Hold the lid by the spindle with the paddle toward you and the inlay ring to the bottom. Look into the aperture through which the investment will flow into the ring, and make sure that the *internal* portion of the wax pattern is visible.

Connect one end of the clear plastic vacuum tubing to the vacuum outlet on the Vac-U-Vestor. Insert the metal connector on the other end of the tubing into the hole in the lid of the Vac-U-Spat (Fig 21-6). Turn on the Vac-U-Vestor briefly. If the gauge shows a vacuum when the lid has not been set on the bowl, the tube is blocked. Turn off the machine and clear the tubing before proceeding. The lumen in the metal nozzle at the end of the tubing and the gauze filter just beyond the nozzle are the most common sites of blockage.

Pour the recommended amount of room-temperature water into the bowl. This must be carefully measured,

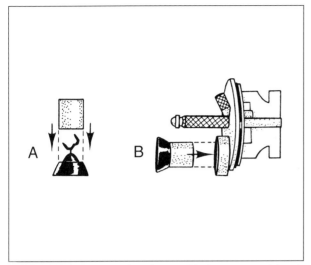

Fig 21-5 The ring is seated on the crucible former (A) and then is placed in the Vac-U-Spat lid (B).

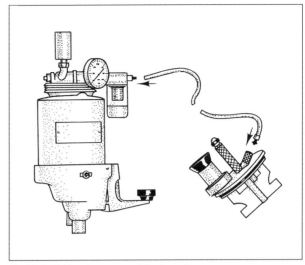

Fig 21-6 Tubing is connected for investing.

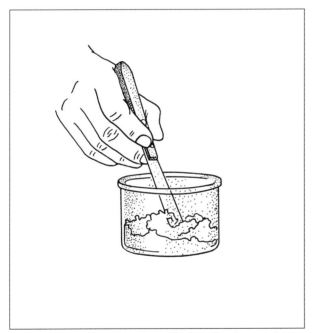

Fig 21-7 Investment is wetted completely by hand spatulation.

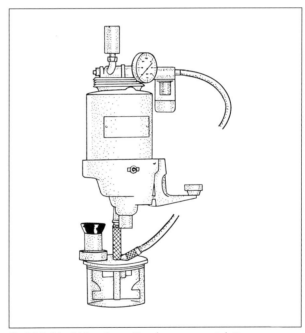

Fig 21-8 Vac-U-Spat in position for power spatulation.

since the water-powder ratio has a critical effect on expansion (more water results in less expansion). Add a package of investment to the water and mix it with a hand-held spatula until all of the investment has become wet (Fig 21-7). Place the lid on the bowl and make sure it is firmly sealed.

Turn on the Vac-U-Vestor and insert the spindle of the lid of the Vac-U-Spat into the smaller of the two drive chucks on the bottom of the unit (Fig 21-8). The gauge should register a vacuum. If it does not, there is probably leakage between the bowl and lid or between the lid and

hose. Power-spatulate for 15 seconds. Since the length of spatulation can affect expansion of the investment, measure the time of spatulation precisely. Overspatulation will increase thermal expansion.[35] Do not introduce another variable into the technique.

Remove the spindle from the drive chuck. Do not turn off the Vac-U-Vestor, and do not disconnect the vacuum at this point. Place the drive nut of the Vac-U-Spat spindle on the vibrator knob. Make sure that the shaft is horizontal and the casting ring is in the lowest position on the circumference of the lid. Hold the Vac-U-Spat in this posi-

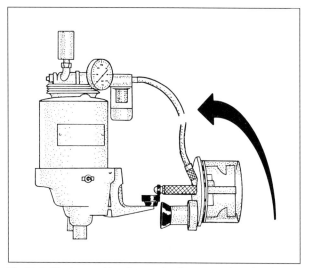

Fig 21-9 Starting position for pouring investment into the ring.

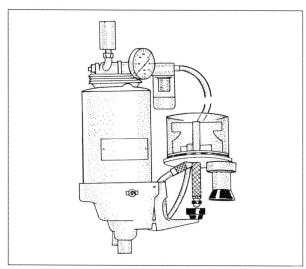

Fig 21-10 Vac-U-Spat inverted after filling the ring.

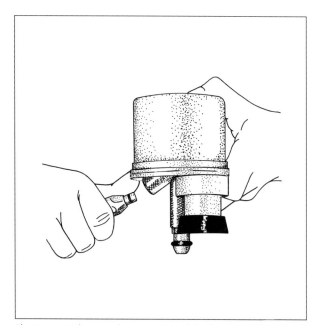

Fig 21-11 Tubing is disconnected while the Vac-U-Spat is still inverted.

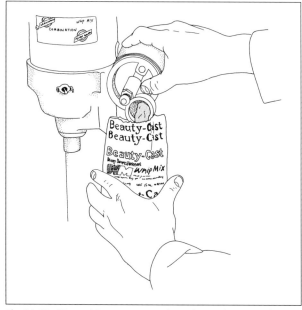

Fig 21-12 Unused investment is vibrated into the original envelope and disposed of in a trash receptacle.

tion for a few seconds until the investment has run to the lower side of the bowl (Fig 21-9).

Slowly invert the Vac-U-Spat until the shaft points straight down, keeping the drive nut in contact with the vibrator (Fig 21-10). It should take slightly less than 30 seconds to traverse the 90-degree arc from the horizontal to the vertical position.

Remove the drive nut from the vibrator knob, keeping the Vac-U-Spat *inverted*. While it is still in this position, turn off the vacuum pump and disconnect the vacuum

hose (Fig 21-11). Then remove the casting ring and crucible former from the Vac-U-Spat lid. Place the crucible former on the vibrator knob for a few seconds to settle any investment that might have spilled during separation of the ring from the lid. Do not overvibrate; this may cause air to slip around the seal between the ring and the crucible former, rising up and lodging on the underside of the pattern.

If a high-temperature (1,200°F, 650°C) burnout technique will be used, place the casting ring and crucible former into a humidor (a covered plastic container or sealed plastic bag with wet paper towels in the bottom) and let set at room temperature. If a low-temperature (900°F, 480°C) burnout technique is to be used, immediately immerse the ring in a 100°F (38°C) water bath to produce expansion of the wax pattern. Allow the investment to set for a minimum of 30 minutes. Leave the ring in the humidor until you are ready for burnout and casting.

To prevent clogging the drains with accumulated investment, empty the unused portion of investment remaining in the Vac-U-Spat bowl into the investment envelope (Fig 21-12). Fold over the top of the package so the waste can be disposed of neatly. Use a brush and running water to clean the bowl, lid, and paddle before the investment hardens on them.

Casting Armamentarium for Types II and III Gold Alloys

1. Casting ring with invested wax pattern
2. Furnace
3. Centrifugal casting machine with crucible
4. Gas-air blowpipe
5. Matches
6. Casting alloy
7. Casting flux
8. Casting tongs
9. Toothbrush
10. Explorer
11. Jel-Pac
12. Porcelain casserole dish
13. Plastic-coated forceps
14. Bunsen burner

Burnout

Burnout prepares the mold for the molten alloy and allows thermal expansion to occur. If thermal expansion alone is to provide the compensation expansion, a high-temperature technique (1,200°F, 650°C) is employed. If a 100° water bath (hygroscopic technique) was used to expand the wax pattern, a lower temperature (900°F, 480°C) can be utilized. Heating must be gradual to allow steam to escape without cracking the mold.

Carefully separate the crucible former from the ring. Check the crater and bottom of the ring for any small chips of investment, and remove any that are found, for they could contaminate the casting later. Place the casting ring, with the crater down, into a 600°F (315°C) oven and leave it for 30 minutes. By burning out in an inverted position, much of the wax will run out of the mold as it is melted, carrying any loose chips of investment with it. With casting tongs, transfer the ring to a hotter furnace (either 900°F [482°C] or 1,200°F [650°C] depending on the technique used) for 1 hour.

As an alternative, the ring can be placed in a cold oven and heated slowly to the casting temperature. The ring should be set crater up about 10 minutes before the casting is made. This allows oxygen to contact the internal area of the mold to insure complete wax residue elimination. A black appearance of the investment surrounding the sprue hole is an indication that there are still carbon particles from the wax permeating the investment. These can impede the escape of gases through the investment as the casting alloy enters the mold and prevent the margins from being completely cast. A bright, clean appearance of the casting is the result of the reducing action of residual carbon and may indicate that it was cast too soon.

Casting for Types II and III Gold Alloys

No more than 30 seconds should be allowed to elapse between the time the ring is removed from the oven and the molten alloy is centrifuged into the mold. Any undue delay will cause heat loss and resultant mold contraction. Therefore, it is imperative that all materials and equipment used in casting be ready ahead of time. It is also helpful to enlist an assistant to transfer the hot ring from oven to cradle until more experience is gained.

Place the crucible in its bracket on the arm of the casting machine (Fig 21-13). Do not melt gold in a crucible that has been used with a base metal alloy. Grasping the counterweight of the casting machine in the right hand, wind it clockwise three times. Raise the pin from the base of the machine in front of the crucible assembly. Slowly release the right hand until the pin rests against the arm, preventing it from unwinding.

Place the casting alloy in the crucible. Enough bulk of metal must be used in casting to fill the mold, the sprue, and part of the crucible former to insure sharp, complete detail in the casting. Four pennyweights (dwt) of gold will usually suffice for most premolar restorations, while six are needed for molar castings. Buttons from previous castings can be reused provided they are well cleaned. Traces of sulfur from investment materials left on used buttons will reduce the alloy's ductility and increase pitting.[46]

Light the gas-air blowpipe and adjust the *red* gas and *green* air knobs to produce a conical flame (Fig 21-14, A). The first cone, the *mixing* zone, is a cool, colorless one. Around this area is a greenish-blue *combustion* zone in which partial combustion takes place; this is an *oxidizing* zone (Fig 21-14, B). Next is a dim blue tip, the *reducing* zone. This is the hottest area in the flame and is the only part of the flame used to heat the casting alloy. Beyond this is another oxidizing zone in which final combustion between the gas and surrounding air occurs.

Neither of the oxidizing zones should be used for heating. They are not as hot as the reducing zone, and if the alloy comes in contact with them, copper and other nonnoble metals will be oxidized, changing the properties of the alloy. This can result in reduced strength and altered solidification shrinkage. The oxides also may become

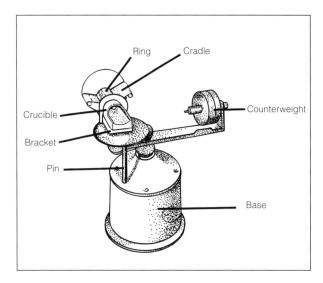

Fig 21-13 Centrifugal casting machine.

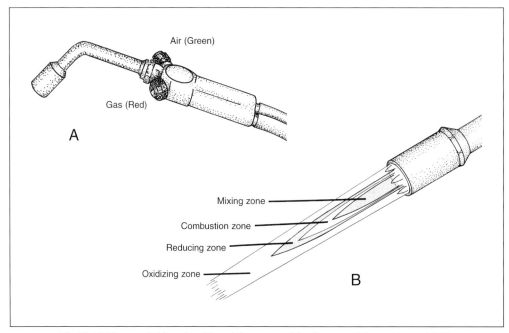

Fig 21-14 The gas-air blowpipe (A) and the zones of the flame used for melting gold (B).

incorporated in the casting as impurities. Practice locating the reducing zone by directing the flame against the crucible to form a glowing hot area. Slowly move the flame closer. When it is too close, a central dark spot will be formed by the cooler combustion zone. Withdraw the torch until the dark spot just disappears. This is the ideal distance the torch should be from the gold.

A small amount of flux should be sprinkled onto the warmed metal (Fig 21-15). Borax, used by itself as a flux, will help to exclude oxygen from the surface of the alloy and dissolve any oxides that are formed. Reducing flux,

which contains carbon in addition to borax, will also reduce back to clean metal any oxides that happen to form. This helps to maintain the original composition of the alloy.[47] Continue heating the gold until it balls up. As it approaches the casting temperature, the gold will become straw yellow in color. It will wiggle easily in the crucible when it is tapped and will follow the flame if it is moved slightly. If the reducing zone has been used properly, the molten gold will appear mirror-like and shiny.

Keeping the flame on the gold, remove the casting ring from the oven with casting tongs and carefully place the

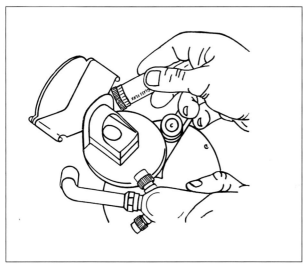

Fig 21-15 Application of casting flux before the ring is placed in the machine.

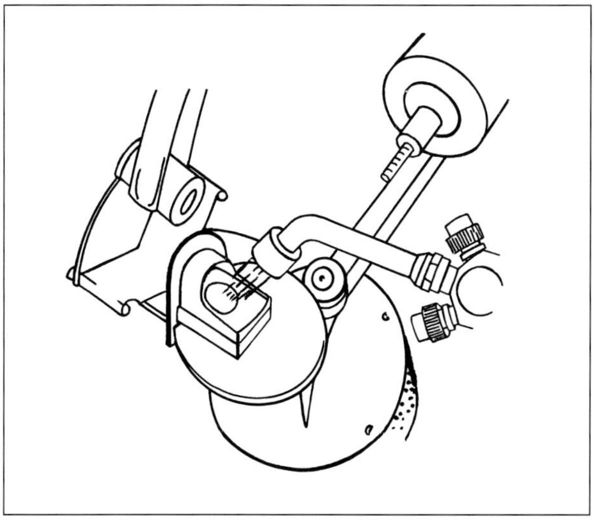

Fig 21-16 Casting ring is set in the cradle with casting tongs.

ring in the cradle (Fig 21-16). Gently slide the platform on which the crucible rests against the ring and cradle. Make sure it fits snugly so that the ring will not roll when the arm is released.

Hold the blowpipe in one hand and apply gentle clockwise pressure on the counterweight with the other hand until the pin drops (Fig 21-17). Jiggle the weight slightly to see that the gold moves freely. Release the weight, allowing the machine to spin. To insure maximum fluidity of the gold, do not lift the torch out of position until the arm of the casting machine has been released. Allow the centrifuge to slow to a stop by itself.

Cleaning the Casting

After the gold button has lost its glow, remove the casting ring with the tongs and thrust it into a pan of cold water. For a casting of Firmilay in a small ring, this quenching should occur about 5 minutes after casting to achieve the best grain structure. If it is quenched while it is too hot, the gold will be softer and weaker. If it is allowed to bench cool completely, the grain structure will be too large.[48] An additional benefit of quenching is the disintegration of the hot investment when it contacts the cold water.

Remove the ring from the water and push the investment and casting out of the ring, if they have not already fallen out. Break off as much of the investment as possible by hand or with an old instrument and then scrub the casting and button with a stiff brush. The casting should appear smooth, with a dull, dark oxide layer. Remove the oxide layer and any remaining particles of investment by lightly sandblasting all surfaces with a 50-μm abrasive, taking care not to abrade thin margins (Fig 21-18).

A process called *pickling* also has been widely used

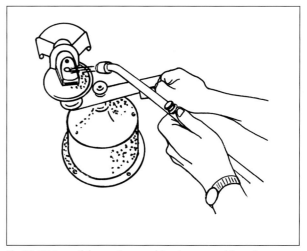

Fig 21-17 Arm of the casting machine is prepared for release.

for cleaning gold castings. This involves soaking the casting in a hot acid solution for several minutes. Jel Pak (JF Jelenko, Armonk, NY) is a much safer and less corrosive pickling agent than the formerly used sulfuric or hydrochloric acid. Still, contact with the skin and inhalation of vapors must be avoided. A porcelain casserole dish is used to contain the pickling solution, and plastic-covered pliers are used to introduce and remove the casting from the solution (Fig 21-19). Metal instruments must not come into contact with gold in strong solution, as electrodeposition may occur on the surface of the casting. Only gold castings may be cleaned by pickling. Because of the health and environmental hazards associated with pickling solutions, air abrasion with small–particle-size abrasives is the preferable means of cleaning castings.

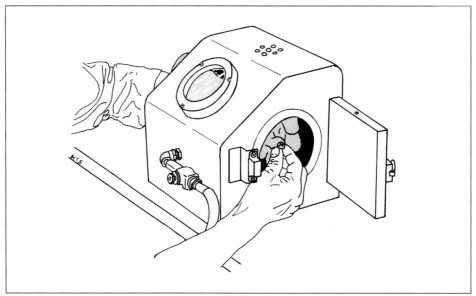

Fig 21-18 Casting is cleaned with a fine air-propelled abrasive.

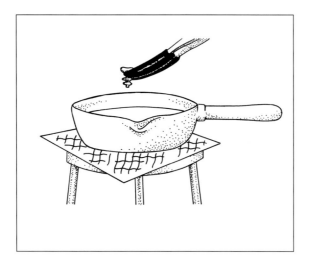

Fig 21-19 Casting is placed in a porcelain casserole dish for pickling.

The casting should be examined closely for casting defects. Figure 21-20 shows some common problems and their causes. A mistake is a failure only if we fail to learn from it.

Investment of Inlay and Dowel-Core Patterns

Less mold expansion is required for dowel cores and inlays than for crowns. If the casting is the least bit larger than the pattern, it will not fit into the tooth. Omitting the ring liner or increasing the investment water-powder ratio by 1.0 mL will result in a slightly undersized casting that will fit more easily into the cavity prepared in the tooth.

The following technique is recommended for investing and casting a dowel-core pattern in a silver-palladium alloy (Albacast, JF Jelenko, Armonk, NY): Invest the pattern in Beautycast (Whip Mix Corp, Louisville, KY) using the standard water-powder ratio, without a ring liner. Burn out at 1,200°F (650°C). Because the casting temperature of Albacast is 2,150°F (1,177°C), a gas-oxygen torch or electric induction casting machine must be used to melt the alloy.

It is possible for an experienced operator to cast and cement gold inlays and dowel cores on the same day that the teeth are prepared by using the following accelerated technique for investment and burnout:

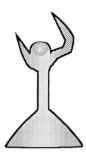

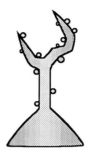

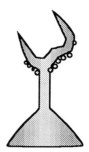

Large nodule—
Air trapped during investing.

Multiple random nodules—
Inadequate vacuum during mixing.

Nodules on underside only—
Prolonged vibration after pouring.

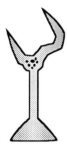

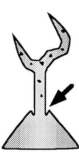

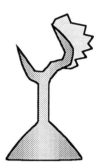

Shrink-spot porosity—
Spue attachment too bulky.
Sprue too long or thin.
Button too small.

Random porosity—
Dirt in wax pattern.
Loose particles of investment
from sharp edges *(arrow)*.

Fins—
Dropped ring, rapid heating
of wet or unhardened mold,
liner flush with end of ring.
excessive casting force.

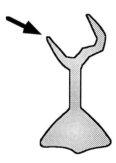

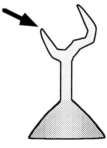

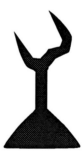

Short, rounded margins with
rounded or lumpy button—
Alloy not hot enough or
insufficient casting force.

Short, rounded margins
with sharp button—
Pattern too far from end of ring
or, if casting is shiny, incomplete
burnout of wax.

Black, rough casting—
Breakdown of investment
from excessive heat.

Fig 21-20 Some common casting defects and their causes.

1. Invest the pattern in a phosphate-bonded investment (Ceramigold, Whip Mix Corp, Louisville, KY) using a ring liner and standard special liquid dilution of 50/50.
2. Allow the investment to harden for 12 to 15 minutes. It should feel firm and warm.
3. Place the invested pattern directly into a 1,300°F (705°C) oven and allow 12 to 15 minutes for burnout.
4. Cast in gold alloy (type II or III for inlays, type III or IV for dowel cores).

In this way, investment, burnout, and casting can be completed in 1 hour, saving the patient an additional appointment.[49]

Phosphate-Bonded Investments

Phosphate-bonded investments are much stronger and withstand much higher temperatures than do gypsum-bonded investments. They are used for investing and casting alloys with higher melting temperatures, eg, silver-palladium, gold-platinum, and nickel-chromium. To obtain sufficient expansion for crowns of these alloys, the mold must be heated to 1,400°F (760°C) or higher, temperatures that would cause decomposition of the calcium sulfate in a gypsum binder with the resultant release of contaminating sulfur into the mold.[50] In general, any alloy with a *casting temperature* in excess of 2,100°F (1,150°C), as differentiated from the *fusion temperature,* which is 100 to 150°F lower, should be cast into an investment with a binder other than gypsum. (Because dowel cores do not require as much expansion of the mold as do crowns, they can be cast with a Ag-Pd alloy into a gypsum-bonded mold heated to only 1,200°F [650°C], as described earlier.)

The powder contains phosphates of magnesium and ammonium, graphite (carbon), and large silica particles, while the special liquid provided with these investments contains an aqueous suspension of colloidal silica. Carbon-free phosphate investments (Hi-Temp, Whip Mix Corp, Louisville, KY) are available for use with base alloys that are made brittle in the presence of carbon.

Magnesium phosphate reacts with primary ammonium phosphate to produce magnesium ammonium phosphate, which gives the investment its strength at room temperature.[51] At higher temperatures, silicophosphates are formed; they give the investment its great strength.

Expansion can be varied by the proportions of silica sol and water:

1. More silica sol and less water = more expansion.
2. Less silica sol and more water = less expansion.

The usual proportion is three parts silica sol liquid to one part distilled water. The overall liquid-powder ratio for Ceramigold investment should remain constant: 9.5 cc liquid to 60 g of powder.

Investing Armamentarium for Phosphate-Bonded Investments

1. 200-cc Vac-U-Spat bowl and lid
2. Vacuum tubing
3. Vac-U-Vestor
4. Rubber crucible former
5. Casting ring
6. Plastic water measure
7. Spatula
8. PKT (Thomas) waxing instruments (no. 1 and no. 4)
9. Cotton pliers
10. Bunsen burner and matches
11. Sticky wax
12. Sprue formers (hollow plastic or wax)
13. One package (60 g) of Ceramigold investment
14. Special liquid
15. Strip of liner 9.5 cm long
16. Small camel's hair brush

Investing With Phosphate-Bonded Materials

Attach a 10-gauge (2.6 mm) plastic sprue former to the tip of the incisal portion of a single crown wax pattern with sticky wax, using a PKT no. 1 instrument to melt and blend the junction. If there is a broad expanse of paper-thin wax between the sprue and the margin, bridge it with a narrow (0.5 mm thick) strip of wax (Fig 21-21) that will serve as an internal sprue. This will provide a channel through which the molten alloy can flow more readily to reproduce the margin. The resulting ridge can be easily trimmed back to the desired thickness after the casting is made.

Carefully remove the pattern from the die and grasp the sprue former with cotton pliers. Seat the sprue former into the soft wax in the center of the crucible former (Fig 21-22). The sprue former's length should be adjusted so that the pattern will be 6.0 mm from the end of the ring when it is in place. Build up the crucible former with wax, if necessary, so that no more than 6.0 mm of the sprue former will be exposed.

Posterior patterns are sprued on the tip of the cusp with the greatest bulk. An 18-gauge wax sprue former (0.8-mm diameter) should connect the other cusp tip (in the veneering area) with the base of the crucible former (attach to the pattern while it is still on the die). The tip of this cusp should be lower than the point of entry of the main sprue (Fig 21-23).

Adapt a layer of dry cellulose liner to the inside of the ring. Immerse the ring briefly in a bowl of water to moisten the liner. Assemble the ring, crucible former, and Vac-U-Spat lid. Place 9.5 cc of the liquid in the Vac-U- Spat bowl and add the contents of a 60-g package of Ceramigold investment. Connect the vacuum tubing and mechanically spatulate under a vacuum for approximately 15 seconds. Disconnect the vacuum and remove the ring from the lid.

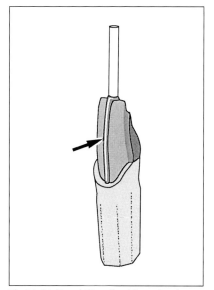

Fig 21-21 Castability of a thin cutback area is improved by the addition of an "internal sprue" *(arrow).*

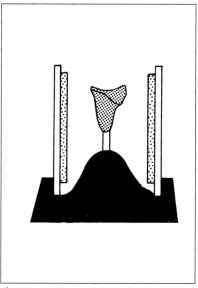

Fig 21-22 Anterior metal-ceramic coping wax pattern ready for investing.

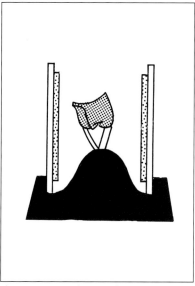

Fig 21-23 Premolar metal-ceramic coping wax pattern ready for investing.

This type of investment possesses poor surface-wetting characteristics. Because of this, the problem of trapping bubbles during investing is even greater than with gypsum investments. Either vacuum or open investing can be used. Allowing the investment to set in a pressure pot will further reduce the size and number of bubbles.[43] If there are small, restricted areas in the interior of a wax pattern (eg, long, thin crowns on incisors), gently brush the investment into the pattern with a small brush (Fig 21-24). Then place the ring over the crucible former and slowly pour the investment down one side of the ring with vibration. You should see a small stream of investment flow over the margin on one side of the pattern, down into the deepest recess, and gradually fill the pattern from the bottom up.

Once the pattern is covered, the ring can be filled the rest of the way with a minimum of vibration. There should be an excess of investment above the end of the ring so the hardened glaze can be easily ground away on a model trimmer. If it is needed, an additional 0.7% expansion can be obtained by placing the investment-filled ring into a 100°F (38°C) water bath before it has hardened.[51] If this is done, the surface of the investment should be protected from the softening effect of water by a thin sheet of rubber or plastic wrap held in place by a rubber band.

Wax patterns for metal-ceramic fixed partial dentures are invested and cast as one unit whenever possible because of the difficulty encountered in soldering the alloys used for this type of restoration. In these situations, the wax pattern should be fabricated on a one-piece die on which the dies of the individual abutment preparations have not been separated. The wax pattern for a fixed partial denture should be invested in a large ring (round

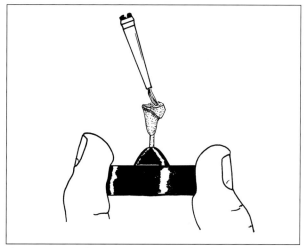

Fig 21-24 It may be necessary to paint phosphate-bonded investment into the wax pattern with a small brush.

or oval, with a diameter of approximately 6.3 cm) to produce the most accurate casting.[52]

For lower-fusing gold alloy castings, sprue formers run directly from crucible former to wax pattern to provide rapid, turbulence-free access of the metal to the mold during casting. Patterns for metal-ceramic fixed partial dentures, however, must be sprued by an indirect method because the alloys used fuse and solidify at much higher temperatures.[53] Because the ambient air is much colder than the molten metal, the exposed button is likely to solidify while the metal at the center of the ring is still liquid. This means that the button cannot serve as a reservoir to prevent shrink-spot porosity. Instead, a

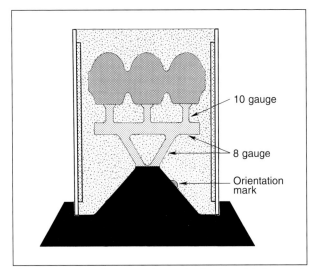

Fig 21-25 Pattern for a metal-ceramic fixed partial denture is sprued indirectly. The feeder sprues and the horizontal runner are 8 gauge, and the manifold sprues are 10 gauge.

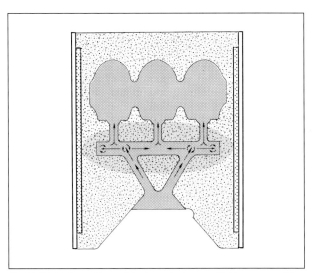

Fig 21-26 Molten alloy swirls through the manifold system, raising the temperature of the surrounding investment *(shaded area).*

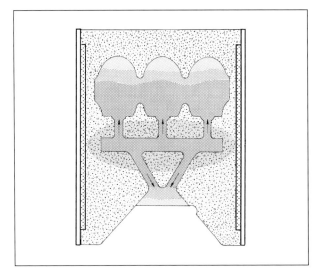

Fig 21-27 As the alloy begins to solidify, the heat around the manifold (dark shading) keeps it molten longer, preventing porosity in the bridge.

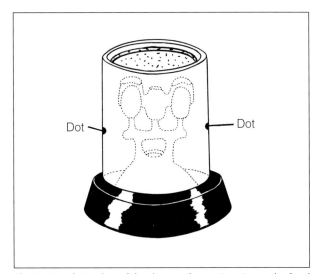

Fig 21-28 Relationship of the dots on the casting ring to the fixed partial denture wax pattern.

bulky horizontal runner bar is placed between crucible former and pattern.

Place a piece of 8-gauge (3.4-mm diameter) hollow plastic sprue former material horizontally into the sprue former network to form a manifold between the crucible former and the wax pattern (Fig 21-25). Be sure to plug both ends of the hollow sprue former with wax to avoid the formation of thin projections of investment that might break off in the mold. As the alloy makes its way through the feeder sprues, runner, and manifold sprues, the temperature of the surrounding investment is elevated (Fig 21-26). The metal farthest from the manifold—the margins, and the surface of the button exposed to ambient

room temperature—will cool first while the feeder bar is still fluid and can serve as a reservoir for solidification contraction in the fixed partial denture (Fig 21-27).

The runner bar also helps to stabilize the pattern against distortion during investing, and it equalizes the flow of metal so that all parts of the mold will be filled evenly and simultaneously during casting.[54]

Orientation of invested fixed partial dentures in the casting machine can affect the flow of metal into the mold. The pattern is placed in a vertical position on the horizontal centrifugal casting machine to insure that all parts of the mold will fill simultaneously. To facilitate proper orientation, a wax dot can be placed on the crucible former. This will leave an imprint on the surface of the investment which can be seen when the ring is placed in the casting machine (see Fig 21-25). As an alternative, two dots can be scribed on the outside of the ring, one directly opposite the other (Fig 21-28). These dots should be aligned with the axis of the pattern before investing.

Casting Armamentarium for Gold-Palladium Alloys

1. Casting ring with invested wax pattern
2. Furnace
3. Centrifugal casting machine with quartz crucible
4. Colored safety glasses
5. Gas-oxygen torch
6. Matches
7. Metal-ceramic alloy
8. Casting tongs
9. Laboratory knife
10. Toothbrush
11. Explorer

Casting Gold-Palladium Alloys

Special gold-palladium alloys are used for metal-ceramic restorations and where greater strength than that provided by type III gold is required. After the investment has set for 1 hour on the benchtop, grind or scrape away some of the excess investment beyond the end of the ring. This will remove the smooth, dense surface layer and allow gases to escape more readily from the mold during casting. Remove the crucible former and place the ring in a 600°F (315°C) oven. After 30 minutes in the low-heat oven, place the ring in a 1,300°F (704°C) oven for 1 hour. If the ring is left at this temperature any longer, the investment will start to break down.

Because of the higher melting temperature of the metal-ceramic alloy, the gas-air blowpipe is inadequate. A single-orifice, gas-oxygen torch should be used. To prevent accidents, exercise caution in the use of this torch. Oxygen always should be added to a gas flame, and the gas flame always should remain on until the oxygen has been turned off. If the gas is turned off first, there will be a small explosion inside the torch when the gas-oxygen ratio reaches a critical level. To start the torch:

1. Turn on gas and ignite.
2. Slowly add oxygen.

To turn off the torch:

1. Turn off the oxygen.
2. Turn off the gas.

A quartz crucible is preferred to a clay crucible. Use no flux with metal-ceramic alloys; it may upset the balance of the alloy and interfere with bonding later. Turn on

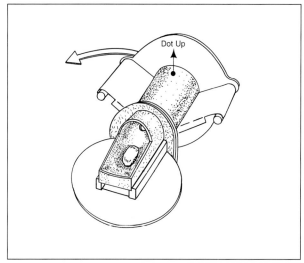

Fig 21-29 Correct positioning of the ring in the casting machine, with one dot facing upward.

the torch and adjust the flame to make the inner cone 0.25 to 0.5 inch (6.0 to 12 mm) long. Wear light blue or other colored protective goggles to protect your eyes from the intense light. Preheat the crucible with the torch and then place the alloy in the crucible.

Heat the alloy until it liquefies. It will go through four stages:

1. Red
2. Orange
3. White (dull)
4. White (mirror-like)

When the gold is orange, transfer the ring from the furnace to the cradle of the casting machine. In casting a fixed partial denture, make sure that one of the dots on the ring is in an up position, indicating that the mold of the framework is vertical (Fig 21-29).

Keep heating the gold. As it becomes white, a light fog or scum forms on the surface. As soon as that scum disappears and the metal is shiny, release the machine and cast. Bench cool the ring to room temperature. Metal-ceramic alloys should not be quenched. When it has cooled, remove the casting and pick off the remnants of the investment. Then wash the casting in water and lightly sandblast it. Do not pickle metal-ceramic alloys.

Casting Base Metal Alloys

These high-fusing alloys experience a high degree of shrinkage on cooling. To achieve the necessary mold expansion, the invested pattern should be placed in a water bath at 100°F (38°C) for 1 hour. Best results are obtained if the investment is allowed to cure overnight before proceeding with burnout. Place the ring in a cold oven and bring it up to 1,500°F (815°C) in approximately

1 hour. Allow it to heat soak at this temperature for approximately 2 hours to eliminate all traces of carbon. The recommended temperature may vary slightly for different alloys. Preheat the quartz crucible in the oven.

Wind the casting machine, giving it one or two extra winds to compensate for the much lighter density of the base metal alloy. Remove the quartz crucible from the oven with casting tongs and place it in the bracket on the casting machine. Place the metal ingots in the crucible.

Wear dark protective goggles for casting. As with gold-palladium alloys, a gas-oxygen torch must be used, but the higher casting temperatures of the base metal alloys require the use of a multiorifice tip. Turn on the gas first, adding oxygen to the gas flame. Adjust the flame to make the inner cones approximately 0.5 inch (12 mm)

long. Heat the alloy evenly by moving the torch around to cover all ingots. They will *not* liquefy. The ingots, glowing a uniform color, will slump, and their edges will round over, but tough oxide skins will prevent them from coalescing. Technicians who are used to melting alloys that form into a shiny pool may overheat the base metal alloys. This common error can burn off lower melting constituents and create bonding problems when the porcelain is later applied.[55] If the alloy is overheated or "burned," throw it out.

Cast immediately to avoid overheating. Bench cool the ring to room temperature. Remove the casting and pick off the remnants of investment. Clean the metal with an air abrasion unit using 50-μm alumina. Do *not* pickle base metal castings.

References

1. Hollenback GM: *Science and Technic of the Cast Restoration.* St Louis, CV Mosby Co, 1964, p 21.

2. Taggart WH: A new and accurate method of making gold inlays. *Dent Cosmos* 1907; 49:1117–1121.

3. O'Brien WJ: Evolution of dental casting. In Valega TM (ed): *Alternatives to Gold Alloys in Dentistry.* DHEW Publ No. (NIH) 77-1227. Washington DC, US Department of Health, Education and Welfare, 1977, pp 2–9.

4. *Dental Technology Reference for Fixed Restorations,* ed 7. 1983. Armonk, NY, JF Jelenko & Co, 1983, p VII–2.

5. Duncanson MG: Nonprecious metal alloys for fixed restorative dentistry. *Dent Clin North Am* 1976; 20:423–433.

6. *Current Dental Terminology,* ed 1. Chicago, American Dental Association, 1991.

7. Council on Dental Materials, Instruments and Equipment: Status report on low-gold-content alloys for fixed prostheses. *J Am Dent Assoc* 1980; 100:237–240.

8. Gourley JM: Current status of semi-precious and conventional gold alloys in restorative dentistry. *J Can Dent Assoc* 1975; 41: 453–455.

9. Kuschner ML: The carcinogenicity of beryllium. *Environ Health Perspect* 1981; 40:101–105.

10. Moffa JP, Guckes AD, Okawa MT, Lilly GT: An evaluation of nonprecious alloys for use with porcelain veneers. Part II. Industrial safety and biocompatibility. *J Prosthet Dent* 1973; 30:432–441.

11. Covington JS, McBride MA, Slagle WF, Disney AL: Quantization of nickel and beryllium leakage from base metal casting alloys. *J Prosthet Dent* 1985; 54:127–136.

12. Tai Y, De Long R, Goodkind RJ, Douglas WH: Leaching of nickel, chromium, and beryllium ions from base metal alloy in an artificial oral environment. *J Prosthet Dent* 1992; 68:692–697.

13. Fisher AA: *Contact Dermatitis,* ed 3. Philadelphia, Lea and Febiger, 1986, p 745.

14. Peltonen L: Nickel sensitivity in the general population. *Contact Dermatitis* 1979; 5:27–32.

15. Mjor IA, Christensen GJ: Assessment of local side effects of casting alloys. *Quintessence Int* 1993; 24:343–351.

16. Wirz J: Was ist dran am Palladium-streit? Ist das Material besser als sein Ruf? [What is the controversy about palladium—Is it better than its reputation?] *Phillip J* 1993; 9:407–408.

17. Moffa JP: Physical and mechanical properties of gold and base metal alloys. In Valega TM (ed): *Alternatives to Gold Alloys in Dentistry.* DHEW Publ No. (NIH) 77-1227. Washington DC, US Department of Health, Education and Welfare, 1977, pp 81–93.

18. Jendersen MD: Non-precious metals and the ceramo-metal restoration. *J Indiana Dent Assoc* 1975; 54:6–10.

19. Preston JD, Berger R: Some laboratory variables affecting ceramo-metal alloys. *Dent Clin North Am* 1977; 21:717–728.

20. Lorey RE, Edge MJ, Lang BR, Lorey HS: The potential for bonding titanium restorations. *J Prosthod* 1993; 2:151–155.

21. Akagi K, Okamoto Y, Matsuura T, Horibe T: Properties of test metal ceramic titanium alloys. *J Prosthet Dent* 1992; 68:462–467.

22. Rekow ED: Dental CAD-CAM systems—What is the state of the art? *J Am Dent Assoc* 1991; 122:42–48.

23. Revised American National Standard/American Dental Association Specification No. 5 for Dental Casting Alloys. New York, American National Standards Institute, 1988.

24. Hollenback GM, Skinner EW: Shrinkage during casting of gold and gold alloys. *J Am Dent Assoc* 1946; 33: 1391–1399.

25. Phillips RW: *Skinner's Science of Dental Materials,* ed 9. Philadelphia, WB Saunders Co, 1991, pp 393–412.

26. Scheu CH: A new precision casting technic. *J Am Dent Assoc* 1932; 19:630–633.

27. Mahler DB, Ady AB: An explanation for the hygroscopic expansion of dental gypsum products. *J Dent Res* 1960; 39:578–589.

28. Hollenback GM: Simple technic for accurate castings: New and original method of vacuum investing. *J Am Dent Assoc* 1948; 36:391–397.

29. Asgar K, Mahler DB, Peyton FA: Hygroscopic technic for inlay casting using controlled water additions. *J Prosthet Dent* 1955; 5:711–724.

30. Mahler DB, Ady AB: The effect of the water bath in hygroscopic casting techniques. *J Prosthet Dent* 1965; 15:1115–1121.

31. Craig RG: *Restorative Dental Materials,* ed 8. St Louis: CV Mosby Co, 1989, p 360.

32. Davis DR, Nguyen JH, Grey BL: Ring volume/ring liner ratio and effective setting expansion. *Int J Prosthodont* 1992; 5:403–408.

33. Verrett RG, Duke ES: The effect of sprue attachment design on castability and porosity. *J Prosthet Dent* 1989; 61:418–424.

34. Mumford GM, Phillips RW: Measurement of thermal expansion of cristobalite type investments in the inlay ring—Preliminary report. *J Prosthet Dent* 1958; 8:860–864.

35. Mahler DB, Ady AB: The influence of various factors on the efective setting expansion of casting investments. *J Prosthet Dent* 1963; 13:365–373.

36. Priest G, Horner JA: Fibrous ceramic aluminum silicate as an alternative to asbestos liners. *J Prosthet Dent* 1980; 44:51–56.

37. Davis DR: Potential health hazards of ceramic ring lining material. *J Prosthet Dent* 1987; 57:362–369.

38. Naylor WP, Moore BK, Phillips RW: A topographical assessment of casting ring liners using scanning electron microscopy. *Quint Dent Technol* 1987; 11:413–420.

39. Earnshaw R, Morey EF: The fit of gold-alloy full-crown castings made with ceramic casting ring liners. *J Dent Res* 1992; 71:1865–1870.

40. Morey EF, Earnshaw R: The fit of gold-alloy full-crown castings made with pre-wetted casting ring liners. *J Dent Res* 1992; 71:1858–1864.

41. Craig RG: *Restorative Dental Materials,* ed 8. St Louis: CV Mosby Co, 1989, p 465.

42. Earnshaw R: The effect of casting ring liners on the potential expansion of a gypsum-bonded investment. *J Dent Res* 1988; 67:1366–1370.

43. Johnson A: The effect of five investing techniques on air bubble entrapment and casting nodules. *Int J Prosthodont* 1992; 5:424–433.

44. Lyon HW, Dickson G, Schoonover IC: Effectiveness of vacuum investing in the elimination of surface defects in gold castings. *J Am Dent Assoc* 1953; 46:197–198.

45. Phillips RW: Relative merits of vacuum investing of small castings as compared to conventional methods. *J Dent Res* 1947; 26:343–352.

46. *Dental Technology Reference for Fixed Restorations,* ed 7. Armonk, NY, JF Jelenko, 1983, ppVIII–4.

47. *Ney Bridge and Inlay Book.* Hartford, CT, JM Ney Co, 1955, p 67.

48. Du Bois LM, Ritnour KL, Weins WN, Rinne VW: The effect of the temperature at quenching on the mechanical properties of casting alloys. *J Prosthet Dent* 1987; 57:566–571.

49. Campagni WV, Majchrowicz M: An accelerated technique for casting post and core restorations. *J Prosthet Dent* 1991; 66:155–156.

50. O'Brien WJ, Nielson JP: Decomposition of gypsum investments in the presence of carbon. *J Dent Res* 1959; 38:541–547.

51. Schnell RJ, Mumford GM, Phillips RW: An evaluation of phosphate bonded investments used with a high fusing alloy. *J Prosthet Dent* 1963; 13:324–336.

52. Saas FA, Eames WB: Fit of unit-cast fixed partial dentures relating to casting ring size and shape. *J Prosthet Dent* 1980; 43:163–167.

53. *Dental Technology Reference for Fixed Restorations,* ed 7. Armonk, NY, JF Jelenko, 1983, p IV–4.

54. Wetterstrom ET: An innovation in sprue design for Ceramico castings. *Thermotrol Technician* 1966; 20:3–4.

55. Weiss PA: New design parameters: Utilizing the properties of nickel-chromium superalloys. *Dent Clin North Am* 1977; 21:769–785.

Chapter 22

Finishing and Cementation

The surface of the casting that is retrieved from investment is too rough for use in the mouth. Five preparatory procedures need to be performed on any type of cemented restoration after it has been fabricated in the laboratory: preliminary finishing, try-in and adjustment, precementation polishing, cementation, and postcementation finishing. With skilled laboratory support, adjustments should be minimal, and the polishing may be done before try-in.

The internal (tooth-facing) and external aspects of a restoration are handled differently. The correct internal configuration allows a restoration to seat completely without binding, provides space for a film of cement, allows the margins to lie in intimate contact with the finish line of the tooth preparation, and provides an internal surface that is conducive to a strong cement bond. Sandblasting leaves a clean, textured surface on metals that is ideal for conventional nonadhesive luting. Special surface treatments are indicated for bonding with resin cements and will be discussed later.

The external surface of a cemented restoration must be smooth, and it should create as nearly a perfect uninterrupted transition from restorative material to tooth as possible. A rough surface accumulates plaque that is injurious to the health of the periodontal tissues,[1] and the amount of plaque is directly related to the roughness of the surface (Fig 22-1).[2] Metallic surfaces may be brought to only a satin finish before try-in, but they must be given a high luster following chairside adjustments. Porcelain that has been roughened by grinding must be polished and may also be reglazed after it is polished, although polishing alone can produce a surface that is as smooth as glazed porcelain[3,4] and slightly less abrasive on opposing enamel.[5]

Finishing and polishing should be accomplished by following a fixed routine, starting with an abrasive that is coarse enough to remove gross irregularities. The particles in any abrasive leave scratches on the surface. The surface is smoothed with abrasives of progressively smaller particle size, thereby substituting increasingly smaller scratches until the scratches are eliminated or reduced to microscopic size. It has been theorized that as a gold surface is polished, minute amounts of the abraded surface material (possibly even of molecular size) are filled into surface irregularities. This results in a microcrystalline surface layer that is known as the Beilby layer.[6]

Abrasives and Polishing Materials

Abrasives are exceptionally hard materials that develop sharp cutting edges when they are chipped. Polishing materials consist of abrasives and softer materials that are reduced to extremely fine particle size. For maximum cutting efficiency, the abrasive must be appreciably harder than the material on which it is used. The Knoop Hardness Numbers of commonly used abrasives, dental materials, and tooth structure are listed for comparison in Table 22-1.[7–10] In determining the effectiveness of an abrasive, factors other than hardness alone can be significant. The toughness of the binder and the ability of abrasive chips to break sharply, rather than rounding, can alter the effectiveness of an abrasive. Some commonly used abrasives and polishing materials are described briefly below:

1. *Diamond*—Chips are bound to a metal shape by a ceramic bond or by metal electroplating. The hardest of all abrasives, diamond should be reserved for use on hard, brittle substances such as enamel or porcelain. When used on ductile substances, such as gold, the abrasive particles become clogged with the material being abraded, and the diamond wheel or point becomes inefficient.
2. *Silicon carbide*—This commonly used laboratory abrasive is the basic material of carborundum. It is pressed into many shapes to form separating discs and the many points and wheels known as green stones.
3. *Emery*—This hard, black natural mineral is a mixture of aluminum oxide and iron oxide. Bound to paper discs with glue or resins, emery can be used on gold or porcelain.
4. *Aluminum oxide*—A synthetic abrasive produced by purifying bauxite to crystalline form in ovens. Coarse

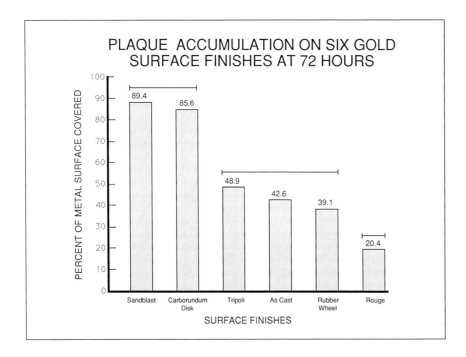

Fig 22-1 Percentage of metal surface covered by plaque (*P* < .05). (From Keenan MP, Shillingburg HT, Duncanson MG, Wade CK: Effects of cast gold surface finishing on plaque retention. *J Prosthet Dent* 1980; 43:168–173.)

Table 22-1 *Knoop Hardness Number (KHN) of Dental Substances and Materials[7–10]*

Substance (Material)	KHN
Cementum	40[7]
Dentin	68[7]
Gold alloy (type III)	145[7†]
Amalgam	155[8]
Gold-platinum MCR* alloy	192[8†]
Gold-palladium MCR* alloy	230[8†]
Ni-Cr MCR* alloy	267[8†]
Enamel	343[7]
Ni-Cr-Be MCR* alloys	367[8†]
Porcelain	460[7]
Pumice	560[8]
Sand (flint)	800[9]
Aluminum oxide	1900[8]
Emery	2000[9]
Silicon carbide	2500[9]
Diamond	8000+[10]

* Metal-ceramic restoration.
† Calculated from Vickers Hardness Number.

grit aluminum oxide is the abrasive in the brown, pink, or "coral" stones used for finishing metal-ceramic copings. A very fine grit (400) is used to manufacture white polishing stones, sometimes called "poly stones."

5. *Garnet* —Available in many grits, or particle sizes, this red abrasive is composed primarily of the silicates of aluminum and iron, with some silicates of magnesium, cobalt, and manganese as well. It will cut both metal and porcelain. Garnet is bound to paper discs with glue.

6. *Sand*—Sandpaper discs are coated with a dense crystalline form of quartz, called flint. Flint is a naturally occurring mineral that chips to form sharp cutting edges. It is not as durable or strong as some other abrasives, but it is a useful abrasive in finishing cast gold. It is available in various grits.

7. *Cuttle*—A fine, relatively soft polishing agent made from the calcified internal shell of the cuttlefish. It is used on paper discs.

8. *Tripoli*— A fine siliceous polishing powder that is combined with a wax binder to form light brown cakes. Tripoli is used in the initial polishing step of gold on either a cloth buff wheel or a soft bristle brush.

9. *Rouge*—Composed of iron oxide (Fe_2O_3), rouge is likewise supplied in cake form. It is the finest of polishing agents used *extraorally* on gold castings. It is applied with a soft bristle brush or a small muslin buff wheel. Rouge is also used to fabricate crocus discs.

10. *Tin oxide*—This is used as a fine powder on a brush or rubber cup for final intraoral polishing of metal restorations. It is the chief ingredient in Amalgloss (LD Caulk Div, Dentsply International, Milford, DE).

These materials are bonded to a paper backing or mixed with a binder and pressed into various shapes to form stone or rubber wheels, discs, and points for specific processes. They are also incorporated into pastes for use on brushes, cloth wheels, or rubber cups. Some commonly used forms are as follows:

1. *Separating discs* ("Joe Dandy" discs) are stiff and will cut on the edges as well as on the sides. They are useful for removing sprues from castings, for sectioning fixed partial dentures, and for contouring embrasures around pontics.
2. *Moore's Discs* (EC Moore Co, Dearborn, MI) are flexible paper discs coated on one side with various grits of garnet, sand, emery, and cuttle, and are used for contouring and smoothing large convex areas on gold and resins. Each disc has a square hole for mounting on a special mandrel, which allows them to be rotated in reverse.
3. *Heatless stones* are extremely coarse stones for bulk removal of metal.
4. *Busch Silent Stones* (Pfingst & Co, South Plainfield, NJ) are large, fine-grained stones for reducing broad areas of porcelain.
5. *Green stones* contain silicon carbide and are manufactured in many different shapes (Fig 22-2). They are permanently mounted to their mandrels and so can be rotated in reverse as well as forward. They are of medium grit and are used for shaping metal and porcelain.
6. *Pink stones* are made of porcelain-bonded aluminum oxide and are to be used only for finishing the areas of metal copings to which porcelain is to be fired.
7. *White stones* contain fine-grained aluminum oxide. They are useful for smoothing the rough surfaces left by green stones and for adapting gold margins to enamel intraorally.
8. *Rubber wheels* and *points* are used for polishing metals and ceramics. Examples of coarser discs are Cratex (William Dixon Co, Carlstadt, NJ), Gold Lustre White (JF Jelenko, Armonk, NY), White Flexie and Brown discs (Dedeco International, Long Eddy, NY). Finer discs that will produce a satin finish include Burlew, Sulci, Gold Lustre Blue (all from Jelenko), and Blue discs (Dedeco). Brownies and Greenies (Shofu Dental Corp, Menlo Park, CA) are fine-grit discs that are capable of producing a fairly high polish.

Preliminary Finishing of Gold Restorations

To minimize the expenditure of valuable chair time, preliminary adjustments using the die and master cast should be completed on the internal and external surfaces of the restoration prior to the cementation appointment. A dentist who can seat a crown that is comfortable with a minimum amount of chairside adjustments will win the confidence of the patient.

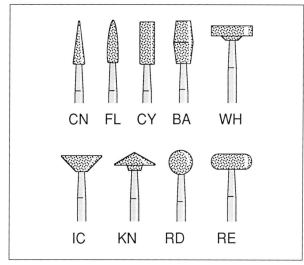

Fig 22-2 Common shapes of abrasive stones are: cone (CN), flame (FL), cylinder (CY), barrel (BA), wheel (WH), inverted cone (IC), knife edge (KN), round (RD), round edge (RE).

Armamentarium

1. High-speed handpiece
2. Straight handpiece
3. Separating disc on mandrel
4. No. 2F Craytex disc on mandrel
5. 5/8-inch Burlew wheel on mandrel
6. Sulci disc on small-head mandrel
7. No. 0 "bud" finishing bur
8. No. 330 friction-grip bur
9. Articulating paper
10. Green stone

Inspect the internal portions of the casting under magnification for small nodules or "bubbles" of gold. Remove any that are found with a no. 330 bur in a high-speed handpiece (Fig 22-3). Trace all of the negative angles on the inside of the occlusal surface with the tip of the bur. When there are no obvious artifacts in the casting, seat it gently on the die. Then remove the casting and inspect the preparation portion of the die. If there are any small scratches on the surface, examine the corresponding areas of the internal portion of the casting and use the side of the 330 bur to relieve any areas of the casting where small particles of stone or smudges of die spacer are found clinging.

Ideally, the casting should touch the die only in the marginal region. There should be a slight gap everywhere else for the future cement film. The optimum film thickness of zinc phosphate cement is approximately 30 to 40 μm.[11–12] The space allows cement to escape as the crown is seated and provides some thermal insulation under metal crowns. If adequate relief has not been created in the laboratory, it can be added by chemical or electrolytic etching until the restoration can be seated

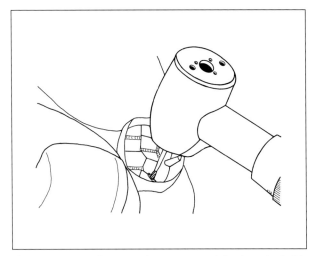

Fig 22-3 No. 330 bur is used to remove nodules from the inside of a casting.

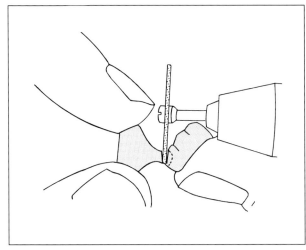

Fig 22-4 Sprue immediately adjacent to the casting is removed with a separating disc.

and removed from the die with gentle finger pressure. Mechanical grinding for this purpose must be done judiciously, because it can easily destroy retentive features or create marginal defects.

When you are satisfied with the fit on the die, the restoration is ready for finishing of the external surface. The procedure described here for finishing the external surface of a gold alloy is essentially the same as that developed by Tanner and described in detail by Troxell.[13]

Use a separating disc to cut the sprues from the casting (Fig 22-4). Diagonal cutting pliers may be used, but the stress generated by them could distort a thin casting.

Hold the handpiece with a firm palm grasp while cutting the sprue next to the casting. Avoid tipping the discs—if a disc binds in the cut groove, it may flip the casting out of your hand. After removing the sprue, use the separating disc to trim the remaining portions of the sprue attachment on the casting until the contour in that area is continuous with the contour of the restoration surrounding the sprue.

Use a coarse rubber disc (Craytex, White Flexie, Gold Lustre White) to smooth away the roughness left by the separating disc. Use light pressure and move the disc about quickly to avoid the formation of facets or flat spots. Use a finer Burlew or Gold Lustre Blue disc in a similar manner after the coarse disc (Fig 22-5, A). The entire external surface of the casting should now be smooth, with a satin finish. The axial surface should be finished to the margin. However, do not extend *over* the margin. To accomplish this, the disc should be rotated parallel with the margin, rather than perpendicular to it (Fig 22-5, B).

Seat the restoration on the mounted working cast. If a separate die and working cast have been used, some of the stone replicating the gingiva may need to be removed to seat the restoration completely. Slowly adjust the gold in the interproximal areas until the restoration

seats completely but still contacts the adjacent teeth. Coarse discs or stones should not be used for this purpose, as an open contact will result when the restoration is given its final polish.

The casting must be completely seated before checking the occlusion on the articulator. Otherwise, it may be ground out of occlusion before it is even tried in the mouth. Adjust any excessive centric and eccentric contacts by using marking ribbon and green stones (Dura-Green, Shofu).

Remove the restoration from the working cast and place it back on the die. Use a no. 0 "bud" finishing bur (Pfingst) to smooth out the grooves on the occlusal surface (Fig 22-6). Smooth the cusp ridges and blend them into the grooves on the occlusal surface with a small rubber sulci disc (Fig 22-7). External gold surfaces should have a satin-like finish produced by a Burlew rubber polishing wheel at try-in. For a novice, a highly polished surface is not desired at this time, because it will make detection of excessive occlusal and proximal contacts more difficult. The inner, or tooth-facing, surface should be air abraded or sandblasted in preparation for try-in.

Try-in and Adjustment of Gold Restorations

If you are careful and gentle, the try-in procedure can be accomplished on many patients without administering an anesthetic. The patient's unimpaired tactile sense can be valuable during the adjustment of the occlusion, and the annoyance of lingering anesthesia is avoided. If the patient is made uncomfortable by the procedure, however, an anesthetic most certainly should be given.

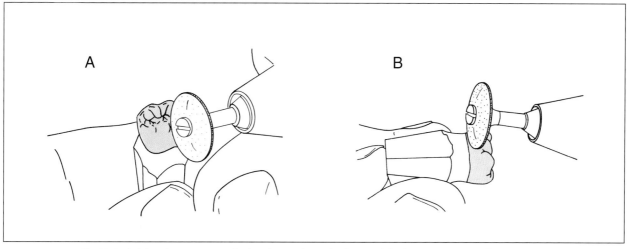

Fig 22-5 Axial surfaces are smoothed with a Burlew wheel (A). While the area very near the margins is being smoothed, the wheel should be turned parallel with the margin (B).

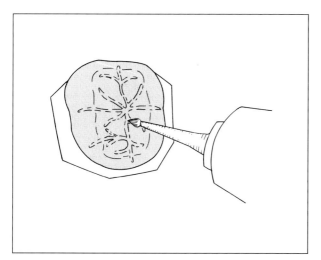

Fig 22-6 Grooves are finished with a small "bud" finishing bur.

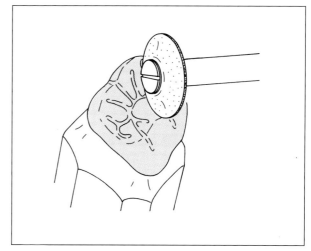

Fig 22-7 Cusp ridges are finished with a small sulci disc.

Cementation should be postponed if the patient reports that the tooth has been hypersensitive under the provisional crown. The tooth would be subjected to even greater chemical and thermal trauma by placement of a metal crown. In these cases, make sure the provisional restoration is not in hyperocclusion and that it covers all prepared tooth surfaces. Recement it for several days. If pulpitis persists, endodontic therapy will be necessary before the permanent restoration can be cemented. Never cement a crown permanently over a symptomatic tooth.

Try-in Armamentarium

1. 2 x 2-inch gauze squares
2. Mallet
3. No. 15 straight chisel
4. Backhaus towel forceps
5. Miller forceps
6. Cotton pliers
7. Cotton pellets
8. Dental floss
9. Plastic bite wafer
10. Articulating paper
11. Silver plastic shim stock (13 mm thick)
12. Straight handpiece
13. 5/8-inch Burlew wheel on mandrel
14. Green stones
15. No. 2 round bur
16. Spratley knife
17. Contra-angle handpiece
18. Tapered white polishing stone
19. Petrolatum
20. 3/8-inch cuttle disc on mandrel

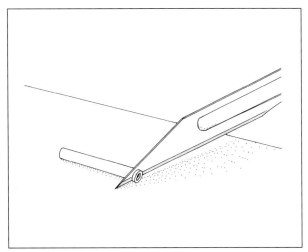

Fig 22-8 A safety ring may be fashioned by cutting a thin slice from a hollow sprue.

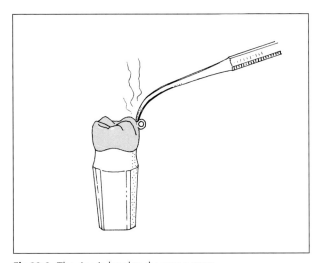

Fig 22-9 The ring is luted to the wax pattern.

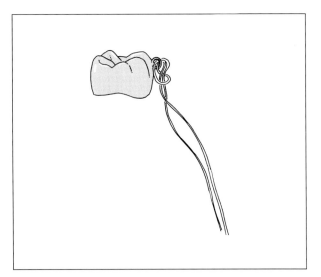

Fig 22-10 A length of dental floss is looped through the ring on the casting.

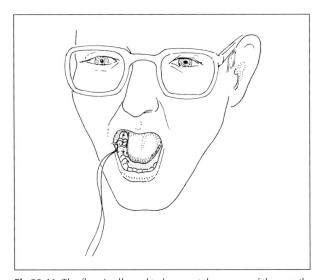

Fig 22-11 The floss is allowed to hang out the corner of the mouth.

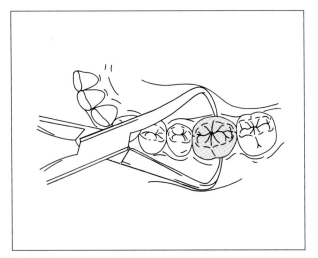

Fig 22-12 The provisional restoration can be removed with a Backhaus forceps.

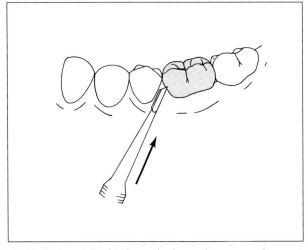

Fig 22-13 A straight chisel can also be used to remove the provisional restoration.

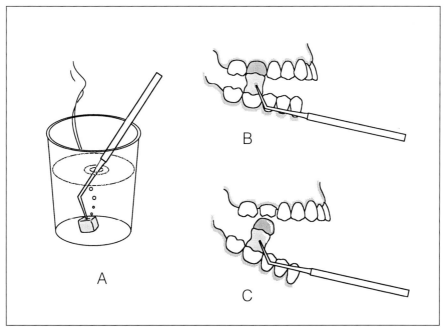

Fig 22-14 A Richwil Crown Remover is soaked in hot tap water for 1 minute (A). The patient closes on the softened cube (B). The patient opens quickly and forcefully to remove the crown (C).

Precautions must be taken during try-in to minimize the risk of the restoration being swallowed or aspirated. This is especially important with patients whose reflexes are diminished, such as those who are elderly or sedated. A small safety ring can be provided on metal crowns by cutting a thin slice from a hollow sprue (Fig 22-8). Attach it to the wax pattern where it will not interfere with the occlusion (Fig 22-9).[14] Thread floss through the ring before trying the casting in the mouth (Fig 22-10). Leave the floss hanging out of the mouth during try-in and adjustments (Fig 22-11). This also makes removal of tightly fitting castings easier. If a safety line is not used, a gauze square should be placed on the floor of the mouth.

Remove the provisional restoration by grasping the buccal and lingual surfaces with the tips of a Backhaus towel forceps and rocking it to the facial and lingual (Fig 22-12). An alternate technique utilizes a small mallet and a straight enamel chisel with a 1.5-mm-wide blade. The tip of the chisel is pointed in an occlusal direction and engaged under a bulge on the buccal surface of the restoration near one of the proximal embrasures (Fig 22-13). The chisel is tapped lightly to loosen the restoration.

Most of the temporary cement will adhere to the inside of the provisional restoration. Carefully pick off any cement left on the surface of the preparation. A dry cotton pellet held in cotton pliers is run over the preparation surface to wipe off small clinging particles. Wash with lukewarm water. Cold water will make the unanesthetized patient uncomfortable.

Evaluation of a restoration should be carried out in the following sequence:

1. Proximal contacts
2. Margins (completeness of seating)
3. Occlusion
4. Contours
5. Esthetics

Adjustment of Proximal Contacts

The proximal contacts of a restoration must be neither too tight nor too light. If they are too tight, they will interfere with correct seating of the restoration, produce discomfort, and make it difficult for the patient to floss. A proximal contact that is too light will allow impaction of strands of food, which is deleterious to the gingiva and annoying to the patient.

Place the restoration on the tooth and seat it with firm finger pressure. Do not mallet or have the patient exert occlusal pressure. Jamming the restoration onto the tooth at this time may make it extremely difficult to remove. You should be able to remove a crown by grasping it with a dry gauze sponge and rocking it slightly. A crown that cannot be removed with the fingers may be removed by using a Richwil Crown Remover (Almore International, Portland, OR), which is a green, sticky cube. The cube is softened in hot water and placed over the crown (Fig 22-14, A). The patient is instructed to bite into the cube and hold for a few seconds (Fig 22-14, B). Then a quick opening movement should remove the crown from the tooth preparation (Fig 22-14, C). Obviously, this requires the presence of firm, natural opposing teeth with no cemented restorations on them.

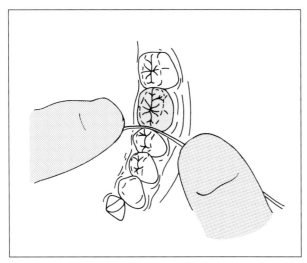

Fig 22-15 Proximal contacts are tested with dental floss.

Using the straight chisel and mallet as described for provisional crown removal may be necessary. Often a crown will be easier to remove after being worn for 24 hours without cement. If all else fails, the restoration must be removed by cutting it off.

A frequent cause for failure of a restoration to seat completely is an overcontoured proximal surface. Hold the restoration firmly in place and test both proximal contacts with waxed floss (Fig 22-15). If you do not hold the crown firmly enough, it may become slightly elevated or tipped, allowing the floss to pass through even though the contact is actually too tight. Each contact should be as tight as the others in the mouth. If floss will not pass through the contact, remove the restoration and examine the proximal surfaces.

At this point, the desirability of leaving a satin finish on a gold restoration becomes apparent, because there will be a shiny burnished area where the tight contact occurred. Use a Burlew or Craytex wheel to remove the shiny mark and try the casting back on the tooth. Repeat until floss can pass through with the same amount of resistance offered by the other contacts. If both proximal contacts feel too tight, adjust only the tighter contact first. Sometimes this will relieve the pressure on the second contact without it needing adjustment.

Care must be taken not to remove too much material from the contact area. If the proximal contact is open or too light, this must be corrected by adding solder before cementation.

Marginal Adaptation (Completeness of Seating)

After the proximal contacts have been corrected, seat the restoration and examine the margins closely. An acceptable margin is not overextended, underextended, too thick, or open (Fig 22-16). A margin is generally considered to be open if the gap is greater than 50 μm, which means the tip of a sharp explorer can be inserted between restoration and tooth. A restoration that rocks perceptibly on the tooth cannot have closed margins on both sides at once. Subgingival marginal discrepancies are the most difficult to detect and the most detrimental to gingival health.

The most common cause of poorly adapted margins is failure of the restoration to seat completely. If the proximal contacts are not too tight and the margins are still short or open, there may be some minute undercut, unseen defect, or distortion preventing seating. A convenient technique for improving the seating of castings of softer gold alloys is to produce a matte surface on the inner surface with a sandblaster or air brush, seat the restoration firmly on the tooth, remove it, and relieve any shiny areas with a no. 330 bur. Be careful not to destroy the metal projections that fit into grooves or boxes.

There are a number of materials that can be used for locating internal discrepancies. The inside of the crown may be painted with chloroform and rouge or thinned typewriter correction fluid, or sprayed with a thin layer of a dry aerosol indicator (Occlude, Pascal Co, Bellevue, WA) (Fig 22-17). Disclosing wax (Kerr Manufacturing Co, Romulus, MI) indicates not only points of interference, but the thickness and configuration of the future cement film, which in turn reveals the completeness of seating and the closeness of adaptation of subgingival margins.[15] Fill the restoration half full of disclosing wax and heat it in a flame just enough to make the wax flow and adhere to the inner surface. The tooth must be wet with saliva to keep the wax from sticking to it. When the wax has resolidified, seat the restoration, hold it in place for approximately 10 seconds, and remove it. Areas of metal-tooth contact will appear inside a crown as shiny spots devoid of wax. Ideally, the margins (where no cement spacer was used on the die) should show intimate contact, and the remainder of the restoration should have a thin coating of wax representing the cement space.

Relief of impinging areas with a no. 330 bur will usually allow the restoration to seat farther. Impression-type materials, such as Fit-Checker (GC Dental Industrial Corp, Tokyo) or alginate can also be used, but they are more time consuming. All disclosing materials must be completely removed from inside the restoration by swabbing with chloroform and sandblasting prior to cementation so that retention will not be diminished. The tooth may be cleaned with Cavilax (ESPE-Premier, Norristown, PA).

Gold Margin Finishing

Type III and softer golds differ from other materials in that they can be burnished against the tooth to some extent. This must not be attempted until you are certain the casting is seated as far as it will go.

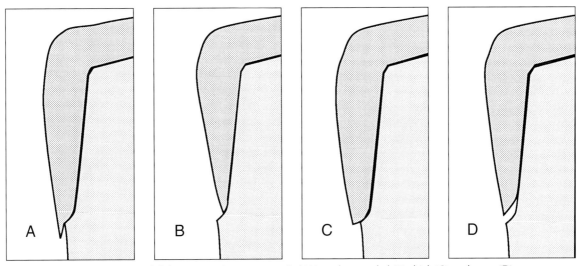

Fig 22-16 Types of defective margins: overextended (A), underextended (B), thick (C), and open (D).

Two types of margins need to be considered. Those margins that will be *subgingival* can be burnished on the die with a beavertail burnisher or fine stone. No intraoral finishing procedure is indicated for subgingival margins because of the risk of damage to the tooth and periodontal structures. *Supragingival margins* of inlays, onlays, and partial veneer crowns can be finished on the tooth. With proper finishing procedures, margins can be adapted to reduce the opening between the margin and tooth to less than the film thickness of the cement.[16]

Place the casting on the prepared tooth and have the patient seat it firmly by closing on a plastic bite wafer or a wooden stick. Verify that the restoration is completely seated and that the margins fit adequately. No attempt should be made to close gross marginal openings, because gold that has been moved or "dragged" by a coarse abrasive forms a soft, granular lip that can be easily broken or deformed during subsequent manipulation.[17]

A burnisher, such as a dull Spratley knife, can be used to press the margins against the tooth surface (Fig 22-18). The restoration must be held in place with another instrument or by having the patient close on a bite wafer during burnishing.

The use of a Spratley knife has been shown to improve marginal adaptation by as much as 30 μm.[18] If a white polishing stone, lubricated with petrolatum, is also used and followed by a cuttle disc, the adaptation of the margin can be improved by nearly 60 μm. Therefore, a white polishing stone and petrolatum are used for finishing after the burnishing. The white stone should always rotate from casting to tooth surface, under heavy pressure and at low speed (Fig 22-19). Cut slight amounts of gold and tooth structure. Check for open margins with an explorer. If slight defects exist, the procedure should be continued until the margin is smooth. Green stones are not recommended, as they may abrade too much tooth

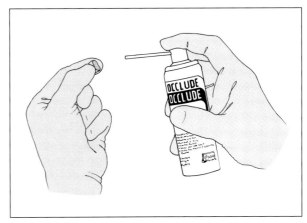

Fig 22-17 Inside of the casting is coated with an indicator that will show the location of areas that prevent complete seating.

structure and gold. A final precementation smoothing can be achieved with a 3/8-inch cuttle disc.

Care should be exercised in removing the casting to prevent damage to the margins. A dull chisel can be placed under a proximal area, and several light taps with a mallet will remove the casting. The Backhaus towel forceps can also be used, taking care not to damage the margins. If there are sound opposing teeth, the Richwil Crown Remover can be used as described previously (page 391). A safety ring made as an integral part of the restoration to prevent aspiration (see Fig 22-8) can also be used as an aid in removing a crown following try-in. When the casting has been removed for the last time, the ring is removed and the area polished.

If a restoration persists in not seating completely, you must recognize that inordinate amounts of time can be

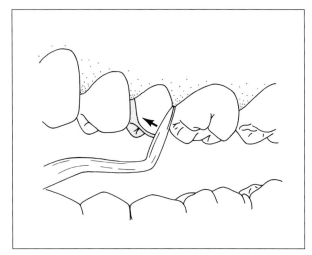

Fig 22-18 All accessible margins are burnished intraorally with a smooth, dull instrument.

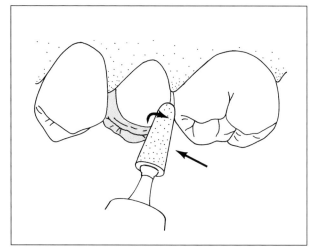

Fig 22-19 Margins are finished with a white stone rotating from gold to tooth.

spent in attempting to make a poor restoration fit. The end result of this expenditure of time will be a mediocre restoration at best. If a restoration will not fit and the cause cannot be quickly determined and corrected, the restoration should be remade. If the discrepancy in fit appears to be similar on the die and on the tooth, a new restoration can be fabricated on the same die, provided the die has not been damaged.

Occlusal Adjustment

Only after you are satisfied that the restoration is seated completely should any occlusal adjustments be performed. To provide a basis for comparison, instruct the patient to close into the customary position of maximum intercuspation with the restoration removed. Note the position of the teeth and the completeness of closure and contact. Locate a pair of teeth near the prepared tooth where the patient can hold a strip of 13-μm (.0005 inch) shim stock (Artus Corp, Englewood, NJ).

Then insert the restoration and see if the patient can still hold the shim between the same pair of nearby teeth. If not, the crown is high in the intercuspal position (Fig 22-20). Place a thumb on the patient's chin and arc the mandible open and closed until the mandible is slowly guided into its most retruded position; have the patient close until the first tooth contact occurs. Ask the patient to point to the tooth touching. If the restoration is indicated, it is high and needs occlusal adjustment.

Ask the patient to close together forcefully and try to make all teeth touch. If the mandible shifts to the side where the restoration is located, the buccal incline of the maxillary lingual cusp or the lingual incline of the mandibular buccal cusp needs adjustment (Fig 22-21). If the mandible shifts to the side away from the restoration, one of two deflective contacts requires correction. There

is a possibility of a heavy contact between the lingual incline of the maxillary buccal cusp and the buccal incline of the mandibular buccal cusp (Fig 22-22). There may also be excessive contact between the lingual incline of the maxillary lingual cusp and the buccal incline of the mandibular lingual cusp that needs correction (Fig 22-23).

Cut a piece of thin articulating paper the width of the restoration and place it in a Miller forceps. Hold it between the restoration and the opposing tooth, and have the patient close. Remove the restoration from the mouth and remove *only* the carbon marks on the *appropriate* surfaces. Ignore other markings on the restoration at this time. This procedure should be continued until no mandibular shift is evident and shim stock can be held between adjacent pairs of teeth. Due to the resiliency of the bones and joints, the patient's ability to hold shim stock on the opposite side of the arch is not a sure indication that the restoration is adequately adjusted.

Care must be taken not to overcorrect the occlusion. This can be monitored by placing a narrow strip of plastic shim stock over the restoration and having the patient close on it. The shim stock should offer the same amount of resistance when tugged from the side as do the adjacent teeth (Fig 22-24). If the shim stock holds on the adjacent teeth and not on the restoration, the restoration has been overadjusted and must be either added to or remade. Ideally, the anterior teeth should not touch in the centric position; they should miss by the thickness of the 13 μm (0.0005 inch) shim stock.

Adjustment of the restoration in excursive movements is essential. This can be tested by again using the narrow strip of plastic shim stock. Place it between the restoration and opposing tooth, and ask the patient to close firmly; then have the patient move into a working relationship on the side of the mouth opposite the restoration. The shim stock should be held tightly in the intercuspal position,

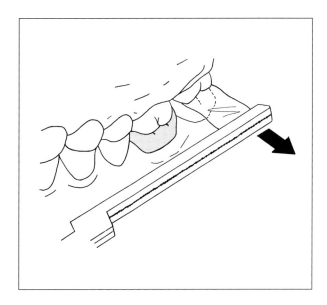

Fig 22-20 If the patient can hold shim stock on adjacent teeth with the crown out, but not with it in, the crown is too high.

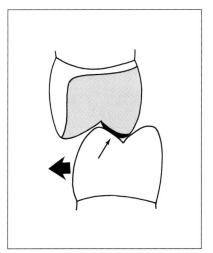

Fig 22-21 A premature contact on the buccal incline of the maxillary lingual cusp produces a buccal shift of the mandible.

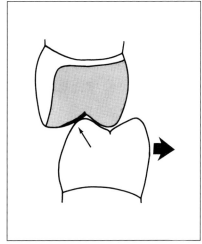

Fig 22-22 A premature contact on the lingual slope of the maxillary buccal cusp produces a lingual shift of the mandible.

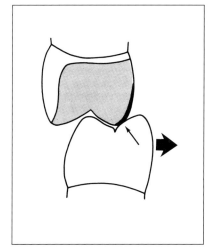

Fig 22-23 A premature contact on the lingual incline of the maxillary lingual cusp produces a lingual shift of the mandible.

but as soon as the nonworking movement starts, it should be able to be removed easily from between the restoration and opposing teeth. If not, replace the shim stock with articulating paper and locate the area of contact.

For adjustment of the nonworking movement, the marks that are found on the buccal inclines of the maxillary lingual cusps and the lingual inclines of the mandibular buccal cusps must be eliminated (Fig 22-25). Working-side interferences on the restoration may be adjusted by having the patient move into a working relationship on the side of the mouth where the restoration is located. For the adjustment of working-side interferences, remove contacts on lingual inclines of maxillary lingual cusps and buccal inclines of mandibular lingual cusps (Fig 22-26).

Contacts between the lingual inclines of the maxillary buccal cusps and buccal inclines of mandibular buccal cusps may or may not be removed depending on the occlusal scheme that is being established. If the goal is a canine-guided or mutually protected occlusion, these contacts should be removed. However, if group function is desired, these contacts are desirable and should be reduced only to the level at which they no longer cause disocclusion of the canine teeth. Teeth that are mobile may move during excursions, giving a false indication on the articulating ribbon. To detect movement, hold a fingernail against the facial surface of the restored tooth and its neighbor during excursions.

Finally, protrusive interferences are identified and re-

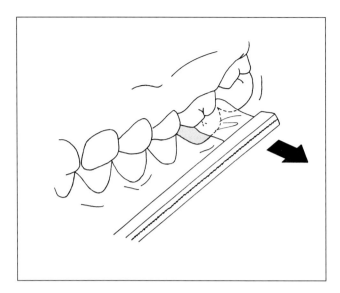

Fig 22-24 If the patient can hold shim stock over the crown, the crown has been correctly adjusted. If not, it has been overadjusted.

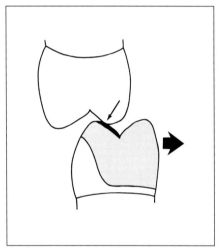

Fig 22-25 Nonworking interference.

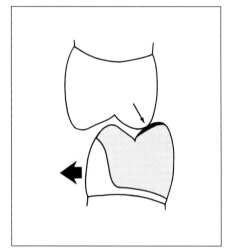

Fig 22-26 Working interference.

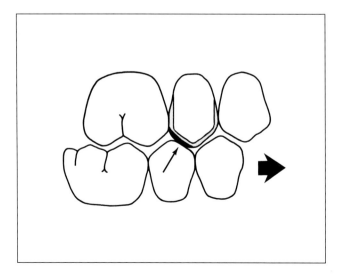

Fig 22-27 Protrusive interference.

moved. Again the patient closes on plastic shim stock in a retruded position and then moves the mandible forward. The distal inclines of the maxillary teeth and the mesial inclines of the mandibular teeth will be adjusted to relieve protrusive interferences (Fig 22-27). Contacts should appear on anterior teeth during excursive movements. Since anterior teeth help to disengage posterior teeth during excursive movements, these are considered desirable contacts. Whenever possible, anterior guidance should be shared by two or more pairs of occluding teeth.

Premature contacts on smooth surfaces can be located with great accuracy by adapting a strip of Occlusal Indicator Wax (Kerr) to the teeth of the restored quadrant with the shiny, adhesive side toward the restoration. Have the patient moisten the wax with saliva to prevent it from sticking to the opposing teeth and then tap the jaws in the maximum intercuspal position several times. The wax over the restoration should appear perforated to the same degree as the wax on the neighboring teeth. Excessive contacts will appear as bright spots uncovered by wax. Relieve these directly through the wax using a large high-speed round bur on metals and a diamond stone on ceramics. After these contacts have been equilibrated, apply more wax and have the patient execute several chewing strokes. Interferences will appear as wax-free areas not present in maximum intercuspation.

Contours

Improper contours may impair gingival health and detract from a natural appearance, as described in Chapter 19. They must be corrected before cementation. Excessive convexity near the gingival margin promotes accumulation of plaque. Surfaces directly occlusal to furcations are usually concave, and the concavity should extend occlusally on the axial surface of the restoration to improve access for a toothbrush.

Esthetics

Step back and view the restoration from a conversational distance to see if its contours harmonize with the rest of the patient's dentition. Let the patient look in a mirror so that any objections to the appearance can be dealt with before the restoration is cemented.

Precementation Polishing of Gold Restorations

After the occlusion has been adjusted and accessible margins have been finished in the mouth, the restoration is polished to a high shine.

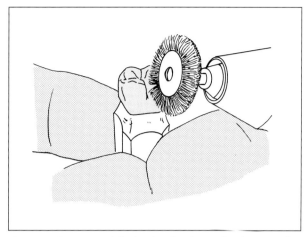

Fig 22-28 Casting is polished with soft Robinson brushes using first tripoli and then gold rouge.

Armamentarium

1. Straight handpiece
2. 5/8-inch Burlew wheel on mandrel
3. Sulci disc on small-head mandrel
4. No. 0 finishing bur
5. Mounted Robinson brushes (soft)
6. Tripoli
7. Gold rouge
8. 1-inch masking tape
9. Sandblaster

Remove any rough spots on the axial surfaces with a 5/8-inch Burlew wheel. Stay 1.0 mm away from any margins that have already been finished in the mouth, as they are fragile and may be bent or polished away with this abrasive wheel. Then polish all the axial surfaces with tripoli on a soft-bristle brush (Fig 22-28). Run the handpiece in reverse to minimize the material thrown back in your face. Polish the axial surface with rouge on a second soft-bristle brush reserved for this purpose only. This should be done with the restoration on a die to avoid rounding over the thin margins. Until this time, manipulation of the gingival margins has been avoided, but now they must be polished to a high shine, especially where they will lie subgingivally. Polishing of supragingival margins that were finished in the mouth may be postponed until after the restoration is cemented.

Occlusal anatomy that has been lost through adjustments is restored with a 171L carbide bur. Then the recreated occlusal grooves are refined with a no. 0 bud-shaped finishing bur. Cusp ridges may be smoothed with a sulci disc, taking care not to destroy the occlusal contacts so carefully developed earlier. From this point, the occlusal surface can be treated in one of two ways: it can be carefully polished to a high shine, or it can be sandblasted to provide a matte finish. The dull matte surface will enable observation of facets or burnishing produced by occlusal contacts after the casting has been in the

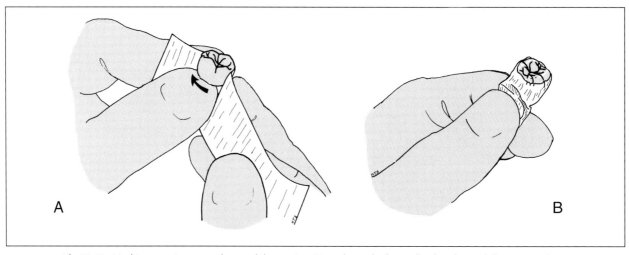

Fig 22-29 Masking tape is wrapped around the casting (A) so that only the occlusal surface is left uncovered (B).

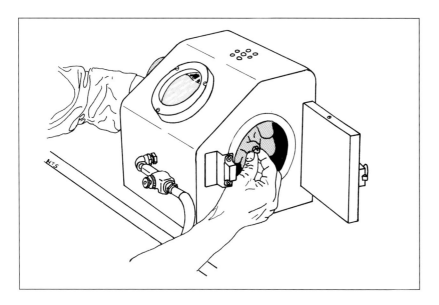

Fig 22-30 Casting is placed in the sandblaster.

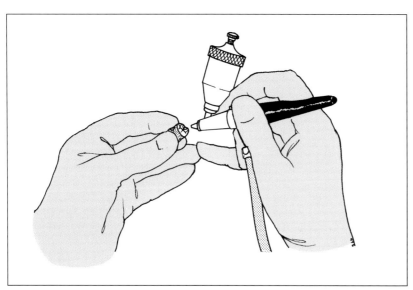

Fig 22-31 An air brush also can be used to apply a matte finish to the occlusal surface of the casting.

mouth for a short time. The use of a matte finish in no way implies that the occlusal surface is unfinished or left in a roughly ground condition.

When a sandblaster is used to produce the matte finish on the occlusal surface, the polished axial surfaces and margins should be protected by wrapping the casting in 1-inch-wide masking tape (Fig 22-29, A). The edge of the tape should be tightly adapted around the marginal ridges and cusp ridges, since any area not covered by the tape will be sandblasted. The excess width of tape left projecting beyond the margin forms a handle by which the casting can be held in the sandblaster (Fig 22-29, B). The casting is placed in the sandblaster (Fig 22-30) and the occlusal surface is given a uniformly dull surface by a stream from the nozzle from a distance of about 3 inches.

A less coarse matte finish can be produced by a handheld air abrasion unit with fine aluminum oxide abrasive (Microetcher II, Danville Engineering, San Ramon, CA; or Air Brush, Paasche Air Brush Co, Harwood Heights, IL) (Fig 22-31). Move the nozzle around until all exposed areas of the crown have been dulled to a uniform matte finish. Rinse the restoration in water and dry with air. Make a final check to be sure there are no remnants of polishing agent or abrasive inside the restoration.

Postcementation Finishing of Gold Restorations

After cementation, the occlusion should be tested again to make sure that there has been no increase in vertical dimension. There also may be excursive prematurities that escaped detection at try-in because of movement of the uncemented restoration. Ask the patient how the restoration feels. Any report of a strange feeling in centric occlusion, or a statement that the restoration "bumps" or "catches" during excursions means that there is a premature contact or an excursive interference. If not corrected, these can cause tooth hypersensitivity, tenderness, and even myofacial disturbances.

As a final check of the occlusion on a polished restoration, use Occlusal Indicator Wax as described on page 397. Then remove the wax, refine the anatomy with pointed stones, and repolish all ground surfaces using fine-grit rubber points.

The white polishing stone lubricated with petrolatum may again be used on the accessible margins of gold castings to reduce any minute projections of gold or enamel. However, after the cement has hardened, no further closing of the margins can be accomplished and the result of attempts to do so is likely to be excessive removal of gold and exposure of even more underlying cement. The white stone may be followed by a fine cuttle disc, which has been lubricated to make it flexible, and several grits of wet pumice on a rubber cup.

Final polishing of the gold restoration can be accomplished intraorally with Amalgloss (LD Caulk) on a rubber cup or brush. An anesthetized tooth can easily be overheated during polishing. To avoid this, use only light intermittent contact and keep one finger resting on the restoration to monitor its temperature.

Preliminary Finishing of Base Metal Restorations

Base metals have grown in popularity in the last couple of decades because they are significantly less expensive than gold alloys. They also provide greater strength than do gold alloys, making them desirable for long-span prostheses. They are commonly used for resin-bonded fixed partial dentures because they provide a strong bond to resin cements when properly etched.

Armamentarium

1. High-speed handpiece
2. Straight handpiece
3. 1.5-inch cutoff disc on mandrel
4. No. 8 coral stone on mandrel
5. No. 330 bur
6. No. 1 round bur
7. Aluminum oxide tapered stone
8. Aluminum oxide inverted cone
9. Blue rubber wheels and mounted points

The technique for finishing castings made of a base metal alloy is similar to that employed for gold alloys. The major difference lies in the use of coarser and harder abrasives on base metals. If the alloy being finished contains beryllium, standards of the Occupational Safety and Health Administration (OSHA) of the US Department of Labor require that it be ground only where there is adequate exhaust ventilation or if the technician is wearing an approved respirator.[19]

Use a 1.5-inch-diameter cutoff disc to remove the sprue(s). Complete the contouring of the surfaces where the sprues were attached with a no. 8 aluminum oxide coral wheel on a mandrel. Examine the internal aspect of the casting for small nodules of metal. Remove them with a no. 330 bur in a high-speed handpiece. When all such defects, as well as all investment, have been removed, try the casting on the working cast. If it binds, remove the casting. Look for particles of stone or smudges of die relief agent on the inside of the restoration and remove them with the no. 330 bur. Reseat the casting for finishing.

Smooth the occlusal grooves with a no. 1 carbide bur. Then do the rough finishing on all accessible areas with the no. 8 aluminum oxide coral wheel. Finish occlusal morphologic features (triangular ridges, cusp ridges, and cusp inclines) with a mounted coral aluminum oxide tapered stone and inverted cone. Smooth the casting with blue rubber wheels and mounted points.

Try-in, Adjustment, and Polishing of Base Metal Restorations

The fit of a base metal restoration is adjusted in much the same way as for a gold restoration. Because of the greater hardness of base metals, sandblasting will not disclose binding areas; therefore, disclosing paints or sprays must be depended on. Smooth, highly polished axial surfaces are of equal importance in castings made of base metals. Because of the hardness of these alloys, some adjustments in technique and materials are required.

Armamentarium

1. Straight handpiece
2. Blue disc on mandrel
3. White disc on mandrel
4. No. 1 round bur
5. Felt wheels
6. Felt cones
7. Ti-Cor
8. Ti-Hi
9. Mounted Robinson brushes (soft)
10. Tripoli
11. Palladius
12. 1-inch masking tape
13. Air abrader

With blue wheels and tips, smooth areas that were roughened during chairside adjustments. Then go over all of the accessible areas with a white rubber wheel. Finish right to the margins by holding the casting so the wheel is running parallel with the margin. The bottom of each groove can be finished with a no.1 carbide bur. Steel burs are not very effective on base metal alloys, so bud finishing burs cannot be used for finishing grooves on base metal castings.

The next step will vary depending on the hardness of the metal used. If it is an extremely hard metal, use Ti-Cor (Ticonium Co, Albany, NY) on a felt disc for axial surfaces and on felt cones for occlusal anatomy. Clean the casting thoroughly and apply the high shine with Ti-Hi (Ticonium) on felt discs and cones. If a somewhat softer base metal alloy such as Rexillium III (Jeneric Industries, Wallingford, CT) is used, the final polish can be achieved by the use of tripoli on a bristle brush, followed by Palladius (Vident, Baldwin Park, CA) on another bristle brush. Rouge can also be used for the final step, although it is not quite as effective. A matte finish on metal occlusal surfaces can be provided with an air abrasion unit if desired. Protect the polished axial surfaces with masking tape if you do.

Because the long-term success of any restoration is strongly influenced by the quality of the patient's oral hygiene, home care instructions and dispensing of appropriate cleaning aids (floss threaders, interproximal brushes, etc) must be considered an essential part of the cementation appointment.

Cements

The gap between an indirect fixed restoration and the tooth is filled with a cement, or luting agent. The mechanisms that hold a restoration on a prepared tooth can be divided into nonadhesive (mechanical) luting, micromechanical bonding, and molecular adhesion. In many cases, combinations of these mechanisms are at work.

Bonding Mechanisms

Nonadhesive Luting. Originally, as the name implies (Latin *lutum* = mud), the luting agent served primarily to fill the gap and prevent entrance of fluids. Zinc phosphate cement, for example, exhibits no adhesion on the molecular level. It holds the restoration in place by engaging small irregularities on the surfaces of both tooth and restoration. The nearly parallel opposing walls of a correctly prepared tooth make it impossible to remove the restoration without shearing or crushing the minute projections of cement extending into recesses in the surfaces (Fig 22-32).

Micromechanical Bonding. Resin cements have tensile strengths in the range of 30 to 40 MPa,[20] which is approximately five times that of zinc phosphate cement. When used on pitted surfaces, they can provide effective micromechanical bonding (Fig 22-33). The tensile strength of such bonds can sometimes exceed the cohesive strength of enamel. This allows the use of less extensive tooth preparation for restorations such as ceramic veneers and resin-bonded fixed partial dentures.

The deep irregularities necessary for micromechanical bonding can be produced on enamel surfaces by etching with a phosphoric acid solution or gel[21]; on ceramics by etching with hydrofluoric acid[22]; and on metals by electrolytic etching, chemical etching, sandblasting, or by incorporating salt crystals into the preliminary resin pattern.[23]

Molecular Adhesion. Molecular adhesion involves physical forces (bipolar, Van der Waals and chemical bonds (ionic, covalent) between the molecules of two different substances (Fig 22-34). Newer cements, such as polycarboxylates and glass ionomers, possess some adhesive capabilities, although this is limited by their relatively low cohesive strength. They still depend primarily on nearly parallel walls in the preparation to retain restorations.

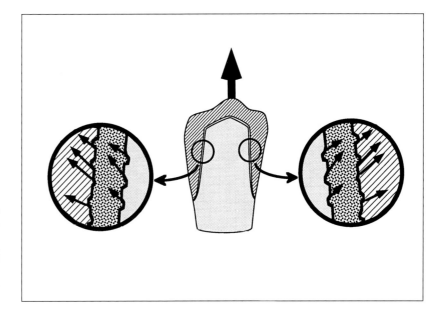

Fig 22-32 Nonadhesive luting. The crown can be removed only along the path *(large arrow)* determined by the axial walls of the preparation. Cement extending into small irregularities of the adjoining surfaces *(shown magnified in the two large circles)* prevents removal along any path more vertical than the sides of the irregularities *(small arrows).*

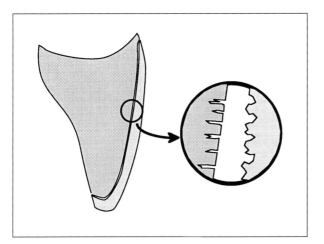

Fig 22-33 Micromechanical bonding. Composite resin cement holds the restoration to the tooth by penetrating into small, deep surface pits.

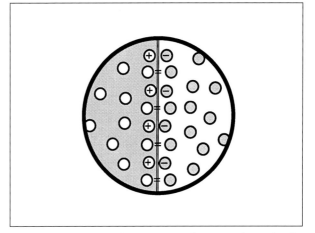

Fig 22-34 Molecular adhesion. True adhesion is the molecular attraction exerted between the surfaces of bodies in contact.

Limited success has been achieved in attempts to develop resin cements and coupling agents that will exhibit strong, durable molecular adhesion to tooth structure, base metals, and ceramics. Noble metal alloys are not well suited for direct molecular bonding. However, a thin layer of silane can be bonded to a gold alloy with special equipment (Silicoater, Kulzer, Irvine, CA; or Rocatec, ESPE-Premier, Norristown, PA) to serve as a coupling agent by bonding chemically to resin cements. Equally effective is a layer of tin electroplated onto the gold alloy.[24]

By applying a silane coupler to roughened porcelain, shear bond strengths in excess of the cohesive strength of the porcelain (approximately 30 MPa) have been achieved in the laboratory. However, such bonds tend to become weaker after thermocycling in water.[25] At this time, molecular adhesion should be looked upon only as a way to enhance mechanical and micromechanical retention and reduce microleakage, rather than as an independent bonding mechanism.

Cement Selection

There are several types of cement available for the permanent retention of indirect restorations. These include zinc phosphate, zinc silicophosphate, polycarboxylate (zinc polyacrylate), glass ionomer, and composite resin cements. Cements based on zinc oxide and eugenol are not indicated for permanent cementation. The properties of various cements are compared in Table 22-2.[26–37]

Table 22-2 Properties of Commonly Used Luting Cements[25-36]

Type	Brand	Form	Composition	Compressive strength (MPa)	Tensile strength (MPa)	Film thickness (μm)	Solubility in water (%)
Composite resin (auto-polymerizing)	All-Bond C&B Luting Composite (*Bisco*)	Paste/paste	Bis-GMA + quartz	220*	43.4*	25*	—
	Biomer (*Dentsply/Caulk*)	Paste/paste	Urethane dimethacrylate + barium glass	186.2*	—	10*	0.09*
	C&B Metabond (*Parkell; Sun Medical*)	Powder/liquid	Powder = PMMA / Liquid = MMA + 4 META	60.1[25]	—	—	—
	Comspan (*Dentsply/Caulk*)	Paste/paste	Bis-GMA	275.9* / 314.1[25]	30.9[26] / 46.9*	20*	0.13*
	Panavia (*Kuraray*)	Powder/liquid	Powder = silanated silica / Liquid = modified bis-GMA + phosphorylated methacrylate	178.5[27] / 255* / 266.9[25]	45.1[27] / 37.2[28]	19*	0.03*
	Panavia 21 (*Kuraray*)	Paste/paste	Modified bis-GMA + barium glass filler	290*	47*	19*	1.4*
	Thin Film Cement (*Den Mat*)	Paste/paste	Bis-GMA + silica and barium glass	117.5[27]	29.4[27]	41.7[29]	—
Composite resin (dual cure)	Dicor LAC (*Dentsply/York*)	Paste/paste	Urethane dimethacrylate	137.7* (shaded) / 251.7* (translucent)	24* (shaded) / 34.5* (translucent)	10–20*	0.15–0.25*
	Dicor LAC with Fluoride (*Dentsply/York*)	Paste/paste	Urethane dimethacrylate, glass with fluoride	180*	45–48*	—	—
	EnForce with Fluoride (*Dentsply/Caulk*)	Paste/paste	Bis-GMA, glass with fluoride	274.5 (auto)* / 293.0 (light)*	42.7 (auto)* / 51.0 (light)*	<25*	0.08*
	Infinity (*Den Mat*)	Paste/paste	Modified bis-GMA, hydrophilic resin, bariofluoroalumino-silicate, quartz	140.7[27]	23.1[27]	20	—
Glass ionomer	Fuji I (*GC America*)	Powder/liquid	Powder = fluoroaluminosilicate glass / Liquid = polyacrylic acid, tartaric acid, citric acid	225* / 175[30] / 186*	13.6*	16*	0.06*
	Glasionomer Type I (*Shofu*)	Powder/liquid	Powder = fluoroaluminosilicate glass / Liquid = polyacrylic acid	122[27] / 196*	—	<25	0.30
	Ketac Cem (*ESPE-Premier*)	Powder/liquid	Powder = glass fillers, sodium, calcium, aluminum, lanthanum, fluorosilicate, dried copolymer of acrylic + maleic acids / Liquid = tartaric acid + water	162.1[27]	17.8[27]	9.5[29]	—
	Ketac Cem Capsule (*ESPE-Premier*)	Powder/liquid	Powder = glass fillers, sodium, calcium, aluminum, lanthanum, fluorosilicate, dried copolymer of acrylic + maleic acids / Liquid = tartaric acid + water	124* / 96.8[27]	12.6[27]	20*	0.1*

Table 22-2 *Continued*

Cements

Type	Brand	Form	Composition	Compressive strength (MPa)	Tensile strength (MPa)	Film thickness (μm)	Solubility in water (%)
Hybrid (glass ionomer + resin)	Advance (Dentsply/Caulk)	Powder/liquid	Powder = glass filler Liquid = OEMA + water	151.7*	34.5*	20*	0–0.07*
	Fuji Duet (GC America)	Powder/liquid	Powder = silane-treated aluminosilicate glass Liquid = HEMA, polyacrylic acid, tartaric acid, water, proprietary resins	155*	24	10*	0.07*
	Vitremer Luting Cement (3M)	Powder/liquid	Powder = Strontium fluoroalumino-silicate glass Liquid = Water + polycarboxylic acid copolymer + 2-HEMA	132.6*	23.3*	19*	0*
Polycarboxylate	Carboxylon (3M)	Powder/liquid	Powder = zinc oxide Liquid = polyacrylic acid	56[31]	6.0[31]	—	—
	Durelon (ESPE-Premier)	Powder/liquid	Powder = zinc oxide, tin oxide, stannous fluoride Liquid = 40% polyacrylic acid	50.7[31] 70[32] 53.3[33] 65[34] 67.4[27]	10* 8.1[31] 12.6[32] 15.1[27]	13* 21.0[29]	0.1*
	Liv Carbo (GC America)	Powder/liquid	Powder = zinc oxide + aluminum oxide + magnesium oxide + polyacrylic acid powder Liquid = polyacrylic acid	79.3*	—	13*	0.01–0.03*
	Shofu Polycarboxylate	Powder/liquid	Powder = zinc oxide Liquid = polyacrylic acid + tannin fluoride	55.0[27] 69.4	10.8[27]	19*	0.04*
	Tylok-Plus	Powder/liquid	Powder = zinc oxide + SnF + dried polyacrylic acid Liquid = water	>69*	>6.9*	19*	—
	Fleck's Zinc Cement (National Keystone Products/Mizzy)	Powder/liquid	Powder = zinc oxide Liquid = orthophosphoric acid	117[32] 56.5[33] 62.1[27]	8.1[32] 9.3[27]	10–20*	<0.2*
	Lee Smith Zinc (Teledyne)	Powder/liquid	Powder = zinc oxide + magnesium oxide Liquid = orthophosphoric acid	96.55–110.3[35]	4.4[36]	25[31]	<0.2
Zinc phosphate	Modern Tenacin (Caulk)	Powder/liquid	Powder = zinc oxide + aluminum phosphate Liquid = orthophosphoric acid	77.5[27] 89.0[32]	9.5[27] 4.3[32]	—	—
	DeTrey Zinc Cement Improved (DeTrey)	Powder/liquid	Powder = zinc oxide Liquid = orthophosphoric acid	150[34] 117[32]	8.1[32]	—	—
	Shofu Zinc Phosphate	Powder/liquid	Powder = zinc oxide Liquid = orthophosphoric acid + tannin fluoride	117*	—	<25*	0.05*

*Manufacturer's data.

Unfortunately, there is no cement that offers superior properties in all areas of concern.

Zinc Phosphate Cement. First introduced in 1878,[38] zinc phosphate cement possesses high compressive strength (96 to 110 MPa).[36] It exhibits a pH of 3.5 at the time of cementation,[39] and it has been widely blamed for contributing to pulpal irritation.[32,40-42] Brännström and Nyborg,[43,44] however, found no irritating effect on the pulp from zinc phosphate, *per se*. Cavity varnishes partially reduce the exposure of the pulp to the cement,[45,46] but unfortunately they also reduce retention.[47] Zinc silicophosphate cement, which also has been in use since 1878,[48] exhibits a high compressive strength (152 MPa) and a moderate tensile strength (9.3 MPa).[49] However, its film thickness can be excessive (88 μm at the occlusal surface under an actual casting),[50] and it also has an acidic pH[39] that may be harmful to the pulp.

Polycarboxylate Cement. While polycarboxylate cement has a higher tensile strength than that of zinc phosphate,[33,37] its compressive strength at 24 hours is significantly lower.[35] Its pH is also low (4.8), but because of the large size of the polyacrylic acid molecule there is apparently little penetration into the dentinal tubules.[33] As a result, it seems to cause little pulpal irritation.[45,51] This cement has shown a moderately high bond strength to enamel (9 MPa) and to dentin (3.3 MPa).[51] Polycarboxylate will also bond to stainless steel, but not to gold.[41]

Zinc Oxide–Eugenol. Cements based on zinc oxide and eugenol cause virtually no pulpal inflammation as long as they make no direct contact with the pulp. They have long been used as temporary cements. Attempts have been made to create more biocompatible permanent cements by adding o-ethoxy-benzoic acid (EBA) to zinc oxide–eugenol and by reinforcing it with aluminum oxide and poly(methyl methacrylate). Based on in vitro tests, this type of cement was reported to have good strength and be less soluble than zinc phosphate cement.[52,53] Unfortunately, its clinical performance was much poorer than its laboratory performance, and in vivo studies have shown that it deteriorates much more rapidly in the mouth than do other cements.[54,55] Zinc oxide–eugenol cements are still used largely for provisional cementation.

Glass Ionomer Cement. Glass ionomer has many properties of an ideal cement. The powder is composed mainly of a calcium fluoroaluminosilicate glass, with fluoride content ranging from 10% to 16% by weight.[56] In some brands the liquid is an aqueous solution of copolymers of polyacrylic acid with itaconic or maleic acid and tartaric acid. In others the polyacrylic acid or copolymer is dried and incorporated into the powder, the liquid consisting only of water or a tartaric acid solution.

Glass ionomer has been in general use as a restorative material in Europe since 1975 and in the United States since 1977, and has gradually gained in popularity as a luting agent. Both its compressive strength (127 MPa) and its tensile strength (8 MPa) are quite good.[49] Its bond to tooth structure is comparable to that of polycarboxylate.[57] Bonding of both glass ionomer and polycarboxy-

late cements to the restoration can be produced by tinplating the inner surfaces of the restoration. A tin–polyacrylic acid product overlying the tin layer on the restoration establishes the bond.[58]

Glass ionomer cement is bacteriostatic during its setting phase,[59] is less soluble than zinc phosphate cement,[55] and releases fluoride at a greater rate than does silicate cement. This has been shown to reduce the solubility of adjacent enamel and therefore should inhibit secondary caries.[60] In one study,[61] glass ionomer was found to be 65% more retentive than zinc phosphate cement. In another,[62] premolars with inlays cemented with glass ionomer were slightly more resistant to fracture than were premolars with inlays cemented with zinc phosphate.

Glass ionomer cement is not without its disadvantages. Its pH is even lower than that of zinc phosphate cement during setting, and some concern has been expressed regarding postcementation hypersensitivity.[63,64] Because the molecules of polyacrylic or polymaleic acid used in glass ionomers are large, it is assumed they are less likely than phosphoric acid to penetrate the dentinal tubules, and varnish is not generally recommended. A calcium hydroxide coating should be applied to areas close to the pulp, however.[65]

Clinical success with glass ionomer cement depends on early protection from both hydration and dehydration.[66] It is weakened by early exposure to moisture, while desiccation, on the other hand, produces shrinkage cracks in the recently set cement.[67] Therefore, the cement at the crown margins must be protected by a coating of petrolatum or varnish.[66] Glass ionomer is more translucent than zinc phosphate, and this property often makes the enamel adjacent to metal castings appear slightly gray, particularly on partial veneer crowns.

This material continues to be improved, but its efficacy is difficult to assess accurately. Tyas[68] sums it up: "Because of constant improvements in glass ionomers, there have been too few studies on any one material, and comparisons between studies are further complicated by differences in evaluation criteria."

Resin Luting Cements. Resin cements are composites composed of a resin matrix, eg, bis-GMA or diurethane methacrylate, and a filler of fine inorganic particles. They differ from restorative composites primarily in their lower filler content and lower viscosity. Resin cements are virtually insoluble and are much stronger than conventional cements. It is their high tensile strength that makes them useful for micromechanically bonding etched ceramic veneers and pitted fixed partial denture retainers to etched enamel on tooth preparations that would not be retentive enough to succeed with conventional cements.

Some of these cements are autopolymerizing for use under light-blocking metallic restorations, while others are either entirely photocured or dual cured (light activated) for use under translucent ceramic veneers and inlays. In dual-cured cements, a catalyst is mixed into the cement so that it will eventually harden within shadowed recesses after a rapid initial hardening is achieved with a curing light.

Problems that have been reported with the use of resin cements for luting full crowns include excessive cement film thickness,[30,69] marginal leakage because of setting shrinkage, and severe pulpal reactions when applied to cut vital dentin. The latter may be related more to bacterial infiltration than to chemical toxicity, however. Use of a dentin bonding agent under a resin cement is critical to its success, unless the preparation has been cut in enamel.

Dentin bonding agents have been reported to reduce pulpal response, presumably by sealing the dentinal tubules and reducing microleakage.[70] Adhesive resin cement was found to produce a better marginal seal than zinc phosphate cement.[71] Even if the problems of film thickness and microleakage should be solved, the problem of adequately removing hardened excess resin from inaccessible margins may preclude the use of resin cement for full crowns with subgingival margins.

A number of systems have been developed, utilizing different mechanisms for bonding to the dentinal surface[72]:

- Tags in dentinal tubules
- Bonding to precipitates on pretreated dentin
- Chemical union with inorganic components
- Chemical union with organic components
- Production of a resin-impregnated layer of dentin

In researching the mechanism of attachment to tooth structure, it was found that resin tags in excess of 200 μm were reported when resin was applied to the dentin surface of extracted teeth. However, the resin penetrated only 10 μm into the dentinal tubules of vital teeth, forming a resin-reinforced layer of tooth structure, the *hybrid layer*.[73]

Chemical bonds are subject to degradation when they are exposed to the oral environment.[74] Microleakage may occur as a result of bond disruption, causing recurrent caries, sensitivity, and pulpal necrosis after restoration placement.[75] The *smear layer,* a 1- to 5-μm-thick,[76] grinding debris–laden layer of dentin produced during the tooth preparation, is a critical barrier that protects the tooth from the oral environment.

If bonding is attempted directly to the smear layer, however, tensile failure can occur between it and the cement, or within the layer itself. Therefore, to enhance bonding to tooth structure, the tooth preparation is usually etched. This step alters the dentin surface by removing the smear layer, opening the tubules, and increasing the permeability of the dentin.[77] If the smear layer is to be removed, an effective dentin bonding agent must be employed, with true adhesion between the restorative material and the tooth.[72]

The practice of "total etching" (etching dentin as well as enamel) was described by Fusayama et al in 1979.[78] Caution has been urged in approaching the pulp with acids, utilizing passive (soaking) rather than active (scrubbing) methods of application and timing them

carefully.[79] Weaker concentrations of acid not only pose less of a risk to the pulp, but they also may produce greater bond strengths.[76] Solutions of 10% phosphoric acid are preferable to those containing nearly 40%.[80] Other etchants effectively used include a 2.5% solution of nitric acid[81]; a 10% citric acid, 20% calcium chloride solution[82]; and a 10% citric acid, 3% ferric chloride solution, called simply "10-3," which dissolves a thin layer of calcium on the surface of the dentin without affecting the collagen.[83] Each system requires a particular acid, so always use the one specified for the dentin bonding agent you are using.

There is controversy about the use of acids, because pulpal damage has been attributed to their application near the pulp.[84,85] Kanca[86] interprets the pulpal irritation as being caused by the eugenol used as a cavity sealer in earlier studies, rather than by the phosphoric acid itself. Brännström[87,88] and Cox et al[89] also have questioned a link between sensitivity and toxicity. Instead they conclude that it is the result of bacterial infection.

Hybrid Ionomer Cements. The recently introduced "hybrid cements," or *resin-modified polyalkenoate cements,* are purported to combine the strength and insolubility of resin with the fluoride release of glass ionomer. They differ from other composite resin cements in that the glass filler particles react with the liquid during the hardening process.

The selection of a cement for the placement of a cast restoration is not a clear-cut decision. Zinc phosphate is a strong cement that has proven itself over many years of use, outliving numerous would-be replacements. When depth of the preparation or history of hypersensitivity raises some concern for the vitality of the pulp, a more biologically compatible cement, eg, polycarboxylate, should be used. Cement deteriorates much more rapidly in some patients than in others.[54] If a particular patient has a history of rapid failure of previous crowns due to washout of zinc phosphate cement and marginal caries, use of a glass ionomer cement might help prevent recurrence. Resin cements are indicated where micromechanical bonding is desired. They are especially useful when the tooth preparation is largely in enamel and all finish lines are accessible.

Cementation

Regardless of the material used, cementation involves a number of steps which, if not carried out meticulously, can result in early failure of an otherwise technically excellent restoration. Some of the problems that can be caused by improper cementation technique are premature occlusion, pulpitis, loosening of the restoration, and recurrent caries.

Many problems are the result of incomplete seating of the restoration. Factors that can influence the completeness of seating are the viscosity of the cement, the mor-

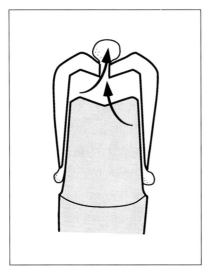

Fig 22-35 A vent hole in the occlusal surface allows cement to escape readily from under crowns. The hole must then be sealed.

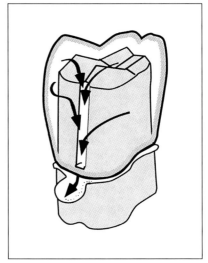

Fig 22-36 A vertical groove in the tooth preparation provides an internal escape channel for cement without perforating the crown.

phology of the restoration, vibration,[90] venting, and seating force.[30] Mesio-occluso-distal onlays seated an average of 34 µm farther than did full crowns in a study by Oliveira et al.[91] In the same study, vibration produced an improvement of 27 µm in the seating of full crowns.

Seating force must be adequate to ensure complete seating, but excessive force of brief duration may produce elastic strains in the dentin, creating a rebound that dislodges the restoration when the force is relaxed.[92] A study by Karipidis and Pearson[93] found that crowns seated on preparations in bovine dentin with a force of 300 N/cm^2 could be removed more easily than those cemented with half the force; the reverse was true when crowns were cemented on more rigid metal dies.

Venting full crowns will facilitate the escape of cement from crowns and allow more complete seating.[94–97] Normally, adequate seating can be achieved without venting. Problems can be encountered, however, over preparations with unusually long, nearly parallel axial walls, or multiple fixed partial denture abutments with greater than normal mobility. The most effective venting is provided by drilling a hole in or near the occlusal surface (Fig 22-35), but that leaves a defect in the crown after cementation.

Various methods have been proposed for sealing the vent hole, including placement of direct filling materials, metal screws, and cemented plugs. Venting can be achieved without perforating the crown by creating an internal escape channel in the form of an unoccupied vertical groove in the axial wall of the preparation (Fig 22-36) or in the internal surface of the crown. The groove should begin at the occlusal surface and end short of the finish line.[98–100]

Techniques for using zinc phosphate, polycarboxylate, glass ionomer, and resin cements follow.

Cementation With Zinc Phosphate Cement

The field must be kept dry during final placement of the restoration and hardening of the cement. The quadrant containing the tooth being restored is isolated with cotton rolls and a suction device such as a saliva ejector for the maxillary arch or a Svedopter for the mandibular arch (Fig 22-37). Inlays should be cemented with a rubber dam in place. If petrolatum was used during finishing of margins, the tooth must be carefully cleaned with Cavilax on cotton pellets.

If the tooth is vital, it is customarily protected from the acidity of the cement. It has been reported that nearly 18% of teeth restored with cores and full crowns later experienced pulpal necrosis.[101] More often than not, a tooth receiving a crown has already been subjected to multiple insults from caries and previous restorations, in addition to the crown preparation and impression procedures. Possible trauma from zinc phosphate cement should be minimized.

Partial protection of the pulp can be provided by the application of two thin layers of copal cavity varnish (Copalite, Cooley and Cooley, Houston, TX). It is applied to the dry tooth with cotton pellets and lightly blown dry after each application. This partially seals the dentinal tubules and protects the pulp from the phosphoric acid. The fact that the cement is irritating to the pulp is evidenced by the pain an unanesthetized patient sometimes experiences when a crown is cemented over a

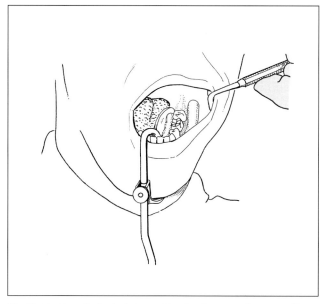

Fig 22-37 Mandibular isolation with a Svedopter and cotton rolls.

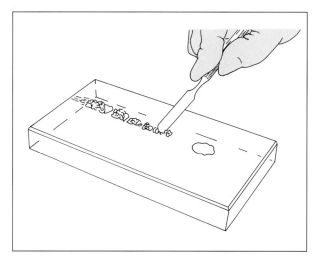

Fig 22-38 Small increments of powder are introduced into the liquid.

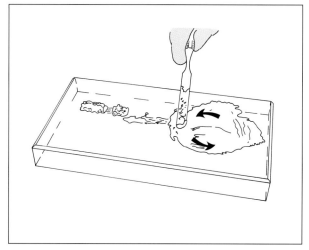

Fig 22-39 Cement is mixed with a circular motion over a wide area.

vital, unvarnished tooth. Because varnish does reduce the retention of a crown,[47] it should not be used on non-vital teeth or with other types of cement. A dentin bonding agent can also be used for this purpose.

Place powder on one end of a glass slab that has been cooled in tap water and wiped dry. At the center of the slab, measure out approximately six drops of liquid for each unit to be cemented. The composition of the liquid may be altered by prolonged exposure to air. Both the loss and gain of water adversely affect the properties of zinc phosphate cement.[102] Therefore, the bottle should be kept capped and the liquid should not be dispensed

until just before it is mixed. Bottles that are less than one-quarter full of liquid should be discarded, as should bottles in which the color of the liquid has changed. It is not "good to the last drop."

Use the spatula to divide the powder into small increments approximately 3 mm on a side. Move one increment across the slab and incorporate it into the liquid, mixing it for 20 seconds across a wide area (Fig 22-38). This will aid in neutralizing the acid and retarding the setting time. Continue to add small increments of powder, mixing each for 10 to 20 seconds using a circular motion and covering a wide area of the slab (Fig 22-39).

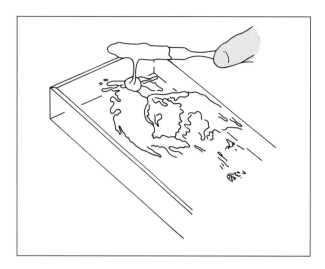

Fig 22-40 Cement that is ready to use will string out from a lifted spatula.

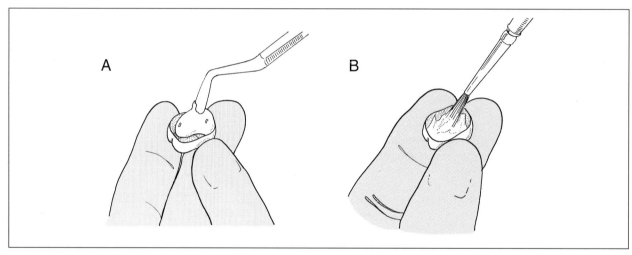

Fig 22-41 The inner walls of the crown are coated with a thin layer of cement, using the small end of an instrument (A) or a brush (B).

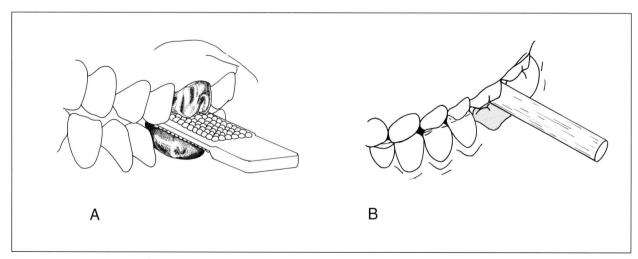

Fig 22-42 While the cement hardens, the patient maintains pressure by biting on a resilient plastic wafer (A) or a wooden stick (B).

During mixing, zinc phosphate cement liberates heat that can unduly accelerate its setting. Therefore, it must be mixed slowly over a wide area on a cool glass slab to insure that a maximum amount of powder can be incorporated into a mix that is still workable. The more powder incorporated into a given amount of liquid, the stronger and less acidic the resulting cement will be.[92] On the other hand, If the mixture becomes too thick, the restoration may be prevented from seating completely.

The setting time can be controlled by the rate at which powder is incorporated into the mix. If powder is added slowly, the setting time will be prolonged. If powder is added more rapidly, the setting time will be shortened, less powder will be incorporated, and the resultant cement will be weaker and more acidic.

Check the consistency by slowly lifting the spatula (Fig 22-40). When the consistency is right, it will string out about 10 mm between the spatula and slab before it runs back onto the slab. If it runs quickly off the spatula, it is too thin, and if it must be nudged off the spatula, it is too thick. A mixture that is too thick cannot be salvaged by adding more liquid. Clean the slab and start over.

Quickly load the clean, dry restoration with cement. Brush or wipe cement on the inner surfaces of the restoration (Fig 22-41, A and B). Brushed-on cement produces a seating discrepancy one-third less than that resulting from filling the crown half full, and more than two-thirds less than that resulting from filling the crown completely full.[103] If there are recessed features on the preparation, such as box forms or grooves, apply some cement directly to the preparation with a plastic applicator (IPPA). Insert cement into pin holes with a small lentulo spiral or the tip of a periodontal probe. Place cement directly into inlay cavity preparations. At this time the tooth should still be dry. If there is persistent contamination from gingival fluids, it may be necessary to place retraction cord in the sulcus for a few minutes and make a fresh mix of cement.

Seat the restoration on the tooth and, if it is a posterior tooth with uniform occlusion, have the patient apply force to the occlusal surface of the restoration by closing on a plastic wafer (E-Z Bite Cementation Wafers, HAL Products, Westlake Village, CA) (Fig 22-42, A). An orangewood stick also can be used for this purpose (Fig 22-42, B). However, the stick may apply force to only one cusp, causing the crown to be crooked. It also requires the patient to open wider to apply seating force, which could cause discomfort in the temporomandibular joint.

Anterior crowns and crowns that occlude on only one corner might become tipped by pressure from the opposing teeth even on a cementation wafer. In these cases it is better to apply force with a finger padded by a cotton roll. The force must be sufficient to seat the crown completely. Vibration can be applied by gently tapping the side of a crown or the wafer with a mirror handle. Vibration will produce more complete seating than static force alone.[91]

Check that the restoration is completely seated by palpating a supragingival margin with an explorer through the soft extruded cement, or by removing the bite stick and having the patient close with shim stock between nearby teeth. This must be done quickly and with cotton rolls in place to avoid contamination of the cement by saliva. If the restoration is not completely seated, remove it before the cement hardens, thoroughly clean both restoration and tooth, and try again. If the restoration cannot be removed intact, it may be ground into occlusion to serve temporarily while a new restoration is fabricated. At the following appointment the unintentional "temporary" restoration will have to be sectioned and removed.

After the restoration is completely seated, keep the field dry until the cement has hardened. The solubility of zinc phosphate is greatly increased by premature contact with moisture.[104] If the patient salivates heavily, the suction device must be left in place during seating of the restoration and hardening of the cement. This makes it necessary to place a thicker object, such as a wooden stick on top of a bite wafer, to maintain pressure on the restoration without allowing the anterior teeth to strike the suction device.

No attempt should be made to remove excess cement while it is still soft. The excess helps protect the margins during setting. Furthermore, large masses of hardened cement will break away more easily and cleanly than will thin, smeared films. Once the cement has completely set, remove all excess with a scaler, explorer, and knotted dental floss. Cement left in the gingival crevice can be very irritating to the tissue. The entire crevice should be checked with an explorer several times to insure that all of the cement has been removed.

Cementation With Polycarboxylate Cement

Use cotton rolls to isolate the quadrant containing the tooth being restored. The tooth should be thoroughly clean. Drying can be accomplished by blotting, since absolute dryness is not required. Following try-in, wash the restoration in water and dip it in alcohol to remove all contaminants. Sandblast the inside of the casting to insure maximum retention. Coat the outside of the casting to be cemented with petrolatum to prevent the cement from sticking where it is not needed.

The powder-liquid ratio for this type of cement is 1.5 parts powder to 1.0 part liquid, which can be dispensed with some degree of accuracy. Dispense one measure of powder for each restoration to be cemented. Pick up the powder by pressing the measuring stick, scoop down, into the bottle of powder. Scrape off the excess and place the powder on a glass slab or a special impermeable mixing pad provided with the cement. Do not use a standard, porous parchment pad.

Express 1.0 mL of liquid from the graduated syringe for each measure of powder and begin mixing immediately. The powder should be incorporated quickly (Fig 22-43)

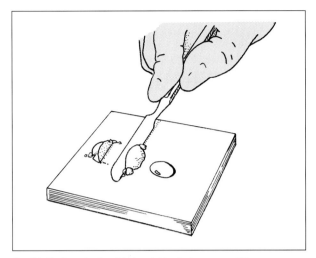

Fig 22-43 Powder is added quickly, in large quantities.

and the spatulation should be completed within 30 seconds. Because the liquid has a honey-like consistency, the cement may seem too viscous. This is normal, and it is not a matter of concern.

Coat the inside of the casting with cement, and place some on the tooth while the cement is still glossy. Place the casting on the tooth with firm finger pressure. Then instruct the patient to bite on a plastic wafer or a wooden stick. If the cement becomes dull in appearance before the casting is cemented, remove the cement from the casting and repeat the procedure. There is approximately 3 minutes of working time after the 30-second spatulation is completed.

Clean the instruments and the slab with water before the cement has set. Remove cement from the casting in the mouth before it becomes rubbery, or after it has set. Removing the cement while it is in its elastic, semi-set stage may pull some out from under the margin of the restoration, leaving a void in the cement near the margin. Keep the restored tooth isolated and dry until the cement has set completely.

Cementation With Glass Ionomer Cement

Complete isolation and protection from moisture is also essential with this type of cement. Isolate the quadrant well with cotton rolls and a saliva ejector or svedoptor. If a dry field cannot be adequately maintained in this way, place a rubber dam. The outside of the crown may be coated with petrolatum to make the hardened cement easier to remove, but care must be taken not to allow any lubricant to contaminate the internal surface.

Clean and dry the tooth. Clean the tooth preparation with wet flour of pumice on a rubber cup (Fig 22-44). It will improve the retention somewhat.[105] Rinse the pumice away (Fig 22-45) and then dry the tooth preparation (Fig

22-46). Do not remove the smear layer with acids as is sometimes done prior to application of the more viscous glass ionomer filling materials.[106] This might have an untoward effect on the pulp, and it has been shown to produce little or no improvement in retention.[105,107,108] Do not apply varnish to the tooth, as that would negate the benefit of the cement's adhesiveness.

Those accustomed to mixing zinc phosphate cement tend to mix glass ionomers too thin, with resultant decreased strength and increased solubility.[109] The manufacturer's prescribed powder-liquid ratio should be rigidly observed. For Ketac Cem (ESPE-Premier) the powder-liquid ratio is 3.4:1 by weight, or one level scoop of powder for two drops of liquid. Shake the powder bottle and then place two level scoops of powder and four drops of liquid onto a glass slab. Mix the cement as quickly as possible.

Glass ionomer cement, unlike zinc phosphate, liberates very little heat during mixing and therefore can be mixed more rapidly over a smaller area. The mix must be completed within 60 seconds and should have a creamy consistency. At first, a properly proportioned mixture will appear too thick, but as the particles dissolve it will become less viscous. Resist the temptation to add more liquid. Too thin a mix may lead to microleakage and washout.[66] Glass ionomer cements are also available in premeasured capsules for mixing on machines designed for mixing amalgam.

Apply the cement to the restoration with a brush. It has been theorized that placing a smaller amount of cement in the crown will prevent a buildup of hydrostatic pressure from excess cement.[66] Seat the crown as described for zinc phosphate cement. Working time is 3 minutes from the start of the mix, so move quickly. If the cement becomes thick or starts to form a skin before the restoration is seated, remove it and start over. The cement must be kept dry until it is hard. Keep the suction device in place and replace cotton rolls as necessary. When the excess cement extruded around the margins has become doughy, cover it with petrolatum to prevent it from dehydrating and cracking.

Wait until the excess cement has become brittle, but before it achieves its full hardness. The excess may then be removed using a scaler, explorer, and floss. The material must be protected from moisture during its early stages of set to prevent weakening. To provide extended protection, cover the margins with the sealing material provided with the cement, varnish, or petrolatum before dismissing the patient.

Cementation With Resin Cements

There are many types of resin cement and each has specific mixing instructions that should be reviewed before use. If resin cement hardens under a restoration that is improperly seated, it is almost always necessary to destroy the restoration in order to remove it. Furthermore, the tooth surface will usually have to be reprepared to

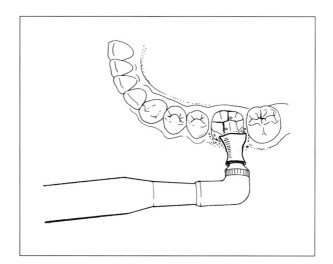

Fig 22-44 The tooth preparation is cleaned with a rubber cup and pumice.

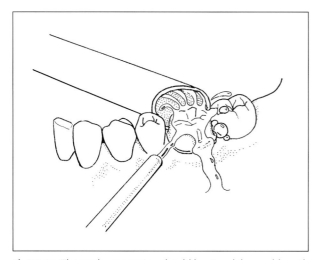

Fig 22-45 The tooth preparation should be rinsed thoroughly with a water syringe.

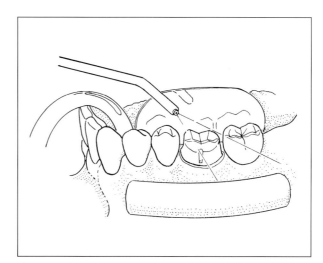

Fig 22-46 The preparation is dried with an air syringe.

remove resin tags projecting into the etched enamel and dentinal tubules. Therefore, it is imperative that the dentist have a clear understanding of the necessary steps and carry them out in an efficient, deliberate manner. Use of a chairside assistant is highly recommended.

The techniques for cementing metal restorations with two autopolymerizing resin cements are described here. Use of a dual-curing cement under translucent ceramic restorations will be discussed in Chapter 24.

Although bonding can be accomplished while using cotton roll isolation,[73] it does require immediate placement of the bonding agent. A delay of as little as 1 minute can reduce the bonding strength by 50%.[110] Barghi et al[111] demonstrated superior results using a rubber dam. Even if the system utilized will tolerate moisture, better control is maintained through the use of a rubber dam.

The first technique is for C&B Metabond (Parkell, Farmingdale, NY), a popular material among practicing dentists. Keep the material and the mixing dish in the refrigerator until time to use them. Air abrade the inside

of the crown with 50 µm aluminum oxide at 80 psi or more. Then rinse it, and dry with compressed air. Clean the tooth preparation with pumice, wash, and dry it. Etch any enamel in the preparation for 30 seconds with a plastic foam pellet saturated with red enamel etchant. Dab; do not rub. Rinse and dry the tooth. Apply green dentin activator to the dentin for 10 seconds, and then rinse and dry lightly. Do not desiccate the dentin.

Place four drops of base into one of the three wells in the chilled (16 to 22°C, or 61 to 72°F) ceramic mixing dish. Add one drop of catalyst from the syringe. Recap each container immediately after its use to prevent evaporation. Mix the two liquids for no more than 5 seconds. Paint both the tooth preparation and the inside of the restoration with the mixture.

Repeat the mixing of four drops of base to one drop of catalyst in a second well of the mixing dish. Use more for a larger casting or for multiple retainers on a fixed partial denture, always maintaining the 4:1 base-catalyst ratio. Again, stir the solution gently for no more than 5 seconds.

Add two level scoops of powder for every unit of liquid (4 drops of base + 1 drop of catalyst). Stir gently for 5 to 10 seconds to produce a creamy mixture. Apply the cement to the restoration. If the restoration or the tooth are no longer wet, apply more liquid to them from the first well *before* placing the mixed cement into the restoration. Seat the restoration quickly, as the normal working time is slightly less than 1 minute. To increase working time to 2.0+ minutes, the base and mixing dish, but *not* the etchants, can be chilled further in the freezer for 15 minutes.

Although the material has a very short working time, it takes at least 10 minutes to set and should be held during that time. Wipe off excess while it is soft with a cotton pellet wetted with a drop of base liquid. Do not remove cement from the casting once it becomes rubbery, because you will tear it out from under the margin of the restoration, creating voids under the margin. Cement remaining after setting must be removed with a scaler.

The second technique described utilizes a bonding agent, All-Bond 2, that works well with most resin luting materials,[112] and a resin cement, All-Bond C&B (Bisco, Itasca, IL). Air abrade the inside of the crown, rinse it, and dry with compressed air. Treat superficial dentin with a dentin bonding agent, while deeper dentin may be protected with a glass ionomer base. Apply 10% phosphoric acid gel (All-Etch, Bisco) to dentin and enamel for 15 seconds, agitating the etchant over the enamel with a brush. Rinse off the acid thoroughly with a water spray. Then air dry very briefly to remove excess moisture, without desiccating the dentin. This particular bonding agent tolerates the presence of some moisture. However, this does *not* mean that contamination by saliva is acceptable.

Mix primer A and B and brush five coats onto enamel and dentin with a disposable brush. Do not dry between any of the five coats. With an air syringe, dry all surfaces for 5 seconds to remove any remaining solvent or water. The tooth surface should have a glossy appearance. Light cure for 20 seconds.

If the dentin bonding agent has been used as a cavity sealer for a nonresin cement, eliminate the following step. If the bonding agent is being used as part of an all-resin luting, brush on a thin layer of Pre-Bond Resin (LD Caulk) immediately before cementation. Blow off excess resin, but do not light cure. Brush two coats of primer B on the inside of the crown and dry with an air syringe.

Mix the base and catalyst of an autopolymerizing resin cement (All-Bond C&B) and quickly spread a thin layer on the inside of the crown. Seat the restoration with gentle pressure and then wipe excess resin from the margin with a cotton roll or cotton pellets. It should be obvious from these two descriptions that techniques vary widely from one brand to another. In the interest of obtaining the best possible result, it is essential that the instructions for the material being used be followed precisely.

Special Considerations

Following is a discussion of the special requirements for inserting gold inlays, custom cast dowel cores, all-ceramic restorations, metal-ceramic crowns, and fixed partial dentures.

Gold Inlays

Because of their smaller size, inlays are more difficult to handle and more readily aspirated by the patient than are crowns. Therefore, trial insertion and cementation should be carried out with a rubber dam in place. Intraoral refinement of occlusal anatomy and margins can be accomplished simultaneously by extending the natural grooves onto the metal with a cone-shaped white stone under heavy pressure. Where space permits, hold the inlay firmly in place with a small blunt instrument. The tip of the stone must be kept sharp by frequently spinning it against a truing stone.

Remove the inlay from its preparation by teasing it loose with an explorer. If difficulty is encountered, try a blast of compressed air. If this fails, soften a corner of a Richwil crown remover in hot water, press it against the inlay for several seconds, and remove.

Place the inlay back on the die for polishing. Follow the white stone with sharp-tipped brown and green rubber points. Give the final polish with tripoli on a rotary brush, followed by gold rouge on a separate brush.

Before cementation, coat the tooth preparation with varnish or dentin bonding agent. Then fill the *cavity preparation* with cement before inserting the inlay. The inlay can be safely carried to the mouth by sticking it to a gloved fingertip in the correct orientation with a small piece of double-sided carpet tape or a spot of tray adhesive.[113]

After the cement has thoroughly hardened, remove the rubber dam and check the occlusion. If adjustments must be made, repolish the occlusal surface with several grades of progressively finer pumice, followed by Amalgloss on a rubber cup or small brush. Again, be careful not to overheat the tooth.

Custom Cast Dowel Cores

The casting is cleaned by sandblasting, and any visible casting nodules are removed with a bur. A longitudinal groove should be cut in the side of the dowel to create a cement escape channel.

If a dowel core is swallowed during try-in, the risk of intestinal obstruction or perforation is even greater than that associated with a full crown. To reduce the risk, a rubber dam can be used. As an alternative, about 2.0 mm of the sprue can be left attached to the casting. This

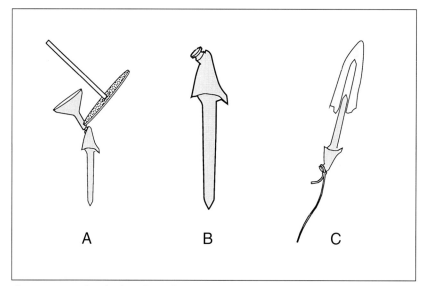

Fig 22-47 A safety knob is formed on a dowel core by leaving a 2-mm stub of sprue attached (A) and notching the stub (B). A floss safety line is then tied to the knob (C).

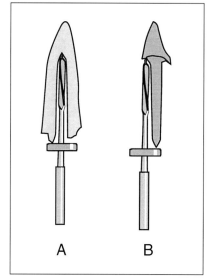

Fig 22-48 To verify that the dowel is as long as the dowel space, the preparation depth is marked on a reamer (A) and this length is compared with that of the dowel (B).

stub is notched with a separating disc, and dental floss is tied to it to act as a safety line (Fig 22-47).

Insert a rubber dam or gauze throat pack. Remove the provisional restoration. Gently rotate a Peeso reamer in the canal with the fingertips to ensure that no cement remains in the dowel space and to measure its length (Fig 22-48, A). Compare the depth of the dowel space with the length of the dowel to be certain that the casting is complete (Fig 22-48, B). Seat the restoration with light force. Never use heavy force, as the root may be split by the wedging action of the dowel. Remove any areas that prevent complete seating.

If the dowel core becomes progressively tighter as it is inserted and resists removal, the interfering area is on the side of the dowel. If it abruptly stops short of seating and offers no resistance to removal, the obstruction is either on the underside of the core or at the tip of the dowel. Once the casting seats completely without binding, remove the safety knob and evaluate the axial and occlusal surfaces. The contours should be those of an ideal crown preparation with adequate occlusal clearance and no undercuts. Adjust if necessary, and then clean all surfaces by sandblasting. Do not polish.

Armamentarium for Dowel Cores

1. High-speed handpiece
2. Straight handpiece
3. Separating disc
4. Cavilax
5. Lentulo spiral

6. Zinc phosphate cement
7. Mixing slab and spatula

Clean the dowel space with paper points or a wisp of cotton wrapped around a reamer and moistened with Cavilax (ESPE-Premier, Norristown, PA). Make a mix of zinc phosphate cement that is slightly thin. If the mix is too thick, or if it sets too rapidly, the dowel may not seat completely. Spin cement into the dowel space by using a lentulo spiral. This has been shown to provide twice as much retention as merely coating the dowel with cement.[114] Seat the dowel core slowly to allow excess cement to escape without building up hydraulic pressure that might "blow out" the apical seal or crack the root. When the cement is hard, remove the excess and place a provisional crown.

All-Ceramic Restorations

Full crowns, labial veneers, and inlays are sometimes made entirely of ceramic materials. The techniques for adjusting, cementing, and finishing these vary significantly from those used for metal restorations and are described in detail in Chapter 24.

Armamentarium for All-Ceramic Restorations

1. Busch Silent Stone on SHP mandrel
2. Fine diamond stones
3. Carborundum stones
4. Porcelain finishing kit

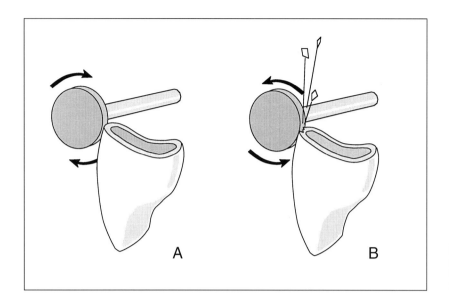

Fig 22-49 Rotation of a stone toward the greatest bulk of porcelain prevents chipping (A). Rotating away from the bulk can lead to fracture (B).

A tight proximal contact will not produce a visible burnished area on porcelain. A thin coating of a pressure indicator such as Occlude (Pascal Co, Belleview, WA) can be applied to these materials before seating to reveal the exact location of the contact. Only gentle forces should be used when inserting and testing ceramic restorations, as fracture may result if forces are too heavy. Internal support for a ceramic crown or onlay can be provided during occlusal adjustment by temporarily "cementing" the restoration to the tooth with a low-viscosity elastomeric impression material.

Broad, relatively flat surfaces are best reduced extraorally with the large, smooth-cutting Busch Silent stone (Pfingst & Co, South Plainfield, NJ), while grooves and ridges are reshaped with smaller pointed diamond stones and green stones. Instruments that have been used on metals should not be used on porcelain, lest particles of metal become imbedded in pores within the porcelain and cause discoloration. When working near an acute edge of porcelain, hold the stone so that it is always moving from the edge toward the greater bulk to reduce the danger of chipping the fragile edge (Fig 22-49). This is the opposite of the technique used in finishing metal margins. It is best to postpone minor grinding adjustments on thin veneers and inlays until after they are permanently bonded to the tooth.

Any roughened ceramic surfaces are smoothed with clean white stones and polished with rubber wheels of progressively finer grit such as those found in the Ceramiste Porcelain Adjustment Kit (Shofu Dental Corp, Menlo Park, CA). These grits are indicated by stripes around the shank of the instrument: no stripe (coarsest), one yellow stripe (medium), and either two yellow stripes or one white stripe (finest). Diamond-impregnated Dialite wheels and points (Brasseler USA, Savannah, GA) may

also be used for this purpose. Pastes containing diamond dust are also available for use on cups and brushes. Porcelain may also be reglazed after it is polished. It is often desirable to leave grooves and ridges on labial surfaces to simulate the texture of young enamel, but surfaces touching the gingiva and opposing teeth should be made as smooth as possible.

Have the patient moisten the ceramic and adjacent teeth with saliva and reevaluate the shade. Always allow the patient to see the completed restoration in a mirror and express approval before cementing it.

Ceramic crowns may be cemented with zinc phosphate, glass ionomer, or composite resin cements. Ceramic crowns that are etched internally and bonded with a composite resin cement have been shown to be 50% stronger than similar crowns cemented with a conventional zinc phosphate cement.[115] Ceramic veneers and inlays should be etched, silaned, and bonded to the underlying enamel with resin cements. This not only provides better retention and color control, but makes the ceramic material less susceptible to fracture than if it were cemented with nonresin cement.[116]

Cement ceramic veneers and inlays with a selected shade of a dual-cure composite resin cement such as Dicor Light-Activated Cement (Dentsply International, York, PA). Store resin cements in a refrigerator to prolong shelf life. Remove the cementation kit from the refrigerator before the appointment to allow it to approach room temperature.

The final appearance of an all-ceramic restoration is affected by the shade of cement used. Determine the correct shade or blend of shades by seating the veneer or inlay on the unetched tooth with water-soluble Dicor try-in paste (white syringe). Opacity can be controlled by varying the proportions of opaque and translucent catalyst. Record the shade or blend of try-in paste selected and clean the veneer thoroughly with a stream of water.

Isolate the tooth and clean it with a mixture of pumice and water. Rinse and dry. Place thin plastic strips interproximally. A piece of heavy black silk suture placed into the sulcus will help prevent contamination by sulcular fluid and will limit the entrance of cement into the sulcus. Etch the enamel for 30 seconds with a phosphoric acid gel. Wash with a stream of water for 15 seconds and dry thoroughly. If areas of exposed dentin are present, a dentin bonding agent should be applied as a very thin layer to seal the tubules.[70]

Place equal amounts of Dicor Light-Activated Cement catalyst (translucent or opaque) and the selected shade of resin cement base from a black syringe onto a paper mixing pad. Mix the components with a clean plastic spatula. Avoid contact with metal instruments. Mix thoroughly to ensure that there are no isolated portions of base or catalyst. Load the veneer with the mixture and carefully seat it on the dry, etched tooth. The plastic interproximal strips may be left in place if they will not interfere with seating of the restoration. Excessive pressure at this time could fracture the veneer. In the case of an inlay, place the cement into the cavity.

Remove the excess cement with cotton pellets, explorer, and floss, leaving a slight amount at the margin to accommodate the oxygen-inhibited layer. Hold the veneer gently against the tooth with a finger and harden the cement with a curing light, first directing the light from the lingual (through the tooth) for 60 seconds so that shrinkage will occur toward the tooth, then directing it from the labial (through the veneer) for an additional 60 seconds.

Adjust any overbulked margins or premature occlusal contacts with a fine diamond stone. If suture material was placed in the sulcus, remove it. Proximal margins of veneers can be polished with fine finishing strips. Polish occlusal surfaces with the rubber wheels and points of a porcelain adjustment kit. Finish the cement margins with carbide finishing burs, fine paper discs, and porcelain polishing paste on a rubber cup.

Metal-Ceramic Crowns

The metal portion is adjusted and finished in the same manner as a full gold crown, except that it is somewhat harder than type III gold. The porcelain portions are handled much the same as all-ceramic restorations, except that there is less risk of breakage and the shade is unaffected by the cement. Normally, ceramic restorations will be received from the laboratory with a glazed surface. If it is anticipated that the contours and color will be modified substantially during try-in, they can be left unglazed until after these adjustments are made.

Check the internal fit in the mouth to be sure there are no heavy contacts on axial walls near porcelain cervical margins. Undue pressure here can cause flaking of the porcelain, either during cementation or later during function. Insufficient contact areas and marginal gaps may be corrected at chairside by adding the appropriate shade of porcelain and firing it in a glazing oven. As an alternative, the restoration can be returned to the laboratory. If the defects are not apparent on the cast, or if the cast has been altered or damaged, new impressions may be necessary.

Each porcelain manufacturer provides a shade modification kit for its porcelain, permitting the alteration of shades at chairside if there is a staining furnace nearby.

If any shade modification or glazing is required, repolish the exposed metal with rubber wheels, beginning with a coarse one, such as Cratex, to remove the black oxide layer. If a film of shading porcelain or glaze extends over the metal surface, it must be removed with a stone before the metal can be polished. Metal-ceramic crowns are cemented in the same manner as gold crowns. Do not have the patient bite on a hard object to seat the crown, as the porcelain may fracture.

Fixed Partial Dentures

Procedures for adjusting, polishing, and cementing a fixed partial denture are the same as for a single crown, except for a few special considerations. A piece of dental floss should be tied around one of the connectors to act as a safety line during try-in and cementation. If the restoration fails to seat properly after removal of internal nodules and adjustment of the proximal contacts, it should be sectioned with a thin separating disc through the connector of the larger retainer, and the two halves tried in separately. If both retainers fit well after sectioning, the fixed partial denture can be reassembled and soldered using a soldering index (see Chapter 27).

References

1. Gildenhuys RR, Stallard RE: Comparison of plaque accumulation on metal restorative surfaces. *Dent Survey* 1975; 51:56–59.

2. Keenan MP, Shillingburg HT, Duncanson MG, Wade CK: Effects of cast gold surface finishing on plaque retention. *J Prosthet Dent* 1980; 43:168–173.

3. Klausner LH, Cartwright CB, Charbeneau GT: Polished versus autoglazed porcelain surfaces. *J Prosthet Dent* 1982; 47:157–162.

4. Raimondo RL, Richardson JT, Wiedner B: Polished versus autoglazed dental porcelain. *J Prosthet Dent* 1990; 64:553–557.

5. Jacobi R, Shillingburg HT, Duncanson MG: Comparison of the abrasiveness of six ceramic surfaces and gold. *J Prosthet Dent* 1991; 66:303–309.

6. Phillips RW: *Skinner's Science of Dental Materials,* ed 7. Philadelphia, WB Saunders Co, 1973, p 631.

7. Craig RG: *Restorative Dental Materials,* ed 8. St Louis, CV Mosby Co, 1989, p 100.

8. O'Brien WJ: *Dental Materials: Properties and Selection.* Chicago, Quintessence Publishing Co, 1989, pp 271, 322, 438.

9. Phillips RW: *Skinner's Science of Dental Materials,* ed 9. Philadelphia, WB Saunders Co, 1991, p 563.

10. Lee PW: *Ceramics.* New York, Reinhold Publishing Corp, 1961, p 143.

11. Cherberg JW, Nicholls JI: Analysis of gold removal by acid etching and electro-chemical stripping. *J Prosthet Dent* 1979; 42:638–644.

12. Campagni WV, Preston JD, Reisbick MH: Measurement of paint on die spacers used for casting relief. *J Prosthet Dent* 1982; 77:606–611.

13. Troxel RR: The polishing of gold castings. *J Prosthet Dent* 1959; 9:668–675.

14. Jacobi R, Shillingburg HT: A method to prevent swallowing or aspiration of cast restorations. *J Prosthet Dent* 1981; 46:642–645.

15. Kaiser DA, Wise HB: Fitting cast gold restorations with the aid of disclosing wax. *J Prosthet Dent* 1980; 43:227–228.

16. Christensen GJ: Marginal fit of gold inlay. *J Prosthet Dent* 1966; 16:297–305.

17. Eames WB, Little RM: Movement of gold at cavosurface margins with finishing instruments. *J Am Dent Assoc* 1967; 75:147–152.

18. Kishimoto M, Hobo S, Duncanson MG, Shillingburg HT: Effectiveness of margin finishing techniques on cast gold restorations. *Int J Periodont Rest Dent* 1981; 1:20–29.

19. Moffa JP, Guckes AS, Okawa MT, Lilly GE: An evaluation of non-precious alloys for use with porcelain veneers. Part II. Industrial safety and biocompatibility. *J Prosthet Dent* 1973; 30:432–441.

20. Kohli S, Levine WA, Grisius UF, Fenster RK: The effect of three different surface treatments on the tensile strength of the resin bond to nickel-chromium-beryllium alloy. *J Prosthet Dent* 1990; 63:4–6.

21. Buonocore MG: A simple method of increasing the adhesion of acrylic filling materials to enamel surface. *J Dent Res* 1955; 34:849–853.

22. Simonsen RJ, Calamia JR: Tensile bond strength of etched porcelain [abstract 1154]. *J Dent Res* 1983; 62:297.

23. Moon PC: Bond strengths of the lost salt proceure: A new retention method for resin-bonded fixed prostheses. *J Prosthet Dent* 1987; 57:435–439.

24. LaBarre E, Belser U, Meyer JM: Shear strength of resins bonded to a precious alloy [abstract 2003]. *J Dent Res* 1990; 69:359.

25. Matsumura H, Kawahara M, Tanaka T, Atsuta M: A new porcelain repair system with a silane coupler, ferric chloride, and adhesive opaque resin. *J Dent Res* 1989; 68:813–818.

26. Kerby RE, Knobloch L, McMillen K: Physical properties of composite resin cements [abstract 1849]. *J Dent Res* 1995; 74:243.

27. Aboush YE, Mudassir A, Elderton RJ: Technical note: Resin-to-metal bonds mediated by adhesion promoters. *Dent Mater* 1991; 7:279–280.

28. White SN, Yu Z: Compressive and diametral tensile strengths of current adhesive luting agents. *J Prosthet Dent* 1993; 69:568–572.

29. Isidor F, Hassna NM, Josephsen K, Kaaber S: Tensile bond strength of resin-bonded non-precious alloys with chemically and mechanically roughened surfaces. *Dent Mater* 1991; 7:225–229.

30. White SN, Yu Z, Kipnis V: Effect of seating force on film thickness of new adhesive luting agents. *J Prosthet Dent* 1992; 68:476–481.

31. Nakajima H, Hashimoto H, Hanaoka K, et al: Static and dynamic mechanical properties of luting cements [abstract 890]. *J Dent Res* 1989; 68:978.

32. Powers JM, Dennison JD: A review of dental cements used for permanent retention of restorations. Part II: properties and criteria for selection. *J Mich Dent Assoc* 1974; 56:218–225.

33. Powers JM, Farah JW, Craig RG: Modulus of elasticity and strength properties of dental cements. *J Am Dent Assoc* 1976; 92:588–591.

34. Drummond JL, Lenke JW, Randolph RG: Compressive strength comparison and crystal morphology of dental cements. *Dent Mater* 1988; 4:38–40.

35. Branco R, Hegdahl T: Physical properties of some zinc phosphate and polycarboxylate cements. *Acta Odontol Scand* 1983; 41:349–353.

36. Swartz ML, Phillips RW, Norman RD, Oldham DF: Strength, hardness, and abrasion characteristics of dental cements. *J Am Dent Assoc* 1963; 67:367–374.

37. Richter WA, Mitchem JC, Brown JD: Predictability of retentive values of dental cements. *J Prosthet Dent* 1970; 24:298–303.

38. Dennison JD, Powers JM: A review of dental cements used for permanent retention of restorations. Part I: Composition and manipulation. *J Mich Dent Assoc* 1974; 56:116–121.

39. Norman RD, Swartz ML, Phillips RW: Direct pH determination of setting cements. 2. The effects of prolonged storage time, powder-liquid ratio, temperature and dentin. *J Dent Res* 1966; 45:1214–1219.

40. Smith DC: Dental Cements. *Dent Clin North Am* 1971; 15:3–31.

41. Grieve AR: A study of dental cements. *Br Dent J* 1969; 127.405–410.

42. Langeland K, Langeland LK: Pulp reactions to crown preparation, impression, temporary crown fixation, and permanent cementation. *J Prosthet Dent* 1965; 15:129–143.

43. Brännström M, Nyborg H: Bacterial growth and pulpal changes under inlays cemented with zinc phosphate cement and Epoxylite CBA 9080. *J Prosthet Dent* 1974; 31:556–565.

44. Brännström M, Nyborg H: Pulpal reaction to polycarboxylate and zinc phosphate cement used with inlays in deep cavity preparations. *J Am Dent Assoc* 1977; 94:308–310.

45. Going RE, Mitchem JC: Cements for permanant luting: A summarizing review. *J Am Dent Assoc* 1975; 91:107–117.

46. Swartz ML, Phillips RW, Norman RD, Niblack BF: Role of cavity varnishes and bases in the penetration of cement constituents through tooth structure. *J Prosthet Dent* 1966; 16:963–972.

47. Chan KC, Svare CW, Horton DJ: The effect of varnish on dentinal bonding strength of five dental cements. *J Prosthet Dent* 1976; 35:403–406.

48. Anderson JN, Paffenbarger GC: Properties of silicophosphate cements. *D Progress* 1962; 2:72–75.

49. Wilson AD, Crisp S, Lewis BG, McLean JW: Experimental luting agents based on the glass-ionomer cements. *Br Dent J* 1977; 142:117–122.

50. Hembree JH, George TA, Hembree ME: Film thickness of cements beneath complete crowns. *J Prosthet Dent* 1978; 39:533–535.

51. Smith DC: A new dental cement. *Br Dent J* 1968; 125:381–384.

52. Brauer GM, McLaughlin R, Huget EF: Aluminum oxide as a reinforcing agent for zinc oxide-eugenol-o-ethoxy-benzoic acid cements. *J Dent Res* 1968; 47:622–628.

53. Phillips RW, Swartz ML, Norman RD, Schnell RJ, Niblack BF: Zinc oxide and eugenol cements for permanent cementation. *J Prosthet Dent* 1968; 19:144–150.

54. Osborne JW, Swartz ML, Goodacre CJ, Phillips RW, Gale EN: A method for assesing the clinical solubility and disintegration of luting cements. *J Prosthet Dent* 1978; 40:413–417.

55. Mesu FP, Reedijk T: Degradation of luting cements measured in vitro and in vivo. *J Dent Res* 1983; 62:1236–1240.

56. Wilson AD, McLean JW: *Glass-Ionomer Cement.* Chicago, Quintessence Publishing Co, 1988.

57. Jemt T, Stalblad PA, Øilo G: Adhesion of polycarboxylate-based dental cements to enamel: An in vivo study. *J Dent Res* 1986; 65:885–887.

58. Smith DC: Polyacrylic acid-based cements: Adhesion to enamel and dentin. *Oper Dent* 1992; 17:177–183.

59. Behen MJ, Setcos JC, Paleik CJ, Miller CH: Antibacterial abilities of various glass ionomers [abstract 626]. *J Dent Res* 1990; 68:312.

60. Maldonado A, Swartz ML, Phillips RW: An in vitro study of certain properties of glass ionomer cement. *J Am Dent Assoc* 1978; 96:785–791.

61. McComb D: Retention of casting with glass ionomer cement. *J Prosthet Dent* 1982; 48:285–288.

62. Kent WA, Shillingburg HT, Duncanson MG, Nelson EL: Fracture resistance of ceramic inlays with three luting materials [abstract 2364]. *J Dent Res* 1991; 70:561.

63. Smith DC, Ruse ND: Acidity of glass ionomer cements during setting and its relation to pulp sensitivity. *J Am Dent Assoc* 1986; 112:654–657.

64. Simmons JJ: Post-cementation sensitivity commonly associated with the "anhydrous" forms of glass ionomer luting cements: A theory. *Tex Dent J* 1988; 10:7–8.

65. Pameijer CH, Stanley HR: Primate response to anhydrous Chembond [abstract 1]. *J Dent Res* 1984; 63:171.

66. McLean JW: Clinical applications of glass-ionomer cements. *Oper Dent* 1992; 17:184–190.

67. Mount GJ, Makinson OF: Clinical characteristics of a a glass ionomer cement. *Br Dent J* 1978; 14:67.

68. Tyas MJ: Clinical studies related to glass ionomers. *Oper Dent* 1992; 17:191–198.

69. White SN, Kipnis V: Effect of adhesive luting agents on the marginal seating of cast restorations. *J Prosthet Dent* 1993; 69:28–31.

70. Qvist V, Stoltze K, Qvist J: Human pulp reactions to resin restorations performed with different acid-etch restorative procedures. *Acta Odontol Scand* 1989; 47:253–263.

71. Tjan AHL, Dunn JR, Brant BE: Marginal leakage of cast gold crowns luted with an adhesive resin cement. *J Prosthet Dent* 1992; 67:11–15.

72. Nakabayashi N: Adhesive bonding with 4-META. *Oper Dent* 1992; 17:125–130.

73. Fusayama T: Total etch technique and cavity isolation. *J Esthet Dent* 1992; 4:105–109.

74. Nakabayashi N, Nakamura M, Yasuda N: Hybrid layer as a dentin bonding mechanism. *J Esthet Dent* 1991; 3:133–138.

75. Cox CF: Effects of adhesive resins and various dental cements on the pulp. *Oper Dent* 1992; 17:165–176.

76. Bertolotti RL: Conditioning of the dentin substrate. *Oper Dent* 1992; 17:131–136.

77. Pashley DH, Michelich V, Kehl T: Dentin permeability: Effects of smear layer removal. *J Esthet Dent* 1981; 46:531–537.

78. Fusayama T, Nakamura M, Kurosaki N, Iwaku M: Non-pressure adhesion of a new adhesive restorative resin. *J Dent Res* 1979; 58:1364–1370.

79. Stanley HR: Pulpal consideration of adhesive material. *Oper Dent* 1992; 17:151–164.

80. Kanca J: Dental adhesion and the All-Bond system. *J Esthet Dent* 1991; 3:129–132.

81. Blosser RL, Bowen RL: Effects of purified ferric oxalate/nitric acid solutions as a pretreatment for the NTG-GMA and PMDM bonding system. *Dent Materials* 1988; 4:225–231.

82. Hosoda H, Fujitani T, Negishi T, Hirasawa K: Effect of a series of new cavity treatment on bond strength and wall adaptation of adhesive composite resins. *Jpn J Conserv Dent* 1989; 32:656–665.

83. Nakabayashi N, Kojima K, Masuhara E: The promotion of adhesion by the infiltration of monomers into tooth substrates. *J Biomed Mater Res* 1982; 16:265–273.

84. Retief DH, Austin JC, Fatti LP: Pulpal response to phosphoric acid. *J Oral Pathol* 1974; 3:114–122.

85. Macko DL, Rutberg M, Langeland K: Pulp response to the application of phosphoric acid to dentin. *Oral Surg* 1978; 45:930–940.

86. Kanca J: An alternative hypothesis to the cause of pulpal inflammation in teeth treated with phosphoric acid on the dentin. *Quintessence Int* 1990; 21:83–86.

87. Brännström M: The cause of postrestorative sensitivity and its prevention. *J Endod* 1986; 12:475–481.

88. Brännström M: Infection beneath composite resin restorations: Can it be avoided? *Oper Dent* 1987; 12:158–163.

89. Cox CF, Keall CL, Keall HJ, Ostro E, Bergenholtz G: Biocompatibility of surface-sealed dental materials against exposed pulps. *J Prosthet Dent* 1987; 57:1–8.

90. Koyano E, Iwaku M, Fusayama T: Pressuring techniques and cement thickness for cast restorations. *J Prosthet Dent* 1978; 40: 544–548.

91. Oliviera JF, Ishikiriama A, Vieira DF, Mondelli J: Influence of pressure and vibration during cementation. *J Prosthet Dent* 1979; 41:173–177.

92. Smith DC: Dental cements. Current status and future prospects. *Dent Clin North Am* 1983; 27:763–792.

417

93. Karipidis A, Pearson GJ: The effect of seating pressure and powder/liquid ratio of zinc phosphate cement on the retention of crowns. *J Oral Rehabil* 1988; 15:333–337.

94. Hembree JH, George TA, Hembree, ME: Film thickness of cements beneath complete crowns. *J Prosthet Dent* 1978; 39:533–535.

95. Jørgensen KD: Factors affecting the film thickness of zinc phosphate cements. *Acta Odontol Scand* 1960; 18:479–490.

96. Van Nortwick WT, Gettleman L: Effect of internal relief, vibration, and venting on the vertical seating of cemented crowns. *J Prosthet Dent* 1981; 45:395–399.

97. Ishikiriama A, Oliveira JF, Vieira DF, Mondelli J: Influence of some factors on the fit of cemented crowns. *J Prosthet Dent* 1981; 45:400–404.

98. Webb EL, Murray HV, Holland GA, Taylor DF: Effects of preparation relief and flow channels on seating full coverage castings during cementation. *J Prosthet Dent* 1982; 49:777–780.

99. Miller, GD, Tjan, AHL: An internal escape channel. A simplified solution to the problem of incomplete seating of full cast-gold crowns. *J Am Dent Assoc* 1982; 104:332–335.

100. Brose MO, Woelfel JB, Rieger MR, Tanquist RA: Internal channel vents for posterior complete crown. *J Prosthet Dent* 1982; 51:755–760.

101. Felton D, Madison S, Kanoy E, Kantor M, Maryniuk G: Long term effects of crown preparation on pulp vitality [abstract 1139]. *J Dent Res* 1989; 68:1009.

102. Norman RD, Swartz ML, Phillips RW, Sears CR : Properties of cements mixed from liquids with altered water content. *J Prosthet Dent* 1970; 24:410–418.

103. Tan K, Ibbetson RJ: The effect of cement volume on crown seating [abstract 169]. *J Dent Res* 1995; 74:422.

104. Swartz ML, Sears, C, Phillips RW: Solubility of cement as related to time of exposure in water. *J Prosthet Dent* 1971; 26:501–505.

105. Button GL, Moon PC, Barnes RF, Gunsolley JC: Effect of preparation cleaning procedures on crown retention. *J Prosthet Dent* 1988; 59:145–148.

106. Council on Dental Materials, Instruments, and Equipment: Using glass ionomers. *J Am Dent Assoc* 1990; 121:181–186.

107. Tamura N, Lim HD, Carroll TD, Woody RD, Nakajima H, Okabe T: Retentive strength of crown by different cleaning procedures [abstract 537]. *J Dent Res* 1990; 69:176.

108. Hewlett ER, Caputo AA, Wrobel DC: Concentration of smear removal agents vs. glass ionomer bond strength [abstract 558]. *J Dent Res* 1989; 68:251.

109. Billington R, Williams J, Pearson G: Glass ionomers: Practice variation in powder/liquid ratio [abstract 629]. *J Dent Res* 1989; 68:945.

110. Nikaido T, Inai N, Satoh M, et al: Effect of an artificial oral environment on bonding of of 4-META/MMA-TBB resin to dentin. *Jpn J Conserv Dent* 1991; 34:1430–1434.

111. Barghi N, Knight GT, Berry TG: Comparing two methods of moisture control in bonding to enamel: A clinical study. *Oper Dent* 1991; 16:130–135.

112. Suh BI: All-Bond—Fourth generation dentin bonding system. *J Esthet Dent* 1991; 3:139–147.

113. Jacobi R, Shillingburg HT: A method to prevent swallowing or aspiration of cast restorations. *J Prosthet Dent* 1981; 46:642–645.

114. Goldman M, DeVitre R, Tenca J: Cement distribution and bond strength in cemented posts. *J Dent Res* 1984; 63:1392–1395.

115. Ludwig K, Joseph K: Untersuchungen zur Bruchfestigkeit von IPS-Empress-Kronen in Abhängigkeit von den Zementiermodalitäten. *Quintessenz Zahntech* 1994; 20:247–256.

116. Dérand T: Stress analysis of cemented or resin-bonded loaded porcelain inlays. *Dent Mater* 1991; 7:21–24.

Chapter 23

Esthetic Considerations

The analysis of natural dentitions and the development of the concept of dental esthetics have been used in the arrangement of denture teeth. To contribute to a pleasing facial appearance, particularly when the patient smiles, contours, size, incisal edges, occlusal plane, and midline must be in harmony. Many of these principles can be applied to fixed restorations in the *appearance zone* (Richter WA: Personal communication, July 1973), that part of the mouth where high visibility requires a restoration or tooth replacement to simulate the appearance of a tooth.

Appearance Zone

A 1984 study of 454 smiles,[1] using both men and women aged 20 to 30 years, noted that when a person smiles, the individual typically displays the maxillary anterior and premolar teeth. The zone frequently also includes maxillary first molars. It varies from person to person, depending upon mouth size, smile width, tooth length, lip size and tightness, and perhaps most importantly, the patient's self-image.

The *smile line* or *incisal curve* is composed of the incisal edges of the maxillary anterior teeth and parallels the inner curvature of the lower lip.[1-3] It is parallel with the interpupillary axis,[2] and it is perpendicular to the midline (Fig 23-1). Nearly 80% of the young subjects in the study by Tjan et al displayed the entire length of the maxillary anterior teeth.[1] Women show nearly twice as much maxillary central incisor as men (3.4 to 1.9 mm, respectively) with the upper lip at rest,[4] and men are 2.4 times more likely to have a low smile line than women.[1]

The length of maxillary incisors cannot be established by esthetics alone, since they play an important role in both anterior guidance and phonetics. If the length is correct, having the patient sound the letter "F" should place the maxillary incisal edges against the inner edge of the vermilion border (the "wet-dry line") of the lower lip (Fig 23-2).[3] The incisal edges of mandibular incisors are established both by occlusal contact with the maxillary incisors and by their position 1.0 mm behind and 1.0 mm

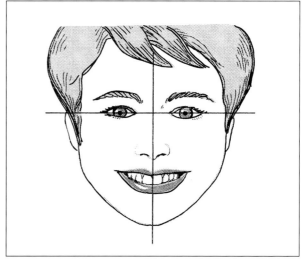

Fig 23-1 The incisal curve should be perpendicular to the midline, which is in the middle of the face, and parallel with the interpupillary line.

below the edges of the maxillary teeth when pronouncing an "S" (Fig 23-3).[3]

Relatively little is seen of mandibular central incisors in people under the age of 30, and the relationship between men and women is the opposite of that seen in the maxillary incisors (1.2 to 0.5 mm, respectively). As time and gravity win out, the tissues surrounding the mouth sag. The length of maxillary incisors exposed diminishes, and the amount of mandibular incisor that is seen increases (Fig 23-4). At the age of 60, the length of maxillary central incisor showing below the upper lip is 0.0 mm, while nearly 3.0 mm of the mandibular incisors is exposed.[4]

The crowns of teeth in "nonorthodontic normal occlusion," from a study of 120 casts of subjects who had not received orthodontic treatment and did not need it, were angled so that the incisal portions of the long axes of the crowns were more mesial than the gingival segments (Fig 23-5).[5] There is likewise a lingual inclination of the incisal or occlusal segment of the facial surfaces of canines, premolars, and especially molars (Fig 23-6).[5] This esthetic requirement necessitates biplanar facial

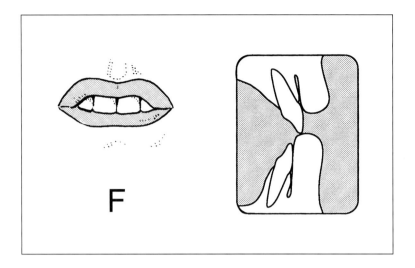

Fig 23-2 The incisal edges of the maxillary incisors touch the inner edge of the vermilion border of the lower lip when making the "F" sound: frontal view *(left)* and midsagittal view *(right)*.

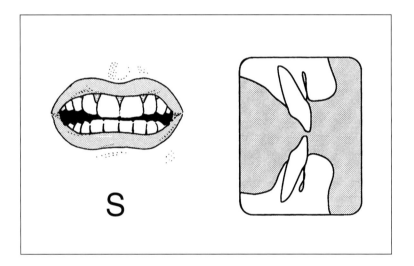

Fig 23-3 The incisal edges of the mandibular incisors are 1.0 mm inferior and 1.0 lingual to the incisal edges of the maxillary incisors when making the "S" sound: frontal view *(left)* and midsagittal view *(right)*.

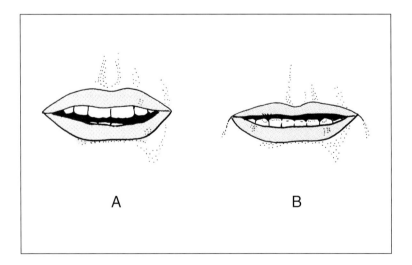

Fig 23-4 In the younger smile, the maxillary incisors are more prominent (A), while the mandibular incisors become more visible as the individual ages (B).

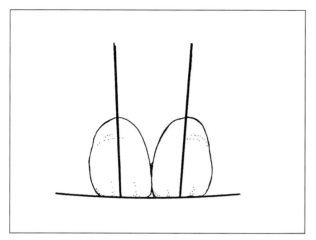

Fig 23-5 The long axes of the maxillary incisor crowns converge slightly toward the midline.

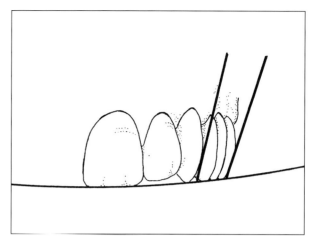

Fig 23-6 The long axes of the crowns of posterior teeth are inclined toward the lingual.

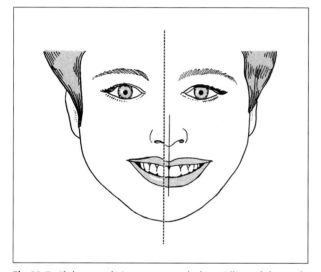

Fig 23-7 If the mouth is not centered, the midline of the smile should be in harmony with facial features nearest the mouth.

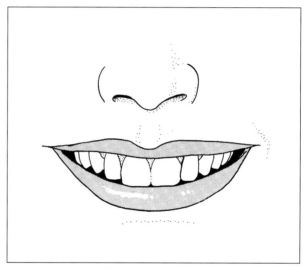

Fig 23-8 There should be slight irregularities on either side of the midline, even though the teeth are similar in size, shape, and alignment.

reduction in tooth preparations for all-ceramic or metal-ceramic crowns on anterior or posterior teeth (described in Chapter 10).

The midline, which is centered on the face,[6] is perpendicular to the interpupillary line.[7,8] It is the focal point of the smile. Total symmetry is rare, and if compromises must be made, the midline of the smile should correspond to the features nearest it, such as the column of the nose or the philtrum (Fig 23-7).[2] The teeth on either side of the midline should be balanced. Perfect *horizontal symmetry* occurs when all anterior teeth have the same shape, looking more or less like central incisors.[9] It is monotonous, and it appears artificial.

If the teeth have different shapes, but the left side is a mirror image of the right, *radiating symmetry* results. A more natural appearance can be produced by introducing slight variations to each side (Fig 23-8).[9] Dentists prefer more irregularities than patients do, and dentists tend to prefer more elongated incisors. Variety in arrangement and shape unquestionably produces a more natural appearance. However, the dentist must discuss the concept beforehand to develop in the patient an appreciation for the role played by subtle irregularities in the creation of a more natural appearance. The patient may have desired "straight, white teeth" for a lifetime. Teeth that do not meet this long-held vision of dental perfection could be rejected by the patient if they suddenly appear in the mouth without warning. It is also quite possible that they may be rejected even if you do attempt to prepare the patient.

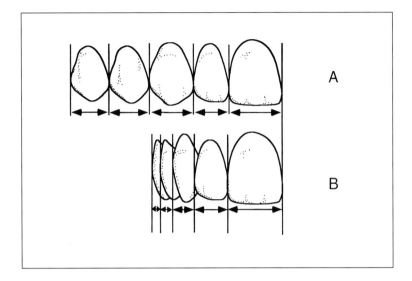

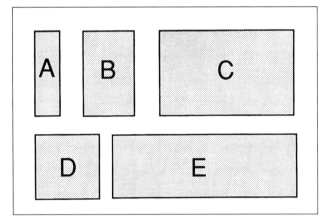

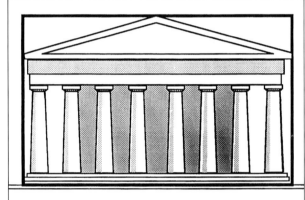

Fig 23-9 When viewed from the facial aspect of each tooth (A), the canines are second in width to the central incisors. However, when viewed from the midline, each tooth is narrower than the tooth mesial to it (B). It is suggested that the apparent width be 60% of the apparent width of the tooth mesial to it.

Fig 23-10 Which of these five rectangles is most pleasing to the eye? Both B and C are golden rectangles.

Fig 23-11 The front of the Parthenon fits within a golden rectangle.

Maxillary central incisors are positioned at the middle of the smile, making them the most prominent teeth. They have crowns that are the widest of the anterior teeth.[10,11] Canines are the next widest, and lateral incisors are the narrowest (Fig 23-9, A).[10,11] However, from a frontal view, the apparent sizes of teeth should become progressively smaller from the midline distally (Fig 23-9, B). It has been suggested that this apparent reduction in size should approximate the proportion of the golden ratio (0.618) as a guide for dental compositions.[7,12,13] Starting at the midline, this geometric formula of proportionality would require that each of the anterior teeth should be slightly less than 40% narrower than the tooth immediately mesial to it.[14]

The ratio of 1.618 to 1.0 is a constant that is designated as ø (phi). *Golden mean,*[15] *golden section,*[16] *golden rectangle,*[17] *golden proportion,*[2] and *divine proportion*[18]

are all terms that have been used to describe various aspects of this proportion. The ratio has been celebrated as the standard of visual esthetics since ancient times. In 1876 Fechner found that 75.6% of the subjects that he tested expressed a preference for rectangles with ratios ranging from 0.57 to 0.67, with 35% selecting the golden rectangle (with a ratio of 0.62) as the most pleasing visually (Fig 23-10).[15,18] The dimensions of the Parthenon, built in Athens in the fifth century BC, fit within the golden rectangle (Fig 23-11).[13,18]

Phi is related to sequences of numbers that are called *Fibonacci* series, in which each number is the sum of the two numbers preceding it: 0, 1, 1, 2, 3, 5, 8, 13, 21, 34, 55, 89... ($n_1 + n_2 = n_3$). The ratio between any number and the number preceding it approximates 1.618 or ø, (eg, 34/21 = 1.6190). Conversely, the ratio of any number and the number following it approximates the reciprocal

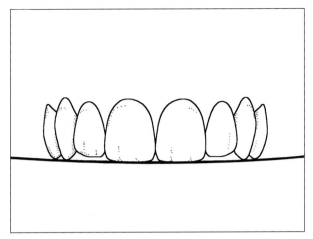

Fig 23-12 Incisal edges of central incisors and cusp tips of canines lie on the same curved line, with the incisal edges of lateral incisors being about 1.0 mm above that same line.

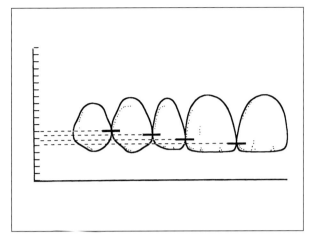

Fig 23-13 Interproximal contacts of the maxillary anterior teeth are situated progressively closer to the gingiva the more distal they are located from the midline.

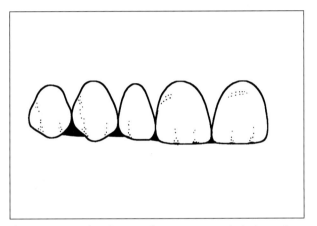

Fig 23-14 Incisal embrasures become progressively larger from central incisor to lateral incisor to canine.

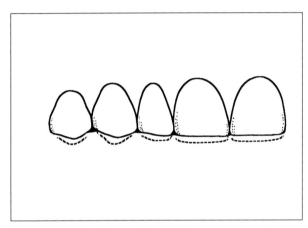

Fig 23-15 Incisal embrasures found in the younger person become smaller, sometimes to the point of disappearing, as the teeth wear.

of 1.618, which is 0.618 (eg, 21/34 = 0.6176). As the numbers in a series become larger, their ratios more closely approximate 1.618 or 0.618. The series appeared as a "brain teaser" in a book, *Liber abaci,* published in 1202 by the mathematician Leonardo of Pisa, also known as Fibonacci.[19] The book eventually came to be regarded as the most influential work on the introduction of the Hindu-Arabic decimal number system to Christian Europe.[19]

This series is one that is seen in nature, occurring in the intertwining equiangular left- and right-handed spirals of a sunflower, in which the number of clockwise and counterclockwise spirals most commonly are the adjacent Fibonacci numbers, 21 and 34. Similar opposing spirals that are also Fibonacci numbers are found in pine cones (5, 8) and pineapples (8, 13).[18] The series is seen again in phyllotaxis, or the arrangement of leaves on the stems of

plants, and in the number of petals of common flowers.[15,18] It would appear that the series is connected to patterns of growth, making it an underlying factor in morphology.[20]

The incisal edges of the maxillary central incisors and the cusp tips of the canines should be on the same gently curved horizontal line, with the lateral incisors approximately 1.0 mm above the line (Fig 23-12). Beginning with the mesial of the central incisors, the interproximal contacts of the maxillary anterior teeth are situated successively more gingivally, all the way to the distal of the canines (Fig 23-13). As the contacts become located farther gingivally, the incisal embrasures become larger, creating a more dynamic and youthful smile (Fig 23-14). With age and increased wear, the incisal embrasures become minimal (Fig 23-15). Solicit the patient's input for which "look" to try to achieve.

In the majority of anterior restorative situations, fewer

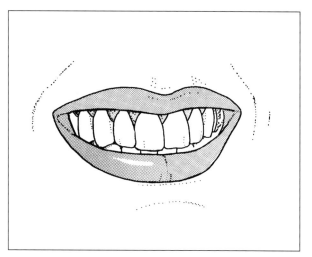

Fig 23-16 If a patient accepts "conversational esthetics," there may be moderate amounts of metal visible when the teeth are viewed critically that will not be seen in normal conversation.

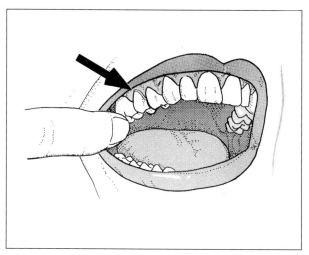

Fig 23-17 Metal collars *(arrow)* and occlusal surfaces will be unacceptable if a patient insists on "absolute esthetics."

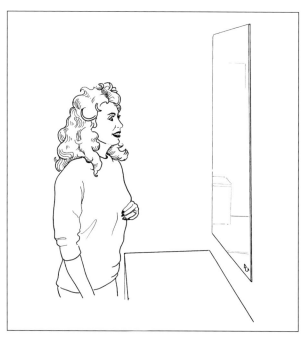

Fig 23-18 Looking at the teeth in a wall mirror shows a patient how the restored tooth will look to others at a normal conversational distance.

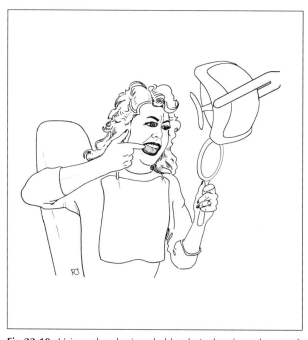

Fig 23-19 Using a hand mirror held only inches from the mouth allows the patient to see the teeth as no one else will.

problems will be encountered if the patient's original tooth position is approximated. However, when the original positions of anterior teeth have been lost through disease or trauma, or if significant changes are to be made for the sake of esthetics, the new tooth position should first be tried in the provisional restoration. Patient satisfaction can be strongly influenced by comments made away from the office by friends or family members. Only after the provisional restoration has passed this "trial by fire" should the changes be incorporated into a final restoration.

Ideal esthetics vary between cultures, generations, and gender, and the dentists view of esthetics must not be the only determinant of the final result.[14] It is important that the patient's esthetic expectations be discussed and understood before a restoration is fabricated. "Absolute esthetics" require that there be no metal visible, even if one were to look carefully. A restoration containing surface metal that is not visible in normal conversation will satisfy "conversational esthetics" (Fig 23-16). On the other hand, if there is metal that can be seen when the

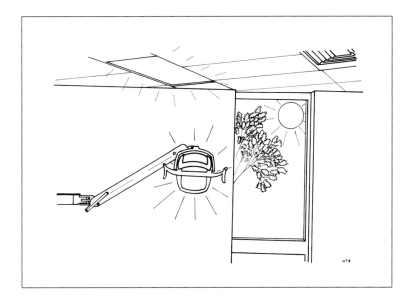

Fig 23-20 The three light sources common to the dental operatory are *(clockwise from top):* fluorescent, natural, and incandescent.

lip is retracted and a strong light shone in the mouth, the restoration or replacement does not meet the requirements of "absolute esthetics" (Fig 23-17).

It may be maddening for the dentist if a patient objects to metal being present even if it is normally not visible. A dentist will do well to remember that the patient is the ultimate judge of an "esthetic" crown or fixed partial denture.[12] It is the patient's mouth, and it is the patient's definition of the appearance zone that must be used. It is far better to learn its boundaries before the restoration is made.

Try, if at all possible, to discuss esthetic requirements in front of a wall mirror (Fig 23-18) and not at chairside, with the patient wielding a hand mirror under a dental unit light (Fig 23-19). Second molars, maxillary or mandibular, are rarely in the appearance zone, and the dentist should be as persuasive as possible to get the patient to permit full metal crowns on these teeth. They are usually short, and reducing them enough to permit a metal-ceramic crown may leave very little tooth structure, with an attendant loss of retention. This could be especially critical if the molar is to serve as a fixed partial denture abutment. The dentist has a responsibility to inform the patient of the disadvantages associated with the use of ceramic materials (greater tooth reduction, increased risk of fracture, and increased abrasion of opposing teeth) to secure a truly informed consent.

Shade Selection

To provide the patient with an esthetic restoration, the dentist must consider the scientific basis of color as well as the artistic aspects of shade selection. Color is a phenomenon of light (red, green, brown, yellow) or visual perception that permits the differentiation of otherwise identical objects.

There are three factors upon which color is dependent: *(1)* the observer, *(2)* the object, and *(3)* the light source.[21] Each of these three factors is a variable and, when any one is altered, the perception of color changes.

Many individuals have some form of color-blindness and are incapable of seeing certain colors. It is well documented that color vision deficiency is more common in men than in women, with a recent study finding 9.3% of the men deficient and 0% of the women.[22] At the 1981 ADA convention, color vision testing of 670 dentists (635 males; 35 females) was included in the Health Assessment Program. Sixty-five (9.8%) men and one (0.1%) woman demonstrated color vision deficiency, and individuals with a red-green deficiency showed lower color vision scores in the yellow region of the visible light spectrum.[23] Since the majority of the dentists in the United States are male, it is important that a dentist be aware of this condition if it exists in himself. If the condition is severe, the dentist can have a laboratory technician or a well-trained assistant match shades.

The object being viewed modifies the light that falls on it by absorbing, reflecting, transmitting, or refracting part or all of the light energy, thereby producing the quality of color. Furthermore, different parts of the same object can exhibit varying amounts of these phenomena. Perception of the object can be influenced by scattered or reflected light from operatory walls, cabinets, and furniture. The walls in a room used for shade selection should be a neutral color, and intense colors should be avoided in selecting cabinets and furniture for this room.

The light source utilized can have a definite effect on the perception of color. There are three light sources commonly found in the dental office: natural, incandescent, and fluorescent (Fig 23-20). The visible portion of the electromagnetic spectrum lies between 380 and 750 μm. Each light source will produce a distinctive distribution of color in the light that it emits.

Natural sunlight itself is extremely variable. The sky appears blue at noon when the sun has less atmosphere to penetrate. There is an uneven distribution of colors in the morning or evening, when the shorter blue and green rays are scattered by the atmosphere surrounding the earth, and the longer red and orange rays of the spectrum are able to penetrate the atmosphere without being scattered. The sky appears red or orange as a result.

Artificial light sources are also lacking in an equal distribution of color. Incandescent light is predominantly red-yellow and lacking in blue. This type of light tends to make reds and yellows stronger and blues weaker. Conversely, under a cool-white fluorescent light source that is high in blue-green energy and low in red, blues are strong and reds are weak.

There are special lights that are "color corrected" to emit light with a more uniform distribution of color. Initial shade selection should be made using color-corrected lights, but any shade should be matched under more than one type of light to overcome the problem of *metamerism*.[21] Metamerism is the phenomenon of an object appearing to be different colors when viewed under different light sources. The different spectrophotometric curves in the light from the surface of a porcelain restoration and from the enamel of an intact tooth may give the appearance of similar colors when viewed under a light source with a particular color distribution. However, they may appear to be different colors when viewed under a light source with a different color distribution. It is better to select a compromise shade that looks reasonably good under all three types of light than to choose one that may look nearly perfect in sunlight, for example, but appear to be badly mismatched in the patient's home or office.

The three characteristics of color are *hue, chroma,* and *value*.[24] To facilitate communication with ceramists, the dentist should be thoroughly familiar with these terms and their definitions. *Hue* is that quality which distinguishes one color from another. It is the name of a color, such as red, blue, or yellow. Hue may be a primary color or a combination of colors. *Chroma* is the saturation, intensity, or strength of a hue. For example, a red and a pink may be of the same hue. The red has a high chroma, while the pink, which is actually a weak red, has a low chroma.

Value, or brightness, is the relative amount of lightness or darkness in a hue. Value is the most important color characteristic in shade matching. If it is not possible to achieve a close match with a shade guide, a lighter shade should be selected since it can be stained more easily to a lower value. It is impossible to stain a tooth to obtain a lighter shade (higher value) without producing opacity. If major changes are attempted in the hue or chroma, there will be an accompanying decrease in value.

A number of related factors must be incorporated in ceramic restorations to achieve natural-appearing results. These factors include: color, translucency, contour, surface texture, and luster.[25] Selecting the basic shade or color of the restoration is merely the first step. Commercially available shade guides do not adequately cover the entire range of tooth color as seen in nature.[26–29] These guides are made of porcelain without a metal backing, and the thickness of the porcelain is much greater than the veneer on a metal-ceramic restoration. The porcelain used for the shade tab is different from that used for fabricating restorations.[30] It is often a higher-fusing porcelain used for denture teeth with extrinsic colorants to develop the desired shade.[31,32] It is easy to see why the color is simply a starting point; natural teeth are much more complicated than shade tabs, and all the individual variations cannot be covered by a commercial guide with approximately 16 selections.

To successfully reproduce natural teeth in ceramic restorations, the various patterns of translucency must be recognized.[33] The translucency pattern contributes to the shade by affecting value: with increasing translucency the value decreases. The amount, location, and quality of translucency varies with individuals and with age. Young teeth often exhibit a great deal of incisal translucency, with the enamel appearing almost transparent at times. Over years of function, the incisal edges wear and this highly translucent enamel is lost.

From daily functions such as eating and toothbrushing, the facial enamel layer becomes thinner allowing the dentin to dominate the shade. In general, older individuals exhibit teeth that are lower in value and higher in chroma than are commonly seen in young adults.[12,14,25] The pattern of translucency will dictate the depth and extent of the enamel and translucent porcelains built into the restoration.[35]

Since tooth color occurs in a very narrow range of the visible light spectrum, the form and contours of the restoration play a major role in esthetics. Matching the outline form is just as important as matching the shade correctly.[36] There can be a slight mismatch in color, but with proper contours, the crown will blend in.[25] The contralateral tooth can provide valuable information regarding the proper contours, embrasure form, and subtle characterizations of the facial surface.

The surface texture of a tooth or a ceramic restoration influences esthetics by determining the amount and direction of light reflected off the facial surface. To harmonize with the natural dentition, the surface texture of a crown must be designed to simulate the reflectance pattern of the adjacent natural teeth.[35,36] Typically, young teeth exhibit a great deal of surface characterization including stippling, ridges, striations, and evidence of developmental lobes. These surface features are gradually worn away with daily function, leaving older teeth with a much smoother, highly polished surface.[37] Communicating the amount and quality of surface texture is very difficult. Some authors suggest the use of sterilized extracted teeth or custom shade tabs as a guide.[36]

The key to the success of natural-appearing restorations is a team approach by the dentist and the technician. Often the ceramist does not participate in the shade selection, making it imperative that the dentist communicate detailed information to the technician. The methods utilized to relay the different factors include a written work

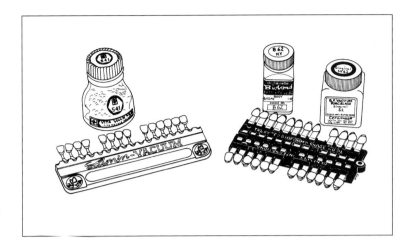

Fig 23-21 The shade guide should match the porcelain: Vita-Lumin for Vita porcelain and Bioform for Biobond and Ceramco.

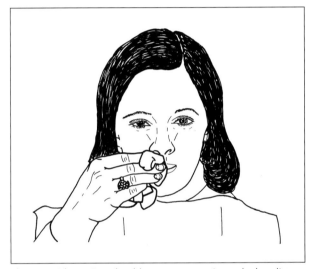

Fig 23-22 The patient should remove cosmetics and other distractions before a shade match is performed.

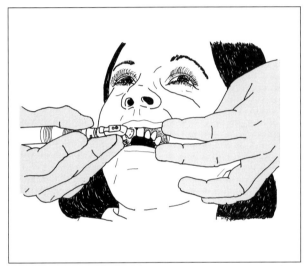

Fig 23-23 Teeth should be clean before an attempt is made to match shades.

authorization with the patient's age and gender, a detailed shade diagram, diagnostic and working casts, and photographs.[35] Custom shade tabs can also aid in the determination of the shade, internal characterization, and surface texture.[36,38] Since ceramists rarely get to see the final result, it is extremely important for the dentist to provide feedback, both positive and negative.

Shade Selection Sequence

There are a few simple guidelines that should be followed by novice and experienced practitioners alike. While following them will not guarantee a perfect match every time, it will eliminate many sources of error and help to standardize the process.

Use the shade guide that matches the porcelain your technician is using (Fig 23-21). Every porcelain is different, and best results are obtained if you use the same guide the manufacturer used in designating the colors of the product. This is preferred to making the technician resort to conversion charts.

The shade should always be matched prior to preparation of the tooth to be restored. Not only can teeth become dehydrated and change color during preparation, but the debris generated in the form of enamel, metal, and cement grindings can coat everything in the mouth.

Ask the patient to remove all distractions before attempting to match a shade. Lipstick in particular should be removed (Fig 23-22). Large, bright items, such as earrings or glasses, can also distract the eye from the intended focus of attention on the teeth. Heavy facial makeup, such as rouge, could also interfere with an accurate match and would need to be removed or masked. Be sure that the teeth are clean and unstained before attempting to match a shade. Perform a quick rubber cup and paste prophylaxis in the area of the mouth where the

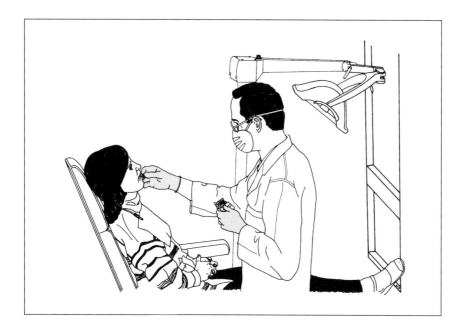

Fig 23-24 When matching a shade, the operator should stand between the patient and the light source.

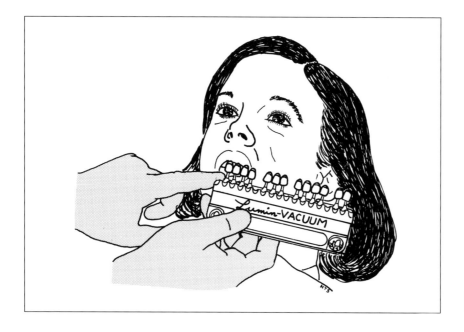

Fig 23-25 The matching process is begun by quickly scanning the guide.

shade is to be matched (Fig 23-23). Rinse the area thoroughly to remove any traces of the prophy paste; otherwise, the prophylaxis will do more harm than good.

Seat the patient in an upright position with the mouth at the operator's eye level (Fig 23-24). Position yourself between the patient and the light source. Observations should be made quickly (5 seconds or less) to avoid fatiguing the cones in the retina.[39,40] The longer the observer's gaze is held, the less ability there is to discriminate, and the cones will become sensitized to the complement of the observed color. Since blue fatigue

accentuates yellow sensitivity, the dentist should glance at a blue object (wall, drape, card, etc) while resting the eyes. The shade should be matched by value, chroma, and hue, in that order.

Scan the entire shade guide quickly, selecting those tabs that are the worst match first and eliminating them (Fig 23-25). By process of elimination, this will leave the few tabs that are the closest matches. Moisten them as they are used.

If a decision cannot be made between two tabs, hold them on either side of the tooth being matched (Fig 23-

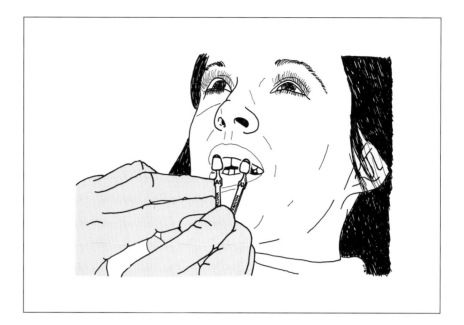

Fig 23-26 The tabs are held on either side of the tooth when making a choice between two closely matching shade tabs.

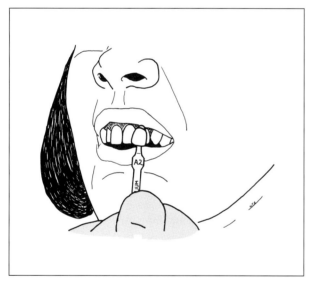

Fig 23-27 The gingival portion of the shade tab is matched with the gingival segment of the real tooth.

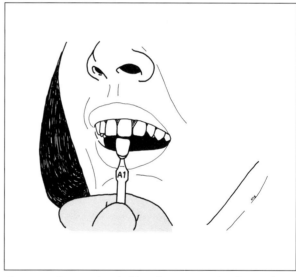

Fig 23-28 The incisal end of the tab is compared with incisal area of the tooth.

26). If no tab will permit a good match, then resort to matching the gingival portion of the shade tabs with the gingival area of the tooth (Fig 23-27).

The necks of the shade tabs often exhibit a great deal of extrinsic colorants. Remove the necks of the tabs to eliminate this very artistic but distracting aspect prior to matching the gingival one-third to one-half of the tooth.[40,41] Complete the matching process by comparing the incisal segments of those tabs which most nearly match with the incisal portion of the tooth (Fig 23-28). Initially select the shade using a color-corrected light (color rendering index

of 90 or greater), then repeat the process under at least one other light source to minimize metamerism.

Since value is the most important dimension of color when selecting porcelain shades, try viewing the tabs through half-closed eyes. Although this decreases the ability to discriminate color, it increases the ability to match value. Arranging the shade guide according to value may also facilitate the correct selection of the tooth's relative lightness or darkness.

Carefully examine the tooth and determine the pattern of translucency and any unique characterizing features

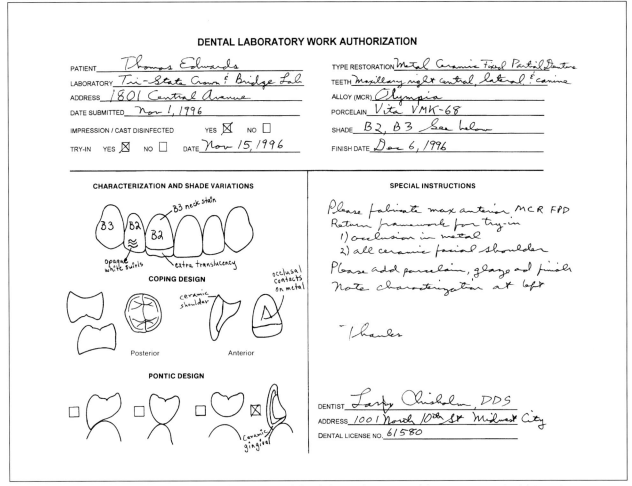

DENTAL LABORATORY WORK AUTHORIZATION

PATIENT *Thomas Edwards*

LABORATORY *Tri-State Crown & Bridge Lab*

ADDRESS *1801 Central Avenue*

DATE SUBMITTED *Nov 1, 1996*

IMPRESSION / CAST DISINFECTED   YES ☒   NO ☐

TRY-IN   YES ☒   NO ☐   DATE *Nov 15, 1996*

TYPE RESTORATION *Metal Ceramic Fixed Partial Denture*

TEETH *Maxillary right central, lateral, & canine*

ALLOY (MCR) *Olympia*

PORCELAIN *Vita VMK-68*

SHADE *B2, B3 See below*

FINISH DATE *Dec 6, 1996*

CHARACTERIZATION AND SHADE VARIATIONS

B3 neck stain

B3 B2 B2

opaque white swirls

extra translucency

occlusal contacts on metal

COPING DESIGN

ceramic shoulder

Posterior   Anterior

PONTIC DESIGN

☐   ☐   ☐   ☒

Ceramic gingival

SPECIAL INSTRUCTIONS

Please fabricate max anterior MCR FPD
Return framework for try-in
1) occlusion in metal
2) all ceramic facial shoulder
Please add porcelain, glaze and finish
Note characterization at left

Thanks

DENTIST *Larry Chisholm, DDS*

ADDRESS *1001 North 10th St Midwest City*

DENTAL LICENSE NO. *61580*

Fig 23-29 The prescription should be precise and detailed in its description of the restoration to be fabricated.

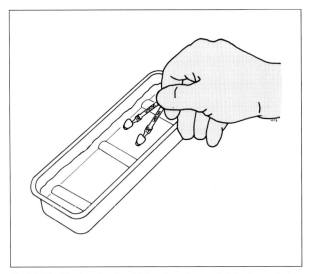

Fig 23-30 Shade tabs should be placed in a disinfecting solution when the shade matching has been completed.

such as craze lines, areas of hypocalcification, etc. Use a periodontal probe or other millimeter measuring device to establish the location and extent of these distinguishing features. Developing color, translucency, and characterizations within the porcelain will create a more lifelike restoration than simply applying extrinsic colorants after the porcelain is fired.

Make a drawing of the facial surface of the tooth in the patient's chart, and record all pertinent information graphically. Indicate different shades if more than one is selected for different parts of the tooth. Transfer this information to the laboratory work authorization, making it as complete as possible (Fig 23-29). It is a good idea, whenever possible, to send the shade lab, a cast including the contralateral tooth, and a photograph to the dental laboratory.

Before putting the shade guide away, *disinfect* it (Fig 23-30). Since parts of most shade guides are made of plastic, avoid the autoclave or other processes involving heat.

References

1. Tjan AHL, Miller GD: The JGP: Some esthetic factors in a smile. *J Prosthet Dent* 1984; 51:24–28.

2. Moskowitz ME, Nayyar A: Determinants of dental esthetics: A rationale for smile analysis and treatment. *Compend Contin Educ Dent* 1995; 16:1164–1186.

3. Heinlein WD: Anterior teeth: Esthetics and function. *J Prosthet Dent* 1980; 44:389–393.

4. Vig RG, Brundo GC: The kinetics of anterior tooth display. *J Prosthet Dent* 1978; 39:502–503.

5. Andrews LF: The six keys to normal occlusion. *Am J Orthod* 1972; 62:296–309.

6. Powell N, Humphreys B: *Proportions of the Aesthetic Face.* New York, Thieme-Stratton, 1984, pp 2, 4–9, 50.

7. Lombardi RE: The principles of visual perception and their clinical application to denture esthetics. *J Prosthet Dent* 1973; 29:358–382.

8. Cipra DL, Wall JG: Esthetics in fixed and removable prosthodontics: The composition of a smile. *J Tenn Dent Assoc* 1991; 71:24–29.

9. Brisman AS: Esthetics: A comparison of dentists' and patients' concepts. *J Am Dent Assoc* 1980; 100:345–352.

10. Black GV: *Descriptive Anatomy of the Human Teeth.* Philadelphia, Wilmington Dental Mfg Co, 1890, p 14–15.

11. Shillingburg HT, Kaplan MJ, Grace CS: Tooth dimensions— A comparative study. *J South Calif Dent Assoc* 1972; 40:830–839.

12. Brisman A, Hirsch SM, Paige H, et al: Tooth shade preferences in older patients. *Gerodontics* 1985; 1:130–133.

13. Levin EI: Dental esthetics and the golden proportion. *J Prosthet Dent* 1978; 40:244–252.

14. Heyman HO: The artistry of conservative esthetic dentistry. *J Am Dent Assoc* 1987; 115:14E–23E.

15. Barratt K: *Logic and Design in Art, Science and Mathematics.* New York, Design Books, 1980, p 108–111.

16. Ricketts RM: The golden divider. *J Clin Orthod* 1981; 15:752–759.

17. Pedoe D: *Geometry and the Visual Arts.* New York, Dover Publications, 1983, pp 69, 70.

18. Huntley HE: *The Divine Proportion—A Study in Mathematical Beauty.* New York, Dover Publications, 1970, pp 23, 62, 64, 161.

19. Gardner M: The multiple fascinations of the Fibonacci sequence. *Scientific Amer* 1969; 220:116–120.

20. Ricketts RM: Divine proportion in facial esthetics. *J Clin Orthod* 1981; 15:752–59.

21. Sproull RC: Color matching in dentistry. Part III. Color control. *J Prosthet Dent* 1974; 31:146–154.

22. Wasson W, Schuman N: Color vision and dentistry. *Quintessence Int* 1992; 23:349–353.

23. Moser JB, Wozniak WT, Naleway CA, Ayer WA: Color vision in dentistry: A survey. *J Am Dent Assoc* 1985; 110:509–510.

24. Sproull RC: Color matching in dentistry. Part I. The three-dimensional nature of color. *J Prosthet Dent* 1973; 29:416–424.

25. Winter RR: Achieving esthetic ceramic restorations. *J Calif Dent Assoc* 1990; 18:21–24.

26. Clark EB: Tooth color selection. *J Am Dent Assoc* 1933; 20:1065–1073.

27. Sproull RC: Color matching in dentistry. Part II. Practical applications of the organization of color. *J Prosthet Dent* 1973; 29:556–566.

28. Preston JD: The metal-ceramic restoration: The problems remain. *Int J Periodont Rest Dent* 1984; 4(5):9–23.

29. Miller LL: Organizing color in dentistry. *J Am Dent Assoc* 1987; 115:26E–40E.

30. Preston JD: Current status of shade selection and color matching. *Quintessence Int* 1985; 16:47–58.

31. Bergen SF: Color in esthetics. *N Y State Dent J* 1985; 51:470–471.

32. Wall JG, Cipra DL: Esthetics in fixed and removable prosthodontics: Shade selection in metal-ceramics. *J Tenn Dent Assoc* 1992; 72:10-12.

33. Yamamoto M: *Metal-Ceramics: Principles and Methods of Makato Yamamoto.* Chicago, Quintessence Publishing Co, 1985, p 350.

34. Bell AM, Kurzeja R, Gamberg MG: Ceramometal crowns and bridges. Focus on failures. *Dent Clin North Am* 1985; 29:763–778.

35. Kessler JC: Dentist and laboratory: Communication for success. *J Am Dent Assoc* 1987; 115:97E–102E.

36. Sorensen JA, Torres TJ: Improved color matching of metal ceramic restorations. Part II Procedures for visual communication. *J Prosthet Dent* 1987; 58:669–677.

37. Pilkington EL: Esthetics and optical illusions in dentistry. *J Am Dent Assoc* 1936; 23:641–651.

38. Seluk LW, Lalonde TD: Esthetics and communication with a custom shade guide. *Dent Clin North Am* 1985; 29:741–751.

39. Yamamoto M: *Metal-Ceramics: Principles and Methods of Makato Yamamoto.* Chicago, Quintessence Publishing Co, 1985, p 240.

40. Sorensen JA, Torres TJ: Improved color matching of metal-ceramic restorations. Part I: A systematic method for shade determination. *J Prosthet Dent* 1987; 58:133–139.

41. O'Keefe KL, Strickler ER, Kerrin HK: Color and shade matching: The weak link in esthetic dentistry. *Compend Contin Educ Dent* 1990; 11:116–120.

Chapter 24

All-Ceramic Restorations

Dental porcelains play an important role in the fabrication of the most esthetic fixed restorations. Translucency, light transmission, and biocompatibility give dental ceramics highly desirable esthetic properties. However, the brittle nature of dental porcelains, which are basically noncrystalline glasses composed of structural units of silicon and oxygen (SiO_4 tetrahedra), limit the use of these materials. Several properties are necessary for their use in the fabrication of dental restorations[1]:

1. Low fusing temperature
2. High viscosity
3. Resistance to devitrification

These properties are obtained by the addition of other oxides to the basic structure.

The fusing temperature is lowered by reducing the cross linkages between oxygen and silicon with glass modifiers, such as potassium oxide, sodium oxide, and calcium oxide. Unfortunately, these modifiers or fluxes also lower the viscosity. Dental porcelains require a high resistance to slumping so that restorations will maintain their basic shape during firing. This is accomplished by the use of an intermediate oxide, aluminum oxide, which is incorporated into the silicon-oxygen lattice.

If too many modifiers are added to the porcelain to disrupt the SiO_4 tetrahedra, the glass tends to devitrify, or crystallize. This becomes a special problem in porcelains with an increased coefficient of thermal expansion, because alkalis are introduced to interrupt the silicon oxygen lattice and raise the expansion. When a porcelain is fired too many times, it may devitrify, becoming milky and difficult to glaze.

Porcelain can be classified by firing temperature[2]:

1. *High-fusing:* 1,290 to 1,370°C (2,350 to 2,500°F)
2. *Medium-fusing:* 1,090 to 1,260°C (2,000 to 2,300°F)
3. *Low-fusing:* 870 to 1,065°C (1,600 to 1,950°F)

High-fusing porcelain is usually used for the manufacture of porcelain teeth, although it has been used to some extent for porcelain jacket crowns. The typical high-fusing porcelain is composed of feldspar (70% to 90%), quartz (11% to18%), and kaolin (1% to 10%). The main

Table 24-1 *Constituents of Dental Porcelains[1]*

	Low-fusing porcelain	Medium-fusing porcelain
Silicon dioxide	69.4%	64.2%
Boric oxide	7.5%	2.8%
Calcium oxide	1.9%	—
Potassium oxide	8.3%	8.2%
Sodium oxide	4.8%	1.9%
Aluminum oxide	8.1%	19.0%
Lithium oxide	—	2.1%
Magnesium oxide	—	0.5%
Phosporous pentoxide	—	0.7%

constituent of feldspar is silicon dioxide, present in the form of $Na_2O \cdot Al_2O_3 \cdot 6SiO_2$ and $K_2O \cdot Al_2O_3 \cdot 6SiO_2$. When it fuses, it forms a glassy material that gives the porcelain its translucency. It acts as a matrix for the high-fusing quartz (SiO_2), which in turn forms a refractory skeleton around which the other materials fuse. It helps the porcelain restoration maintain its form during firing. Kaolin, a clay, is a sticky material that binds the particles together when the porcelain is "green" or unfired.

Low- and medium-fusing porcelains are manufactured by a process called *fritting*. The raw constituents of porcelain are fused, quenched, and ground back to an extremely fine powder. When fired again in the fabrication of the restoration, the powder fuses at a lower temperature and undergoes no pyrochemical reaction. The constituents of typical low- and medium-fusing porcelains are shown in Table 24-1.[1]

The addition of certain metallic oxides (zirconium oxide, titanium oxide, and tin oxide) will make the porcelain opaque. A layer of opaque porcelain is used to mask the metal coping of a metal-ceramic restoration. Certain other metallic substances are added to the frit during manufacturing to produce color in the porcelain[1]: indium (yellow); chromium, tin (pink); iron oxide (black); cobalt salts (blue).

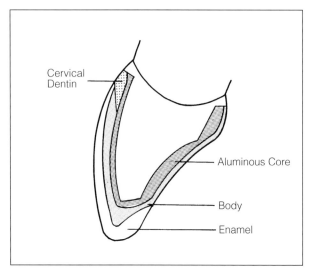

Fig 24-1 The layers of an aluminous porcelain jacket crown (after McLean and Hughes[4]).

All-Ceramic Crowns

The first all-ceramic crown was developed by Land[3] in 1886 and was known as the *porcelain jacket crown* (PJC). For many decades it was the most esthetic full-veneer restoration dentistry had to offer. The PJC was once made from high-fusing porcelains utilizing platinum foil for support during firing. It relied on the support of the underlying tooth preparation during function. Because of the tendency of this type of restoration to fracture, its use usually is limited to single anterior teeth, primarily incisors.

As the demand for more natural-looking crowns has increased in recent years, dentists and porcelain manufacturers have investigated a variety of methods to reinforce ceramics with the ultimate goal of a ceramic material that possesses not only a high level of esthetics and soft tissue acceptance, but sufficient strength to allow the fabrication of fixed partial dentures.

In 1965 McLean and Hughes developed a porcelain jacket crown with an inner core of aluminous porcelain containing 40% to 50% alumina crystals to block the propagation of cracks (Fig 24-1).[4] The reinforcing inner core of the restoration that surrounds the preparation is layered with conventional porcelain, resulting in a restoration approximately twice as strong as the traditional PJC. The use of this type of reinforcement revived the use of porcelain jacket crowns. Unfortunately, the strength was still insufficient for anything but single anterior crowns.

Fracture resistance in the aluminous porcelain jacket crown was improved by a technique in which the platinum matrix was left in the completed restoration.[5,6] The strength of the crown was augmented even more by the "twin foil" technique.[7] The platinum foil matrix not only provided additional support of the porcelain, it allowed a chemical bond between the tin-plated foil and oxides in the porcelain. However, the residual platinum foil did decrease the amount of light transmitted, which diminished somewhat the esthetic advantage of an all-ceramic restoration.

In the last two decades, research has focused on strengthening dental ceramics by modification of the porcelain's microstructure. The typical "glassy" matrix of feldspathic porcelain is manipulated to include a unique crystalline structure that alters both optical and mechanical properties of the ceramic. Strength and fracture toughness can be directly compared in materials with similar surface flaws.[8] Three mechanisms strengthen ceramics, and they all require incorporation of a second phase of heat-generated crystal production to increase the energy necessary for crack propagation:

1. *Crack-tip interactions*. Obstacles in the microstructure impede crack motion by reorienting or deflecting the plane of fracture.
2. *Crack-tip shielding*. Events triggered by the high stresses in the crack tip region act to reduce the stress; ie, transformation toughening (often associated with zirconium) and microcrack toughening.
3. *Crack bridging*. Second-phase crystalline structure acts as a "bandage" to prevent a crack from opening further.[9,10] The 1980s saw the introduction of several "new" all-ceramic restorations that relied on the introduction of a second-phase crystalline structure to reinforce the porcelain. They included two castable glass-ceramics (Dicor, Dentsply International, York, PA,[11] and Cerapearl, Kyocera, San Diego, CA[12]) and a shrink-free ceramic crown (Cerestore Non-Shrink Alumina Ceramic, Coors Biomedical Co, Lakewood, CO[13,14]).

These systems were appealing because they used the lost wax technique in crown fabrication. Their esthetics were better than metal-ceramic restorations, and the reinforcement method offered the potential of greater strength. Unfortunately, the improvements they offered were not great enough to outweigh the disadvantages of each system. A big problem was the necessity of purchasing expensive equipment and materials, which in turn necessitated charging higher laboratory fees to the dentist. The ceramics were not strong enough for fixed partial dentures, so each system essentially became another way of doing a PJC—at a higher cost. Coupled with cost were technique sensitivity and high fracture/failure rates. These systems of fabricating all-ceramic crowns have fallen victim to the demands of the market.

In the Cerestore system, a core, or coping, was waxed for marginal integrity and porcelain support. Following investing, a ceramic material with a high alumina crystal content was melted and flowed into the mold. The mold was heated overnight, the core was divested, and conventional porcelain was applied to the core. The core could distort during firing of the porcelain veneer, and esthetics could be compromised by the opaque nature of the core, especially in the marginal area.

The idea of casting ceramics is not new. In 1923 Wain described a method for casting glass in a refractory mold similar to the lost wax technique of casting gold.[15] In 1968 MacCulloch fabricated denture teeth from a glass-ceramic used to make cookware (Pyrosil) and suggested the possibility of using glass-ceramics for inlays and crowns.[16] The strength of certain glasses can be increased by adding a small amount of nucleating agent (metal phosphate) to the molten glass and heating the glass after solidification. During the reheating phase, *ceramming,* crystals form on the small metal nuclei, greatly increasing the strength of the ceramic.

The Dicor system, utilizing a castable glass-ceramic, was introduced in the 1980s. This glass-ceramic material was composed of SiO_2, K_2O, MgO, fluoride from MgF_2, minor amounts of Al_2O_3 and ZrO_2 incorporated for durability, and a fluorescing agent for esthetics.[17,18] The fluoride acts as a nucleating agent (as a source of fluoride ions), a necessary agent in the crystalline phase, and it improves the fluidity of the molten glass.[17]

Fabrication of Dicor restorations was immediately familiar, since it was built around waxing the crown to full anatomic contour with precise control of the occlusion and axial contours.[19] The wax pattern was invested in a phosphate-bonded investment, burned out, cast in molten glass, and divested following solidification. The casting was embedded in investment and reheated to allow nucleation and growth of the crystalline phase. After ceramming, the material is approximately 55% crystalline and contains tetrasilicic fluormica crystals $(K_2Mg_5Si_8O_{20}F_4)$.[19]

These crystals are similar to mica, and the microstructure consists of many small, interlocking, randomly oriented crystals. The cerammed casting is achromatic, and shade is developed by adding external colorants. Although the lack of internal color was criticized, its translucency led to a variation in which Dicor was used as a coping material. Conventional porcelain was applied to achieve the desired contours and color. Despite significant start-up costs, Dicor experienced popularity for partial veneer and complete-coverage restorations in all areas of the mouth. Unfortunately, a high failure rate in the posterior regions of the mouth, as well as the development of other materials, led to the phasing out of this product.

Cerapearl, another castable glass-ceramic, also employed the lost wax technique to produce the initial stage of the restoration and a reheating phase to develop a crystalline microstructure. The microstructure in this ceramic contained $CaP_2O_5SiO_5$, a crystal similar to the hydroxyapatite of enamel.[12,20] The brief availability of this system made it relatively unknown in the United States.

Perhaps the greatest contribution of glass-ceramics was reinforcement of the microstructure by the secondary crystalline phase. In the newest generation of high-strength ceramics for all-ceramic restorations, crystalline-reinforced composite materials employ a variety of reinforcing crystals (Table 24-2). Two materials, IPS-Empress (Ivolclar North America, Amherst, NY) and In-

Table 24-2 *Reinforcing Crystals Used in Brands of Dental Porcelain*

Reinforcing crystal	Brand	Manufacturer
Alumina	*Vitadur-N core*	Vident, Brea, CA
	In-Ceram	Vident
Alumina and zirconium	*In-Ceram (recent)*	Vident
Leucite	*Cerinate*	Den-Mat Corp, Santa Maria, CA
	IPS-Empress	Ivolclar North America, Amherst, NY
	Optec HSP	Jeneric/Pentron, Wallingford, CT
	Vita VMK 68	Vident
Magnesium aluminous spinel	*In-Ceram Spinell*	Vident
Sanidine	*Mark II*	Vident
Zirconia whiskers	*Mirage II fiber*	Myron International Kansas City, KS

Ceram (Vident, Brea, CA), stand out for their unique technology and popularity.

The IPS-Empress system is indicated for inlays, onlays, veneers, and complete-coverage crowns. The system relies on a leucite-reinforced glass-ceramic that is heat-pressed into a phosphate-bonded investment, forming either a core or a completed restoration. Unlike previous glass-ceramics, the IPS-Empress system does not require a second heating cycle to initiate the crystalline phase of leucite crystals. Instead, they are formed within the glass matrix of feldspathic porcelain throughout various temperature cycles.[21]

When the restoration is retrieved from the investment, heavily pigmented colorants and glaze can be painted on the surface of the achromatic material to form the completed restoration. A popular option uses an Empress core or "dentin structure" veneered with ceramic. A wide range of shades and translucency similar to natural tooth structure provide excellent esthetics.[22]

Fatigue parameter testing indicates that IPS-Empress is less fatigue-susceptible and has a greater 12-year failure stress than feldspathic porcelain.[23] However, it exhibits lower compressive strength than metal-ceramic crowns or In-Ceram crowns.[24] In comparisons of flexural strength of current ceramic materials, IPS-Empress exhibited less fracture resistance and less fracture toughness than alumina-reinforced ceramics.[10,25] Low flexural strength precludes IPS-Empress from consideration for fixed partial dentures, but it offers considerable versatility for single-tooth restorations with high translucency.

In-Ceram shows promise for all-ceramic crowns and fixed partial dentures. This system has evolved from

research by Sadoun[26] in 1985, using alumina as the core material. A suspension of finely ground material *(slip)* mixed to a thin, creamy consistency, is brushed onto the die in a method called *slipcasting.* The alumina is fired, or *sintered,* in a furnace, fusing particles together without completely melting them.[2] In a second firing process, glass is applied to the surface of the porous core and is *infused,* or absorbed into the porous core material, by capillary action. The densely packed alumina crystals limit crack propagation, and glass infiltration eliminates residual porosity.[27]

A comparison of the flexural strength of alumina core material, infusion glass, the infused alumina core, feldspathic porcelain (VMK 68), and glass-ceramic (Dicor) revealed that the infused alumina core was 2.5 times stronger than glass-ceramic and feldspathic porcelain.[28]

Although the sintered alumina core is relatively weak, there is a marked elevation of strength following glass infusion.[28] The design of the core resembles the coping of a metal-ceramic restoration. It provides a strong substructure that resists flexure and supports the veneer. Conventional porcelain (Vitadur-N or Alpha porcelain, Vident) is applied to the core to develop the final contours and color.

Research in Europe and the United States confirms the desirable physical properties of In-Ceram. When uniform premolar crowns were loaded in a "crushing" manner on axial surfaces, In-Ceram crowns demonstrated greater fracture resistance than two other all-ceramic systems (Hi-Ceram and veneered glass-ceramic). Although the fracture resistance of the In-Ceram did not differ significantly from the metal-ceramic restorations (control), the authors had standardized the number of firings between groups by eliminating the application of opaque porcelain in the control group.[29]

Another study compared the compressive strength of In-Ceram and IPS-Empress to that of metal-ceramic crowns. This study found that In-Ceram possessed greater compressive strength than IPS-Empress, but less than the metal-ceramic control.[25] Evaluations of flexural strength and fracture toughness appear more relevant to clinical performance.

In comparing flexural strength of six new-generation ceramics, all of the In-Ceram core materials (alumina reinforced, alumina and zirconia reinforced, and magnesium aluminous spinel) were significantly stronger than all other ceramic systems. A spinel is a natural oxide of magnesium (Mg++) and aluminum (Al+++) in which other metals can be substituted for the two named here. These compounds are commonly used for refractory purposes. Crack deflection appears to be the principle strengthening mechanism in the highly crystalline materials.[10] In evaluating fracture toughness and hardness, alumina was the most effective reinforcing agent.[21]

Ceramic strength is influenced by flaw size, number, and distribution, especially in areas of high tensile stress. Voids and flaws at the interface between the core and porcelain would allow crack propagation and failure, leaving the core intact.[30] Due to its high strength and toughness, In-Ceram has been used to fabricate fixed partial dentures, but the manufacturer recommends only short-span (three-unit) anterior restorations.

In a study evaluating 20 experimental (in vitro) and 9 clinical (in vivo) unsuccessful fixed partial dentures, failure occurred in the connector areas of all specimens. Approximately 70% to 78% originated from the core-veneer interface.[31] All of the experimental restorations and the majority of the clinical examples replaced posterior teeth, supporting the manufacturer's suggested use on anterior fixed partial dentures only. The development of the newest core material with 33% zirconia may strengthen the core material sufficiently for use in posterior fixed partial dentures.

Early evaluations of In-Ceram restorations were more anecdotal than scientific. However, initial longitudinal clinical studies are favorable. In one study, 63 In-Ceram crowns were observed over 24 to 44 months (average time of 37.6 months). In this time frame, the success rate was 98.4%, with one crown failing due to improper tooth preparation.[32] Another study included a total of 76 restorations distributed over single crowns and fixed partial dentures. Single-tooth restorations did very well over the 35-month trial period. Failures occurred only in fixed partial dentures. It is interesting to note that as a result of "extensive tooth preparation," 3 of 68 teeth required endodontic treatment.[33]

One disadvantage of metal-ceramic restorations is the absence of light transmission due to the metal coping. The improved esthetics of all-ceramic restorations is partially due to the ability of porcelain to transmit light. Recent developments in all-ceramic crowns have greatly improved this esthetic requirement. When light transmission was measured in a variety of dimensions and shades of In-Ceram discs, there was an inverse relationship between thickness and light transmission. Light transmission also decreased as shade intensity increased.[34]

Alumina-reinforced ceramic systems significantly improve the light reflection characteristics of crowns when compared to conventional metal-ceramic restorations.[35] However, opaque aluminum oxide diminishes translucency when compared to leucite-reinforced systems (Optec, IPS-Empress). To improve light transmission and reflection in single anterior crowns where maximum strength is not required, a magnesium aluminous spinel may be utilized. The transilluminating qualities seem to be similar to those of natural teeth.[36]

With a variety of core materials for diverse clinical situations, and reported strength and longevity, In-Ceram is a system worthy of consideration when all-ceramic restorations are planned for a patient. A description of the fabrication of a typical restoration follows. Strict adherence to instructions and specified materials is essential to the success in the clinical application of the system.[37]

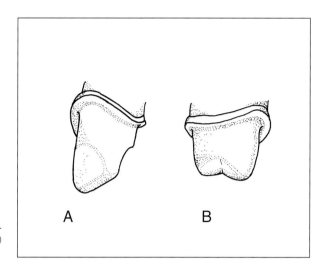

Fig 24-2 Tooth preparations for all-ceramic crowns: (A) anterior; (B) posterior.

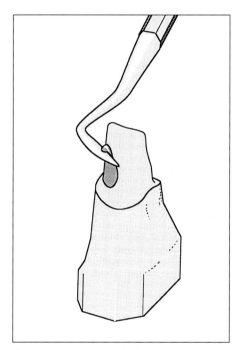

Fig 24-3 Undercuts are blocked out in axial walls.

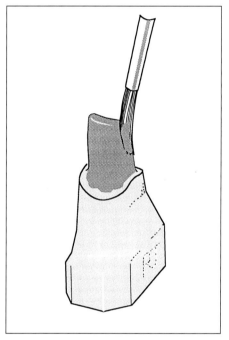

Fig 24-4 Die spacer is applied to the preparation, staying away from the finish line.

Crown Fabrication

All-ceramic crowns demand a significant amount of tooth reduction to allow for a minimum thickness of core material, development of internal shade characterization, and the ability to maintain biologically acceptable contours. Tooth preparation for In-Ceram restorations should provide a minimum overall reduction of 1.0 mm.[27] However, 1.5 mm on the facial and 1.5 to 2.0 mm on the occlusal aspects are preferred. All line and point angles should be rounded.[26,28] (See Chapter 10 for a complete description of the tooth preparation for an all-ceramic crown.)

The finish line is a 1.0-mm-wide radial shoulder on the facial and 0.5 to 0.7 mm in other areas (Fig 24-2).[26] A study comparing the marginal adaptation of In-Ceram crowns with varying finish lines found that all three of the configurations tested (chamfer, 50-degree shoulder, and 9-degree shoulder) yielded acceptable results.[38]

Following the impression of the prepared tooth, a master cast with removable dies is constructed. Trim the dies and block out any undercuts (Fig 24-3). Apply cement spacer to the dies, staying 0.5 to 1.0 mm from the finish line (Fig 24-4). An addition silicone impression material is utilized in duplicating the master cast (Fig 24-5) and

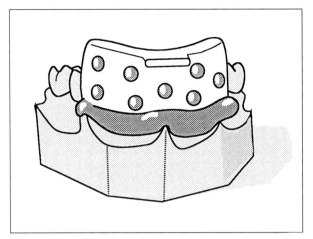

Fig 24-5 A sectional impression of the master cast is made with an addition silicone material.

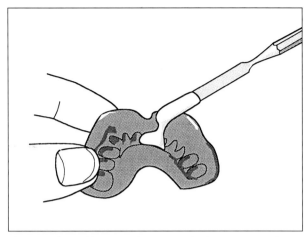

Fig 24-6 The mold is poured in a special refractory material.

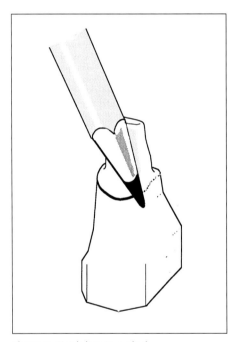

Fig 24-7 Finish line is marked.

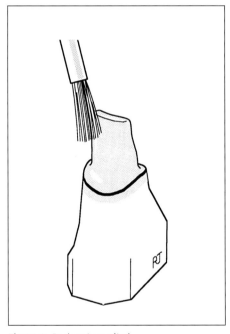

Fig 24-8 Sealant is applied.

poured in a specially formulated stone (Fig 24-6). The expansion of this stone corresponds to the contraction of the slipcasting material during the initial sintering process. After trimming the duplicate dies, mark the finish line (Fig 24-7). Apply a sealant , which will act as a surface wetting agent, decreasing absorption of liquid slip by the die (Fig 24-8).

An ultrasonic device (Vitasonic, Vident) is utilized for the preparation of the aluminous oxide slip material (Fig 24-9). Liquid, alumina powder, and an additive are combined and mixed on a vibrator (Fig 24-10) until becoming an homogenous mass. The slip should exhibit *rheopex*

properties; ie, the liquid mass stiffens under pressure. This property may cause the ceramist a few moments of frustration and require some additional practice.

Rapidly apply the slip with a synthetic brush, building up the desired coping configuration (Fig 24-11). The die readily absorbs the fluid, aiding the condensation of alumina particles. The consistency of the applied slip materials resembles wax and carves easily. Use a scalpel and other carving instruments for initial shaping of the coping (Fig 24-12). Allow the completed aluminous oxide coping to dry for 30 minutes. Then apply a liquid stabilizer to the framework to facilitate corrections after firing.

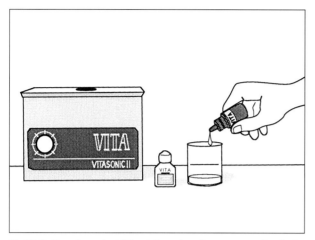

Fig 24-9 One drop of additive is introduced to one ampule of mixing fluid.

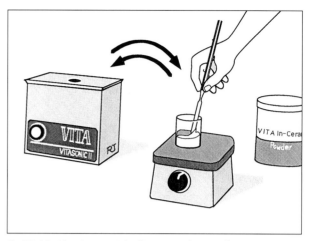

Fig 24-10 Aluminum oxide slip is mixed in an ultrasonic unit. As liquid is added to the container, the mixture is vibrated.

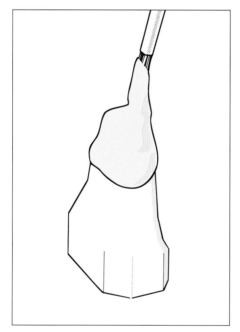

Fig 24-11 The slip is applied with a synthetic brush.

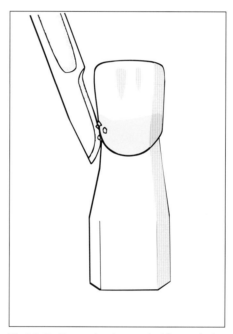

Fig 24-12 The coping is carved with a scalpel.

The framework is sintered in a furnace designed for long-duration firing (Fig 24-13). During the 10-hour firing cycle temperatures reach 1,120°C. When the cycle reaches its maximum temperature, the copings are held at 1,120°C for 2 hours to allow the development of aluminous oxide crystals. During the sintering process the duplicate dies shrink, making the removal of the copings extremely easy (Fig 24-14). Final shaping of the framework is accomplished with rotary stones and diamond burs.

Glass infiltration provides the coping with its final shade, translucency, and strength. The glass powders are coordinated with the shades in the Vita-Lumin shade guide. Mix the desired shade of glass powder with distilled water. Generously apply the mixture to the coping (Fig 24-15), leaving a small area uncovered to facilitate an escape of air as the glass fills the porosities. Place the coping on platinum foil in preparation for firing (Fig 24-16). The infiltration firing cycle at 1,100°C requires 4 hours for single crowns and 6 hours for fixed partial denture frameworks.

During this cycle the glass infiltrates the alumina core materials via capillary action, very much like coffee soaks into a lump of sugar. When infiltration is complete, re-

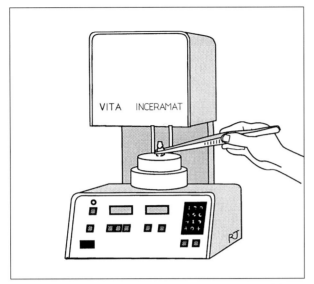

Fig 24-13 The coping is placed in the furnace and sintered for 10 hours.

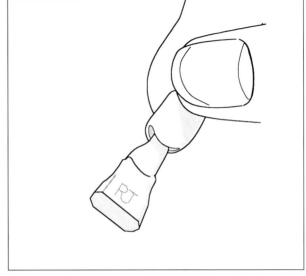

Fig 24-14 The coping is easily removed from the die, which shrinks during the heat treatment.

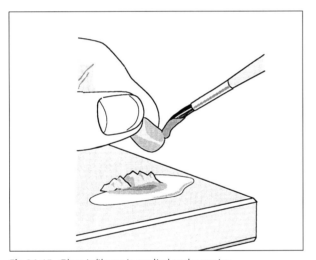

Fig 24-15 Glass infiltrate is applied to the coping.

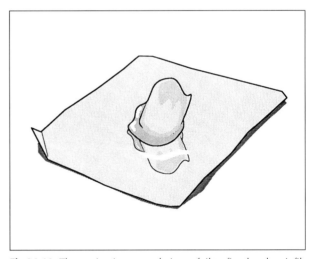

Fig 24-16 The coping is set on platinum foil to fire the glass infiltrate.

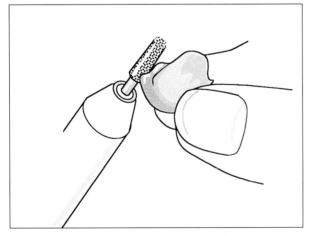

Fig 24-17 After firing the glass infiltrate, excess is removed with a diamond.

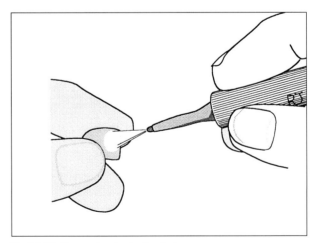

Fig 24-18 The coping is air abraded.

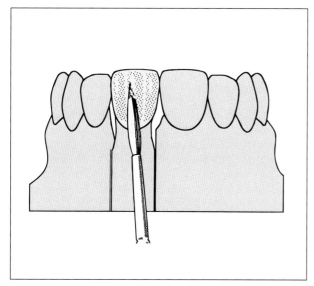

Fig 24-19 Crown form is built up with feldspathic porcelain.

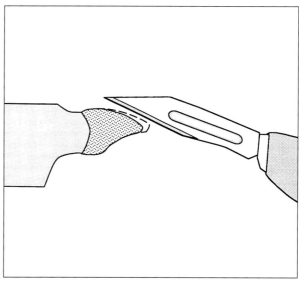

Fig 24-20 Incisal area is cut back.

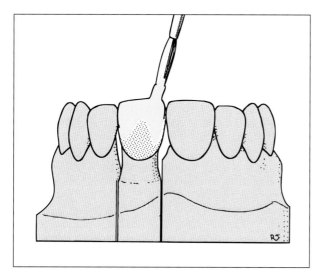

Fig 24-21 Incisal porcelain is added to the part of the buildup that has been cut back.

move excess bulk of glass with diamond burs (Fig 24-17). Then air abrade the coping (Fig 24-18). Excess infiltration glass (0.1 to 0.3 mm) on the surface of the core does not appear to adversely affect the compressive strength of In-Ceram crowns.[39] However, it could increase the chroma of the restoration and decrease light transmission.

Following glass infiltration, conventional porcelain (Vitadur-Alpha) is added to the coping, restoring the correct anatomic form and occlusal function (Fig 24-19). Cut back the incisal area in "green" porcelain (Fig 24-20). Add back to full contour with incisal porcelain (Fig 24-21). After necessary correction bakes, the crown is glazed and ready for cementation.

Porcelain Laminate Veneers

The laminate veneer is a conservative alternative to full coverage for improving the appearance of an anterior tooth.[40] Laminate veneers have evolved over the last several decades to become one of esthetic dentistry's most popular restorations. A porcelain laminate veneer is an extremely thin shell of porcelain applied directly to tooth structure.[41] This restoration may be used to improve the color of stained teeth, alter contours of misshapen teeth, and close interproximal spaces. Tooth preparation is minimal, remaining within enamel. The restoration derives its strength from the ability of a composite resin luting agent, with a silane coupling agent, to bond with etched porcelain and etched enamel.

The idea of porcelain veneers is not new. In the 1930s and 1940s Dr Charles Pincus used thin porcelain veneers to improve the esthetics of movie stars' teeth.[42] Unfortunately, he had to use denture adhesive to hold the veneers in place. The development of bis-GMA and composite resin restorative materials provided innovative opportunities to restore discolored or malposed teeth.

In the mid-1970s and early 1980s the composite resin laminate veneer, with or without a facing, evolved. At first composite resin was added directly to the facial surface of a tooth to restore fractured, discolored, and malformed permanent incisors in a procedure commonly known as "bonding."[43] The early composite resin bonding presented several problems, including a monochromatic appearance, with staining and a loss of luster occurring over time. Early composite resin veneers typically did not employ any tooth preparation, and a bulk of material was necessary to obtain a pleasing appearance.[44] Unfortunately, the overcontoured restorations contributed to gingival inflammation.

The second evolution of veneers involved the development of preformed veneers or crown forms that were joined to the etched tooth structure. Constructing a veneer (without regard to the material) and bonding it to etched tooth structure is referred to as "laminating."[44] Indications for these laminate veneers included use as an interim restoration for esthetic improvement of badly discolored anterior teeth, especially in young patients.[45] The application of preexisting facings became a popular practice. The three types of facings commonly used were hollow-ground denture teeth, preformed stock laminates, and custom-fabricated laminates of processed acrylic resin.[40,46]

The preformed veneers were a definite improvement over bonding. However, color instability, surface staining, loss of surface luster, low abrasion resistance, biologic incompatibility, and a poor bond between the veneer and the tooth still persisted.[47,48] The bond between the acrylic resin laminate and the composite resin was weak, allowing the veneer to be removed easily or simply to fall off. Surface pretreatments helped, but the effectiveness was technique sensitive.[46] These problems eventually led to the diminished use of acrylic resin and/or composite resin veneers.

Glazed porcelain is nonporous, resists abrasion, possesses esthetic stability, and is well-tolerated by gingiva.[47,48] In the early 1980s a method of bonding porcelain to acid-etched enamel was developed. Etching the porcelain, usually with hydrofluoric acid or a derivative, is the most important factor in determining bond strength between the composite resin luting agent and the porcelain veneer.[49,50] The mechanical retention obtained by etching the porcelain increases the shear bond strength by a factor of four when compared to unetched porcelain.[51]

The application of a silane coupling agent also improves the bond strength.[52] The silane coupling agent initiates a weak chemical bond[53] between the SiO_2 of the porcelain and the bis-GMA polymer of the composite resin.[40] Scanning electron microscope examination of the porcelain-resin interface exhibits a smaller gap when the etched porcelain is treated with a silane coupling agent.[51] Thermocycling does not significantly reduce the strength of etched enamel/composite/etched porcelain bonding when a silane coupling agent is first applied to the porcelain.[54]

The improved shear bond strength of etched porcelain/silane/resin/etched enamel permits an expanded use of veneers, but sufficient enamel must remain to achieve an adequate bond. Indications for porcelain laminate veneers include enamel hypoplasia, tooth discoloration, intrinsic staining (such as tetracycline staining), fractured teeth, closure of diastemas, and correction of anatomically malformed anterior teeth.[43] Porcelain laminate veneers can be considered a conservative approach to restoring anterior guidance, especially on worn mandibular incisors. An increase in incisal length up to 2.0 mm does not significantly change the fracture resistance of either the restoration or the tooth.[55] The

popularity of this restoration has increased significantly over the last several years.

Tooth Preparation

Porcelain laminate veneers require preparation of the tooth. Although this preparation is minimal and limited to the enamel of the tooth, sufficient enamel thickness must be removed to provide adequate space for a correctly contoured restoration.[56] The preparation should provide a reduction of approximately 0.5 mm.[53,56,57] Ideally, the finish line should be a slight chamfer placed within enamel at the level of the gingival crest or slightly subgingival.

Enamel provides a better seal and more effectively diminishes marginal leakage than a finish line in either cementum or glass ionomer.[58] Due to the relatively thin enamel in the gingival half of the labial surface of most anterior teeth,[59] the desired reduction in that area is 0.3 mm. The minimal thickness for a porcelain laminate veneer is 0.3 to 0.5 mm. The required uniform reduction can be achieved by following an orderly progression of steps.

Facial Reduction. Since the amount of enamel decreases at the cementoenamel junction,[59] some teeth (eg, mandibular incisors) permit less reduction at the gingival finish line. The standard reduction is 0.3 mm. The optimal reduction for the incisal half of the labial surface and incisal edge is 0.5 mm. Tooth preparation is facilitated by using instruments designed specifically for the task. A diamond depth cutter with three 1.6-mm-diameter wheels mounted on a 1.0-mm-diameter noncutting shaft (Model 834-016, Brasseler USA, Savannah, GA) creates the correct depth-orientation grooves in the gingival half of the labial surface. The radius of the wheel extending from the noncutting shaft is 0.3 mm. If the wheels are made to penetrate the enamel until the shaft is flush with the tooth surface, a depth-orientation groove of 0.3 mm is produced (Fig 24-22).

A second three-wheeled diamond depth cutter (Model 834-021, Brasseler USA) produces the correct reduction in the incisal half of the facial surface (Fig 24-23). The wheels extend from the noncutting shaft to a diameter of 2.0 mm, with a 0.5-mm radius from the shaft to the perimeters of the wheels. Once again, the wheels cut through the enamel until the shaft is flush with the surface, and 0.5-mm-deep grooves are created.

Remove tooth structure remaining between the depth-orientation grooves with a round-end tapered diamond (Model 856-016, Brasseler USA). This completes the gingival portion of the facial reduction while the tip of the diamond establishes a slight chamfer finish line at the level of the gingiva (Fig 24-24).

Proximal Reduction. Proximal reduction is simply an extension of facial reduction. Using the round-end tapered diamond, continue the reduction into the proxi-

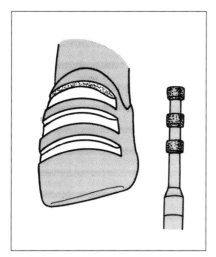

Fig 24-22 Depth-orientation grooves (gingival half): three-wheel diamond depth cutter (0.3 mm).

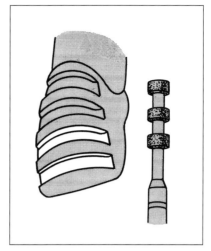

Fig 24-23 Depth-orientation grooves (incisal half): three-wheel diamond depth cutter (0.5 mm).

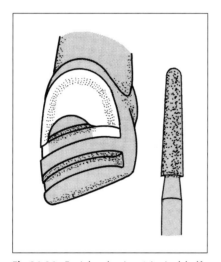

Fig 24-24 Facial reduction (gingival half): round-end tapered diamond.

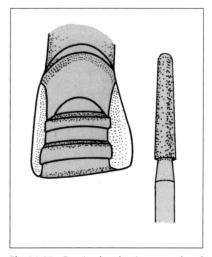

Fig 24-25 Proximal reduction: round-end tapered diamond.

mal area, being sure to maintain adequate reduction, especially at the line angle (Fig 24-25). As the diamond is carried into the interproximal embrasure, it is easy to lift the instrument slightly toward the incisal, creating a "step" at the gingival. This "step" should be eliminated, since that tooth structure, although small, could create an unsightly dark shadow when the veneer is placed.

To correct an uneven finish line, make sure the diamond is parallel with the long axis of the tooth. This will guarantee that the gingival extension in the interproximal area is equal to the reduction of the proximal surface at the incisal. The proximal reduction should extend into the contact area, but it should stop just short of breaking the contact. When multiple adjacent teeth are prepared for veneers, the contacts should be opened to facilitate separation of the dies without damaging the interproximal finish line.

Incisal Reduction. There are two techniques for placement of the incisal finish line. In the first, the prepared facial surface is terminated at the incisal edge. There is no incisal reduction or preparation of the lingual surface. In the second technique, the incisal edge is slightly reduced and the porcelain overlaps the incisal edge, terminating on the lingual surface. In a retrospective clinical evaluation of 119 veneers, the two techniques were used equally and provided clinically acceptable results for an average period of 18 months.[60] Faciolingual thickness of the tooth, the need for esthetic lengthening, and occlusal considerations will help to determine the design of the incisal edge.

Porcelain is stronger in compression than in tension. Wrapping the porcelain over the incisal edge and terminating it on the lingual surface places the veneer in compression during function. A slight incisal overlap provides

443

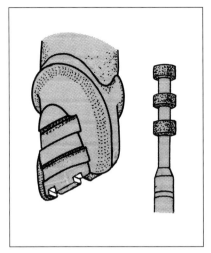

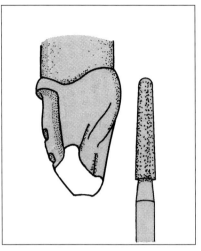

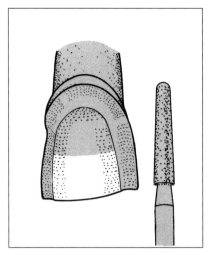

Fig 24-26 Depth-orientation grooves (incisal): three-wheel diamond depth cutter (0.5 mm).

Fig 24-27 Incisal reduction: round-end tapered diamond.

Fig 24-28 Facial reduction (incisal half): round-end tapered diamond.

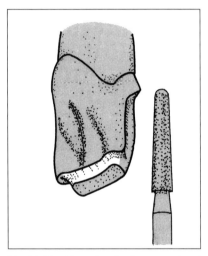

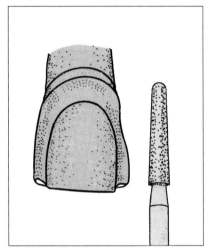

Fig 24-29 Lingual reduction: round-end tapered diamond.

Fig 24-30 Incisal notches: round-end tapered diamond.

a vertical stop that aids in the proper seating of the veneer.[48] Photoelastic studies indicate that the stress concentration within the laminate veneer is diminished by covering the incisal edge, providing a wide vertical stop to resist vertical loads.[61] For most patients, coverage of the incisal edge will be the preferred design.

The multiple-wheel diamond bur (Model 834-021, Brasseler USA) is used to make 0.5-mm-deep orientation grooves in the incisal edge (Fig 24-26). The wheels will penetrate the enamel until the shaft touches the incisal edge. Remove tooth structure between the grooves with a round-end tapered diamond (Fig 24-27). The diamond parallels the incisal edge of the tooth, maintaining that configuration. With the same diamond, complete the facial reduction (Figs 24-28).

Lingual Reduction. Create the lingual finish line with the round-end tapered diamond. Hold the instrument parallel to the lingual surface, with its end forming a slight chamfer 0.5 mm deep. The finish line should be approximately one-fourth the way down the lingual surface, preferably 1.0 mm from centric contacts, and connecting the two proximal finish lines (Fig 24-29). The creation of the lingual finish line often produces a notch at the mesial and distal incisal corners (Fig 24-30). Besides placing the porcelain in compression, extension onto the lingual surface will enhance mechanical retention and increase the surface area for bonding.

Placement of the lingual finish line for a laminate veneer will depend on the thickness of the tooth and the patient's occlusion. Whenever possible, the finish line

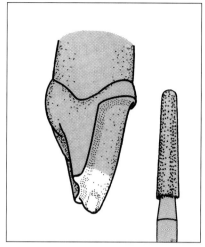

Fig 24-31 Incisal finishing: round-end tapered diamond.

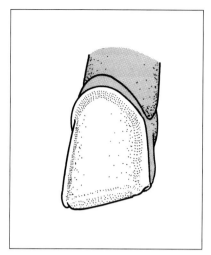

Fig 24-32 Completed laminate veneer preparation.

should be placed on the lingual surface. An extremely thin tooth may require that the finish line be on the incisal edge. Placing it on the lingual surface may expose dentin and overshorten the tooth preparation.

Finishing the Preparation. Be sure to remove any sharp angles that might serve as a focal point for stress concentration, particularly at the junction of the incisal angle and the lingual surface (Fig 24-31). At the completion of the lingual reduction, use the round-end tapered diamond to remove the sharp features that may have formed where the facial, proximal, and lingual planes of reduction meet. The completed preparation has no sharp angles (Figs 24-32).

Impression

Gingival retraction is usually necessary for making an impression of laminate veneer preparations because the cervical finish line is terminated at or slightly below the gingival margin. Some patients may require anesthesia for cord placement, while others will tolerate the procedure without it. This is an individual judgment. Small-diameter retraction cord will reduce or eliminate discomfort.

Any impression material suitable for fixed prosthodontics can be employed. If the impression will be sent to the laboratory for pouring, a stable material such as polyvinyl siloxane or polyether should be used. In most cases, porcelain laminate veneers will play a role in some aspect of the patient's occlusal scheme by providing protrusive or lateral guidance. For this reason, the casts should be made from full-arch impressions and they should be articulated.

Provisional Restorations

Since the preparation remains in enamel, most patients will not require a provisional restoration.[42] For patients who insist upon a "temporary" veneer, light-activated microfilled composite resins may be utilized.[56] Place one or two dots of etchant on the facial surface, then build up the lost tooth structure with composite resin with or without the use of a clear stint. Be very careful to avoid the finish line when removing excess composite resin. Provisional restorations for veneer preparations are time-consuming, and the results can be disappointing. Avoiding provisional restorations in this situation will decrease frustrations.

Fabrication of Working Casts and Dies

Many laboratories use a removable die system that is a modification of a plastic tray with internal orientation grooves and notches (eg, Accutrak, JF Jelenko, Armonk, NY). Pour the impression in die stone, with a minimum base of 20 mm. After the stone has set, remove the cast from the impression and trim it to a height of 15 mm and a faciolingual width of 10 mm on a model trimmer and arbor band. The trimmed cast should fit loosely in the tray. Score the base of the die stone. Mix stone and vibrate it into the assembled tray. Seat the trimmed cast with a jiggling motion until the cervical areas of the teeth are approximately 5.0 mm above the edge of the tray. Remove excess stone and allow the stone to set until it is hard and dry.

Next the tray is disassembled to allow separation of the die(s). Use a saw to separate the die from the base of the cast to avoid damage to the interproximal finish lines (Fig 24-33). The saw cut should extend through the interden-

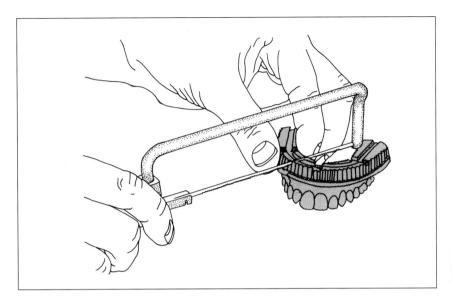

Fig 24-33 The base of the cast is sawed through on both sides of the prepared tooth.

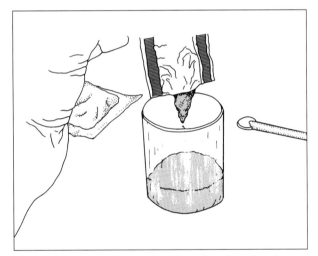

Fig 24-34 Packets of duplicating paste, liquid, and catalyst are emptied into the plastic cup.

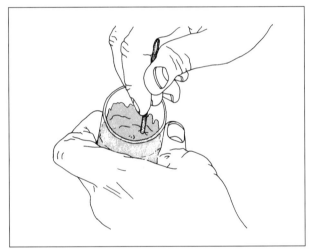

Fig 24-35 Duplicating paste is mixed in the cup.

tal papillae and stop 1.0 mm short of the interproximal finish line. Use finger pressure to break the die and attached teeth from the cast by squeezing the two pieces together. Repeat the process to separate the die from the teeth attached to it. Trim the die and mark the finish line with a red pencil. Apply a minimum of two coats of cement spacer to the die, staying 1.0 mm away from the finish line. Then reassemble the die and working cast in the tray.

Fabrication of the Refractory Die

Use low-viscosity polyvinyl siloxane duplicating material (Vita Hi-Ceram Duplicating Material, Vident) to reproduce the die(s); the low viscosity allows registration of minute details. It is supplied in packets of paste, liquid, and catalyst (Figs 24-34) that are mixed in a clear plastic cup (Fig 24-35). Adapt putty to the working cast and die(s) to limit the flow of the mold material. It should extend several teeth beyond the die(s) and beyond the edge of the tray on both the facial and lingual sides (Fig 24-36). To avoid air entrapment, fill the putty reservoir by pouring the mixture (Fig 24-37). The duplicating material should be at least 3.0 mm thick, and it should extend 3.0 mm beyond the incisal edges of the teeth to provide adequate support for the refractory material.

The setting time may vary due to room temperature and humidity, but the minimum time before separation is 30 minutes (Fig 24-38). When the duplicating medium has set, remove the silicone putty reservoir (Fig 24-39) and disassemble the plastic tray (Fig 24-40). By applying

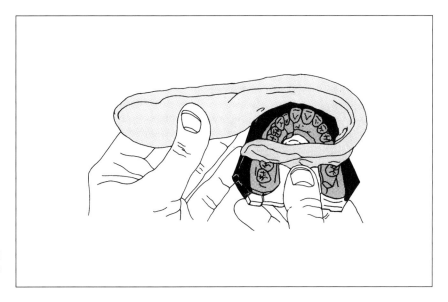

Fig 24-36 A strip of putty is wrapped around the part of the cast that contains the die of the prepared tooth.

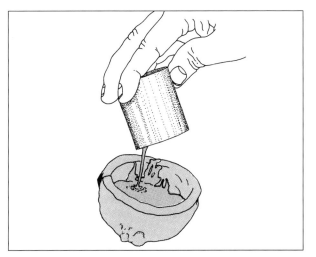

Fig 24-37 Duplicating paste is carefully poured into the area encircled by the strip of putty.

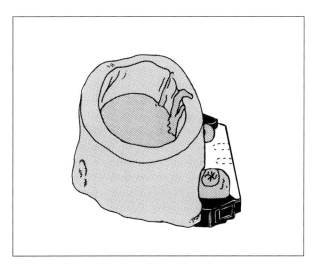

Fig 24-38 The mold is allowed to set for at least 30 minutes.

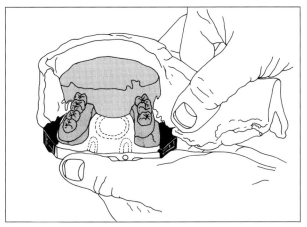

Fig 24-39 The strip of putty is removed from the mold.

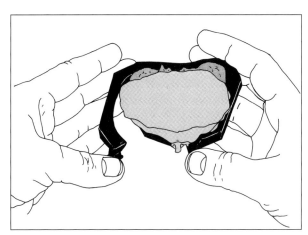

Fig 24-40 The tray is carefully disassembled.

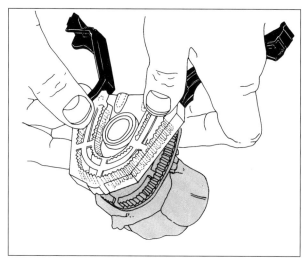

Fig 24-41 The tray is removed from the cast without disturbing the mold.

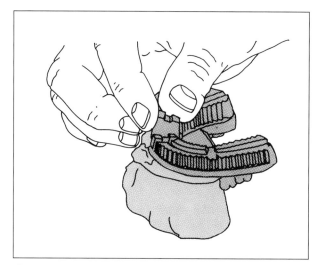

Fig 24-42 The master die is removed from the mold.

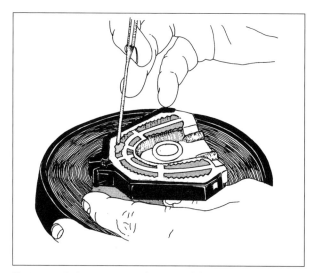

Fig 24-43 Refractory material is poured through openings in the underside of the die tray.

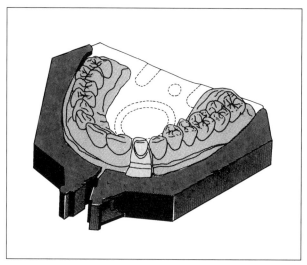

Fig 24-44 The refractory die duplicates the master die in relation to other teeth as well as in configuration.

pressure to the base of the tray, the master cast is loosened with the duplicating material intact (Fig 24-41). The master die of the prepared tooth can then be removed from the cast (Fig 24-42) and then from the duplicating material.

At this point it is easy to see that the larger the area duplicated, the greater the stability of the cast in the duplicating material. The plastic tray is reassembled without the bottom articulating plate. The absence of this plate allows access for pouring the refractory material in the area of the missing die(s), while maintaining the stability and orientation of the cast in the duplicating material.

A number of refractory investments suitable for porcelain laminate veneer fabrication are commercially available. Selection will depend on porcelain compatibility and personal preference. The refractory material should

be mixed according to the manufacturer's directions, and the recommended liquid-powder ratio must be followed. Deviation from this precise ratio may cause uncontrolled expansion or shrinkage during setting and possibly a weakened die.

Mix and carefully vibrate the refractory die material through the opening in the base of the tray to fill the space vacated by the die (Fig 24-43). Since the orientation and stability of the die depend on the grooves and notches of the tray, the entire opening must be filled with refractory material. Allow the refractory die to set for the manufacturer's recommended time, which is usually 1 to 2 hours. When the duplicating mold is removed, the refractory die(s) should occupy the exact location and orientation of the master die(s) (Fig 24-44).

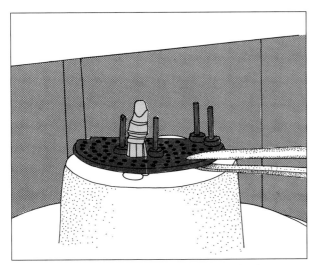

Fig 24-45 After preheating in a burnout furnace, the die is transferred to a porcelain furnace.

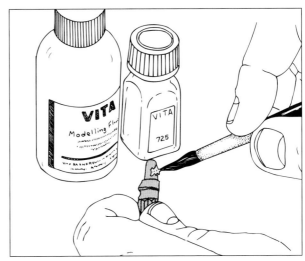

Fig 24-46 The die is sealed by applying dentin porcelain and glaze to it.

Preparation of the Refractory Die

Prior to porcelain application, degas the refractory die to eliminate ammonia and sulfur gases that would contaminate the porcelain. These noxious gases also can contaminate the muffle of a porcelain furnace. Therefore, the initial stage of the degassing process is completed in a casting burnout oven. Place the die in a room-temperature oven, and heat and hold it to a specified temperature. Then transfer the die to a preheated porcelain furnace and continue the heating cycle without vacuum (Fig 24-45). Allow the refractory die to cool to room temperature.

Following burnout, the refractory die should appear uniform in color with no dark-gray streaks. Mark the finish line with an underglaze clay pencil. Soak the die in water until no more bubbles are emitted. To seal the die, apply a thin wash of half glaze, half dentin porcelain to it and fire (Fig 24-46). Two applications of this mixture may be necessary to completely seal the die. Without a sealant, the porous refractory material will absorb water from the porcelain, making it difficult to apply and shape the porcelain.

Porcelain Application

To produce a natural-looking porcelain laminate veneer, the technician must have information regarding the shade of the unprepared tooth, the desired shade, and the location of discolored areas. Discoloration associated with intrinsic staining often appears more intense following tooth preparation. The technician should receive diagrams and photographs of the teeth prepreparation and postpreparation to facilitate the fabrication of customized porcelain veneers.[62]

Perhaps one of the greatest challenges of porcelain veneers is maintaining a natural appearance while masking discolorations. Opaque porcelains or luting agents can be used to mask the colors but produce a dull, whitish result. There are two methods of adding color to porcelain veneers: *(1)* by adding color and characterization to the porcelain itself, or *(2)* by adding tints to the luting agent.[62]

The addition of tints to the luting agents requires knowledge of the subtractive color system and the use of complements to "neutralize" the discolored areas.[62,63] The tinted resin is applied directly to the tooth in thin layers, followed by enhancers to raise the value. A cement spacer must be applied to the master die to allow for this additional luting agent.

The use of complementary colors to mask discolorations also has been applied to porcelain addition. Special complementary-color porcelain (a mixture of dentin and modifier porcelain) neutralizes the existing prepared tooth color. This produces a grayish tone that requires a white modifier to increase the value.[64]

Another technique utilizes a masking dentin porcelain to block the color of the underlying tooth structure before dentin, enamel, and translucent porcelains are added. The masking dentin is effective in a very thin layer (0.1 mm) and acts as internal shading and light diffuser.[65] The other porcelains continue to develop the color and translucency of the restoration. The dentist and technician must communicate to select the technique of color modification. With a cooperative effort, the desired esthetic result can be achieved.

The application of the porcelain is similar to a layered buildup of a conventional ceramic restoration. First apply the dentin porcelain (Fig 24-47) and then build it up to the full contour. Use a sable brush or spatula to apply and shape the porcelain to the desired contour (Fig 24-48).

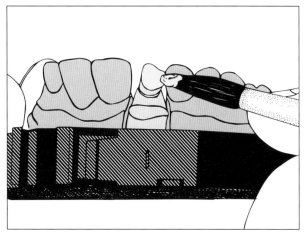

Fig 24-47 Dentin porcelain is applied first.

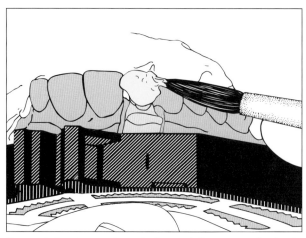

Fig 24-48 Dentin porcelain is built up to full contour with a brush.

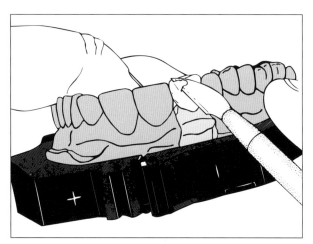

Fig 24-49 Mesioincisal area is cut back with a sharp knife.

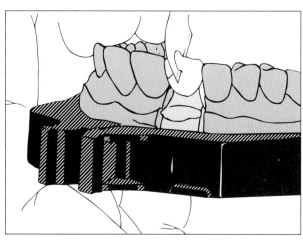

Fig 24-50 The same is done to the distoincisal area.

Using a tissue and a slight amount of condensation, remove the excess moisture. The porcelain should remain slightly damp, but it should carve easily.

Finalize gingival contours and use a sharp blade to cut back the incisal one-third to one-half to allow for the enamel porcelain (Figs 24-49 and 24-50). The desired amount of translucency determines the depth and extent of the cutback. The enamel porcelain should be supported by the dentin porcelain. If the cutback is straight across the incisal edge without any supporting dentin, the fired porcelain will be too translucent and it will lack color and vitality as well.

Like dentin porcelain, enamel porcelain is applied with either a damp sable brush or a spatula (Fig 24-51). It should be blended with the dentin porcelain on the facial, and the incisal edge should be slightly overbuilt to compensate for shrinkage. Use a tissue and a small amount

of condensation to remove any excess moisture. Finalize and smooth the axial contours of the porcelain (Fig 24-52). Remove the die from the working cast and add porcelain to the proximal contours. Carefully examine the margins and remove even the slightest amount of excess porcelain.

Place the refractory die with the porcelain buildup on a sagger tray in front of the muffle to dry. Then fire the porcelain according to manufacturer's recommendations. Allow the die to cool completely to room temperature. Then reseat it in the working cast. After evaluating the contours and occlusion of the fired porcelain, corrections may be made by grinding with a fine-grit diamond or green stone or by adding an appropriate porcelain and refiring at a slightly lower temperature.

When the desired contours, margins, and occlusion have been produced, glaze the porcelain veneer on the

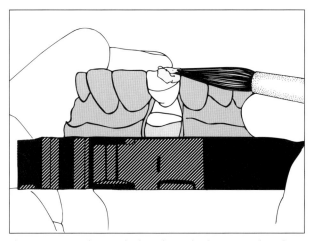

Fig 24-51 Enamel is applied to the cutback areas with a damp sable brush.

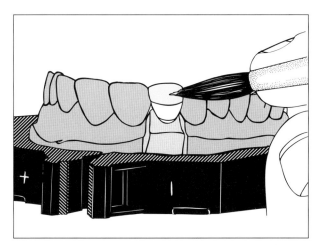

Fig 24-52 Contours of the porcelain are smoothed with a brush.

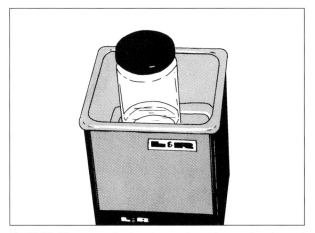

Fig 24-53 The veneer is placed on a piece of gauze in a jar, and the jar is placed into an ultrasonic cleaner.

refractory die. After cooling, carefully remove the die from the veneer by glass-bead air abrasion on the die. Confirm marginal integrity of the veneer on the original stone die. Place the veneer in a jar in the ultrasonic cleaner (Fig 24-53). The veneer should rest on a piece of gauze to prevent its fracture against the hard glass bottom of the jar.

To bond the porcelain laminate veneer to the composite resin luting agent, it is necessary to acid-etch the internal aspect of the glazed veneer. Apply 5% hydrofluoric acid solution and let it remain in contact with the porcelain for 30 seconds. A gel etchant is easily confined to the internal aspect of the veneer. If a liquid etchant is used, the glazed porcelain should be protected. When applied to porcelain, the acid produces microstructural pits that enhance the mechanical interlocking with the composite resin.

Cementation and Finishing of All-Ceramic Restorations

The techniques for adjusting, cementing, and finishing all-ceramic crowns, labial veneers, and inlays vary significantly from those used for metal restorations.

A tight proximal contact will not produce a visible burnished area on porcelain. A thin coating of a pressure indicator such as Occlude (Pascal Co, Bellevue, WA) can be applied to these materials before seating to reveal the exact location of the contact. To avoid fracture, only gentle forces should be used for inserting and testing ceramic restorations. Internal support for a ceramic crown or onlay can be provided during occlusal adjustment by temporarily "cementing" the restoration to the tooth with a low-viscosity elastomeric impression material.

Broad, relatively flat surfaces are best reduced extraorally with a large, smooth-cutting Busch Silent stone (Pfingst & Co, South Plainfield, NJ), while grooves and ridges are reshaped with smaller pointed diamond stones and green stones. Instruments that have been used on metals should not be used on porcelain. Metal particles become embedded in pores in the porcelain and cause discoloration. When working near an acute edge of porcelain, apply the stone so that it is moving from the edge toward the greater bulk to prevent chipping the fragile edge. This is opposite of the technique used in finishing metal margins. It is best to postpone minor grinding adjustments on thin veneers and inlays until after they are permanently bonded to the tooth.

Roughened ceramic surfaces are smoothed with clean white stones and polished with rubber wheels of progressively finer grit such as those found in the Ceramiste Porcelain Adjustment Kit (Shofu Dental Corp, Menlo Park, CA), or diamond-impregnated wheels and points (Dialite, Brasseler USA). Grit in the Ceramiste kit is indicated by stripes around the shank of the instrument: no stripe is coarse, one yellow stripe is medium, and either two yellow stripes or one white stripe is fine. Pastes containing diamond dust are available for use on cups and brushes. Porcelain also may be reglazed after it is polished.

At try-in, have the patient moisten the ceramic and adjacent teeth with saliva. Evaluate the shade under incandescent, fluorescent, and natural light. To minimize the effects of metamerism, it is better to accept a shade that matches reasonably well under all lighting conditions than one that matches perfectly under natural light but appears discolored under artificial light. Allow the patient to look at the completed restoration in a wall mirror and approve it before cementation.

Crown Cementation

Ceramic crowns may be cemented with zinc phosphate, glass ionomer, or a dual-polymerizing resin cement such as Enforce with Fluoride (LD Caulk Div, Dentsply International, Milford, DE). The cement comes in four shades (A2, C2, B1, and B3), permitting some influence on the final shade of transluscent crowns. Ceramic crowns that have been etched internally and bonded with a composite resin cement are 50% stronger than similar crowns cemented with zinc phosphate cement.[66]

The crown should be clean, etched, and silaned. Remove any organic debris with ethanol or acetone, followed by placing the restoration in an ultrasonic cleaner. Further cleaning can be accomplished by applying liquid phosphoric acid etchant. If the crown was not silaned at the laboratory, it can be done at this time with Silane Coupling Agent (LD Caulk). Dispense one drop of Silane Primer and one drop of Silane Activator into a dappen dish. Stir the liquid in the dish for 10 to 15 seconds with a brush. Set the mixture aside for no less than 5 minutes, nor more than 10 minutes before application. Apply it to the internal surface of the crown, and gently air dry. Repeat once. Avoid application of the activated silane to the external surface of the crown by covering the outside of the crown with wax. Remove the cement and mixing dish from the refrigerator and allow it to warm to room temperature.

Rinse the crown and dry it with compressed air. Clean the tooth preparation with a rubber cup and flour of pumice. Then wash and dry it. Etch enamel on the preparation for 30 seconds with 37% phosphoric acid on a foam pellet. Dab, do not rub. Rinse for 20 seconds and air dry the tooth.

Apply ProBOND Primer to dentin and keep moist for 30 seconds. Air dry. Apply a thin layer of ProBOND adhesive over the entire preparation with a brush. Thin the bonding agent with compressed air for 15 seconds. Use a second clean brush to remove excess adhesive. Polymerize the adhesive for 20 seconds with a light. Do not apply any primer or adhesive to the crown.

Dispense equal amounts of Enforce base from the syringe and catalyst from the tub. Mix for 10 to 20 seconds with a flat-ended plastic mixing stick. Apply a thin

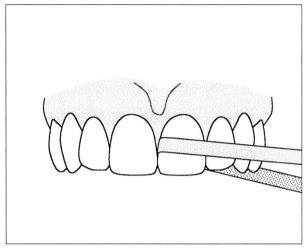

Fig 24-54 Proximal margins are polished with a finishing strip.

layer of cement to the internal surfaces of the crown. Seat the crown and remove excess cement from the marginal areas with an explorer and a clean brush. Leave a slight excess to avoid ditching the cement at the margin. Aim the light cure at marginal areas from facial, lingual, and occlusal directions for 40 seconds. When light activation is not utilized, allow 6 minutes for autopolymerization. Adjust bulky margins or premature occlusal contacts with a fine diamond stone. Polish occlusal surfaces with wheels from a porcelain adjustment kit.

Veneer Cementation

Ceramic veneers and inlays should be etched, silaned, and bonded to the underlying enamel with a selected shade of dual-polymerizing hybrid composite resin cement such as Vita Luminbond (Vident). This type of composite resin has a superior coefficient of thermal expansion, low water absorption, and a surface smoothness similar to microfilled composite resins. The luting agent comes in several shades coordinated with the shade of porcelain selected. Other kits that include colored modifiers and opaque modifiers may be used for special needs. This not only provides better retention and color control, but it makes the ceramic material less fragile than if it were cemented with nonresin cement.[68]

Clean the prepared tooth with nonfluoride pumice and try in the porcelain veneers. Verify the marginal fit. A drop of water or glycerine will help the veneer stay in place on the tooth during the try-in. If there is an overhang, trim it with a fine-grit diamond. After verifying the marginal fit, evaluate the proximal contacts.

The final appearance of a veneer is affected by the shade of cement used. Isolate the teeth with Mylar strips. Determine the correct shade or blend of shades by seating the veneer or inlay on the unetched tooth with resin cement. Avoid exposure to high-intensity light to prevent bonding at this time.

After try-in and shade determination, clean the veneer with a solvent such as acetone. Pumice the teeth to remove any traces of polymerized composite resin. Apply a 30% phosphoric acid etchant gel to the prepared tooth and allow it to remain 1 minute. Thoroughly rinse the tooth with a steady stream of water for 30 seconds and dry with air. Check that the tooth surface has the dull, frosted-white appearance of properly etched enamel.

Apply the silane coupling agent or primer to the internal surface of the veneer and allow it to remain in contact with the etched porcelain for 1 minute. At the end of that time, dry the veneer with an air syringe by blowing the air parallel to and slightly above the veneer.

Apply a small amount of the previously selected composite resin luting agent to the internal surface of the veneer and use a brush to evenly distribute it over the surface. Carefully seat it on the dry, etched tooth. In the case of an inlay, place the cement into the cavity. The plastic interproximal strips may be left in place if they do not interfere with seating of the restoration. Using finger pressure, gently seat the veneer from the labial surface. Excessive pressure at this time could fracture the veneer.

When the veneer is positioned correctly, hold it gently against the tooth with a finger and apply a visible-light curing unit for 10 seconds. Verify that the veneer is placed correctly on the tooth. After the initial set, the flash may be carefully removed before the resin is completely polymerized. Continue polymerizing for an additional 45 to 60 seconds, directing the light from the lingual (through the tooth) so that shrinkage will occur toward the tooth. Then direct the light from the labial (through the veneer) for an additional 60 seconds.

Once the luting agent is polymerized, fine-grit flame diamonds may be used to trim excess composite resin. The occlusion should be checked and adjusted only after the veneer is bonded to the tooth. Final finishing procedures can be accomplished with porcelain polishing agents, including rubberized abrasives and diamond polishing paste. The proximal areas can be finished with finishing strips (Fig 24-54).

References

1. McLean JW: *The Science and Art of Dental Ceramics,* vol I: *The Nature of Dental Ceramics and Their Clinical Use.* Chicago, Quintessence Publ Co, 1979, p 30–37.

2. Phillips RW: *Skinner's Science of Dental Materials,* ed 9. Philadelphia, WB Saunders Co, 1991, p 505–527.

3. Land CH: A new system of restoring badly decayed teeth by means of an enamelled coating. *Independent Pract* 1886; 7:407.

4. McLean JW, Hughes TH: The reinforcement of dental porcelain with ceramic oxides. *Br Dent J* 1965; 119:251–267.

5. McLean JW, Sced IR: The bonded alumina crown. Part I. Bonding of platinum to aluminous porcelain using tin oxide coating. *Aust Dent J* 1976; 21:119–127.

6. Sced IR, McLean JW, Hotz P: The strengthening of aluminous porcelain with bonded platinum foils. *J Dent Res* 1977; 56:1067–1069.

7. Munoz CA, Goodacre CJ, Moore BK, Dykema RW: A comparative study of the strength of aluminous porcelain jacket crowns constructed with the conventional and twin foil techniques. *J Prosthet Dent* 1982; 48:271–281.

8. Green DJ: Microcracking mechanisms in ceramics. In: Bradt RC, Evans AG, Lange FF, Hasselman DP (eds): *Fracture Mechanics of Ceramics,* vol 5. New York: Plenum Press, 1983, pp 457–478.

9. Green DJ, Hannink RHJ, Swain MV: *Transformation Toughening of Ceramics.* Boca Raton, Fl: CRC Press, 1989, pp 57–91.

10. Seghi RR, Sorensen JA: Relative flexural strength of six new ceramic materials. *Int J Prosthodont* 1995; 8:239–246.

11. Adair PJ, Grossman DG: Esthetic properties of lost tooth structure compared with ceramic restorations [abstract 1025]. *J Dent Res* 1982; 61:292.

12. Hobo S, Iwata T: Castable apatite ceramics as a new biocompatible restorative material. I. Theoretical considerations. *Quintessence Int* 1985; 16:135–141.

13. Sozio RB, Riley EJ: The shrink-free ceramic crown. *J Prosthet Dent* 1983; 49:182–187.

14. Riley EJ, Sozio RB, Shklar G, Krech K: Shrink-free ceramic crown versus ceramometal: A comparative study in dogs. *J Prosthet Dent* 1983; 49:766–771.

15. Wain D: Porcelain casting. *Br Dent J* 1923; 44:1364.

16. MacCulloch WT: Advances in dental ceramics. *Br Dent J* 1968; 89:361–365.

17. Adair PJ, Grossman DG: The castable ceramic crown. *Int J Periodont Rest Dent* 1984; 4(2):32–45.

18. Malament KA, Grossman DG: The cast glass-ceramic restoration. *J Prosthet Dent* 1987; 57:674–683.

19. Grossman DG. Cast glass ceramics. *Dent Clin North Am* 1985; 29:725–739.

20. Hobo S, Iwata T: Castable apatite ceramics as a new biocompatible restorative material. II. Fabrication of the restoration. *Quintessence Int* 1985; 16:207–216.

21. Seghi RR, Rosenstiel DF: Relative fracture toughness and hardness of new dental ceramics. *J Prosthet Dent* 1995; 74:145–150.

22. Wohlwend A, Schärer P: The Empress technique: A new technique for the fabrication of full ceramic crowns, inlays and veneers. *Quintessenz Zahntech* 1990; 16:966–978.

23. Nixon RL: IPS Empress: The ceramic system of the future. *Signature* 1994; Fall:10–15.

24. Myers ML, Ergle JW, Fairhurst CW, Ringle RD: Fatigue failure parameters of IPS-Empress porcelain. *Int J Prosthodont* 1994; 7:549–553.

25. Pröbster L: Compressive strength of two modern all-ceramic crowns. *Int J Prosthodont* 1992; 5:409–414.

26. Levy H, Daniel X: Working with the In-Ceram porcelain system. *Prothèse Dentaire* 1990; 44-45:1–11.

27. Pröbster L, Diehl J: Slip-casting alumina ceramics for crown and bridge restorations. *Quintessence Int* 1992; 23:25–31.

28. Giordano RA, Pelletier L, Campbell S, Pober R: Flexural strength of an infused ceramic, glass ceramic, and feldspathic porcelain. *J Prosthet Dent* 1995; 73:411–418.

29. Castellani D, Baccetti T, Giovannoni A, Bernaedini UD: Resistance to fracture of metal ceramic and all-ceramic crowns. *Int J Prosthodont* 1994; 7:149–154.

30. Yoshinari M, Dérand T: Fracture strength of all-ceramic crowns. *Int J Prosthodont* 1994; 7:329–338.

31. Kelly JR, Tesk JA, Sorensen JA: Failure of all-ceramic fixed partial dentures in vitro and in vivo: Analysis and modeling. *J Dent Res* 1995; 74:1253–1258.

32. Scotti R, Catapano S, D'Elia A: A clinical evaluation of In-Ceram crowns. *Int J Prosthodont* 1995; 8:320–323.

33. Pröbster L: Survival rate of In-Ceram restorations. *Int J Prosthodont* 1993; 6:259–163.

34. Ironside JG: Light transmission of a ceramic core material used in fixed prosthodontics. *Quintessence Dent Technol* 1993; 103–106.

35. Sieber C: Illumination in anterior teeth. *Quintessence Dent Technol* 1992; 15:81–88.

36. Paul SJ, Pietrobon N, Schärer P: The new In-Ceram Spinell system—A case report. *Int J Periodont Rest Dent* 1995; 15:521–527.

37. Claus H: VITA In-Ceram: A new system for producing aluminum oxide crown and bridge substructures. *Quintessenz Zahntech* 1990; 16:35–46.

38. Pera P, Gilodi S, Bassi F, Carossa S: In vitro marginal adaptation of alumina porcelain ceramic crowns. *J Prosthet Dent* 1994; 72:585–590.

39. Carrier DD, Kelly JR: In-Ceram failure behavior and core-veneer interface quality as influenced by residual infiltration glass. *J Prosthod* 1995; 4:237–242.

40. Horn HR: Porcelain laminate veneers bonded to etched enamel. *Dent Clin North Am* 1983; 27:671–684.

41. McLaughlin G: Porcelain fused to tooth—A new esthetic and reconstructive modality. *Compend Contin Educ Dent* 1984; 5:430–435.

42. Ibsen RL, Strassler HE: An innovative method for fixed anterior tooth replacement utilizing porcelain veneers. *Quintessence Int* 1986; 17:455–459.

43. Goldstein R: Diagnostic dilemma: To bond, laminate or crown? *Int J Periodont Rest Dent* 1987; 5:9–29.

44. Faunce FR, Myers DR: Laminate veneer restoration of permanent incisors. *J Am Dent Assoc* 1976; 93:790–792.

45. Faunce FR: Tooth restoration with preformed laminate veneers. *Dent Survey* 1977; 1:30–32.

46. Boyer DB, Chalkley Y: Bonding between acrylic laminates and composite resin. *J Dent Res* 1982; 61:489–492.

47. Horn H: A new lamination: Porcelain bonded to enamel. *NY State Dent J* 1983; 49:401–403.

48. Calamia JR: Etched porcelain facial veneers: A new treatment modality based on scientific and clinical evidence. *NY J Dent* 1983; 53:255–259.

49. Simonsen RJ, Calamia JR: Tensile bond strength of etched porcelain [abstract 1154]. *J Dent Res* 1983; 62:297.

50. Stangel I, Nathanson D, Hsu CS: Shear strength of the composite bond to etched porcelain. *J Dent Res* 1987; 66:1460–1465.

51. Hsu CS, Stangel I, Nathanson D: Shear bond strength of resin to etched porcelain [abstract 1095]. *J Dent Res* 1985; 64:296.

52. Calamia JR, Simonsen RJ: Effect of coupling agents on bond strength of etched porcelain [abstract 79]. *J Dent Res* 1984; 63:179.

53. Calamia JR: Etched porcelain veneers: The current state of the art. *Quintessence Int* 1985; 16:5–12.

54. Stacey G: A shear stress analysis of the bonding of porcelain veneers to enamel. *J Prosthet Dent* 1993; 70:395–402.

55. Wall JG, Reisbick MH, Johnston WM: Incisal-edge strength of porcelain laminate veneers restoring mandibular incisors. *Int J Prosthodont* 1992; 5:441–446.

56. Jordan RE: *Esthetic Composite Bonding*. Philadelphia, DC Decker Inc, 1987, Ch 3.

57. Quinn F, McConnell RJ, Byrne D. Porcelain laminates: A review. *Br Dent J* 1986; 161:61–65.

58. Lacy AM, Wada C, Du W, Watanabe LP: In vitro microleakage at the gingival margin of porcelain and resin veneers. *J Prosthet Dent* 1992; 67:7–10.

59. Shillingburg HT, Grace CS: Thickness of enamel and dentin. *J South Calif Dent Assoc* 1973; 41:33–36.

60. Karlsson S, Landahl I, Stegersjo G, Milleding P: A clinical evaluation of ceramic laminate veneers. *Int J Prosthodont* 1992; 5:447–451.

61. Highton R, Caputo AA, Mátyás J: A photoelastic study of stresses on porcelain laminate veneers. *J Prosthet Dent* 1987; 58:157–161.

62. Robbins JW: Color characterization of porcelain veneers. *Quintessence Int* 1991; 22:853–856.

63. Reid JS: Tooth color modification and porcelain veneers. *Quintessence Int* 1988; 19:477–481.

64. Yamada K: Porcelain laminate veneers for discolored teeth using complementary colors. *Int J Prosthodont* 1993; 6:242–247.

65. Hobo S: Porcelain laminate veneers with three-dimensional shade reproduction. *Int Dent J* 1992; 42:189–198.

66. Ludwig K, Joseph K: Untersuchungen zur Bruchfestigkeit von IPS-Empress-Kronen in Abhängigkeit von den Zementiermodalitäten. *Quintessenz Zahntech* 1994; 20:247–256.

67. Qvist V, Stolze K, Qvist J: Human pulp reactions to resin restorations performed with different acid-etch restorative procedures. *Acta Odontol Scand* 1989; 47:253–263.

68. Dérand T: Stress analysis of cemented or resin-bonded loaded porcelain inlays. *Dent Mater* 1991; 7:21–24.

Chapter 25

Metal-Ceramic Restorations

Metal-ceramic restorations combine the strength and accuracy of cast metal with the esthetics of porcelain. Their use has grown markedly in the last 30 years as a result of technical improvements. However, restraint should be exercised in the selection of this type of restoration, as there is a tendency to overuse it. Metal-ceramic restorations should not be substituted for less destructive types of restorations when the latter will serve as well. A 1986 survey of 80 dentists revealed that 70% of them placed metal-ceramic crowns on their patients' posterior teeth 70% to 100% of the time, but the same dentists indicated a preference for partial veneer gold crowns in their own mouths.[1]

The metal-ceramic crown has gone by a variety of names since its introduction to dentistry nearly four decades ago. It was called, at different times and in different parts of the US, a "Ceramco crown" (for one of the first brands of porcelain used for fabricating this type of restoration), a "porcelain veneer crown" (PVC), "porcelain fused to gold" (PFG), as well as "porcelain fused to metal" (PFM), a term commonly used in the dental literature during the 1970s and '80s.

Metal-ceramic is a more precise term scientifically, and it is compatible with the terminology used to describe *all-ceramic* crowns, inlays, veneers, etc. Because there seems to be a proclivity in the English language for three-letter abbreviations (rhythm, trinity connection, who knows?), *MCR* appears to be a reasonable abbreviation for metal-ceramic restoration.

The metal-ceramic restoration is composed of a metal casting, or coping, which fits over the tooth preparation and ceramic that is fused to the coping. The coping may be little more than a thin thimble, or it may be clearly recognizable as a cast crown with some portion cut away. The contours in the area that has been cut away will be replaced with porcelain that will mask or hide the metal coping, produce the desired contours, and make the restoration esthetically pleasing.

The metal coping in a metal-ceramic restoration is covered with three layers of porcelain (Fig 25-1):

1. *Opaque porcelain* conceals the metal underneath, initiates the development of the shade, and plays an important role in the development of the bond between the ceramic and the metal.

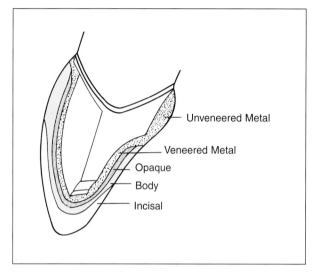

Fig 25-1 Layers of a metal-ceramic restoration.

Labels: Unveneered Metal / Veneered Metal / Opaque / Body / Incisal

2. *Dentin,* or *body, porcelain* makes up the bulk of the restoration, providing most of the color, or shade.
3. *Enamel,* or *incisal, porcelain* imparts translucency to the restoration.

Other porcelains, such as opaque or dentin modifiers, or clear porcelain, are utilized within the three basic layers for special effects and characterization.

There are two principal reasons for the acceptance of metal-ceramic restorations. First, they are more resistant to fracture than the traditional all-ceramic crown, the *porcelain jacket crown* (PJC), because the combination of ceramic and metal bonded together is stronger than the ceramic alone. The strength of metal-ceramic restorations depends on the bond between the ceramic and the metal substructure, the design and rigidity of the metal coping, and the compatibility of the metal and the porcelain. Second, the MCR is the only dependable means of fabricating an esthetic fixed partial denture when full coverage is required on one or both retainers.

Bonding Mechanisms

Four mechanisms have been described to explain the bond between the ceramic veneer and the metal substructure:

1. Mechanical entrapment
2. Compressive forces
3. Van der Waal's forces
4. Chemical bonding

Mechanical entrapment creates attachment by interlocking the ceramic with microabrasions in the surface of the metal coping, which are produced by finishing the metal with noncontaminating stones or discs and air abrasion. When compared with unprepared metal, surface finishing enhances the metal-ceramic bond.[2] Air abrasion appears to enhance wettability, provide mechanical interlocking, and increase the surface area for chemical bonding.[3] The use of a bonding agent, such as platinum spheres, 3 to 6 μm in diameter, also can increase bond strength significantly.[4]

Compressive forces within a metal-ceramic restoration are developed by a properly designed coping and a slightly higher coefficient of thermal expansion for the metal coping than for the porcelain veneered over it. This slight difference in coefficients of thermal expansion will cause the porcelain to "draw" toward the metal coping when the restoration cools after firing.

Van der Waal's forces comprise an affinity based on a mutual attraction of charged molecules. They contribute to bonding, but they are a minor force that is not as significant as was once thought.[5] Although the molecular attraction makes only a minor contribution to overall bond strength, it is significant in the initiation of the most important mechanism, the chemical bond.

Chemical bonding is indicated by the formation of an oxide layer on the metal,[6,7] and by bond strength that is increased by firing in an oxidizing atmosphere.[8,9] When fired in air, trace elements in the gold alloy, such as tin, indium, gallium, or iron, migrate to the surface, form oxides, and subsequently bond to similar oxides in the opaque layer of the porcelain. A gold alloy containing minute amounts of tin and iron creates a significantly stronger bond with porcelain than a pure gold alloy does.[10] The bond strength of true adhesion is such that failure or fracture will occur in the porcelain rather than at the porcelain-metal interface.[11] The clean separation of porcelain from the metal coping is evidence of bond failure from contamination of the coping surface, or an excessive oxide layer. Base metal alloys readily form chromium oxides that bond to the porcelain without the addition of any trace elements.

Alloys Used for Fabricating Metal-Ceramic Restorations

High noble
Gold-platinum-palladium
Gold-palladium-silver
Gold-palladium

Noble
Palladium-silver
High palladium

Predominantly base
Nickel-chromium
Nickel-chromium-beryllium
Cobalt-chromium

Alloys Used

The properties of the porcelain cannot be considered alone. The porcelain and metal used for a restoration must have compatible melting temperatures and coefficients of thermal expansion. Conventional gold alloys have a high coefficient of thermal expansion ($14 \times 10^{-6}°C$) while conventional porcelain possesses a much lower value ($2 \sim 4 \times 10^{-6}°C$). A difference of only $1.7 \times 10^{-6}°C$ can produce sufficient shear stress to produce failure of the bond.[11] The optimum difference between the two would be no greater than $1 \times 10^{-6}°C$. The coefficient of thermal expansion of porcelain can be increased to as much as $7 \sim 8 \times 10^{-6}°C$ by the addition of an alkali such as lithium carbonate. At the same time, the coefficient of the metal can be lowered to $7 \sim 8 \times 10^{-6}°C$ by adding palladium or platinum.

The melting range of the alloy used in the coping must be 170 to 280°C (300 to 500°F) higher than the fusing temperature of the porcelain applied to it. A similar melting range of the two materials would result in the distortion or melting of the coping during the firing and glazing of the porcelain. The greater the difference, the fewer the problems that are encountered during firing. A noble metal coping is subject to flow, or creep, when it is heated to 980°C (1,800°F).[12] The porcelain used must not require that the metal be heated much beyond this point. Porcelains most commonly used for this purpose have a fusing temperature of nearly 980°C (1,800°F), and noble alloys melt at near 1,260°C (2,300°F).

Many alloys have been used for metal-ceramic restorations. A classification system proposed by the American Dental Association is based on noble metal content (see box above).[13] *High noble alloys* have a noble metal (gold, platinum, palladium) content greater than 60%, with at least 40% gold. *Noble alloys* have a noble metal content of at least 25%, and *predominantly base alloys* have less than 25% noble metal content.

Major constituents also are used to further describe an alloy, eg, a *gold-palladium alloy.* The choice of an alloy will depend on a variety of factors, including cost, rigidity, castability, ease of finishing and polishing, corrosion resistance, compatibility with specific porcelains, and personal preference. No alloy system is superior in all aspects.

Alloys that have proven most satisfactory for metal-ceramic crowns and fixed partial dentures are composed of gold (44% to 55%) and palladium (35% to 45%) with small amounts of gallium, indium, and/or tin. Disadvantages most often attributed to gold-palladium alloys are cost and incompatibility with certain types of porcelains. Other systems developed over the past 20 years also have been successful. The choice of an alloy must be made after weighing all factors.

The skyrocketing cost of gold in the late 1970s stimulated the development of alloys containing little or no gold. A logical transition was the application of materials commonly used in the fabrication of removable partial denture frameworks to fixed prosthodontics. These alloys possess desirable properties such as low cost, increased strength and hardness, high fusion temperatures, and greater resistance to distortion during porcelain firing. However, there are inherent problems with these alloys when used as an integral part of a metal-ceramic system. The disadvantages include excessive oxide formation, difficulty in finishing and polishing, and questionable biocompatibility.

Beryllium, which is added to alloys to control oxide formation, is a carcinogen. It can pose a hazard to laboratory personnel who may inhale it as dust in improperly ventilated work areas.[14] Approximately 5% of the general population is sensitive to nickel, and that sensitivity is 10 times as prevalent in women as in men.[15] Contact dermatitis from nickel-containing prostheses appears to be a risk to some patients.[16] Dissolution and occlusal wear affect the amount of nickel and beryllium released in an artificial oral environment.[17] Nickel sensitivity should be considered in the diagnosis of any soft tissue changes that occur after crown placement.[16]

Another cost-cutting alternative to traditional alloys is the modification of existing noble metal alloys by using less-expensive metals, such as copper or cobalt, in the alloy. Unfortunately, the addition of these elements caused dark oxide formation and poor high-temperature strength.[18] Subsequent formulations replaced the copper or cobalt with a small amount of gold and silver. One of the most common disadvantages of the silver-containing alloys is the potential of porcelain discoloration, most commonly described as "greening." No system is without disadvantages, whether they be financial or technical.

Coping Design

The metal coping is an important part of the metal-ceramic restoration, and one that unfortunately is often overlooked. Its design can have an important effect on the success or failure of the restoration. To provide structural integrity in function, the coping must reflect the unique relationship of the two dissimilar materials used to fabricate metal-ceramic restorations. Since the kaolin content must be reduced to allow translucency, dental porcelains may behave more like glass than a true ceramic. Like glass, dental porcelains are significantly stronger in compression than in tension.

The coping must allow the porcelain to remain in compression by supporting the incisal region, the occlusal table, and the marginal ridges. Otherwise, occlusal forces will create a situation similar to applying a load to a pane of glass suspended between two sawhorses. Without any underlying support, the glass would break—and so will unsupported porcelain on a restoration.

There are four features of importance to be considered when designing the metal coping for a metal-ceramic restoration:

1. Thickness of metal underlying and adjoining the porcelain
2. Placement of occlusal and proximal contacts
3. Extensions of the area to be veneered for porcelain
4. Design of the facial margin

Thickness of Metal

Porcelain should be kept at a minimum thickness that is still compatible with good esthetics. Relatively thin porcelain, of uniform thickness and supported by rigid metal, is strongest. The absolute minimum thickness of porcelain is 0.7 mm, and the desirable thickness is 1.0 mm. Deficiencies in the incisal edge, interproximal areas, or occlusal surface of the tooth preparation that have been caused by caries or previous restorations should be blocked out in the preparation or compensated for with extra thickness of the coping in those areas.

An evenly flowing convex contour of the veneering area distributes stress best. Sharp angles and undercuts should be avoided. The outer junction of porcelain to metal should be at a right angle to avoid burnishing of the metal and subsequent fracture of the porcelain. An acute angle of metal at the metal-porcelain interface is more likely to produce porcelain crazing than an angle of 90 or 135 degrees.[19] On the other hand, if the edge of metal at the porcelain-metal junction line is beveled or rounded, the porcelain will end in a feathered edge, through which the oxidized metal or opaque will show.

Maximum restoration strength and longevity is achieved by coping rigidity. The metal must not flex during seating or under occlusal forces, because flexure places the porcelain in tension and leads to its shearing. The metal

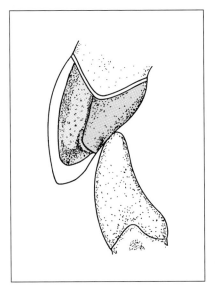

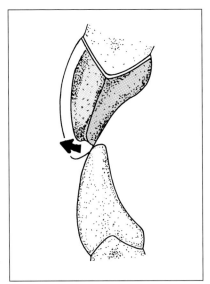

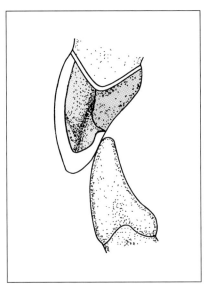

Fig 25-2 Metal occlusal contact on the lingual surface of a maxillary incisor.

Fig 25-3 Porcelain may fracture if the metal extends too far incisally.

Fig 25-4 Porcelain occlusal contact on the lingual surface of a maxillary incisor.

must be as hard as practical, and the coping design must insure an optimum bulk for rigidity.

For adequate strength and rigidity, a noble metal coping should be at least 0.3 to 0.5 mm thick.[20] A base metal alloy with a higher yield strength and elevated melting temperature may be as thin as 0.2 mm.[21] The thickness of the coping may vary, depending on the configuration of the preparation. These values are only minimum thicknesses for different alloy systems. The ultimate goal of achieving a uniform thickness of approximately 1.0 mm of porcelain will dictate the thickness of the metal coping.

Occlusal and Proximal Contacts

If the coping is designed to place occlusal contacts on unveneered metal surfaces, their location and the area covered by ceramic can be more precisely controlled, with less resultant wear on opposing teeth. Studies and clinical experience have documented the highly abrasive nature of dental porcelain and its deleterious effects on enamel or gold.[22–25] Jacobi et al[24] found that glazed porcelain removes 40 times as much opposing tooth structure as gold. Therefore, occlusal contacts should occur on metal whenever possible, well away from the porcelain-metal junction line. Contact near the junction can lead to metal flow and subsequent porcelain fracture. The porcelain-metal junction should be placed 1.0 mm from occlusal contacts at the position of maximum intercuspation (Fig 25-2).

To minimize stress resulting from occlusal contacts on the lingual surface of maxillary anterior restorations, the porcelain-metal junction should not be placed in the vicinity of those contacts with the mandibular teeth.[26] The porcelain-metal junction must not be placed too close to the incisal edge. Incisal translucency will be destroyed and the chances of porcelain fracture will be increased greatly because the porcelain is no longer supported by metal. When occlusal forces are exerted, the porcelain will be placed in tension, a condition that it does not resist well (Fig 25-3).

When there is inadequate vertical overlap to place the contact on metal, the porcelain-metal junction is placed far enough gingivally for the contact to occur on porcelain close to the junction line (Fig 25-4). A constant application of increasing compressive force on the porcelain-metal junction line, irrespective of its angulation, produces failure less readily than a load applied to porcelain 1.0 or 2.0 mm from the junction.[27] Anterior metal-ceramic restorations with guidance in lateral excursions and protrusion on porcelain will abrade opposing natural teeth. The patient should be cautioned that the opposing teeth eventually will require restorations.

The collar of exposed metal on the lingual should be at least 3.0 mm wide incisogingivally. Wherever there will be porcelain on the lingual surface, there must be greater tooth reduction. Proximal contacts for anterior teeth should be on porcelain, which the dentist must facilitate during the tooth preparation by adequate reduction of the interproximal areas. The cosmetic effect is improved by placing the metal lingually, so that proximal porcelain has greater depth and translucency. Interproximal metal tends to darken the unrestored proximal surfaces of adjacent teeth. An optimum stress distribution also occurs when the porcelain-metal junction is lingual to the proximal contact areas.[28]

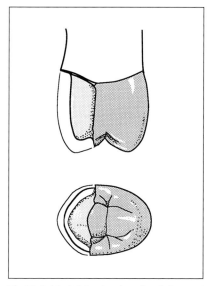

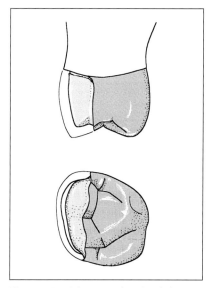

Fig 25-5 Mesial *(top)* and occlusal *(bottom)* views of a standard metal-ceramic coping design for a maxillary premolar.

Fig 25-6 Mesial *(top)* and occlusal *(bottom)* views of a standard metal-ceramic coping design for a maxillary first molar.

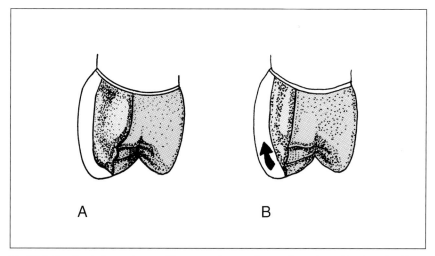

Fig 25-7 Proximal views of a maxillary posterior metal-ceramic coping with (A) and without (B) proper metal support under the facial cusp.

Extent of Veneered Area

To place occlusal contacts in metal, the porcelain on the facial surface extends over the cusp tip and about half of the way down the lingual incline of the facial cusp on maxillary premolars (Fig 25-5) and molars (Fig 25-6).[29] There must be a rounded ledge of metal under the facial cusp to support the porcelain (Fig 25-7, A). Without a supporting ledge, the ceramic will fracture (Fig 25-7, B). This configuration will satisfy the cosmetic requirements of most patients and provide longevity if the porcelain-metal junction is kept away from the occlusal contacts.

This design is more resistant to fracture than those in which the porcelain extends to the central groove or covers the entire occlusal surface.[30] Variants for maxillary teeth include porcelain coverage of the mesial marginal ridge up to the middle of the triangular ridge (Fig 25-8), or for those patients who demand absolute esthetics, complete coverage with porcelain of the occlusal surface of premolars (Fig 25-9) and molars (Fig 25-10).

Mandibular first premolars will require complete porcelain coverage of the occlusal surfaces of metal-ceramic crowns placed on them (Fig 25-11). The degree of porcelain occlusal coverage on metal-ceramic crowns for

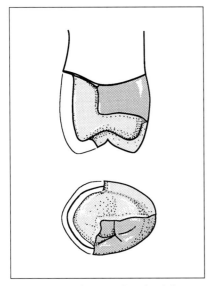

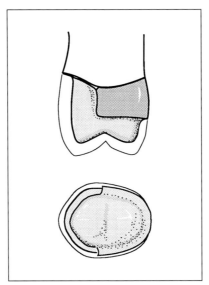

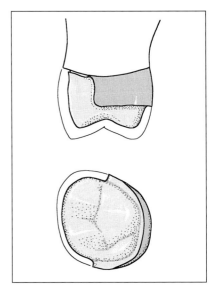

Fig 25-8 Mesial *(top)* and occlusal *(bottom)* views of a modified metal-ceramic coping design for a maxillary premolar.

Fig 25-9 Mesial *(top)* and occlusal *(bottom)* views of a maxillary premolar metal-ceramic coping design with full porcelain occlusal coverage.

Fig 25-10 Mesial *(top)* and occlusal *(bottom)* views of a maxillary first molar metal-ceramic coping design with full porcelain occlusal coverage.

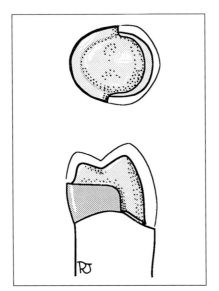

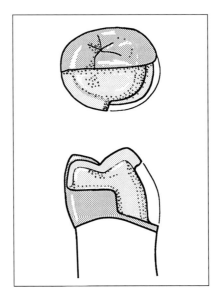

Fig 25-11 Occlusal *(top)* and mesial *(bottom)* views of a mandibular premolar metal-ceramic coping design (standard for first premolar, optional for second premolar).

Fig 25-12 Occlusal *(top)* and mesial *(bottom)* views of a standard mandibular second premolar metal-ceramic coping design.

mandibular molars and second premolars will be dictated by patient wishes, occlusal restoration of the opposing arch, and the presence or absence of bruxism. The distal half of premolars (Fig 25-12) and molars (Fig 25-13) can be unveneered to allow more occlusal contacts to be on metal, if the patient can be satisfied with a tooth-colored veneer on the mesial marginal ridge, proximal contact, fossa, and cusp incline.

If the patient is extremely concerned about esthetics, the occlusal surfaces of mandibular molars can be covered with porcelain (Fig 25-14). A 1.0- to 2.0-mm-wide metal collar can be used on the facial surface to minimize the destruction of tooth structure for a facial shoulder. The patient should be informed of the potential damage to opposing teeth and the necessity for a more destructive crown preparation to provide adequate

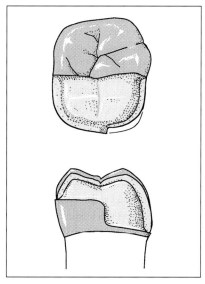 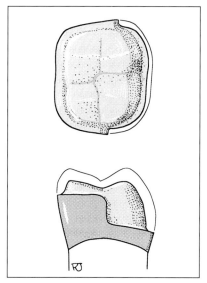

Fig 25-13 Occlusal *(top)* and mesial *(bottom)* views of a standard mandibular first molar metal-ceramic coping design.

Fig 25-14 Occlusal *(top)* and mesial *(bottom)* views of an optional mandibular first molar metal-ceramic coping design.

space for the porcelain. In the final analysis, it is the patient's mouth, and the final decision is the patient's. Be sure that it is an informed one.

A posterior crown with porcelain occlusal coverage should have a 3.0-mm metal collar on the lingual, with metal support under the marginal ridges. Although the greater portion of the crown will be veneered with porcelain, it should still be waxed to a full contour and then cut back to insure a uniform thickness of porcelain and correct contours. A "thimble" coping may result in unsupported, fracture-prone porcelain.

Facial Margins

For many years, the conventional facial margin for a metal-ceramic crown was a narrow metal collar. To avoid an unesthetic display of metal on highly visible teeth, the facial finish line often was placed subgingivally, which may contribute to chronic gingival inflammation or more serious periodontal problems. Gingival recession may occur from the trauma of tooth preparation, impression-making, or an improperly contoured provisional restoration. Following cementation, 60% of subgingival margins become visible within a 2-year period.[31] The association of subgingival crown margins and detrimental effects on the periodontium is well-documented.[32-35]

To avoid showing an unsightly band of metal, porcelain was extended onto the collar itself. This can create an overcontoured gingival margin; thin, fracture-prone porcelain; or an undetected open margin. Frustration with the esthetics of the conventional metal collar led to the use of the all-porcelain facial margin, which can be

even with the gingiva or even slightly supragingival. An improvement in periodontal health was an unexpected bonus.

Improved esthetics and periodontal health made the all-porcelain margin popular, and the demand spawned many ways of fabricating one. The first was a transition from a technique used for porcelain jacket crowns, in which a platinum foil matrix supports the porcelain margin during firing.[36] Another technique employs a refractory die to support the porcelain margin during firing.[37,38]

In an effort to simplify the fabrication of all-porcelain shoulders even more, direct-lift techniques were tried. Correction porcelain was added to the margin, after a full-contour buildup of the crown. The porcelain was condensed by compression and fired to produce the final margin.[39] In 1979 Vyronis[40] described a method which required a tooth preparation with a 90-degree shoulder finish line and a metal coping that terminated at the gingivoaxial line angle. Opaque porcelain was applied to the metal coping and the shoulder on a sealed stone die, forming the margin. After obtaining a satisfactory margin, dentin and enamel porcelains were added to complete the crown.

A blend of dentin and enamel porcelains was substituted to form the margin.[41] However, margins of conventional porcelain tend to round or slump during subsequent firings because the fusion temperatures are identical. To correct this problem, manufacturers created special shoulder porcelains containing aluminous porcelain that fuse at temperatures 30 to 80°C higher than the dentin or enamel porcelains. The higher-fusing porcelain allows repeated firings of the crown buildup with no effect on the completed margin.[42] In addition to stability during the firing cycle, shoulder porcelains are stronger

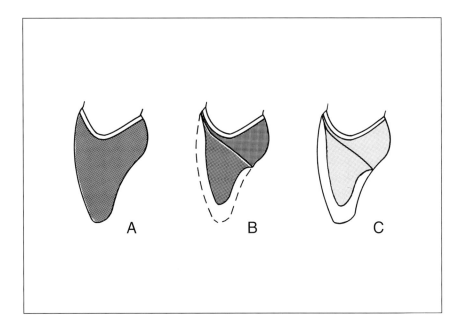

Fig 25-15 The correct steps in the fabrication of a metal-ceramic restoration: A, full-contour wax pattern; B, coping wax pattern cut back; C, porcelain addition to metal coping.

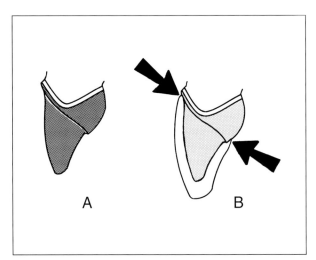

Fig 25-16 If the coping pattern (A) is the first step in fabrication, the porcelain veneer on the final restoration may have contours that are not continuous with those of the unveneered coping (B).

binders indicates that the quality of the margins is directly related to the skill of the ceramist. If a talented and conscientious ceramist is not available, all-porcelain facial margins are definitely contraindicated.

Single Coping Wax Pattern

Before a coping can be fabricated for a metal-ceramic crown, the wax pattern should be made to the complete contour of the finished restoration (Fig 25-15). Then the areas to be veneered with porcelain are cut back. Only by following this procedure can there be a smooth continuation of the lingual and proximal contours between the unveneered metal and the porcelain. If only the portion of the wax pattern that later will be unveneered metal is made, it is difficult to be sure that the contours of the unveneered portion of the coping will match the contours of the porcelain (Fig 25-16).

in flexure than conventional porcelains, making the margin more resistant to fracture.[43]

A number of studies have shown the accuracy of all-porcelain margins to be quite acceptable.[44–48] Early studies utilized conventional porcelains for the margins. Recent studies using shoulder porcelains and the direct-lift technique have produced a consistent level of marginal adaptation with mean marginal openings of 15 to 23 μm[49] and 8 to 11 μm.[50]

The demonstration of acceptable porcelain margins with a wide assortment of techniques, porcelains, and

Waxing Armamentarium

1. PKT (Thomas) waxing instruments (nos. 1, 2, 3, 4, and 5)
2. Beavertail burnisher
3. No. 7 wax spatula
4. Discoid carver
5. Large spoon excavator
6. Sable brush
7. No. 2 pencil

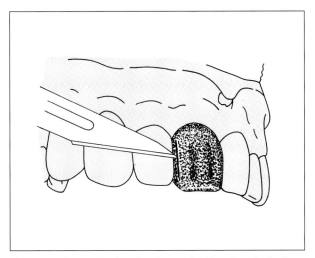

Fig 25-17 The proximal outline is traced with a sharp knife tip.

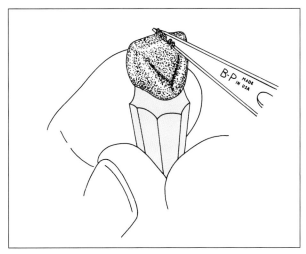

Fig 25-18 From the incisal portion of the pattern, 1.5 mm is cut.

8. Laboratory knife with no. 25 blade
9. Iwanson thickness gauge
10. Cotton pliers
11. Bunsen burner and matches
12. Inlay casting wax
13. Zinc stearate
14. Die lubricant

All-Wax Technique

Wax is first applied to the lubricated die with a hot no. 7 wax spatula. Trim the wax back from the margins and transfer the wax thimble to the articulated working cast. Build up the axial contours, including the proximal contacts, in harmony with the adjacent teeth. Establish the proper occlusal relationships with the opposing teeth. If the wax pattern is for a posterior tooth, use the PKT instruments to build up the occlusal surface with cones and ridges to obtain good occlusion (see Chapter 19).

When the full-contour wax pattern is completed, make an impression of it with a resilient condensation silicone putty impression material. This impression can be poured to produce a stone cast, providing a visual guide to the desired contours, or it can be sectioned horizontally to allow assessment of the amount and contours of the cutback.

The first step in forming the veneering area is sketching of the outline of that area on the wax pattern. Place the no. 25 blade on the proximal surface of the adjacent tooth. Using this guide, scratch a line on the proximal surface of the pattern, placing it as far lingual as possible (Fig 25-17).

After drawing the outline on the pattern, place it on the

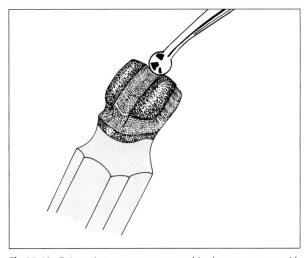

Fig 25-19 Orientation grooves are carved in the wax pattern with a discoid carver.

die. Remove 1.5 mm from the incisal portion of an anterior pattern with the knife (Fig 25-18). Place the proximal porcelain-metal junction 0.5 mm to the lingual of the proximal contacts (which will be nearly 1.0 mm lingual to the proximal line drawn earlier). Use a discoid carver to finish the wax that will form the porcelain-metal junction on the proximal surface. Carve a vertical groove in the center of the labial surface with the discoid carver (Fig 25-19). Cut similar grooves on the mesial and distal. From an incisal view, these grooves should be about 1.0 mm deep. They are used to gauge the depth of wax to be removed from the veneering area.

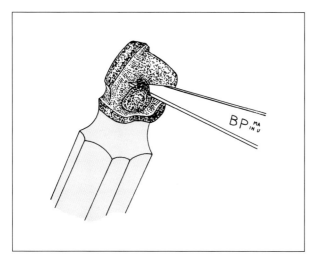

Fig 25-20 Wax is removed with a sharp knife to the desired depth.

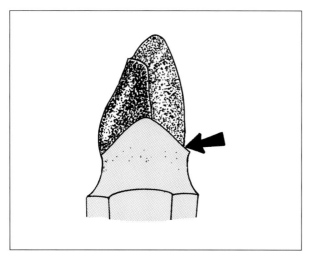

Fig 25-21 The facial axial wall of a wax pattern for a crown with an all-porcelain shoulder ends at the gingivofacial angle *(arrow)*.

The design of the facial margin must be decided before preparing the tooth, because it will be dictated by the facial finish line. For a metal collar, the bulk of the wax is removed with the knife, leaving a collar of wax 1.0 mm wide at the facial margin to reinforce it during investing and to insure an adequate bulk to cast the margin (Fig 25-20). The collar will be narrowed to approximately 0.3 mm in metal. For an all-porcelain facial margin, the wax pattern terminates at the junction of the facial axial wall and the facial shoulder (Fig 25-21). Adapt the margins with a warm beavertail burnisher.

Check the thickness of the wax pattern with a thickness gauge. It should be 0.4 to 0.5 mm thick in the veneering area. It will be thinned to about 0.3 mm after it has been cast. If it is made too thin at this point, it may not cast completely.

Plastic Shell Technique

Thinning the wax in the areas to be veneered with porcelain can create problems. The wax becomes very fragile and breaks easily; forces generated during the cutback may distort the adaptation of the wax, and it is difficult to judge the thickness of the coping wax pattern. The use of a plastic shell coping can overcome the problems encountered in fabricating wax patterns for single units and fixed partial dentures. Techniques utilizing plastic shells to form the underlying structure of coping patterns have been in use for nearly 25 years.

Shells for multiple dies can be made with the use of machines to apply compressed air to the plastic shell[51] or vacuum-forming machines. Shells for single dies can be formed in hand-held frames without the need for machines.[52] Another convenient and reliable method for making a plastic shell coping is to compress a plastic sheet to fit a die (Adapta, BEGO GmbH & Co, Bremen, Germany). This technique is especially useful in small laboratories or in training programs, where the volume of work does not require large numbers of copings to be made at once. The commercially available kit contains sheets of coping material, thinner sheets of material used as a cement spacer, a frame for holding the materials during heating, and a molding apparatus containing silicone putty.

Plastic Shell Armamentarium

In addition to items listed for waxing:

1. 4.0-cm spacer disks
2. 4.0-cm coping disks
3. Wire holding frame
4. Putty-filled jar
5. Iris scissors

The technique[53] is simple and easily mastered. Lay a 4.0-cm-diameter spacer disk, 0.1 mm thick, over a 4.0-cm-diameter disk of coping material, 0.6 mm thick (Fig 25-22). Place the coping material and spacer disks onto a wire holding frame (Fig 25-23). Heat the disks slowly and evenly by holding them, approximately 10 cm (4 inches) above a Bunsen burner flame (Fig 25-24). The plastic sheets are flammable, so heat the material cautiously. The material will first buckle and then slump, becoming transparent.

Place the heated coping disk and spacer over the mouth of the molding apparatus, a plastic jar filled with silicone putty. The spacer should be facing upward (Fig 25-25). Press the trimmed die forcefully against the softened spacer and coping disks until the finish line of the preparation is completely submerged (Fig 25-26). This closely adapts the two disks over the tooth preparation. Continue to exert pressure against the disks with the die until the sheet becomes cloudy, which will take approximately 10 seconds. The heating and adaptation of the coping disk stretches it to the desired thickness of 0.3 mm.

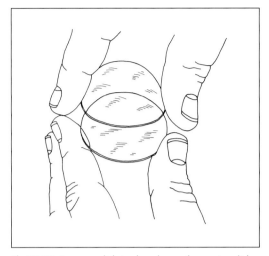

Fig 25-22 A spacer disk is placed over the coping disk.

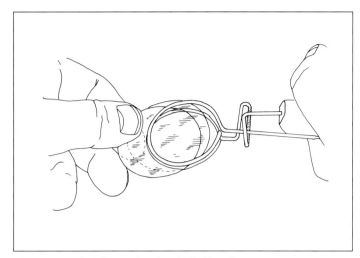

Fig 25-23 Both disks are placed in the holding frame.

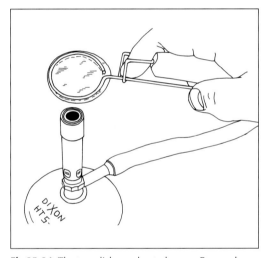

Fig 25-24 The two disks are heated over a Bunsen burner flame.

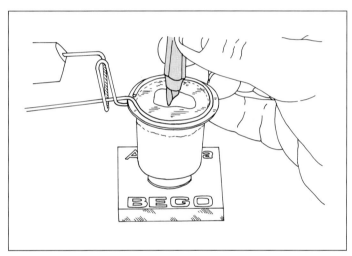

Fig 25-25 The disks are held over the mouth of the jar filled with silicone.

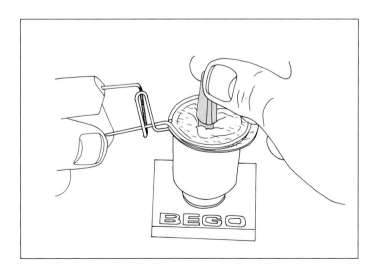

Fig 25-26 The die of the tooth preparation is plunged into the heat-softened disks over the putty.

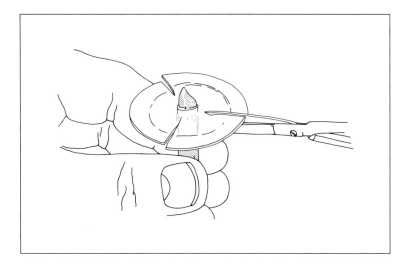

Fig 25-27 Three cuts are made in the unadapted skirt of the disks with a pair of iris scissors.

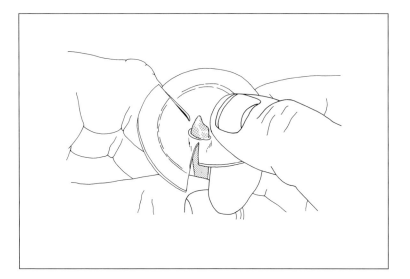

Fig 25-28 The disks are pulled off the tooth preparation die.

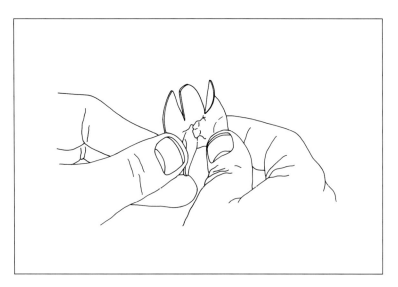

Fig 25-29 The spacer disk is peeled out of the coping shell.

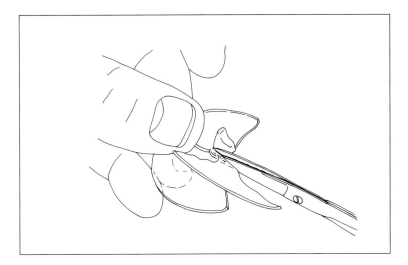

Fig 25-30 Excess border material is cut off 1.0 mm above the preparation finish line.

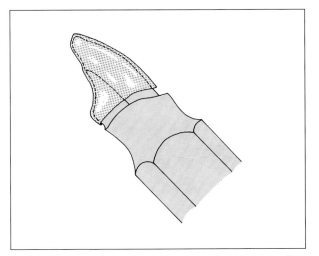

Fig 25-31 The trimmed shell is placed on the die. The edges of the coping are about 1.0 mm short of the finish line on the die.

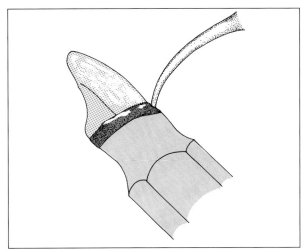

Fig 25-32 The 1.0-mm gap between the shell and finish line is filled with wax.

Remove the die with the adapted spacer and coping disks from the silicone putty in the molding apparatus with a sharp movement. Use a small, sharp-nosed scissors with straight blades to make three or four lateral cuts in the unadapted skirt of the coping disk (Fig 25-27). Remove the adapted coping and spacer disks from the die (Fig 25-28). Because the coping material is well-adapted to the tooth preparation, it will offer some resistance to removal. Separate the spacer from the inside of the coping (Fig 25-29). Use cotton pliers or a hemostat, if necessary, to accomplish the task.

This is an important step, not only because the spacer provides room for the cement in the completed restoration, but also because it will not burn out. Use the scissors to trim the margin of the coping shell (Fig 25-30). At this point the margin should be about 1.0 mm short of the gingival finish line when the coping is replaced on the die (Fig 25-31).

Add wax to the gap between the edge of the coping and the preparation finish line (Fig 25-32). If any of the wax runs under the coping, remove the plastic shell from the die and scrape it clean. The only wax in contact with the die should be the 1.0-mm-wide band immediately occlusal to the finish line. Any other contact defeats the relief provided previously by the spacer disk. The well-adapted coping is now ready for the application of wax.

Complete the full-contour wax pattern in the usual fashion (Fig 25-33) and make a silicone index. Determine and mark the outline of the cutback area on the wax pattern. Use a PKT no. 4 carver to remove the wax down to the level of the plastic shell on those areas of the pattern where porcelain is to be applied later (Fig 25-34). A large spoon excavator is ideally suited for creating the deep chamfer at the porcelain-metal junction line around the area to be veneered with porcelain (Fig 25-35). If there is to be an all-porcelain shoulder on the finished crown,

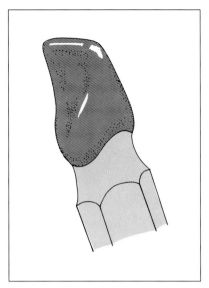

Fig 25-33 The pattern is waxed to full contour.

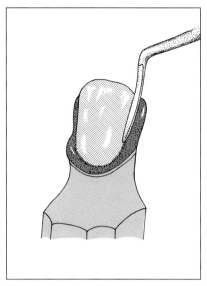

Fig 25-34 With a PKT no. 4 carver, those portions of the pattern that will be veneered with porcelain later are cut back to the shell.

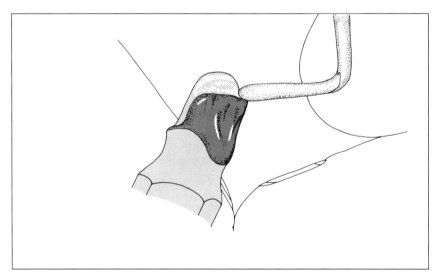

Fig 25-35 A large spoon excavator is used to shape the porcelain-metal junction line in wax.

carefully remove the wax collar at the gingival area of the facial surface using a laboratory knife with a no. 25 blade (Fig 25-36).

The benefit of using the plastic shell coping becomes apparent during the cutback stage. The plastic coping provides rigidity and resists distortion during the removal of wax. When the cutback is complete, use the silicone index of the full-contour wax pattern to verify the adequacy of the cutback. Adapt the margins with a warm beavertail burnisher (Fig 25-37) and smooth the wax pattern. Carefully inspect the wax pattern, paying particular attention to the lingual margins (Fig 25-38). Then sprue

and invest the pattern in the customary manner. The resulting casting should be well-adapted internally, with a uniform relief for cement.

Alloy Surface Treatment

The surfaces of a coping that are to receive porcelain must be properly finished to assure a strong bond and an esthetic restoration. Surface irregularities and small particles of investment may be embedded in the surface of

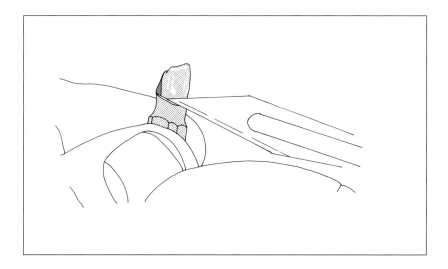

Fig 25-36 The wax overlying the shoulder is cut back to permit fabrication of an all-porcelain shoulder.

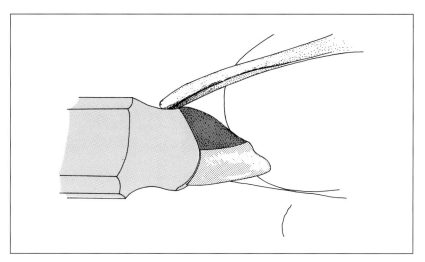

Fig 25-37 The margin is melted and adapted on the rest of the pattern with a hot beavertail burnisher; burnishing is continued as the instrument cools.

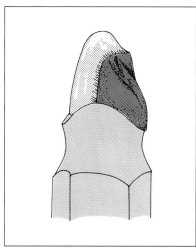

Fig 25-38 The lingual surface of the completed pattern is checked for marginal adaptation.

the casting. Finishing can remove much of this residue while producing uniform striations in one direction to decrease the possibility of gas entrapment during the initial firing cycles.

Surface Treatment Armamentarium

1. Straight handpiece
2. Carborundum separating disc on mandrel
2. Aluminum oxide separating disc on mandrel
3. Aluminum oxide stones
4. Craytex disc on mandrel
5. Burlew disc on mandrel
6. Fine cuttle disc on mandrel

Place the casting on the die. Remove the sprue with a carborundum separating disk. To finish the veneering area, use only new, clean burs and noncontaminating stones and discs. Instruments that have been previously used on other types of metal will contaminate the veneering area.

Use aluminum oxide stones (Forum Brown Abrasives, Unitek Corp, Monrovia, CA; or Lab Series Coral Stones, Shofu Dental Corp, Menlo Park, CA) for rough finishing of the veneering area (Fig 25-39). If a disc must be used, it also must be aluminum oxide since it will not contaminate the veneering area (Dura-Thin Disc, National Keystone Products Co, Cherry Hill, NJ). The demarcation line between the veneered and unveneered areas of the coping should be distinct, with an external angle of 90 degrees and a rounded internal angle.

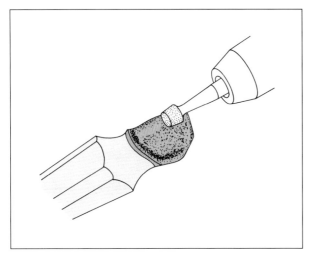

Fig 25-39 The veneering area is prepared with aluminum oxide stones.

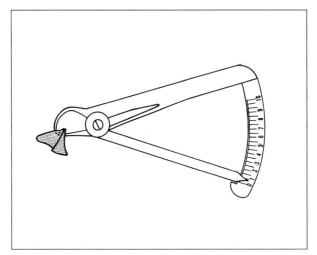

Fig 25-40 The coping thickness is checked with an Iwanson thickness gauge.

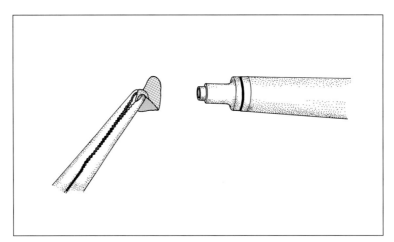

Fig 25-41 The final step in metal preparation is reduction of the oxide layer on the part of the coping to be veneered with porcelain by air abrading with 50 μm aluminum oxide.

Check the thickness of the metal to be veneered with a thickness gauge (Fig 25-40). On noble metal castings it should measure at least 0.3 mm, while on base metal copings it can be 0.2 mm. Narrow the cervical collar, if there is one, from 1.0 mm to about 0.3 mm. Be careful not to run over the margin. Use Craytex and Burlew discs on the unveneered area, and finish the face of the collar with a fine cuttle disc. Do not use any polishing compounds, as they may contaminate the surface of the metal to be veneered later.

Novices would be wise to try the casting in the patient's mouth. Experienced operators will usually bypass this step unless there are a large number of single castings being done at one time, or a long-span fixed partial denture. Check the marginal adaptation of the casting and make any occlusal or contour adjustments that are necessary.

Heat Treatment

Any remaining investment or abrasive particles embedded in the surface of the casting could oxidize and release gases during firing. Oils from the skin left during handling of the casting are another serious form of contamination. "Live steam" is effective in removing residual contamination caused by surface deposits of abrasive particles.[54]

The coping is ready for the *oxidation cycle.* Metal surface treatments are unique for each porcelain-alloy combination, and manufacturer's recommendations should be followed. Bond strength varies with the surface treatment. Unaltered, as cast, gold-palladium and silver-palladium specimens produce low bond values.[2] Typically, a coping is placed in a furnace at a relatively low temperature and the temperature is raised 300 to 400°C at a

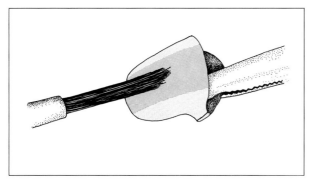

Fig 25-42 The veneering surface of the coping is wetted with distilled water or special liquid recommended by the manufacturer.

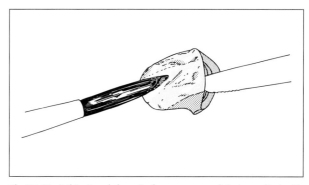

Fig 25-43 A thin "wash layer" of opaque porcelain is applied with a brush.

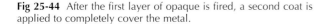

Fig 25-44 After the first layer of opaque is fired, a second coat is applied to completely cover the metal.

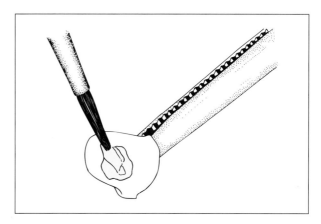

designated rate of climb. The atmosphere (air or vacuum) during this heating process, as well as the length of time at temperature, is dictated by the alloy.

Heat treatment of noble metal alloys causes the trace quantities of tin, gallium, indium, and zinc in the alloy to form oxides that enhance bonding with the porcelain.[55] Base metal alloys, on the other hand, readily oxidize, so oxide formation must be carefully controlled. Following oxidation, most alloys require air abrasion with 50 μm aluminum oxide to reduce the layer of oxide (Fig 25-41), as excess oxide weakens the porcelain-to-metal bond.

Oxidation is only one of the functions of the initial firing. During casting, hydrogen gas is incorporated into the molten alloy. This gas, if left in the coping, can weaken the bond between porcelain and metal,[5] causing the formation of bubbles in the porcelain.[56] The hydrogen is released during the oxidation cycle, degassing the alloy as well as forming the important oxide layer.

Porcelain Addition

The buildup of porcelain is a skill that requires a great deal of practice to develop. Therefore, only a brief description for the sake of familiarization is given here.

Opaque Porcelain Application

The casting is now ready for the actual placement of porcelain. Opaque porcelain is applied first to mask the metal, to give the restoration its basic shade, and to initiate the porcelain-metal bond. The prepared coping is painted with a thin coating of distilled water or special liquid (Fig 25-42). A small amount of the appropriate opaque powder is mixed with distilled water or the specially formulated liquid, forming a thin wash which is applied with a brush (Fig 25-43).

No attempt should be made to thoroughly mask the metal with this initial application. It is intended to completely wet the metal and penetrate the striations created by finishing. The coping is dried and fired under vacuum to a specific temperature. The vacuum is broken and the coping held at the temperature under air for 1 minute.

The second application of opaque porcelain should mask the metal (Fig 25-44). The powder and liquid are mixed to a creamy consistency and applied to the coping with a brush in a vibrating motion. The opaque layer should be applied as thinly as possible to still mask the metal. The coping is gently vibrated to condense the porcelain, and excess water is removed with a dry tissue. The second layer of opaque is fired using the same firing cycle. The opaque layer of porcelain should be approximately 0.3 mm thick.

All-Porcelain Margin Fabrication

Restorations with a metal collar facial margin are now ready for the application of dentin and enamel porcelains following opaque application. For restorations with an all-porcelain facial margin, a few extra steps are necessary at this point. The additional time and skill required to fabricate a direct-lift porcelain margin will often translate into a higher laboratory fee for the restoration.

To fabricate an all-porcelain margin using the direct-lift technique, mark the shoulder finish line on the die using the side of a red pencil (Fig 25-45). Then seal the porous surface of the gypsum die by brushing on a special sealing material (Cera-Seal, Belle de St Claire, Chatsworth, CA) or by squeezing a thin layer of cyanoacrylate cement (Permabond 910 Adhesive, Buffalo Dental Mfg Co, Brooklyn, NY) onto the finish line area of the die (Fig 25-46). Blow off the excess liquid with compressed air to insure a uniformly thin layer of sealant (Fig 25-47).

Apply a special lubricant, or *porcelain release agent* (Cera-Sep, Belle de St Claire), to the facial shoulder of the sealed die with a brush (Fig 25-48). Then seat the opaqued coping on the die. Shoulder porcelain powder should be mixed with distilled water or the manufacturer's recommended liquid. There are techniques utilizing high-temperature investment liquid as the binder for direct-lift porcelain margins. The investment liquid hardens as the wet porcelain mixture dries on the die, making it easier to remove the coping from the die without fracturing the margin. However, after firing, residual silica particles act as inclusions in the porcelain, weakening it and making it more prone to fracture.[50]

Add the initial increment of shoulder porcelain to the facial shoulder; it should extend approximately 2 to 3 mm onto the coping (Fig 25-49). Condense the porcelain and blot it dry with tissue (Fig 25-50). Carve the porcelain with a large spoon excavator or a small cleoid (Fig 25-51) to produce a slight bevel or undercontour. This produces space for a narrow layer of dentin porcelain over the shoulder porcelain.

Lightly smooth the shoulder porcelain at the margin with a no. 10 sable condensing brush (Fig 25-52). Carefully tease the coping from the die (Fig 25-53). Inspect the inside of the casting for any specks of porcelain and remove any found (Fig 25-54). Although they can be ground out after firing, they are more easily seen and removed in the prefired state. Gently place the coping on a sagger tray (Fig 25-55).

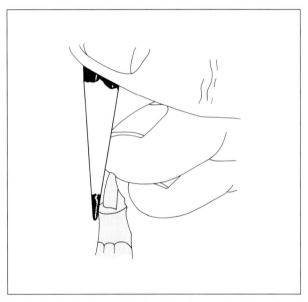

Fig 25-45 The facial shoulder finish line is marked with the side of a red pencil.

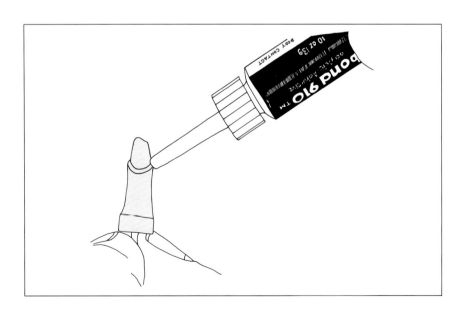

Fig 25-46 Cyanoacrylate cement is applied to seal the die in the area of the facial shoulder.

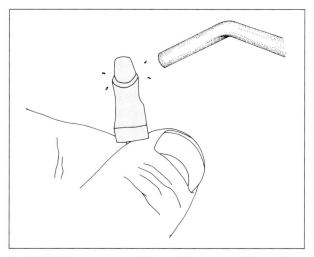

Fig 25-47 Excess cement is blown off to insure a thin, uniform coat.

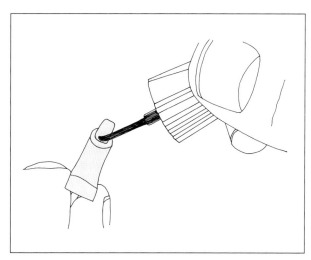

Fig 25-48 Porcelain release agent is applied to the die around the facial shoulder to prevent porcelain from sticking to the die.

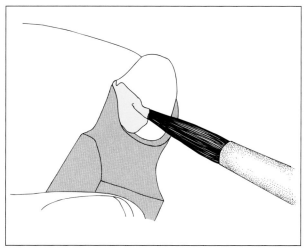

Fig 25-49 The first shoulder porcelain is applied to the facial shoulder of the die with a brush. It should extend 2 to 3 mm onto the metal coping.

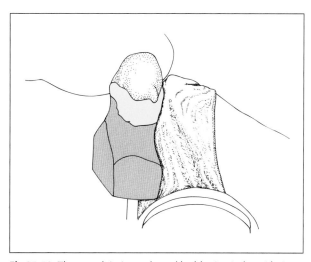

Fig 25-50 The porcelain is condensed by blotting it dry with tissue until no more liquid comes to the surface.

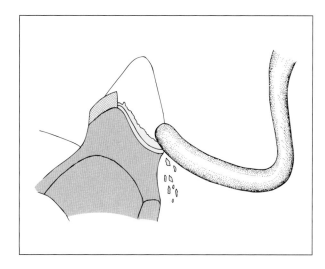

Fig 25-51 A large spoon excavator or a discoid carver is used to remove the excess "green" shoulder porcelain. Only the material directly over the shoulder and a slight extension (1.0 mm or less) onto the coping is left in place.

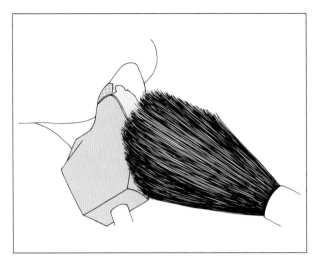

Fig 25-52 A large no. 10 sable brush is used to smooth the margin and remove excess bulk.

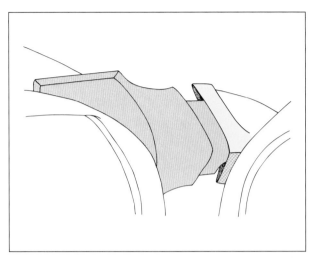

Fig 25-53 The coping is gently teased off the die and the shoulder porcelain is inspected for defects.

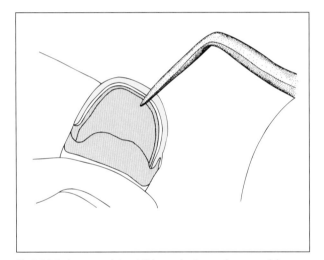

Fig 25-54 Any porcelain visible on the internal aspect of the coping is removed.

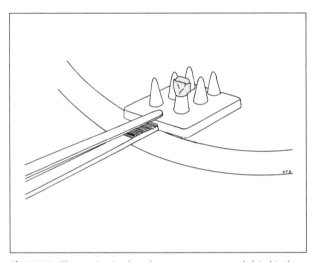

Fig 25-55 The coping is placed on a sagger tray and dried in front of the oven door.

Thoroughly dry the porcelain in front of the furnace. Then fire it under vacuum at a temperature approximately 30°C higher than the corresponding dentin and enamel porcelains. When the initial increment of shoulder porcelain is inspected on the die after firing, a small opening may be apparent at the facial margin (Fig 25-56). More shoulder porcelain can be added to the discrepancy with the crown seated on the die. Vibrate it into the opening with a small vibrating sable brush.

Some ceramists prefer to add a very small amount of shoulder porcelain of a runny consistency to the gingival aspect of the fired margin to correct the discrepancy (Fig 25-57). Place the coping back onto the die, alternately applying firm seating pressure (Fig 25-58) and vibrating the die. Be sure that the metal margin on the lingual of the casting seats completely. If it doesn't, remove the coping from the die and scrape away some of the newly added "correction porcelain." Condense and smooth the porcelain (Fig 25-59). Use the same firing cycle for the correction bake as used in the initial application. When the margin is satisfactory (Fig 25-60), proceed with the dentin and enamel buildup.

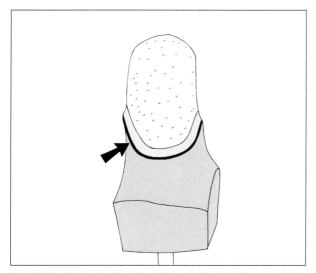

Fig 25-56 Following the first firing of the shoulder porcelain, porcelain shrinkage will cause a slight marginal gap *(arrow)*.

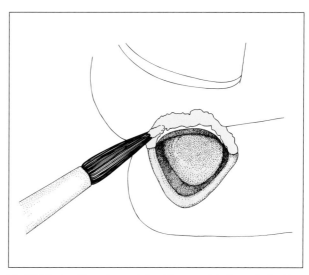

Fig 25-57 A uniform layer of shoulder porcelain is applied with a brush to the underside of the already fired porcelain.

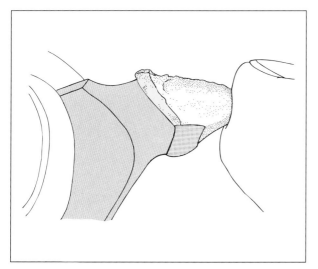

Fig 25-58 The coping is placed back on the die, maneuvering it to completely seat it.

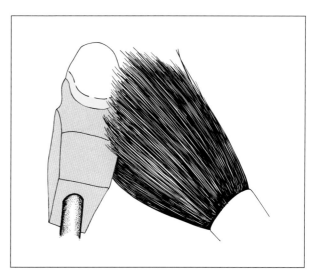

Fig 25-59 The corrected porcelain application is condensed and smoothed with a large condensing brush.

Fig 25-60 The marginal gap between the shoulder porcelain and the finish line must be closed before proceeding.

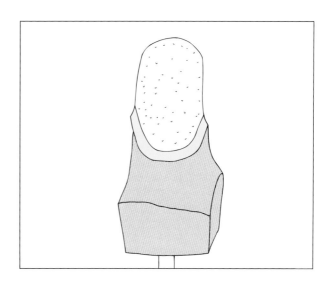

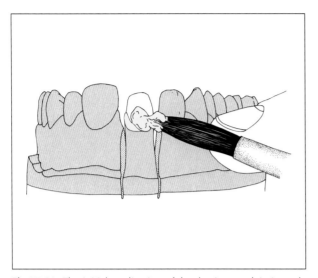

Fig 25-61 The initial application of the dentin porcelain is made with a brush.

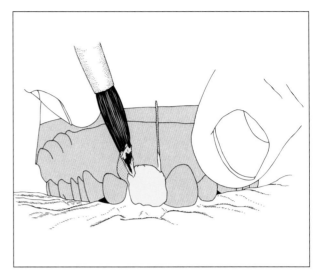

Fig 25-62 Buildup of the dentin porcelain is continued with the brush while holding a piece of tissue behind the incisal edge to absorb water.

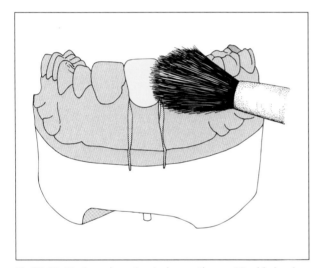

Fig 25-63 Final condensation is done with a no.10 sable brush.

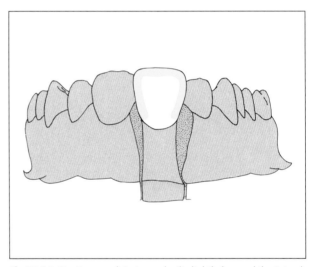

Fig 25-64 Dentin porcelain is overbuilt slightly beyond the intended final contour of the crown.

Dentin and Enamel Porcelain Application

Mix dentin porcelain to a creamy consistency with distilled water or the manufacturer's recommended liquid. Then apply it over the opaque with a sable brush or small spatula, starting at the gingivofacial of the coping, which is seated on the working cast (Fig 25-61). First develop the full contour of the crown in dentin porcelain with a brush. Vibrate the porcelain to condense it, absorbing the liquid with tissue (Fig 25-62). Then brush it with a no. 10 sable condensation brush (Fig 25-63). The completed buildup should be overcontoured (Fig 25-64). When the porcelain is condensed and dried to a consistency of wet sand, carve the dentin back to allow the placement of the enamel porcelain.

The desired translucency pattern dictates the amount and design of the cutback. It will commonly produce some form of bevel on the incisofacial segment of the buildup in dentin porcelain (Fig 25-65). Frequently the cuts at the incisoproximal corners overlap in the center (Fig 25-66). Apply the enamel porcelain to restore the full contour of the restoration (Fig 25-67). Use carving instruments or brushes to shape the porcelain to its final contours (Fig 25-68). Condense the porcelain by blotting from the lingual (Fig 25-69, A) and the facial (Fig 25-69, B).

Commercially available porcelains exhibit significant linear firing shrinkage, with a typical central incisor metal-ceramic crown shrinking 0.9 mm at the incisal edge.[57] When completed, the restoration should be slightly larger incisally to compensate for this shrinkage (Fig 25-70).

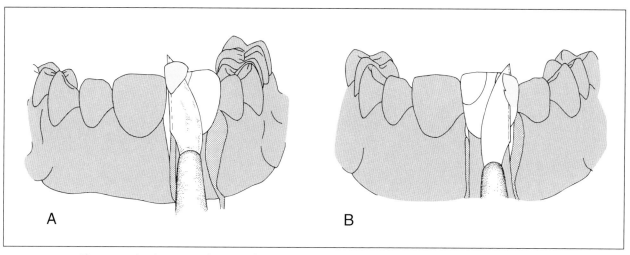

Fig 25-65 The dentin porcelain is cut back to allow placement of the incisal porcelain (A). The amount and extent are dictated by the translucency pattern desired for the restoration. It could require the removal of nothing more than the corners (B).

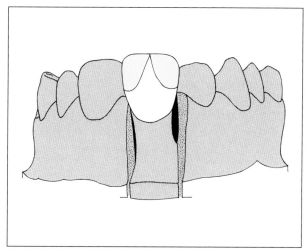

Fig 25-66 Completion of cutback for the incisal porcelain.

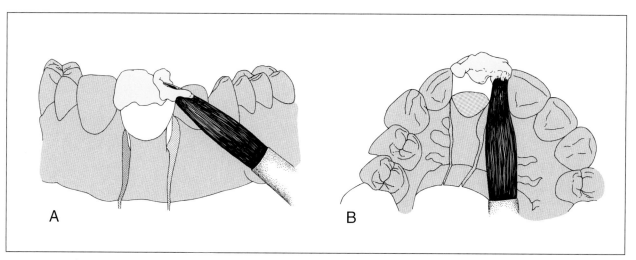

Fig 25-67 Enamel porcelain is added with a brush to the cutback areas: frontal view (A) and incisal view (B).

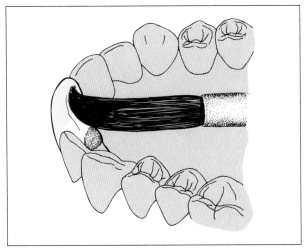

Fig 25-68 The enamel porcelain is carried onto the lingual surface. The lingual fossa is shaped with a brush.

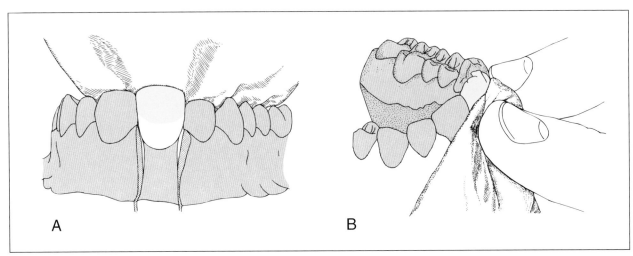

Fig 25-69 The newly added porcelain is shaped by blotting it from the lingual (A) and from the facial (B).

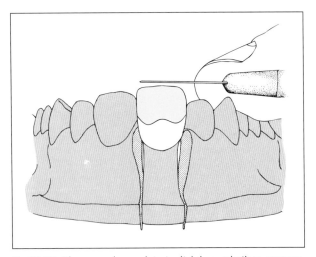

Fig 25-70 The enamel porcelain is slightly overbuilt to compensate for shrinkage during firing.

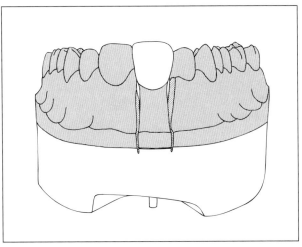

Fig 25-71 Facial view of completed porcelain buildup on the working cast.

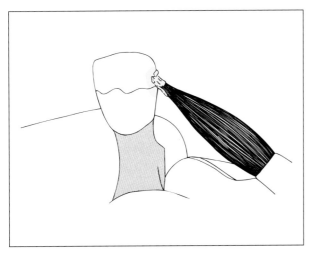

Fig 25-72 The die is removed from the cast and a small amount of porcelain is added to the two interproximal surfaces.

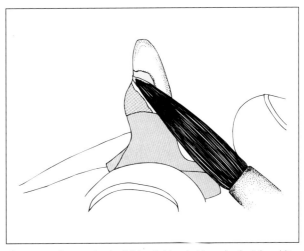

Fig 25-73 The proximal addition is blended into the facial and lingual contours.

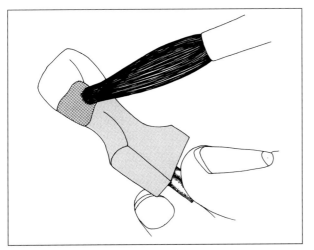

Fig 25-74 Any porcelain that extends onto the metal is removed prior to firing.

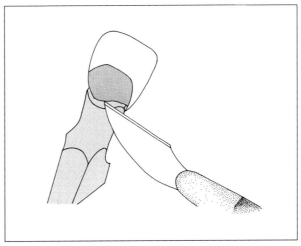

Fig 25-75 The completed crown is carefully removed from the die.

Overall, make the crown about one-fifth larger than the desired size to compensate for the 20% shrinkage that will occur during firing (Fig 25-71).

Cautiously remove the restoration from the working cast and add porcelain to the interproximal areas (Fig 25-72). Blend the proximal addition into the surrounding contours of the crown (Fig 25-73). Remove excess porcelain from the unveneered metal at the porcelain-metal junction (Fig 25-74). Tease the crown off the die by placing the tip of a sharp instrument under the lingual metal margin (Fig 25-75). Avoid any ceramic margin while removing the crown.

Complete the condensation by vibrating the forceps holding the crown with the serrations on a Roach carver (Fig 25-76). Blot up any moisture brought to the surface by this process. With a brush, remove any bits of porcelain that may have strayed into the crown (Fig 25-77). The initial buildup is dried in front of the furnace for several minutes, and then it is fired under vacuum and carried to the temperature specified by the manufacturer of that porcelain.

Try the restoration back on the working cast and evaluate contours. The proximal contacts will often be open (Fig 25-78). Insufficient contours can be corrected by adding the appropriate porcelain. Remove the crown from the die, and grasp it on the unveneered metal in the beaks of a modified mosquito hemostat, which prevents damage to the margin.[58] Add porcelain to the proximal contacts and blend in the contours (Fig 25-79). Fire the restoration at a temperature about 10 to 20°C lower than the initial bake. The higher-fusing porcelain forming the facial margin should not be affected by these subsequent firings.

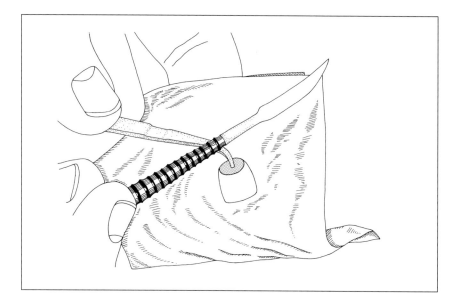

Fig 25-76 The condensation of the porcelain is completed, using a tissue to absorb the excess moisture.

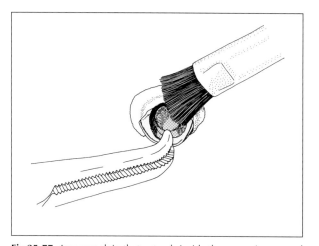

Fig 25-77 Any porcelain that extends inside the crown is removed with a dry brush.

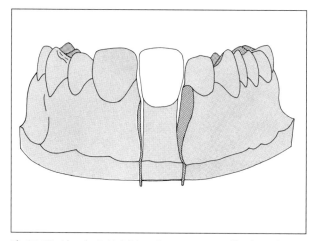

Fig 25-78 After the initial firing, the crown is tried back on the cast and the contours are evaluated.

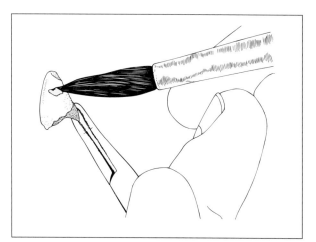

Fig 25-79 A small amount of porcelain is added to the proximal surfaces to restore contact.

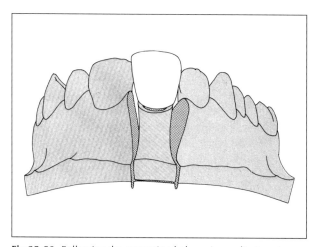

Fig 25-80 Following the correction bake, minor adjustments may be necessary, such as the heavy proximal contact demonstrated here.

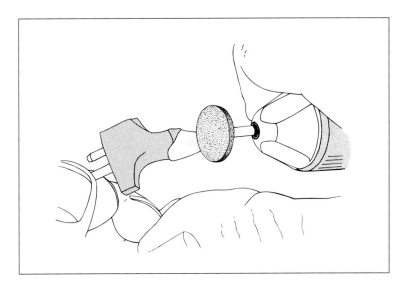

Fig 25-81 A clean green stone or diamond is used to recontour the porcelain.

Following the correction bake, the crown may not seat completely, or it may have other minor deficiencies (Fig 25-80). Adjustments are made on the porcelain with diamond discs, aluminum oxide stones, or carborundum stones (Fig 25-81).

Porcelain Surface Treatment

Once the desired contours and occlusion have been achieved, the restoration must receive a surface treatment. Three commonly used treatments include: *(1)* natural or autoglaze, *(2)* applied overglaze, or *(3)* polishing. Commercially available kits of rubberized abrasives and polishing compounds are available to polish porcelain.

Porcelain has the ability to glaze itself when held at its fusing temperature under air for 1 to 4 minutes. Many ceramists prefer this treatment, feeling that it preserves the surface character and texture of the porcelain. Applied overglaze is a low-fusing clear porcelain that is painted on the surface of the restoration and fired at a fusing temperature much lower than the fusing temperature of the dentin and enamel porcelains.

Since porcelain loses its ability to form a natural glaze after multiple firings, an applied overglaze may be indicated on large restorations that have required numerous corrections. However, caution must be exercised not to overfire the porcelain. It may return to a more crystalline state and become milky or cloudy in appearance, a condition known as *devitrification*. Devitrification causes a loss of natural appearance, and no surface treatment can revive the porcelain.

Polishing lends itself to use on relatively small areas of adjustment such as proximal contacts and limited areas of occlusal contact. Traditionally, polished porcelain has been regarded as a rougher surface than glazed porcelain.[59] However, recent qualitative and quantitative evaluations of polished porcelain surfaces indicate that an acceptable surface may be obtained by using a commercially available system (Truluster, Brasseler USA, Savannah, GA; Porcelain Adjustment Kit, Shofu Dental Corp, Menlo Park, CA).[60] Jacobi et al showed polished porcelain to be less destructive of tooth structure in the opposing arch than glazed porcelain.[24]

Finishing and Cementation

The metal portion is adjusted and finished as described on page 397. Ceramic portions are handled much the same as all-ceramic restorations. If the contours or shade will be modified substantially during try-in, the restoration can be left unglazed until after the adjustments are made. Insufficient proximal contacts and marginal gaps may be corrected at chairside or the restoration may be returned to the laboratory.

Shade Modification

If the shade of a metal-ceramic crown is too dark (its value too low) it is almost impossible to lighten it by custom staining without making the tooth appear too opaque. However, if it is too light (its value too high), it can be modified. Fracture lines and areas of discoloration also can be simulated to give a more natural appearance.

References

1. Christensen GJ: The use of porcelain-fused-to-metal restorations in current dental practice. A survey. *J Prosthet Dent* 1986; 56:1–3.

2. Jochen DG, Caputo AA, Matyas J: Effect of metal surface treatment on ceramic bond strength. *J Prosthet Dent* 1986; 55:186–188.

3. Carpenter MA, Goodkind RJ: Effect of varying surface texture on bond strength of one semi-precious and one non-precious ceramo-alloy. *J Prosthet Dent* 1976; 42:86.

4. Gavelis JR, Lim SB, Guckes AD, Morency JD, Sozio RB: A comparison of the bond strength of two ceramometal systems. *J Prosthet Dent* 1982; 48:424–428.

5. McLean JW, Sced IR: Bonding of dental porcelain to metal—I. The gold alloy/porcelain bond. *Trans Br Ceram Soc* 1973; 72:229–233.

6. Knap FJ, Ryge G: Study of bond strength of dental porcelain fused to metal. *J Dent Res* 1966; 45:1047–1051.

7. Anusavice KJ, Horner JA, Fairhurst CW: Adherence controlling elements in ceramic– metal systems. I. Precious alloys. *J Dent Res* 1977, 56:1045–1052.

8. von Radnoth MS, Lautenschlager EP: Metal surface changes during porcelain firing. *J Dent Res* 1969; 48:321–324.

9. Dent RJ, Preston JD, Moffa JP, et al: Effect of oxidation on ceramometal bond strength. *J Prosthet Dent* 1982; 47:59–62.

10. Vickery RC, Badinelli LA: Nature of attachment forces in porcelain-gold systems. *J Dent Res* 1968; 47:683–689.

11. Shell JS, Nielson JP: Study of the bond between gold alloys and porcelain. *J Dent Res* 1962; 41:1424–1437.

12. Phillips RW: *Skinner's Science of Dental Materials*, ed 9. Philadelphia, WB Saunders Co, 1991, p 505–527.

13. Council on Dental Materials, Instruments, and Equipment: Classification system for cast alloys. *J Am Dent Assoc* 1984;109:838–850.

14. Moffa JP, Guckes AD, Okawa MT, Lilly GE: An evaluation of nonprecious alloys for use with porcelain veneers. Part II. Industrial safety and biocompatibility. *J Prosthet Dent* 1973; 30:432–441.

15. Peltonen L: Nickel sensitivity in the general population. *Contact Dermatitis* 1979; 5:27–32.

16. Kelly JR, Rose TC: Nonprecious alloys for use in fixed prosthodontics: A literature review. *J Prosthet Dent* 1983; 49:363–370.

17. Tai Y, De Long R, Goodkind RJ, Douglas WH: Leaching of nickel, chromium and beryllium ions from base metal alloy in an artificial environment. *J Prosthet Dent* 1992, 68:692–697.

18. Naylor WP: *Introduction to Metal Ceramic Technology.* Chicago, Quintessence Publishing Co, 1992, pp 33–34.

19. Fisher RM, Moore BK, Swartz ML, Dykema RW: The effects of enamel wear on the metal-porcelain interface. *J Prosthet Dent* 1983, 50:627–631.

20. Mumford G: The porcelain fused to metal restoration. *Dent Clin North Am* 1965; 9:241–249.

21. Weiss PA: New design parameters: Utilizing the properties of nickel-chromium superalloys. *Dent Clin North Am* 1977; 21:769–785.

22. Monasky GE, Taylor DF: Studies on the wear of porcelain enamel and gold. *J Prosthet Dent* 1971; 25:299–306.

23. Mahalik JA, Knap FJ, Weiter EJ: Occlusal wear in prosthodontics. *J Am Dent Assoc* 1971; 82:154–159.

24. Jacobi R, Shillingburg HT, Duncanson MG: A comparison of the abrasiveness of six ceramic surfaces and gold. *J Prosthet Dent* 1991; 66:303–309.

25. Wiley MG: Effects of porcelain on occluding surfaces of restored teeth. *J Prosthet Dent* 1989; 61:133–137.

26. Craig RG, El-Ebrashi MK, Peyton FA: Stress distribution in porcelain-fused-to-gold crowns and preparations constructed with photoelastic plastics. *J Dent Res* 1971; 50:1278–1283.

27. Woods JA, Cavazos E: Effects of porcelain-metal junction angulation on porcelain fracture. *J Prosthet Dent* 1985; 54:501–503.

28. Craig RG, El-Ebrashi MK, Farah JW: Stress distribution in photoelastic models of transverse sections of porcelain-fused-to-gold crowns and preparations. *J Dent Res* 1973; 52:1060–1064.

29. Hobo S, Shillingburg HT: Porcelain fused to metal: Tooth preparation and coping design. *J Prosthet Dent* 1973; 30:28–36.

30. Marker JC, Goodkind RJ, Gerberich WW: The compressive strength of nonprecious versus precious ceramometal restorations with various frame designs. *J Prosthet Dent* 1986; 55:560–567.

31. Weir D, Stoffer W, Irvin D, Navarro R, Cwynar R, Schlimmer S, Morris H: The stability of crown margin placement vs. time [abstract 1154]. *J Dent Res* 1986; 65:297.

32. Waerhaug, J: Histologic considerations which govern where the margins of restorations should be located in relation to the gingiva. *Dent Clin North Am* 1960; 4:161–176.

33. Silness J: Periodontal conditions with patients with dental bridges III: The relationship between the location of the crown margin and the periodontal condition. *J Periodont Res* 1970; 5:225.

34. Silness J: Fixed prosthodontics and periodontal health. *Dent Clin North Am* 1980; 24:317–329.

35. Loe H: Reactions of marginal tissue to restorative procedures. *Int Dent J* 1968; 18:759–775.

36. Goodacre CJ, Van Roekel NB, Dykema RW, Ullmann RB: The collarless metal ceramic crown. *J Prosthet Dent* 1977; 38:615–622.

37. Schneider DM, Levi MS, Mori DF: Porcelain shoulder adaptation using direct refractory dies. *J Prosthet Dent* 1976; 36:583–587.

38. Sozio RB, Riley EJ: A precision ceramic-metal restoration with a facial butted margin. *J Prosthet Dent* 1977; 37:517–521.

39. Toogood GD, Archibald JF: Technique for establishing porcelain margins. *J Prosthet Dent* 1978; 40:464–466.

40. Vryonis P: A simplified approach to the complete porcelain margin. *J Prosthet Dent* 1979; 42:592–593.

41. Vryonis P: *A Manual for the Fabrication of the Complete Porcelain Margin.* Adelaide, Stock Journal Publishers Pty, 1982, p 27.

42. Kessler JC, Brooks TD, Keenan MP: The direct lift technique for constructing porcelain margins. *Quint Dent Technol* 1986; 10:145–150.

43. Prince J, Donovan T: The esthetic metal ceramic margin: A comparison of techniques. *J Prosthet Dent* 1983; 50:185–192.

44. Belser UC, MacEntee MI, Richter WA: Fit of three porcelain-fused-to-metal marginal designs in vivo: A scanning electron microscope study. *J Prosthet Dent* 1985; 53:24–29.

45. Hunt JL, Cruickshanks-Boyd DW, Davies EH: The marginal characteristics of collarless bonded porcelain crowns produced using a separating medium technique. *Quint Dent Technol* 1978; 2(9):21–26.

46. West AJ, Goodacre CJ, Moore BK, Dykema RW: A comparison of four techniques for fabricating collarless metal ceramic crowns. *J Prosthet Dent* 1985; 54:636–643.

47. Arnold HN, Aquilino SA: Marginal adaptation of porcelain margins in ceramometal restorations. *J Prosthet Dent* 1988; 59:409–417.

48. Wanserski DJ, Sobczak KP, Monaco JG, McGivney GP: An analysis of margin adaptation of all-porcelain facial margin ceramometal crowns. *J Prosthet Dent* 1986; 56:289–292.

49. Boyle JJ, Naylor WP, Blackman RB: Marginal accuracy of metal ceramic restorations with porcelain facial margins. *J Prosthet Dent* 1993; 69:19–27.

50. Brackett SE, Leary JM, Turner KA, Jordan RD: An evaluation of porcelain strength and the effect of surface treatment. *J Prosthet Dent* 1989; 61:446–451.

51. Scheu R: Kunstoff ersetztwachs-Rationelle fromebung fur stumpf- and kronenhulsen. *Zahntecnik (Zur)* 1970; 28: 359–362.

52. Hauser HJ: Technical fabrication of caps for crown preparation (II). *Quint Dent Technol* 1978, 2(3):43–47.

53. El-Sherif MH, Shillingburg HT, Smith KS: A plastic shell technique for fabricating porcelain-fused-to-metal coping patterns. *Quint Dent Technol* 1987; 11:383–388.

54. Stein RS, Kuwata M: A dentist and a dental technologist analyze current ceramo-metal procedures. *Dent Clin North Am* 1977; 21:729–749.

55. McLean JW: *The Science and Art of Dental Ceramics, Vol I. The Nature of Dental Ceramics and the Clinical Use.* Chicago, Quintessence Publishing Co, 1979, p 71.

56. McLean JW: *The Science and Art of Dental Ceramics, Vol II. Bridge Design and Laboratory Procedures in Dental Ceramics.* Chicago, Quintessene Publishing Co, 1980, p 242.

57. Rosenstiel SF: Linear firing shrinkage of metal ceramic restorations. *Br Dent J* 1987; 162:390–392.

58. Brooks TD: Instrumentation that facilitates porcelain restoration construction. *J Prosthet Dent* 1983; 49:446.

59. Klausner LH, Cartwright CB, Charbeneau GT: Polished versus auto-glazed porcelain surfaces. *J Prosthet Dent* 1982; 47:157–162.

60. Goldstein GR, Barnhard BR, Penugonda B: Profilometer, SEM, and visual assessment of porcelain polishing methods. *J Prosthet Dent* 1991; 65:627–634.

Chapter 26

Pontics and Edentulous Ridges

The pontic, or artificial tooth, is the *raison d'être* of a fixed partial denture. Its name is derived from the Latin *pons,* meaning bridge. It is not a simple replacement, because placing an exact anatomic replica of the tooth in the space would be hygienically unmanageable. The design of the prosthetic tooth will be dictated by esthetics, function, ease of cleaning, maintenance of healthy tissue on the edentulous ridge, and patient comfort.[1]

Pontics may be metal-ceramic, cast metal, or, less commonly today, resin processed to metal (Fig 26-1). Several clinical studies have indicated that all materials used for pontics are tolerated equally, although some inflammation can occur in the gingival tissue in response to any of them.[2-4] Porcelain has been observed to be easily cleanable and hygienic,[3,4] and many clinicians have advocated glazed porcelain as the preferred, or only, material that should touch the edentulous ridge.[5-10] Because of the porous nature of resin, and the difficulty in maintaining a highly polished surface on it, resins should not be used on pontics near the tissue.[11] Glazed or highly polished porcelain and gold with a mirror-like finish are preferred for tissue contact.

Proper design is more important to cleanability and good tissue health than is the choice of materials.[12] The surrounding tissues change with the loss of a tooth so that a pontic cannot exactly duplicate the lost tooth. Alveolar resorption and remodeling reshapes the edentulous area, rounding over sharp edges and filling the socket itself. If there is trauma or periodontal disease associated with the loss of the tooth, the final healed ridge shape may be an even greater departure from the original configuration. Because some of the supporting tissues are lost when the tooth is removed, and because the pontic lies over the tissue instead of growing from it, modifications must be made in basic tooth morphology to insure that the pontic will be cleanable and noninjurious to soft tissues.

The contours in the apical half of the facial surface cannot match those of the tooth that originally occupied the space, or of the remaining natural teeth (Fig 26-2). If they do, the facial surface will be too long and it will look artificial (Fig 26-3). The pontic must be shortened apically, but it cannot simply be clipped off, as the result would be an uncleanable gingivofacial ledge (Fig 26-4). The facial surface must be altered to curve gently from the gingivofacial angle to the middle of the facial surface (Fig 26-5).

Tissue Contact

The extent and shape of the pontic contact with the ridge is very important. Excessive tissue contact has been cited as a major factor in the failure of fixed partial dentures.[5] There is widespread agreement that the area of contact between the pontic and the ridge should be small (Fig 26-6, A),[2,9,11,13] and the portion of the pontic touching the ridge should be as convex as possible.[2,6,9,14] However, if there is contact along the gingivofacial angle of the pontic, there must be no space between pontic and soft tissue on the facial side of the ridge (Fig 26-6, A). If the tip of the pontic extends past the mucogingival junction,[15] an ulcer will form there (Fig 26-7, A). The pontic should contact only attached keratinized gingiva (Fig 26-7, B).[5,15]

The once-popular practice of scraping the ridge on the cast to obtain close adaptation of the pontic with tissue compression is not indicated, because the resultant pressure on the ridge is likely to cause inflammation.[9] It is generally accepted that the pontic should exert no pressure on the ridge.[2,3,16] One author has gone so far as to suggest that the contact be with the film of saliva on the ridge.[13] Others flatly state that the pontic should not contact the tissue at all.[12,17] However, pontics not contacting the ridge at the time of insertion of a prosthesis may become surrounded by hypertrophied tissue after a time in the mouth.[18]

Although one study has shown that the tissues under a pontic can be maintained in an inflammation-free state if the patient flosses vigorously at least once a day,[19] there will be an imprint, or "footprint," of the pontic on the ridge even without inflammation. There is an increased risk of clinical failure if success depends too much on a patient's cooperation.

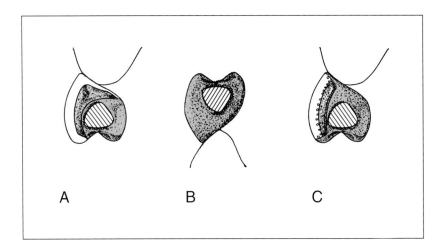

Fig 26-1 Proximal views of a metal-ceramic pontic (A), an all-metal pontic (B), and a resin-processed-to-metal pontic (C).

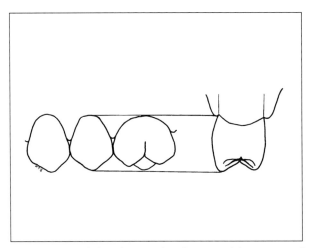

Fig 26-2 Facial *(left)* and proximal *(right)* views of the contours of a maxillary second premolar.

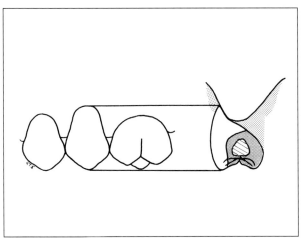

Fig 26-3 Because a ridge resorbs after extraction of a tooth, an attempt to follow the exact contours of the original tooth will result in an elongated pontic. Dotted area shows contours of tooth and soft tissue before extraction.

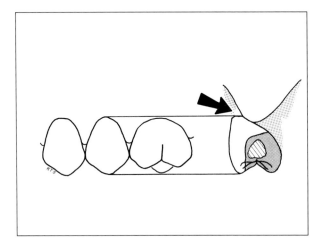

Fig 26-4 Cutting off the apical end of the pontic would solve the length problem, but an unacceptable debris-trapping shelf would result.

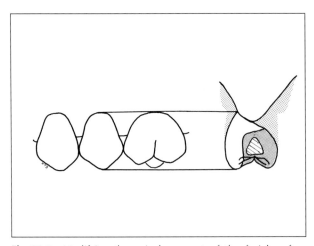

Fig 26-5 Modifying the apical segment of the facial surface will help the pontic blend in without compromising hygiene or esthetics.

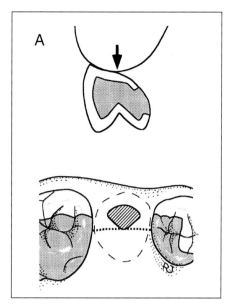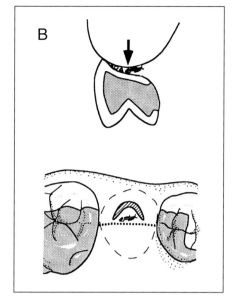

Fig 26-6 Pontic contact with the ridge should be compact, facial to the crest of the ridge, slightly wider mesiodistally at the facial, and narrower at the lingual aspect (A). Contact with the tissue should not fall just along the gingivofacial line angle; if there is a space between it and the crest, a debris trap will result (B).

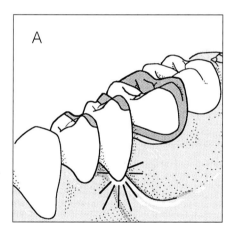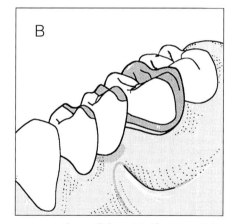

Fig 26-7 If the pontic encroaches on unattached mucosa, an ulcer will form (A). The tip must be restricted to keratinized gingiva (B).

Postinsertion Hygiene

The mesial, distal, and lingual gingival embrasures of the pontic should be wide open to allow the patient easy access for cleaning,[3,5,12,16,20] and the contact between pontic and tissue must allow the passage of floss from one retainer to the other. After the fixed partial denture is cemented, teach the patient appropriate technique(s) that can be mastered. Motivate the individual to practice good hygiene around and under the pontic with dental floss (Fig 26-8), interproximal brushes (Fig 26-9), or pipe cleaners. The method used will depend on embrasure size, accessibility, and patient skill.

Give the patient time to learn the techniques and demonstrate the ability to clean the underside of the pontic and the adjacent areas of the abutment teeth. Evaluate home care at each appointment and reinforce the necessity for good hygiene and the skills to accomplish it. Even the smoothest pontic surface must be cleaned well and often to prevent the accumulation of plaque.[21] If cleaning is not done at frequent, regular intervals, the tissue around the pontic will become inflamed.[18]

Pontics designed for placement in the *appearance zone* (areas of high visibility [Richter WA: personal communication, July 1973]) must produce the illusion of being teeth, esthetically, without compromising clean-

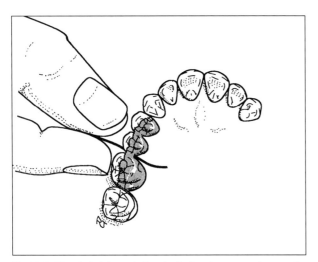

Fig 26-8 Floss is fed through the gingival embrasure and run under the pontics and connectors by the patient. If the space is tight, a monofilament floss threader can be used.

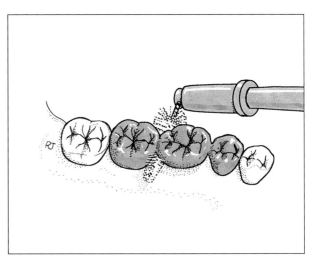

Fig 26-9 Interproximal brushes are excellent for cleaning the gingival embrasures around pontics.

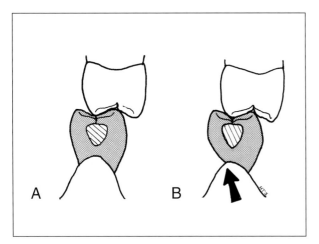

Fig 26-10 A classic saddle, or ridge lap pontic (A). A linguogingival ridge *(arrow)*, or extension past the crest of the ridge, although less severe, still constitutes a saddle (B).

ability. Those pontics placed in the *nonappearance zone* (usually mandibular posterior replacements) are there to restore function and prevent the drifting of teeth. Since esthetics is usually a minor consideration in this area of the mouth, it may not be necessary to utilize materials or contours that suggest the presence of a tooth.

The pontic should be on as straight a line as possible between the retainers to prevent any torquing of the retainers and/or abutments. The pontic will be slightly narrower than the natural tooth, partly because of the effort to place it on the interabutment axis. The pontic may also be somewhat narrower at the expense of the lingual surface in an effort to avoid the formation of an uncleanable, overhanging shelf in the pontic overlying the lingual aspect of the ridge. However, no attempt is made to make the pon-

tic narrower by a set percentage (eg, 10% per pontic). Doing so does not alter the plaque index.[1] Narrowing the pontic is not practical if an effort is being made to maintain occlusal contacts on cusps or in fossae.

Pontic Designs

There are several designs available for our use in situations requiring pontics in the fabrication of fixed partial dentures. These include: saddle (ridge lap), modified ridge lap, hygienic, conical, ovate, prefabricated pontic facings, and metal-ceramic pontics.

Saddle

This pontic looks most like a tooth, replacing all the contours of the missing tooth. It forms a large concave contact with the ridge (Fig 26-10, A), obliterating the facial, lingual, and proximal embrasures. It is also called a *ridge lap,* because it overlaps the facial and lingual aspects of the ridge. A contact with the ridge that extends beyond the midline of the edentulous ridge, or a sharp angle at the linguogingival aspect of the tissue contact, constitutes a ridge lap (Fig 26-10, B). This design has long been recognized as being unclean and uncleanable.[22] It still is.[23,24] The saddle is impossible to clean, because floss cannot traverse the tissue-facing area of the pontic because it bridges across the linguogingival and faciogingival angles of the pontic. The saddle causes tissue inflammation, and it should not be used.[25]

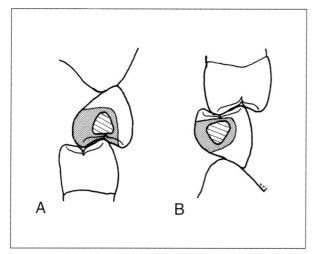

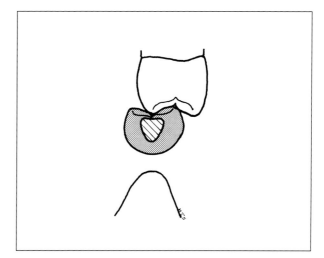

Fig 26-11 Modified ridge lap pontics: A, maxillary; B, mandibular.

Fig 26-12 Hygienic or sanitary pontic.

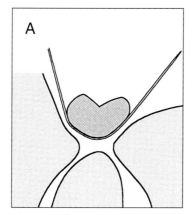

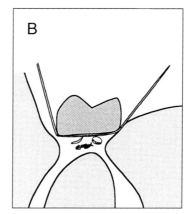

Fig 26-13 Floss passes over a smooth, round surface (A) more easily than over a flat surface and sharp angles (B).

Modified Ridge Lap

This design gives the illusion of a tooth, but it possesses all or nearly all convex surfaces for ease of cleaning. The lingual surface should have a slight deflective contour to prevent food impaction and minimize plaque accumulation.[14] There may be a slight faciolingual concavity on the facial side of the ridge, which can be cleaned and tolerated by the tissue as long as the tissue contact is narrow mesiodistally and faciolingually.

Ridge contact must extend no farther lingually than the midline of the edentulous ridge, even on posterior teeth. Whenever possible, the contour of the tissue-contacting area of the pontic should be convex, even if a small amount of soft tissue on the ridge must be surgically removed to facilitate it. This design, with a porcelain veneer, is the most commonly used pontic design in the appearance zone for both maxillary and mandibular fixed partial dentures (Fig 26-11).

Hygienic

The term hygienic is used to describe pontics that have no contact with the edentulous ridge (Fig 26-12). This pontic design is frequently called a "sanitary pontic," which in years past was the trade name for a prefabricated, convex facing with a slot back, used for mandibular molar pontics.

The hygienic pontic is used in the nonappearance zone, particularly for replacing mandibular first molars. It restores occlusal function and stabilizes adjacent and opposing teeth. If there is no requirement for esthetics, it can be made entirely of metal. The occlusogingival thickness of the pontic should be no less than 3.0 mm, and there should be adequate space under it to facilitate cleaning. The hygienic pontic is frequently made in an all-convex configuration, faciolingually and mesiodistally.

Making the undersurface of the pontic round without angles allows for easier flossing (Fig 26-13, A). It is more

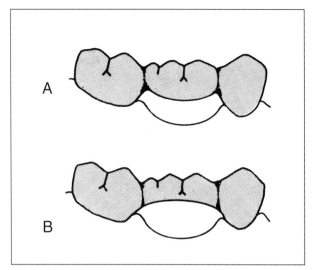

Fig 26-14 Facial view of hygienic, or sanitary, pontics: A, conventional ("fish belly"); B, modified (Perel).

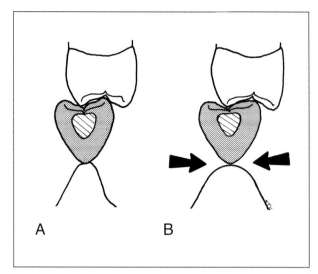

Fig 26-15 Conical pontic used correctly with a thin ridge (A) and incorrectly with a broad, flat ridge (B). Arrows indicate debris-trapping embrasure spaces.

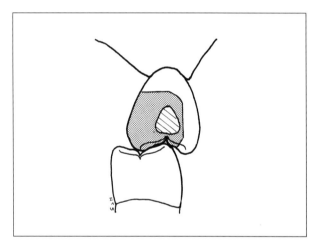

Fig 26-16 The round-end ovate pontic fits into a depression in the ridge.

difficult to get floss to pass over a flat undersurface evenly, or to get over sharp faciogingival and linguogingival line angles (Fig 26-13, B). The round design has been described as a "fish belly" (Fig 26-14, A).

An alternative design, in which the pontic is made in the form of a concave archway mesiodistally (Fig 26-14, B), has been suggested. The undersurface of the pontic is convex faciolingually, giving the tissue-facing surface of the pontic the configuration of a hyperbolic paraboloid. There is added bulk for strength in the connectors, and access for cleaning is good.[26] Stress is reduced significantly in the connectors, and deflection is diminished in the center of the pontic, with less gold used.[27] An esthetic version of this pontic can be created by veneering with porcelain those parts of the pontic that are like-

ly to be visible: the occlusal surface and the occlusal half of the facial surface, which happens to be all of the facial surface on this pontic. This design has been called an "arc-fixed partial denture,"[23] a "modified sanitary pontic,"[27] or simply a "Perel pontic."

Conical

The conical pontic is rounded and cleanable, but the tip is small in relation to the overall size of the pontic. It is well suited for use on a thin mandibular ridge (Fig 26-15, A). However, when used with a broad, flat ridge, the resulting large triangular embrasure spaces around the tissue contact have a tendency to collect debris (Fig 26-15, B).[10] This pontic is related to the "sanitary dummy" described by Tinker in 1918.[28] Its use is limited to replacement of teeth over thin ridges in the nonappearance zone.

Ovate

The ovate pontic is a round-end design currently in use where esthetics is a primary concern.[25] Its antecedent was the porcelain root-tipped pontic,[22,28–32] which was used considerably before 1930 as an esthetic and sanitary substitute for the saddle pontic. The tissue-contacting segment of the ovate pontic is bluntly rounded, and it is set into a concavity in the ridge (Fig 26-16). It is easily flossed. The concavity can be created by placement of a provisional fixed partial denture with the pontic extending one-quarter of the way into the socket immediately after extraction of the tooth. It also can be creat-

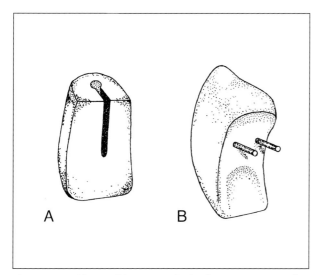

Fig 26-17 Prefabricated facings: A, slot-back; B, Harmony pin facing.

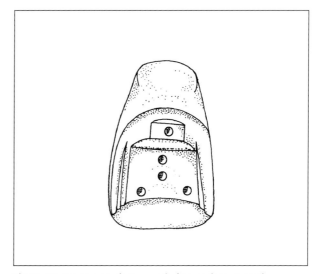

Fig 26-18 Reverse pin facing made from a denture tooth.

ed surgically at some later time.[25] This pontic works well with a broad, flat ridge, giving the appearance that it is growing from the ridge.

Prefabricated Pontic Facings

At one time, preformed porcelain facings were popular for fabricating pontics.[33] They required adaptation to a specific edentulous space,[16,34] after which they were reglazed. Some, such as *Trupontics, Sanitary pontics,* and *Steeles facings* (Franklin Dental Co, Columbus, OH), relied on a lug in a custom cast metal backing to engage a slot in the occlusal or lingual surface of the facing (Fig 26-17, A). The large bulk of porcelain could result in a thin gold backing susceptible to flexing. *Harmony* and *Trubyte* facings used horizontal pins that fit into the gold backing (Fig 26-17, B). They were difficult to use in patients with limited occlusogingival space, and refitting the pins into a backing after casting was demanding.

Porcelain denture teeth also were modified to use as pontic facings. Multiple pin holes, 2.0 mm deep, were made with a drill press in the lingual surface of the reverse pin facing (Fig 26-18).[34] The pins came out of the backing, providing retention where a deep overbite would have overshortened conventional pins. Unfortunately, the pin holes in the facing were stress points that led to fracture.

Metal-Ceramic Pontics

With the widespread use of metal-ceramic restorations, metal- ceramic pontics have replaced other types of pontics employing porcelain. Metal-ceramic pontics have the greatest esthetic potential as prosthetic replacements for missing teeth.[35] Additionally, metal-ceramic pontics are stronger, since the porcelain is bonded to the metal substrate rather than cemented to it. They are easier to use because the backing is custom made for a space (no need to adapt a premade porcelain facing to the space).

The Edentulous Ridge

Before a fixed partial denture is undertaken, the edentulous ridge should be examined carefully. The type and amount of destruction will play a role in selecting the pontic to be used and also may indicate the necessity for reshaping the ridge surgically.

Classification

Ridge deformities have been grouped into three categories by Siebert (Fig 26-19),[36] and this classification has been widely accepted[11,37]:

- *Class I.* Loss of faciolingual ridge width, with normal apicocoronal height.
- *Class II.* Loss of ridge height, with normal width.
- *Class III.* Loss of both ridge width and height.

If a "normal" classification (Class N) with minimal deformity is added, there are four classes of ridge contours. In a study of 416 diagnostic casts, Abrams et al[28] showed Class I defects to constitute 32.4% of the edentulous ridges, with 2.9% being Class II, 55.9% being Class III, and only 8.8% having no defects.

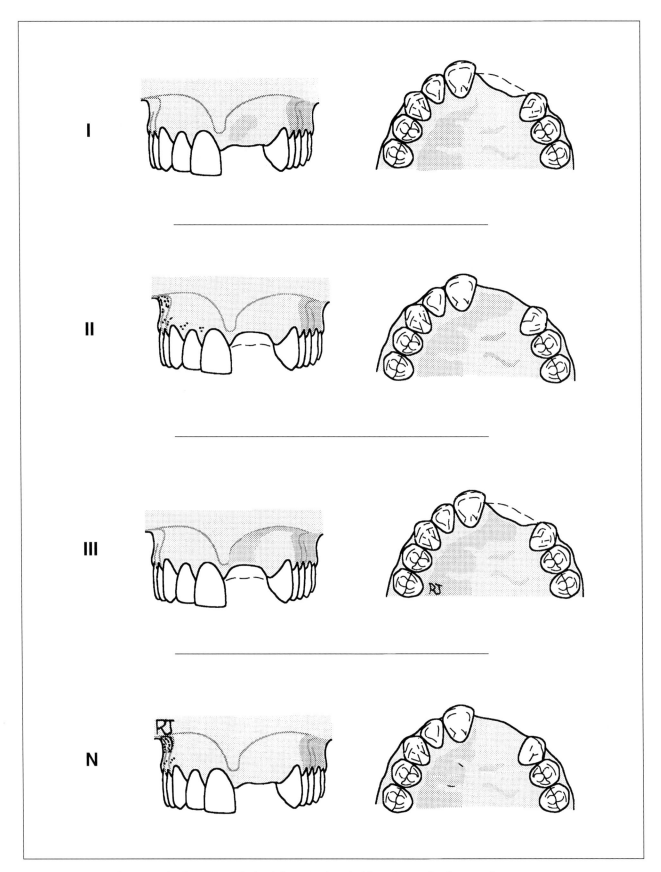

Fig 26-19 The three types of ridge deformities described by Siebert[36] plus the normal category (N).

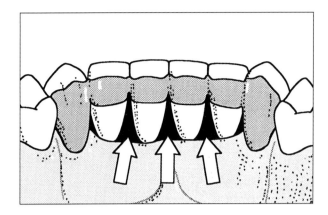

Fig 26-20 Lingual view of open gingival embrasures ("black triangles") on a fixed partial denture replacing mandibular incisors.

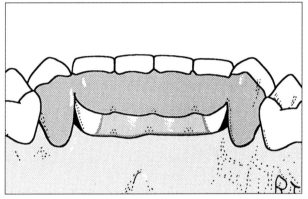 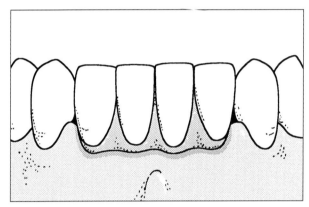

Fig 26-21 Lingual *(left)* and facial *(right)* views of fixed partial denture with embrasure filled with pink porcelain. This is esthetic as long as the patient does not show the porcelain-gingiva junction.

Pontic Modification

At one time it was common to modify a pontic to fit an edentulous space, no matter what the esthetic consequences were. Developments in surgical techniques have made it simpler to change the configuration of a ridge to create a more esthetic and a more easily cleanable shape. It has become more common to modify the ridge than to suffer the rigors of "making do" with a deficient ridge.

There are nonetheless situations in which a more conservative approach may be desired. The patient's inability to undergo surgery, or an unwillingness to consider it, will force the consideration of an alternative form of pontic. In ridges with severe defects, where two or more pontics must be used to fill the space, it is not uncommon to eliminate gingival embrasure spaces between the pontics.

"Black triangles" can be very unesthetic (Fig 26-20), and they serve no useful purpose. They collect plaque, interfere with the passage of floss, and may reduce the rigidity of the pontic span.[39,40] Pink porcelain can be added to the gingival embrasure area of the pontic to simulate interdental papilla (Fig 26-21),[41,42] although the shade rarely matches the particular hue of the patient's gingiva. The gingival extension of porcelain must be supported by the metal framework. If not, all of the gingival

porcelain, as well as much of the facial porcelain, is at risk of fracturing.[43] Elimination of interpontic gingival embrasures in a multitooth pontic may limit or eliminate soft tissue proliferation.[44]

Embrasure spaces filled with porcelain can be satisfactory when replacing mandibular molars[39] and mandibular incisors,[40,43] where the gingival area is not subject to close scrutiny. However, it is more difficult to achieve an esthetic result simply by modification of the embrasure spaces in a high-profile area such as the maxillary incisor region (Fig 26-22). In the presence of a large deformity, an unmodified pontic would leave large, unsightly gingival embrasures (Fig 26-23), and the addition of a gingival flange may be too conspicuous (Fig 26-24).

One solution used in the restoration of large ridge defects, particularly in the anterior segment, is the Andrews bridge system.[45] It utilizes fixed retainers that are connected by a rectangular bar that follows the curve of the ridge under it (Fig 26-25). The prosthesis consists of teeth set in a patient-removable flange of gingiva-colored acrylic resin that clips over and is stabilized by the rectangular bar. Unfortunately, the flange is a food and plaque trap that is difficult to keep clean. In spite of its drawbacks, it still may be the best way of handling some large ridge defects.[45]

493

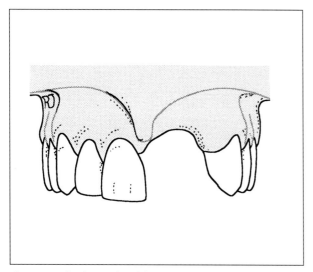

Fig 26-22 This large ridge defect in the maxillary anterior region is not a good candidate for pontic modification.

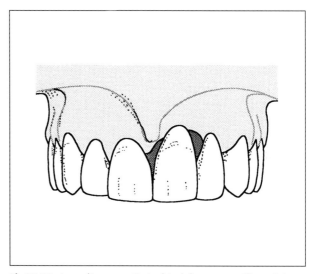

Fig 26-23 An ordinary pontic in this defect space will result in an elongated pontic with large, highly visible embrasures.

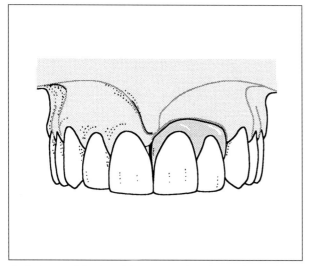

Fig 26-24 Modification of the pontic with pink porcelain in this situation will be conspicuous.

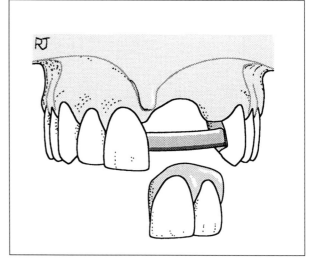

Fig 26-25 In some cases, larger anterior defects may be better managed by an Andrews bridge system with a removable acrylic insert that clamps down over a bar linking the abutments.

Surgical Correction

Ridge augmentation can be accomplished by the addition of either soft or hard tissue, although filling a ridge defect with bone is not essential unless the ridge is to be used for implants.[46] Excellent esthetic results in Class I defects can be obtained by connective tissue plastic surgery,[47] in the form of a subepithelial or submucosal connective tissue graft.[47,48]

The technique for a connective tissue graft is based on procedures described by Langer and Calagna[48] and Kaldahl et al.[47] A horizontal incision is made on the palate 1.0 mm apical to the free gingival margin of the molars. The length of the incision is dependent on the size of the

defect being repaired. Vertical releasing incisions are made at both ends of the incision to allow the reflection of a split-thickness flap from the underlying connective tissue. The connective tissue base is dissected from the flap and removed for later use as the donor material. The incision is then sutured.

Incisions are made 1.0 mm on either side of the defect in the edentulous ridge. An incision paralleling the crest of the ridge joins them (Fig 26-26). A partial-thickness pedicle flap is dissected to a depth of 1.5 to 2.0 mm in the palatal area. On the facial it can remain a partial-thickness flap,[47] or it can become a full-thickness flap (Fig 26-27).[48] The donor tissue is placed into the defect under the base of the flap on the facial side of the ridge

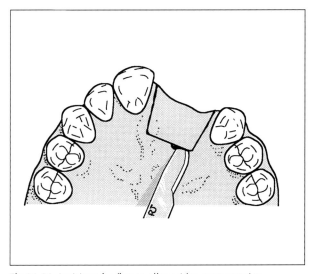

Fig 26-26 Incisions for flap to allow ridge augmentation.

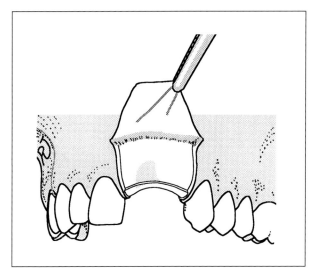

Fig 26-27 Reflection of flap.

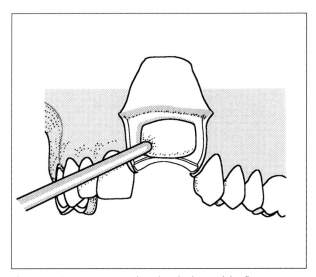

Fig 26-28 Donor tissue is placed at the base of the flap.

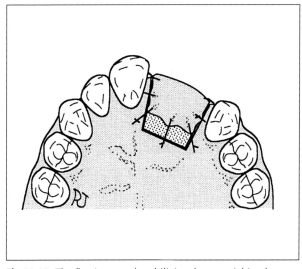

Fig 26-29 The flap is sutured, stabilizing the material in place.

(Fig 26-28) until the defect is filled. The flap is sutured, stabilizing the donor material in position (Fig 26-29).

Unfortunately, apicocoronal Class II and III defects cannot be adequately treated by a pouch type of ridge augmentation. This type of defect is better treated using an onlay graft, which Seibert describes as a "thick free gingival graft."[45,49] The surface of the edentulous ridge is planed with a no. 15 scalpel blade to remove as much epithelium as possible (Fig 26-30), followed by parallel striations cut into the exposed lamina propria 1.0 mm apart and perpendicular to the curvature of the alveolar ridge (Fig 26-31).[36]

These cuts create bleeding, which is highly desirable for the graft to "take." Anesthetic for the procedure should be of a type providing minimal vasoconstriction and as far from the surgical site as possible, so as not to interfere with bleeding. The full-thickness donor tissue is harvested from the gingival zone or the palatal area of the tuberosity. The more fatty tissue that is included, the more the graft will shrink over time as the tissue is resorbed.

The premolar/first molar vault area is an excellent donor source. It provides the greatest volume, and the gingiva there is pliable and easily adapted.[50] The graft is placed over the prepared area and sutured in place (Fig 26-32). The procedure is limited by donor site availability. Ridges with severe defects may require more than one surgery, allowing 8 weeks before repeating the procedure.[11,49] The patient should be forewarned of this possi-

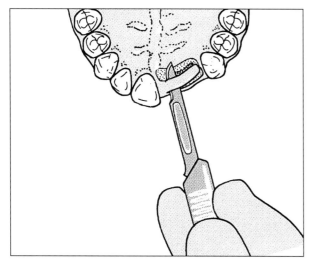

Fig 26-30 As much epithelium as possible is planed off from the crest of the ridge.

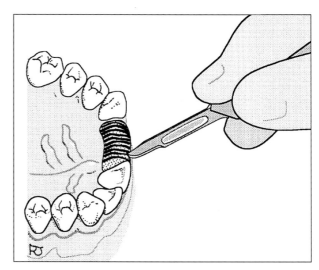

Fig 26-31 Striations are cut in the ridge to encourage bleeding.

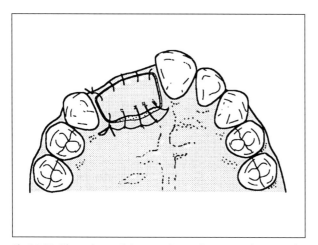

Fig 26-32 The onlay graft is sutured over the prepared area on the ridge.

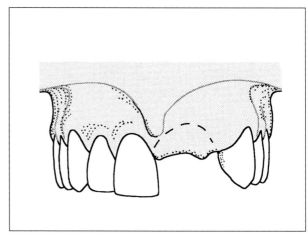

Fig 26-33 The healed, augmented ridge. It may be necessary to do more than one surgical procedure to achieve the desired contour in the ridge.

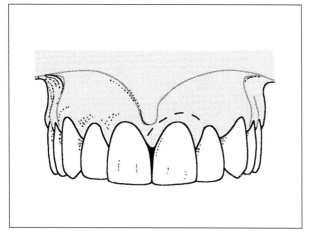

Fig 26-34 Pontics over the surgically enhanced ridge should have a natural appearance.

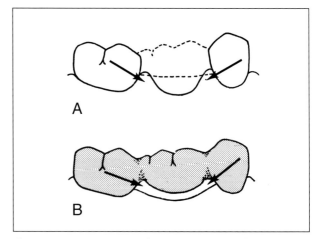

Fig 26-35 Excessive gingival tissue adjacent to the edentulous space (A) is removed by electrosurgery before the fixed partial denture is made (B).

bility before the first surgery. After the graft has healed (Fig 26-33), the final fixed partial denture can be fabricated with a natural-looking pontic (Fig 26-34).

If the facial contour of a ridge has a convex shape or irregularities that will prevent the use of a convex pontic, the soft tissue may be recontoured surgically to provide an easily cleanable and esthetic pontic. Another problem frequently encountered is a large "cuff" of tissue adjacent to the edentulous space. If left there, this tissue will force the connectors to be made too small occlusogingivally and will probably result in uncleanable embrasures under the solder joints after the fixed partial denture is seated (Fig 26-35, A). This roll of gingival tissue should be removed before the impressions are made for fabrication of the fixed partial denture (Fig 26-35, B).

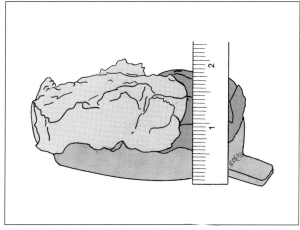

Fig 26-36 Full-arch impression poured to a thickness of approximately 1.5 inches.

Pontic Fabrication

Following are the techniques for waxing *(1)* an all-metal mandibular posterior fixed partial denture with a hygienic pontic and *(2)* a metal-ceramic maxillary posterior fixed partial denture[34] with a modified ridge lap pontic.

Armamentarium

1. Sable brush
2. Plaster bowl
3. Spatula
4. Quick-setting plaster
5. Bunsen burner and matches
6. PKT (Thomas) waxing instruments (no. 1, no. 2, no. 3, no. 4, no. 5)
7. Beavertail burnisher
8. No. 7 wax spatula
9. Inlay casting wax
10. Die lubricant
11. Zinc stearate
12. Cotton pliers
13. Hollow plastic sprue

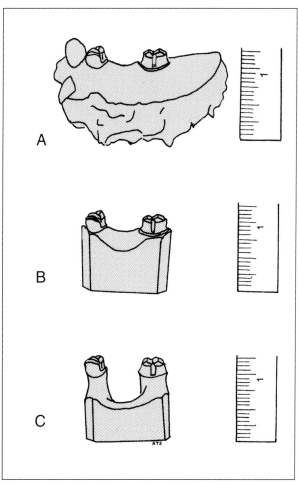

Fig 26-37 An untrimmed die should measure approximately 1.25 inches from preparation to base (A). Everything but the prepared teeth is trimmed from the poured cast (B). The edentulous segment between preparations is reduced to allow access to finish lines from an apical direction (C).

All-Metal Hygienic Pontic Fabrication

Pour the full-arch impression, filling the prepared teeth and one tooth on either side of them to a height of 3.8 cm (1.5 inches) off the tabletop (Fig 26-36). Trim the die to an overall height of about 3.2 cm (1.25 inches). Leave the dies attached with a common base, which will retain the exact relationship of the two preparations. Trim away the stone 1.2 cm (0.5 inch) apical to the finish line (Fig 26-37) to produce a U-shaped die. Coat the dies with cement spacer and lubricant.

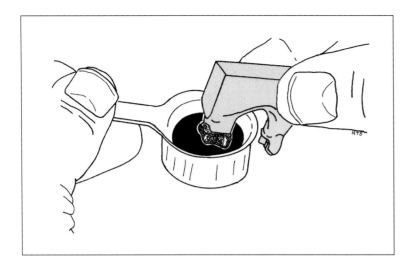

Fig 26-38 The wax coping can be started by dipping the die into molten wax.

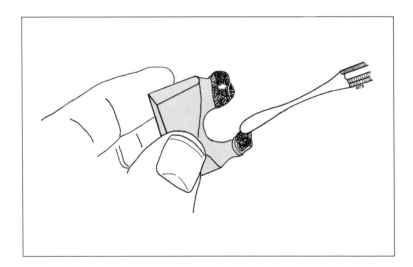

Fig 26-39 The coping can also be started by adding wax with the wide end of a no. 7 wax spat-

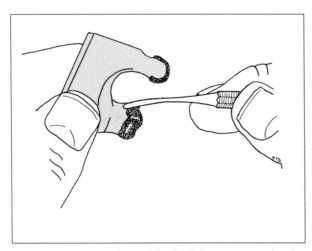

Fig 26-40 Excess wax beyond the finish lines is removed with a warm beavertail burnisher.

Place wax on the lubricated dies either by dipping them in a small container of molten wax (Fig 26-38) or adding dollops of wax with the large end of a no. 7 wax spatula (Fig 26-39). Use a warm beavertail burnisher to trim off excess wax beyond the retainer margins on the die (Fig 26-40). Place the wax patterns on the working cast and correct axial contours as needed (Fig 26-41). Replace the retainer patterns onto the die and connect them with a short stick of inlay wax (Fig 26-42).

With a hot beavertail burnisher, carve wax off the "top" (occlusal aspect) of the stick of wax connecting the two retainers (Fig 26-43). Turn the die over and deposit the molten wax on the undersurface of the pontic (Fig 26-44). Carve the undersurface of the pontic to produce the totally convex "fish belly" (Fig 26-45). Smooth and round the undersurface of the pontic with instruments and a clean cotton roll dipped in die lubricant (Gator Die Lube, Whip Mix Corp, Louisville, KY) (Fig 26-46).

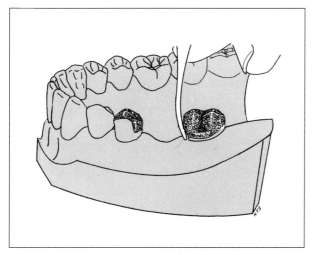

Fig 26-41 Axial contours are adjusted on the working cast.

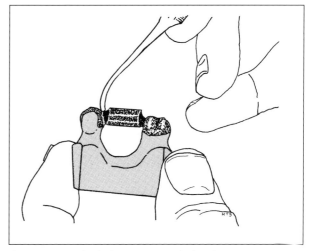

Fig 26-42 A stick of inlay wax is attached to the retainer wax patterns.

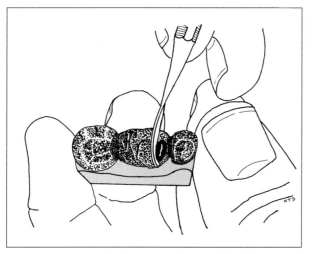

Fig 26-43 Excess wax is removed from the occlusal aspect of the stick wax "pontic" with a hot beavertail burnisher.

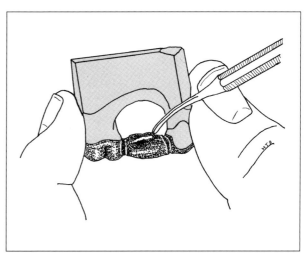

Fig 26-44 Wax removed in the previous step is added to the underside of the pontic.

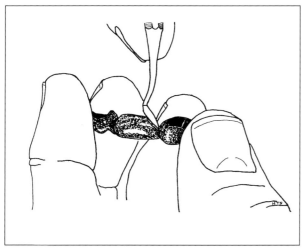

Fig 26-45 A PKT no. 4 is used to define the gingival embrasure and to smooth the undersurface of the pontic.

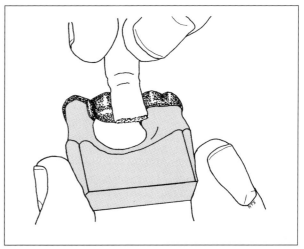

Fig 26-46 Die lubricant on a cotton roll is used to finish smoothing the underside of the pontic.

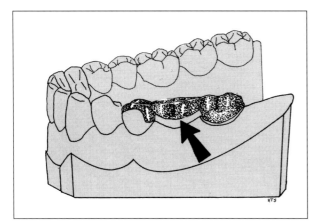

Fig 26-47 The pattern is placed on the working cast, and the contours of the pontic are checked one last time.

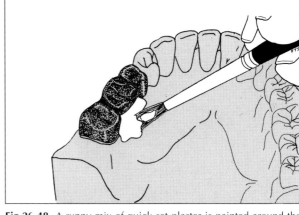

Fig 26-48 A runny mix of quick-set plaster is painted around the undersurface of the pontic.

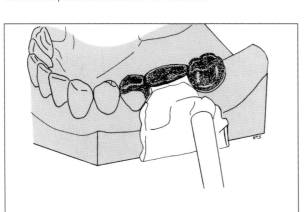

Fig 26-49 More plaster is added to the facial surface of the pontic.

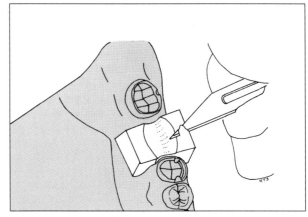

Fig 26-50 When the plaster has set, the wax pattern is removed and the plaster matrix is trimmed so that the occlusal surface is free of plaster.

Plaster Matrix. Place the fixed partial denture wax pattern on the working cast and evaluate the configuration of the underside of the pontic in relation to the edentulous ridge (Fig 26-47). Check for clearance with the ridge, impingement on the interdental papilla adjacent to the edentulous space, smoothness, and degree of curvature on the undersurface of the pontic. If any aspect requires adjustment, remove the wax pattern from the working cast and make the necessary changes. Then replace the pattern on the cast.

Lubricate the area of the cast adjacent to the edentulous ridge with a light coating of petrolatum. Construct a matrix on the facial and lingual surfaces of the cast with quick-setting plaster. Use a sable brush or instrument to place the plaster in the embrasure spaces around the lingual (Fig 26-48) and facial aspects of the wax pattern to insure complete support of the pontic and connectors later. Apply a *thin* mixture of plaster over the facial surface of the cast and the pontic (Fig 26-49).

Be sure to wash the brush before the plaster sets on it. When the plaster has set on the cast, remove the wax

pattern and trim the matrix so that none of it overlaps the prepared teeth (Fig 26-50). The edge of the matrix should be about 1.0 mm below the occlusal edge of the pontic.

With the wax pattern on the cast, close the articulator and reproduce all functional mandibular movements to test opposing cusp relationships. The occlusal surface is developed by the placement of cones and ridges, as are utilized for the waxing of any occlusal surface (Fig 26-51). If the fixed partial denture is to be cast as two pieces with assembly following after try-in, saw through the larger connector with a piece of 3-0 suture silk (Fig 26-52). Finish the margins on the U-shaped die (Fig 26-53).

Investing and Casting. Attach a 10-gauge hollow plastic sprue to a nonfunctional cusp of each of the fixed partial denture retainer wax patterns. Place one sprue on each of the pontic nonfunctional cusps (Fig 26-54). Connect the free ends of the multiple sprues with sticky wax. Remove the wax pattern from the die by grasping the facial and lingual surfaces of the pontic wax pattern between the thumb and forefinger (Fig 26-55). *Do not* use

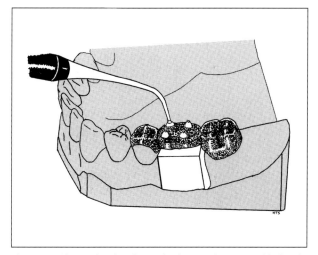

Fig 26-51 The occlusal surface is built up with a wax-added technique.

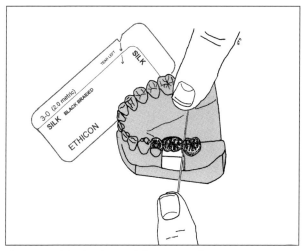

Fig 26-52 If the fixed partial denture is to be cast in two pieces, 3-0 suture silk can be used to saw through the connector.

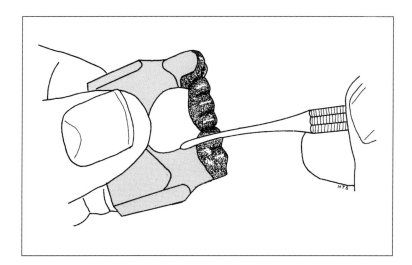

Fig 26-53 The margins are finished on the U-shaped die with a beavertail burnisher.

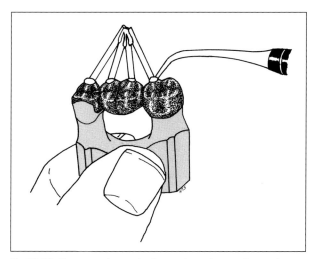

Fig 26-54 One sprue is attached to each retainer and to each cusp of the pontic.

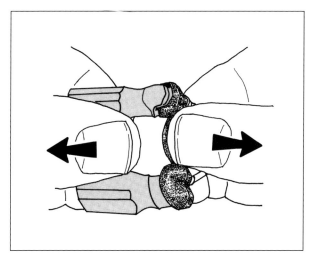

Fig 26-55 The pattern is removed by grasping the facial and lingual surfaces of the pontic.

501

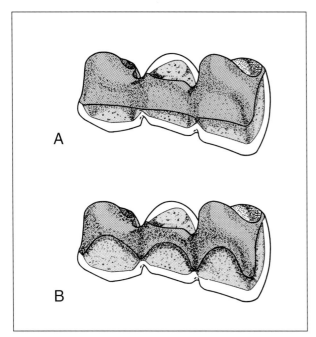

Fig 26-56 The unveneered metal strip extending from retainer to retainer on the lingual surface of a metal-ceramic fixed partial denture is straight across at the incisal aspect (A). If occlusion requires the metal strip to be narrower, the connectors can be bolstered by increasing the length of the struts incisally (B).

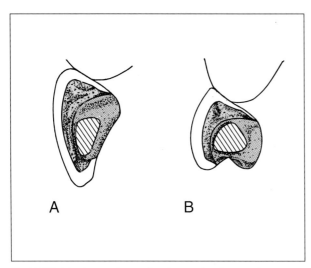

Fig 26-57 Metal-ceramic pontics: A, anterior; B, posterior.

the sprue as a handle to loosen the pattern from the die. Carefully take the wax pattern by the sprue between the thumb and forefinger of the left hand. The tips of the fingers should support the pattern without distorting it. Attach the sprues to the crucible former. Do not try to hold the pattern by the proximal surfaces.

Invest and cast the fixed partial denture wax pattern in the usual manner. Remember to use more casting alloy than would be used for crowns, since the pontic is solid. After the casting is retrieved from the investment, scrub it clean. Cut off the sprues and finish the casting. Remove the plaster matrix from the working cast and place the casting on the working cast. It is now ready for try-in.

Metal-Ceramic Fixed Partial Dentures

Metal frameworks or copings for metal-ceramic fixed partial dentures should be constructed with these requirements in mind: (1) there must be an adequate bulk of metal to insure rigidity for strength and (2) porcelain should be of nearly equal thickness throughout to avoid the possibility of weakening the porcelain through uneven stress concentrations. To meet these requirements, there should be a continuous strip of exposed metal on the lingual surface, extending from the metal portion of one retainer, across the lingual of the pontic, to the metal portion of the other retainer.

The incisal configuration of the lingual aspect of the coping may be straight, if occlusion permits (Fig 26-56, A), or scalloped (Fig 26-56, B).[51] The scalloped or "trestle" design is indicated when the connector is diminished in its faciolingual dimension to allow for the porcelain in the embrasures. By increasing the height of the strut incisogingivally, the strength of the connector will increase.[52] This provides a bulk of metal for rigidity in the connector areas between the pontic and the respective retainers; if soldering should be necessary, it provides adequate metal for a strong solder joint.

Porcelain coverage of the retainers is the same as that for single units, except in the area adjacent to the pontic. The porcelain veneer on the pontic is continuous with the porcelain veneering of the retainers. It covers the incisal portion of the lingual surface, the labial surface, and the entire area adjacent to or contacting the ridge. Porcelain terminates against the metal on the lingual surface, about 1.0 mm incisal to the ridge (Fig 26-57). Porcelain tissue contact allows for better esthetics and removes the potentially rough porcelain-metal junction from contact with the tissue, where it could cause irritation.[53]

The metal coping on the underside or gingival aspect of the pontic follows the same contours that the porcelain will, rather than being just a straight bar of metal between the retainer copings. This makes the pontic esthetically similar to the retainers in the gingival area and provides support for the porcelain. The tissue contact of the porcelain should be a modified ridge lap on the facial aspect of the ridge. There must be no saddle contact.

An exception to the recommended porcelain coverage on the gingival aspect of a pontic occurs in those situations where an all-porcelain occlusal surface is used and the occlusogingival space is limited. To ensure rigid support for the porcelain, the gingival aspect of the pontic should remain in metal, with the porcelain-metal junction located on the gingivofacial aspect of the pontic.

An attempt at producing an esthetic posterior fixed partial denture will require the use of all-porcelain occlusal surfaces, especially in the mandibular arch, since only the occlusal aspect of premolars and molars is seen, if, in fact, any part is seen. Any time that an all-porcelain occlusal surface is used on a pontic, a judgment must be made regarding the occlusogingival thickness of the metal in the pontic. To insure adequate rigidity, the undersurface of the pontic may have to be metal to compensate for the metal removed from the occlusal (Fig 26-58).

Fixed Partial Denture Coping Wax Pattern. Portions of any metal-ceramic fixed partial denture will remain unveneered and, in the posterior region, unveneered metal may constitute the majority of the surface area of the fixed partial denture. To produce a continuous contour between metal and porcelain and to provide a uniform thickness of porcelain, it is important to fabricate the wax pattern to full contour and then cut it back.

Fabricate copings on the lubricated die of the abutment preparations with a no. 7 wax spatula. Trim the excess from the margins and transfer the copings to the working cast. Form the axial contours facially, lingually, and interproximally. On posterior teeth, develop the occlusion in the usual manner (see Chapter 19).

Cut off a short section of a stick of blue inlay wax and heat one end of it in a Bunsen burner flame until the wax has been softened. Place the piece of wax into the edentulous space on the cast, pressing the softened end against the lubricated edentulous ridge. When the wax has hardened, flow wax into the interproximal areas to attach it to the retainer wax pattern on either side of it. Using wax addition and carving, produce the desired axial contours in the pontic.

Check the alignment of the pontic in a mesiodistal direction to prevent any "leaning" (Fig 26-59). Remember

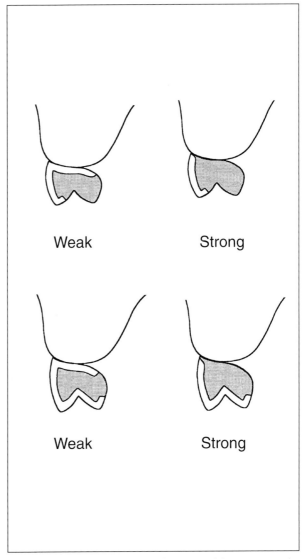

Fig 26-58 A pontic with a short occlusogingival dimension may be too weak with a ceramic ridge contact *(upper left);* it could be strengthened by changing the ridge contact to metal *(upper right).* A pontic may be weakened by covering the occlusal surface with porcelain *(lower left).* The loss of metal bulk can be compensated by using a metal ridge contact *(lower right).*

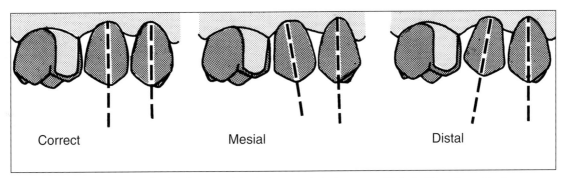

Fig 26-59 The mesiodistal inclination of the facing must be in harmony with that of the adjacent teeth.

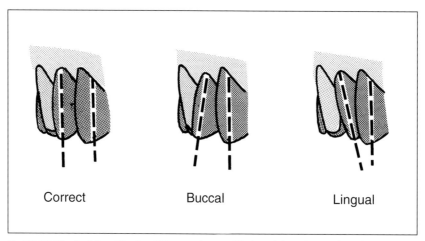

Correct   Buccal   Lingual

Fig 26-60 The facial profile should be consistent with that of the other teeth in the quadrant.

also to check the alignment of the occlusal two-thirds of the facial surface to make sure that it is in harmony with the facial surfaces of the other teeth in the arch (Fig 26-60).

Remove the assembled wax pattern to carve the tissue side of the pontic to produce the desired open embrasures in the mesiogingival, distogingival, and linguogingival aspects. In the appearance zone, the pontic should be a modified ridge lap design. When completed, duplicate the full-contour wax pattern with a resilient impression putty material, such as condensation silicone. This impression can be poured to produce a stone cast, providing a visual guide to the desired contours, or it can be sectioned horizontally to allow assessment of the amount and contours of the cutback.

Replace the pattern on the working cast and sketch the outline of the area to be veneered with a no. 25 blade in a laboratory knife (Fig 26-61). Place the mark as far to the lingual as possible in the interproximal areas. Remove the fixed partial denture wax pattern from the working cast and place it on the single-piece die of the abutment preparation. Use a discoid carver to place a groove adjacent to the outline of the boundaries of the veneering area. Place the groove just buccal to the proximal contact on a pattern for a posterior tooth so that the contact will be on metal. On a pattern for an anterior tooth, place the groove lingual to the contact so that the contact will be on porcelain.

Use a discoid carver to place grooves on the facial surface of the pontic and on any retainers that are to be veneered (Fig 26-62). These grooves should be 0.7 to 1.0 mm deep. With grooves it is possible to gauge the depth of the wax that will be removed from the veneering area to make room for porcelain. A similar groove is placed on the lingual surface of the pontic to mark the linguogingival porcelain-metal junction line (Fig 26-63).

Use a sharp no. 25 blade to remove the bulk of wax left between the grooves (Fig 26-64). Leave a 1-mm-wide collar of wax at the gingival margin to insure an adequate bulk to be invested and cast accurately. The collar will be thinned markedly after casting. Use the discoid carver to blend in all cuts made near the porcelain-metal junction line (Fig 26-65).

The cutback of the pontic should follow the general contours of the original full-contour wax-up, with a bulk of wax underlying the cusp tip and gingival tip of the pontic so that the porcelain which will ultimately be placed over those contours will be supported by metal (Fig 26-66, A). On maxillary posterior teeth, be sure that there is a ledge of smoothly contoured wax underlying the eventual location of the buccal cusp tips on both the pontic and retainers (Fig 26-66, B).

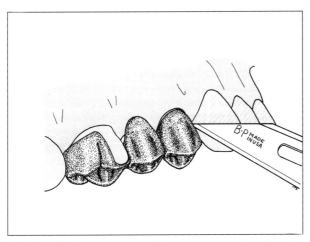

Fig 26-61 Proximal extensions of the porcelain-metal junction line are marked on the wax pattern with a knife tip.

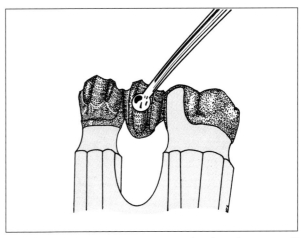

Fig 26-62 Orientation grooves are cut with a discoid carver on all surfaces of the retainer and pontic that are to be veneered.

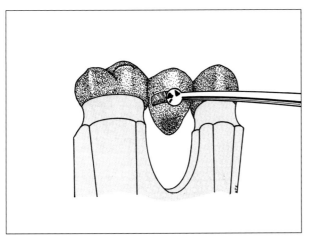

Fig 26-63 An orientation groove is carved along the location of the linguogingival porcelain-metal junction line on the pontic.

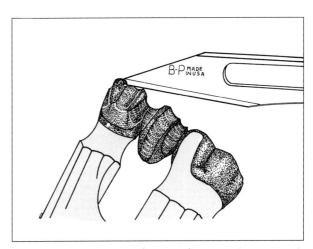

Fig 26-64 Wax remaining between the orientation grooves is removed with a sharp knife.

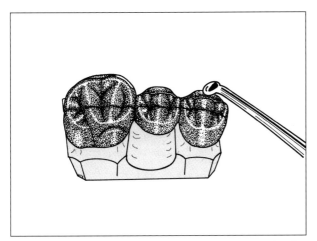

Fig 26-65 The porcelain-metal junction line is accentuated with a discoid carver.

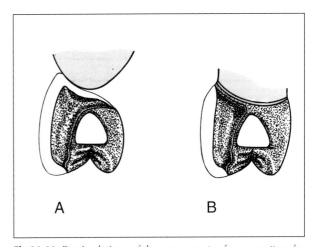

Fig 26-66 Proximal views of the components of a wax pattern for a maxillary posterior metal-ceramic fixed partial denture: A, the pontic; B, the retainer.

There should not be any sharp angles in the area to be veneered. The porcelain-metal junction line should have the configuration of a deep chamfer with a crisp 90-degree angle in the wax pattern at the porcelain-metal junction. Smooth the veneering area with a cotton pellet dipped in die lubricant. Wash off the excess and blow dry. Place the pattern of the fixed partial denture on the working cast and carefully inspect the area to be veneered from the facial (Fig 26-67, A), the occlusal (Fig 26-67, B), and the lingual (Fig 26-67, C) aspects. Be sure that all angles which will be covered with porcelain are rounded, all contours are smoothed, and all aspects of the porcelain-metal junction line are sharply defined. Return the pattern to the freshly lubricated die and readapt the margins. Prepare the pattern for investing by attaching the sprues (see Chapter 21).

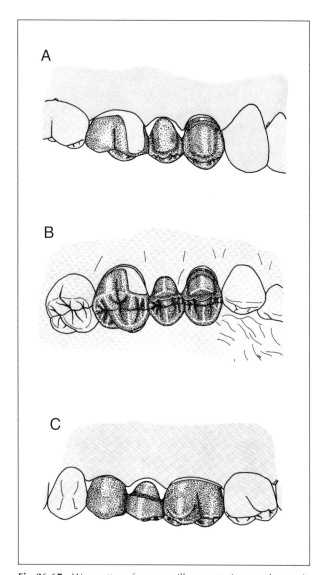

Fig 26-67 Wax pattern for a maxillary posterior metal-ceramic fixed partial denture from the facial (A), the occlusal (B), and the lingual (C) aspects.

References

1. Parkinson CF, Schaberg TV: Pontic design of posterior fixed partial prostheses: Is it a microbial misadventure? *J Prosthet Dent* 1984; 51:51–54.

2. Stein RS. Pontic-residual ridge relationship: A research report. *J Prosthet Dent* 1966; 16:251–285.

3. Henry PJ, Johnston JF, Mitchell DF: Tissue changes beneath fixed partial dentures. *J Prosthet Dent* 1966; 16:937–947.

4. Podshadley AG: Gingival response to pontics. *J Prosthet Dent* 1968; 19:51–57.

5. Smith DE, Potter HR: The pontic in fixed bridgework. *Dent Digest* 1937; 43:16–20.

6. Klaffenbach AO: Biomechanical restoration and maintenance of the permanent first molar space. *J Am Dent Assoc* 1952; 45:633–644.

7. Boyd HR: Pontics in fixed partial dentures. *J Prosthet Dent* 1955; 5:55–64.

8. Harmon CB. Pontic design. *J Prosthet Dent* 1958; 8:496–503.

9. Cavazos E: Tissue response to fixed partial denture pontics. *J Prosthet Dent* 1968; 20:143–153.

10. Eissmann HF, Radke RA, Noble WH: Physiologic design criteria for fixed dental restorations. *Dent Clin North Am* 1971; 15:543–568.

11. Johnson GH, Leary JM: Pontic design and localized ridge augmentation in fixed partial denture design. *Dent Clin North Am* 1992; 36:591–605.

12. Schield HW: The influence of bridge pontics on oral health. *J Mich Dent Assoc* 1968; 50:143–147.

13. Reynolds JM: Abutment selection for fixed prosthodontics. *J Prosthet Dent* 1968; 19:483–488.

14. Hirshberg SM: The relationship of oral hygiene to embrasure and pontic design—A preliminary study. *J Prosthet Dent* 1972; 27:26–38.

15. Tjan AH: Biologic pontic designs. *Gen Dent* 1983; 31:40–44.

16. Johnston JF: Pontic form and bridge design: A new survey (Part I). *Ill Dent J* 1956; 25:272–279.

17. Roid GH, Wilson LG, Grenfell J, Ueno H: *Bridging the Gap: An Instructional Program in Pontic Design.* Monmouth, OR Teaching Research, 1973, p 16.

18. Silness J, Gustavsen F, Mangernes K: The relationship between pontic hygiene and mucosal inflammation in fixed bridge recipients. *J Periodont Res* 1982; 17:434–439.

19. Tripodakis A-P, Constantinides A: Tissue response under hyperpressure from convex pontics. *Int J Periodont Rest Dent* 1990; 10:408–414.

20. Becker CM, Kaldahl WB: Current theories of crown contour, margin placement and pontic design. *J Prosthet Dent* 1981; 45:268–277.

21. Clayton JA, Green E: Roughness of pontic materials and dental plaque. *J Prosthet Dent* 1970; 23:407–411.

22. Ante JH: Construction of pontics. *J Can Dent Assoc* 1936; 2:482–486.

23. Tjan AHL: A sanitary "arc-fixed partial denture": Concept and technique of pontic design. *J Prosthet Dent* 1983; 50:338–341.

24. Yamashita A: Practical construction procedure for a new type of bridge pontic. *Quintessence Int* 1985; 16:743–753.

25. Garber DA, Rosenberg ES: The edentulous ridge in fixed prosthodontics. *Compend Contin Educ Dent* 1981; 2:212–224.

26. Perel ML: A modified sanitary pontic. *J Prosthet Dent* 1972; 28:589–592.

27. Hood JA: Stress and deflection of three different pontic designs. *J Prosthet Dent* 1975; 33:54–59.

28. Tinker ET: Sanitary dummies. *Dent Rev* 1918; 32:401–408.

29. Dobson NJ: The value of porcelain in artificial root insertion. *Dent Cosmos* 1921; 63:247–248.

30. Budde CC: Porcelain baked roots in fixed bridgework. *J Am Dent Assoc* 1928; 15:1914–1916.

31. Bowles RO: Fixed bridges with special reference to tissue contact pontics and inlay abutments. *J Am Dent Assoc* 1931; 18:1521–1537.

32. Dewey KW, Zugsmith R: An experimental study of tissue reactions about porcelain roots. *J Dent Res* 1931; 13:459–472.

33. Boyd I IR: Pontics in fixed partial dentures. *J Prosthet Dent* 1955; 5:55–64.

34. Shooshan ED: The reverse pin-porcelain facing. *J Prosthet Dent* 1959; 9:284–301.

35. Faucher RR: A system for localizing pontics. *J Prosthet Dent* 1984; 52:643–647.

36. Seibert JS: Reconstruction of deformed, partially edentulous ridge, using full thickness onlay grafts. Part I. Technique and wound healing. *Compend Contin Educ Dent* 1983; 4:437–453.

37. Hawkins CH, Sterrett JD, Murphy HJ, Thomas JC: Ridge contour related to esthetics and function. *J Prosthet Dent* 1991; 66:165–168.

38. Abrams H, Kopczyk RA, Kaplan AL: Incidence of anterior ridge deformities in partially edentulous patients. *J Prosthet Dent* 1987; 57:191–194.

39. Behrend DA: The mandibular posterior fixed partial denture. *J Prosthet Dent* 1977; 37:622–638.

40. Behrend DA: The design of multiple pontics. *J Prosthet Dent* 1981; 46:634–638.

41. Schregle M: Firing of gingiva-colored ceramic powders. *Quintessence Dent Technol* 1981; 3:245–252.

42. Vryonis P: Esthetics and function in multiple unit bridges. *Quintessence Dent Technol* 1981; 3:237–241.

43. Porter CB: Anterior pontic design: A logical progression. *J Prosthet Dent* 1984; 51:774–776.

44. Crispin BJ: Tissue response to posterior denture base-type pontics. *J Prosthet Dent* 1979; 42:257–261.

45. Siebert JS, Cohen DW: Periodontal considerations in preparation for fixed and removable prosthodontics. *Dent Clin North Am* 1987; 31:529–555.

46. Siebert JS, Nyman S: Localized ridge augmentation in dogs: A pilot study using membranes and hydroxyapatite. *J Periodontol* 1990; 61:157–165.

47. Kaldahl WB, Tussing GJ, Wentz FM, Walker JA: Achieving an esthetic appearance with fixed prosthesis by submucosal grafts. *J Am Dent Assoc* 1982; 104:449–452.

48. Langer B, Calagna L: The subepithelial connective tissue graft. *J Prosthet Dent* 1980; 44:363–367.

49. Siebert JS: Ridge augmentation to enhance esthetics in fixed prosthetic treatment. *Compend Contin Educ Dent* 1991; 12:548–560.

50. Orth CF: A modification of the connective tissue graft procedure for the treatment of type II and type III ridge deformities. *Int J Periodont Rest Dent* 1996; 16:267–277.

51. Stein RS, Kuwata M: A dentist and a dental technologist analyze current ceramo-metal procedures. *Dent Clin North Am* 1977; 21:729–749.

52. Miller LL: Framework design in ceramo-metal restorations. *Dent Clin North Am* 1977; 21:699–716.

53. Hobo S, Shillingburg HT: Porcelain fused to metal: Tooth preparations and coping design. *J Prosthet Dent* 1973; 30:28–36.

Chapter 27

Solder Joints and Other Connectors

Soldering is the joining of metal components by a filler metal, or solder, which is fused to each of the parts being joined. Strictly speaking, if the filler metal has a melting temperature greater than 450°C (840°F), the process is *brazing*.[1] The term soldering, as commonly used in dentistry, will be used in this chapter. Bonding is contingent on *wetting* of the joined surfaces by the solder, and not on melting of the metal components. When a solder joint is done properly, there should be no fusion or alteration of the two components joined.[2] Soldering differs in that respect from welding, another means of joining metals. In fusion welding, the pieces that are joined are melted or fused together, without solder.

Solder can be used for *joining,* as in the fabrication of a fixed partial denture, or it can be used for *building,* as when an addition is made to the proximal surface of a crown. Cleanliness is the prime prerequisite of soldering,[3] inasmuch as the soldering process depends on wetting of the surface to achieve bonding. Corrosion products, such as oxides and sulfides, that are present as a result of the casting process or that occur on the surface of metals when they are heated, interfere with bonding.

Flux is placed on the surfaces to be soldered before they are heated. Fluxes may provide surface protection, reduce oxides, or dissolve oxides.[1] Flux is displaced by solder, which then can form an interface with and bond to the surface being soldered. Soldering fluxes for noble metals are based on borate compounds. They form low-fusing glasses that protect the metal surface, and they also reduce oxides such as copper oxide. They often are too fluid for preceramic soldering.[1] Fluorides are used on base metal alloys to dissolve the stable oxides of chromium, cobalt, and nickel. In addition to acting as solvents, these fluxes also serve a protective role.[1]

Flux is more easily applied if it is in paste form. While a flux paste can be made with alcohol, the most popular form for use with noble metal alloys employs petrolatum as a vehicle, since it is more easily handled. It keeps air from the flux, and when heated, the petrolatum burns off without leaving any residue. Fluxes made from common borax, or pastes made with water, tend to effloresce when they are heated, producing pits in the solder joint.

Antiflux is a material used to outline the area to be soldered in order to restrict the flow of solder. The most common antiflux is the mark of a soft graphite pencil, which works best on surfaces that do not have a high polish. Polishing rouge (iron oxide) suspended in chloroform can also be painted around the area of the solder joint to prevent undesired spread of the solder.

Gold solders are classified by fineness and by carat. *Fineness* refers to parts per thousand of the solder that is gold. For example, a 600 fine solder would be 600 parts gold per 1,000, or 60% gold. When used to designate a casting alloy, carat refers to parts per 24 of a metal that are gold. As an example, an alloy that is 18 K is 18 parts gold per 24, or 75% gold. When used with solder, however, carat has a different meaning. A solder that is designated as 18 K does *not* have a 75% content of gold. Instead, the 18 K designation means that it was formulated to be used with 18 K casting alloys. The actual noble-metal content of the solder would be given by its fineness rather than by its carat. The higher the fineness of a solder, the higher will be its melting range and the greater its corrosion resistance. While a solder with a lower fineness has a lower melting range, it also has poorer flow characteristics.[3]

Dental solder should be[4]:

1. *Corrosion resistant.* Restorations, such as fixed partial dentures, which are permanently placed in the mouth require the use of a solder of high fineness to resist corrosion. The minimum fineness that should be used is 580 fine, and a higher number would be better for preventing tarnish and discoloration.

2. *Lower fusing than alloy.* The solder should possess a fusion temperature that is about 60°C (100 to 150°F) below that of the metal being soldered.[3]

3. *Nonpitting.* Pitting in solder is not desirable. More pitting occurs when there is an increased amount of base metal in the solder, which may vaporize when the gap between the components is too narrow or when the solder is overheated.

4. *Strong.* Solder should be as strong as the alloy with

which it is used. The hardness of the solder decreases as the fineness (gold content) increases.

5. *Free-flowing.* The solder should flow freely. Silver in the solder tends to make it adhere to metal and to flow more freely. Copper, on the other hand, makes it more sluggish. Solders that melt at higher temperatures have a lower surface tension and flow easily through narrow gaps. Low-fusing solders flow poorly through narrow gaps.[5]

6. *Same color.* The color of the solder should match that of the alloy being soldered.

As is the case with many aspects of dentistry and life in general, soldering is much more complicated today than it was a relatively few years ago. Crowns and fixed partial dentures were made of a gold alloy, solders were gold, fluxes were borates, and, at least from a dental perspective, it was a fairly simple process. With the nearly 1,500 alloys available for use in dentistry today, a dentist cannot be proficient in every aspect of soldering.

However, soldering is still not in the exclusive domain of the dental laboratory. There are occasions when being able to solder in the office can be a great convenience for dentist and patient alike. An otherwise acceptable gold restoration may not have an adequate proximal contact. Adding that proximal contact is a simple procedure that can and should be done in the office. It usually does not require investing.

If a fixed partial denture must be sectioned because it does not seat completely, or if it was constructed in segments for intraoral try-in, the dentist must at least be able to index the components to insure that the technician who does the actual soldering will have an accurate starting point. The components that are to be joined with solder must be stabilized in soldering investment to maintain the exact relationship throughout the soldering process.

The soldering procedures to be considered are:

• Gold alloy fixed partial denture soldering
• Adding proximal contact
• Repairing casting voids
• Breaking solder joints
• Preveneer metal-ceramic alloy soldering
• Postveneer metal-ceramic alloy soldering

Gold Alloy Fixed Partial Denture Soldering

There are two ways in which a three-unit fixed partial denture can be fabricated. It can be made as a single casting, with the pontic wax pattern attached to that of each of the retainers. The fixed partial denture may be cast as two units, with the pontic wax pattern attached to that of one of the retainers and cast with it. The two units are then assembled by soldering.

Single-Piece Casting

Certainly it is possible to achieve an accurately fitting fixed partial denture by use of a single-piece casting.[6] If this is to be attempted, a one-piece die in which the abutment preparations have not been separated from each other offers the greatest accuracy. (Refer to Chapter 26 for a discussion of this type of die.) To achieve maximum accuracy, the wax pattern should be invested in a large-diameter casting ring (60 mm or larger) to assure uniform expansion.[7] Either a round or an oval casting ring can be used. Both investment expansion and pattern distortion can affect the accuracy of multiunit castings.[8] There is less pattern distortion when investment is allowed to bench set rather than using the hygroscopic technique.[8]

As the length of a single-piece fixed partial denture casting increases, so does its inaccuracy.[9–11] Distortion is three-dimensional, as though the pattern has elongated and twisted. Schiffleger et al found the discrepancies greatest at the mesiogingival aspect of the anterior retainer and the distolingual aspect of the posterior retainer.[11] Four- and five-unit fixed partial dentures joined by soldering have better-fitting margins than do one-piece castings of the same length.[12] Any fixed partial denture larger than three units should still be cast in two pieces and soldered.[13]

A single-piece casting must be tried in the mouth with an awareness of some of the problems inherent in the technique. The single-piece casting offers no opportunity to verify the fit of the individual retainers. In an effort to make a nonfitting casting seat, there is a tendency to relieve the internal surfaces of the retainers so drastically that all retention is lost. In that event, the fixed partial denture cannot be saved even if it is later separated, indexed, and soldered. If the fixed partial denture will not seat totally after routine adjustments have been made, use a thin (0.009 inch or 0.23 mm) separating disc (Ultra Thin Abrasive Disks, Dedeco International, Long Eddy, NY) to cut through one connector and then try the separate pieces of the fixed partial denture back in the mouth.

Indexing

A two-piece casting can be used to fabricate a fixed partial denture with a solid pontic, such as a hygienic. The technique described is used for soldering three-unit posterior fixed partial dentures. The pontic is cast with the smaller retainer. Then the retainer-pontic unit is soldered to the larger retainer, utilizing an index of the relationship of the fixed partial denture components in the patient's mouth. This provides for the most accurate relationship between the retainers and between each retainer and its abutment tooth.

The index must accurately maintain that relationship until the parts of the fixed partial denture have been embedded in soldering investment. Numerous materials have been described for transferring the relationship of

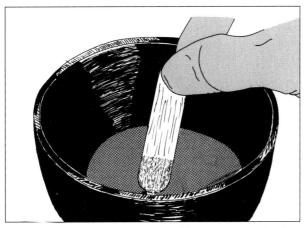

Fig 27-1 The tongue depressor is soaked before using it to hold the plaster index.

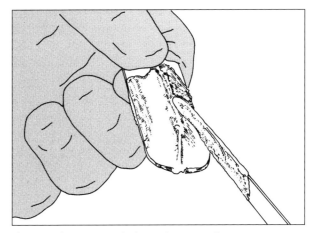

Fig 27-2 Plaster is troweled onto the tongue depressor to create a ridge that extends from one end of the index to the other.

the fixed partial denture components from mouth to laboratory bench: plaster,[14–16] sticky wax,[3,17] autopolymerizing acrylic resin (Duralay),[18] 4-META adhesive resin,[19] and zinc oxide–eugenol,[20] which has been shown to be a highly accurate material for indexing.[20]

If plaster is used, the most accurate and consistent results will be obtained if the castings are not removed from the index prior to investing.[21] Resin indices (Duralay, Reliance Dental Manufacturing Co, Worth, IL) are as accurate as those made of plaster if the components are separated from and reseated in the plaster. However, excess bulk of a resin index will diminish accuracy because of additional polymerization shrinkage.[22]

Armamentarium

1. Plaster bowl, spatula
2. Impression plaster
3. Bite registration paste, mixing pad
4. Index tray or tongue blade
5. Petrolatum
6. Laboratory knife with no. 25 blade
7. PKT (Thomas) waxing instruments: no. 1, no. 2
8. Straight handpiece, no. 8 round bur
9. Explorer
10. Sticky wax, utility wax, boxing wax
11. Soldering investment
12. Vibrator
13. No. 2 pencil
14. Fisher burner, matches
15. Tripod, screen
16. Solder (650 fine), soldering flux
17. Blowpipe, casting tongs
18. Toothbrush

Remove the provisional restoration from the patient's mouth and make certain that there are no traces of temporary cement left on the tooth preparations. Try in the single retainer first and then the retainer-pontic combina-

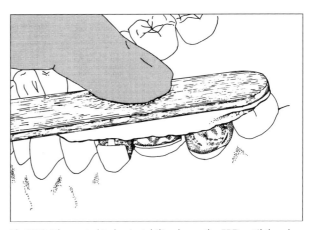

Fig 27-3 The seated index is stabilized over the FPD until the plaster sets.

tion. On the first try-in for each, do not leave the other unit in place. Verify the marginal fit of each retainer first. Make sure that there is a small gap between the pontic and the retainer to which it has not yet been soldered.

Adjust the occlusion with green stones or other appropriate abrasives. Perform preliminary finishing procedures on the retainer margins, if they are accessible. Smooth off the occlusal surface with a rubber sulci disk. The rough surface left on the casting by a green stone could create problems in seating the castings into the index. Do not polish the castings at this point, since polishing rouge is iron oxide, a specific antiflux for soldering.

Mix a small amount of fast-setting impression plaster. Place it on a plastic index tray (Index Tray, Crown Enterprises, Oklahoma City, OK) or a thoroughly wet tongue depressor (Fig 27-1). Arrange the index material on the carrier so that a sharp ridge of material runs the length of the depressor (Fig 27-2) or tray. This ridge facilitates getting index material into the central grooves of the casting. Carefully position the index on the occlusal surface of the castings, vibrating it gently as you seat it (Fig 27-3).

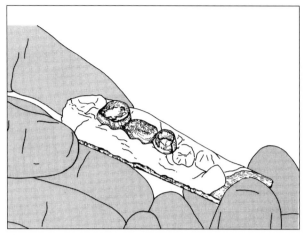

Fig 27-4 Plaster index with components trapped in it.

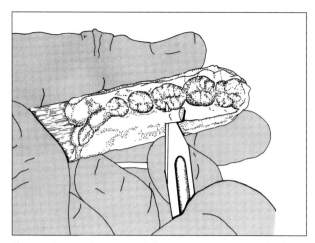

Fig 27-5 Excess plaster around the FPD imprint is trimmed off with a sharp knife.

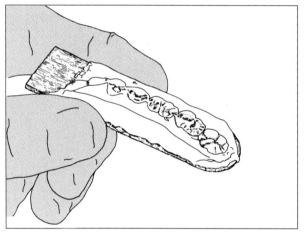

Fig 27-6 The trimmed index exhibits shallow imprints of the FPD components.

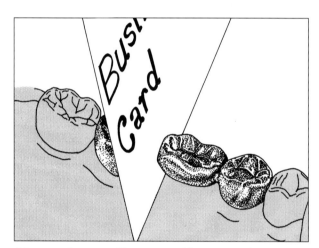

FFig 27-7 The gap width is measured by passing a business card through it.

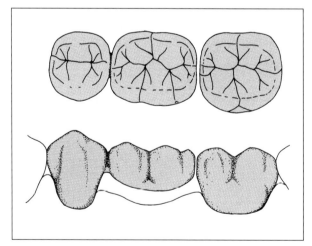

Fig 27-8 When the two surfaces to be soldered are parallel, there is less likelihood of distortion. Occlusal view *(top)* and facial view *(bottom)*.

When the material has set, remove the index. If the castings come out with it, so much the better (Fig 27-4). A plaster index is most accurate when the crowns stay in it.[21] Carefully trim it with a laboratory knife with a no. 25 blade so that all margins are exposed by at least 1.0 mm (Fig 27-5). The index should extend at least 3.0 mm mesially and distally past the crowns being soldered. This guarantees a symmetric, uniform bulk of investment surrounding the units to be soldered and should minimize distortion.[15] The plaster index should be approximately 6 mm (0.25 inch) thick.

If the crowns separate from the index when it is removed from the cast, trim off excess that might prevent the castings from seating completely back into the imprints. Trim the area around the imprints enough so that a substantial part of the axial walls will be covered by investment (Fig 27-6). Then clean the index thoroughly with compressed air. The slightest bit of debris between the index and crown will keep the crown from seating in the index and will make the relationship inaccurate. Scrub the occlusal surfaces of the crowns and clean them in the ultrasonic cleaner before repositioning them in the index. Place the index on the bench and carefully try the castings in their respective imprints.

If the castings touch, there is a likelihood of increased distortion.[3,14,23] For this reason, it has been suggested that there be a gap of at least 0.005 inch (0.13 mm) between the pontic and the retainer.[3,14] A conflict arises in determining the proper gap dimension for a solder joint. The wider the solder joint gap, the stronger the joint, apparently because there is less porosity in the joint.[13] Therefore, a gap width of 0.012 inch (0.30 mm) is recommended for strength.

In another study, however, it was determined that increased gap width produces an increase in distortion. A gap width of 0.006 inch (0.15 mm) is recommended for greatest accuracy.[24] Obviously there is a need for some compromise. A gap width of 0.008 inch (0.20 mm) would appear to be optimum, since it is intermediate between the narrow, undistorted joint and the wide, strong joint. Indeed, some investigators have used this distance as a standard.[25] Furthermore, it can be determined easily by inserting a business card into the gap (Fig 27-7), since the average card is 0.008 inch thick.

The opposing surfaces of the retainer and pontic on either side of the solder joint should parallel each other (Fig 27-8). If these surfaces diverge, the resulting wedge shape of the solder joint may produce distortion.[26] In addition, wherever there is contact, there will not be space for the solder and there will be no bonding. On the other hand, if the gap is too wide, it will be harder to solder, since capillary action is more difficult to achieve. As a result, solder will be more likely to stick to one surface or the other, instead of filling the gap and adhering to both surfaces.

Investing

Pontics and retainers that have come off the index should be luted back on the index with sticky wax. It is often necessary to use a no. 8 round bur to cut a small "well" on the facial and lingual edges of each imprint in the index (Fig 27-9). This permits space for a bulk of sticky wax without forcing it over the margins. Separate the tongue depressor from the index if they have not already come apart. Use a cast trimmer to remove excess from the edge of the index, leaving approximately 3.0 mm all around the perimeter (Fig 27-10). Allow the index to dry, and apply sticky wax to each casting using the PKT no. 1 instrument (Fig 27-11). Do not allow the sticky wax to cover occlusal margins (if any) on the facial surfaces.

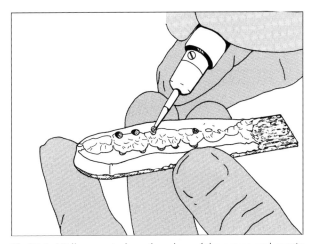

Fig 27-9 Wells are cut along the edges of the crown and pontic imprints to provide space for sticky wax.

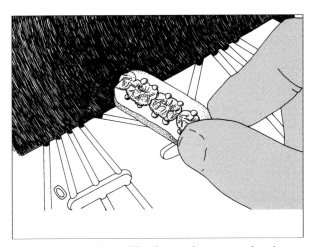

Fig 27-10 The periphery of the plaster index is trimmed on the cast trimmer so that there will be a 3.0-mm apron around the imprint of the FPD.

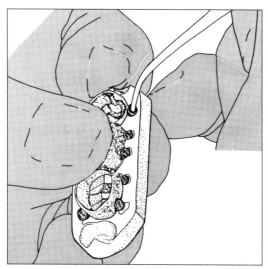

Fig 27-11 Sticky wax is used in the wells to attach the FPD to the index.

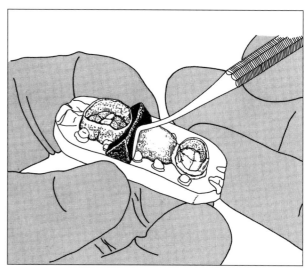

Fig 27-12 A triangular-shaped piece of utility wax is extended facially and lingually from the solder joint area. There must be no gaps.

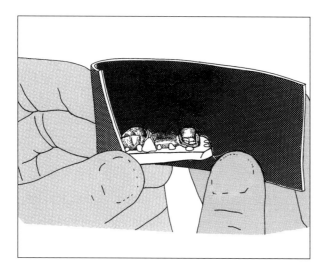

Fig 27-13 A strip of boxing wax 2.5 cm (1.0 inch) wide is wrapped around the index.

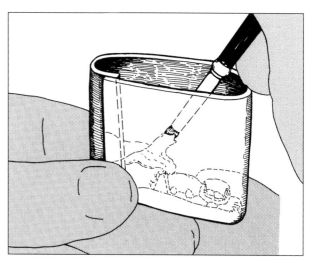

Fig 27-14 Investment is brushed into the retainers.

Flow utility wax into the joint with a PKT no. 2 instrument to prevent the joint area from being filled with investment. The waxed area should be slightly larger than the solder joint will be. Any margin covered by wax at this point will not be covered by soldering investment. This could cause the margin to melt when heated by the blowpipe during soldering. Run a triangular-shaped extension of utility wax from the lingual side of the solder joint area of the index (Fig 27-12). There should be a slightly smaller one on the facial. These wax wedges will be narrower in the solder joint area than at the edge of the index. Check again to make sure that the castings are completely seated.

A separating medium (Super-Sep, Kerr Dental Manufacturing Co, Romulus, MI) may be painted over the index outside the castings to insure easy separation later. Place boxing wax around the index (Fig 27-13). There should be 3.0 mm of space between the castings and the boxing wax. Mix a small amount of soldering investment (Soldering Investment, Whip Mix Corp, Louisville, KY) . Paint it into the castings and carefully vibrate it into the boxed area (Fig 27-14). Hold the index so that there is a finger between it and the vibrator. Overzealous vibrating could jar one of the castings loose.

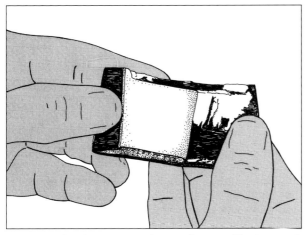

Fig 27-15 After the investment has set, the strip of boxing wax is removed from the index.

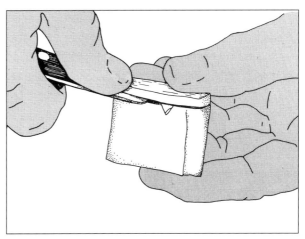

Fig 27-16 The index is pried loose from the block of investment.

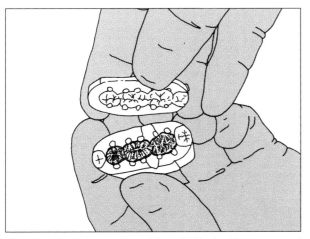

Fig 27-17 The index is separated from the block of investment and inspected.

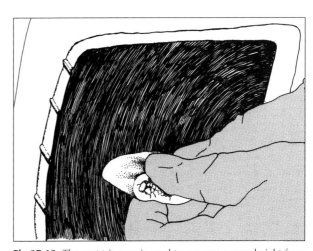

Fig 27-18 The cast trimmer is used to remove excess height from the block of investment.

Allow the investment to set for 1 hour and then remove the boxing wax (Fig 27-15). Run hot water over the investment and index to soften the sticky wax. Separate the index and the investment with a heavy laboratory knife (Fig 27-16). Inspect the block of investment containing the fixed partial denture castings (Fig 27-17). The investment should measure 2.5 cm (1.0 inch thick) top to bottom. If it is more, trim off the excess from the bottom on a cast trimmer (Fig 27-18). Use a laboratory knife with a no. 25 blade to cut a V-shaped notch buccal and lingual to the solder joint (Fig 27-19).

The wax extension placed on the lingual earlier will facilitate this step. The lingual notch is larger than the facial, because the solder will be fed into the joint area from the lingual. The facial notch is necessary to gain access for heating the castings during soldering. If either of these notches is not placed, an incomplete solder joint is likely to result. Flush out the remaining wax with boiling water

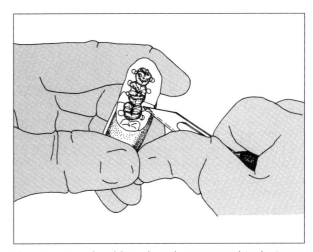

Fig 27-19 Buccal and lingual notches are carved in the investment.

515

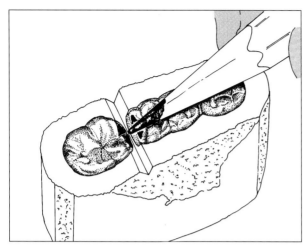

Fig 27-20 Pencil marks are used as an antiflux on the occlusal surface of the castings.

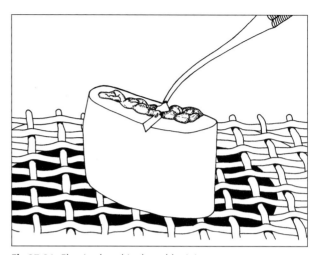

Fig 27-21 Flux is placed in the solder joint area.

from a boil-out tank. Use a no. 2 pencil to draw a heavy line across the marginal ridges adjacent to the solder joint area (Fig 27-20). This will act as an antiflux and will prevent solder from flowing onto the occlusal surfaces.

While the castings are still warm, add flux paste with an explorer (Fig 27-21). It will melt, and capillary action will draw it through the entire solder joint. If flux is applied later when the castings are hot, it will bubble up and stick where it is applied rather than flowing into the joint where it is needed. Also, surface oxidation may occur before the protective flux is applied.

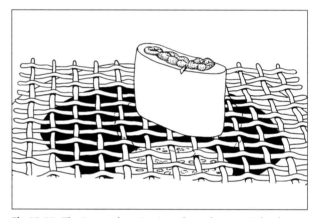

Fig 27-22 The invested casting is preheated over a Fisher burner for 10 to 15 minutes.

Soldering

The invested castings should be preheated to insure even heating. If the castings are not preheated, the uneven heat distribution that will occur when the blowpipe is applied to a cold block may produce distortion of the finished joint.[14,23] The investment block can be placed in an oven and brought from room temperature to 815°C (1,500°F).[17] In an alternative method of preheating the invested castings, they are set on a tripod and screen over a Fisher burner. Continue to preheat the castings for 10 to 15 minutes (Fig 27-22).

Begin heating with the blowpipe, and brush the flame over the entire investment block repeatedly until it is so hot that the castings glow red when the flame is held on them for 2 or 3 seconds (Fig 27-23). Leave the burner on throughout this process. Wedge two or three pieces of solder, 2 × 3 mm, covered with flux, into the lingual embrasure of the joint area (Fig 27-24). They will be melted by the heat of the castings, and not by the blowpipe. If too much solder is used, it may run onto the occlusal surface, and a larger bulk of solder is more likely to produce distortion.

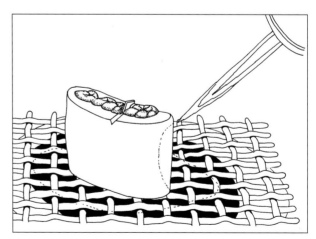

Fig 27-23 The flame is directed against the investment from all sides until it glows if the flame is left in one place for a few seconds.

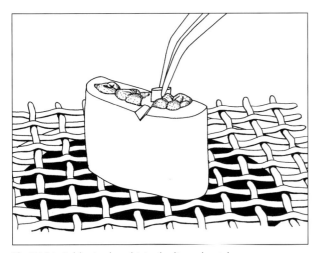

Fig 27-24 Solder is placed into the lingual notch.

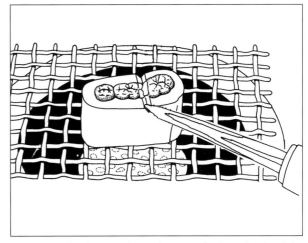

Fig 27-25 The flame is directed against the buccal side of the investment and into the buccal notch when the block is hot enough for soldering.

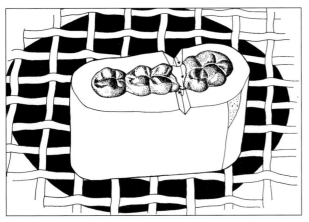

Fig 27-26 When the solder in the joint appears to "roll," the flame is taken away.

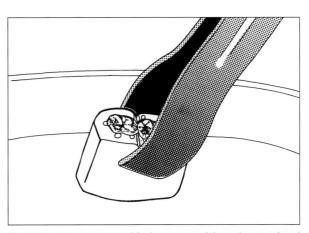

Fig 27-27 The investment block is removed from the tripod and put in a casting well.

If the blowpipe is used to melt the solder directly, the following difficulties can be expected: the solder will "ball up" and not flow at all, or it will not flow through the entire joint.

Aim the blowpipe obliquely at the investment, since an obliquely directed flame results in more even heating and less distortion.[14] Concentrate the tip of the blue cone on the buccal side of the block near the open space between retainer and pontic (Fig 27-25). The solder on the lingual side of the castings will flow toward the source of heat on the facial. When the solder starts to flow, direct the torch into the buccal notch and keep it there while the solder flows through the joint. Leave the flame there a few seconds longer while the solder shimmers and appears to "roll" in the joint. Turn off the flame (Fig 27-26).

Remove the investment block from the tripod with casting tongs and place it someplace where there is no chance of someone picking it up and getting burned.

The bottom of a casting well is good for this purpose (Fig 27-27). If you must place it on a benchtop, select an area where there is little traffic and be sure the surface is heat resistant. Leave a conspicuous sign to warn off "lab lizards" who wander around picking up other people's work. Do not quench immediately. Quenching shortly after soldering will produce thermal stresses that will result in distortion.[26]

On the other hand, allowing the investment block to cool slowly to room temperature may produce excessive recrystallization and grain growth.[3] The resulting solder joint will be weaker. If the invested fixed partial denture is allowed to bench cool for 5 minutes and is then quenched, distortion should be minimized. This allows time for the gold and solder to respond to an ordering heat treatment, which will increase hardness and strength while reducing elongation.

Place the invested block in water and remove the

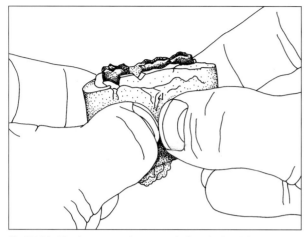

Fig 27-28 The investment is removed after placing it in water.

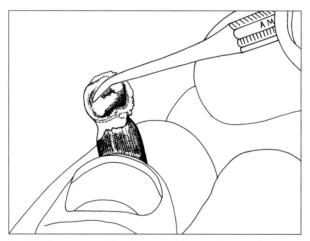

Fig 27-29 Any remaining investment is picked out with a sharp instrument.

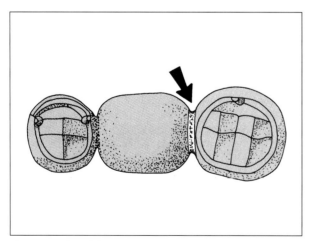

Fig 27-30 The solder joint *(arrow)* is inspected for size and completeness.

investment (Fig 27-28). That which does not flake off should be picked off with a sharp instrument and an old toothbrush (Fig 27-29). Examine the solder joint to make sure that it is pit free. Evaluate its size (Fig 27-30). If it is too bulky, it can be trimmed down with a carborundum disc. Inadequate bulk or the presence of pits requires reinvestment and resoldering. Air abrade the castings with 50 μm aluminum oxide. The fixed partial denture is ready to be finished and tried in the patient's mouth.

Adding Proximal Contacts

The addition of solder to a proximal contact area is done to build up a contour that may be deficient for any number of reasons. It can easily be done freehand on a single restoration. A fixed partial denture must be invested before the addition.

Armamentarium

1. Straight handpiece
2. 5/8-inch Burlew disc
3. Bunsen burner, matches
4. No. 2 pencil
5. Locking soldering pliers
6. Solder (650 fine), soldering flux

Finish the proximal area to be soldered with a Burlew disc. Outline the interproximal surface to be soldered with a no. 2 pencil. The area to be soldered must be wider than the contact. It should extend across the entire proximal surface, just apical to the marginal ridge. The periphery of this new bulk will be blended into the contours of the crown, rather than being a pimple on the side of the crown. A 1.5-cm-long piece of ceramic ring lining material can be rolled and packed into the restoration, leaving some to overlap the crown margins.[27] This step will be of greater benefit for smaller crowns.

Bend one tip of a pair of locking soldering pliers so that a crown can be held by its axial wall without the pliers touching the margin (Fig 27-31). Grasp the crown with the locking soldering pliers. The bent beak should be inside the casting, and there should be no contact at any other point (Fig 27-32). Wrap a wet paper towel around the handle of the soldering pliers.

Warm the casting slightly and place a small drop of soldering flux on the contact to be soldered, staying within the pencil outline. Dip a 2 × 4-mm piece of solder (± depending on the size of the casting) into the flux. Place the solder on the proximal surface (Fig 27-33). Holding the soldering pliers with the wet towel, place the casting over the burner, keeping the casting in the blue reducing tip of the flame (Fig 27-34). Keep it there until the casting glows a bright red, allowing the solder to melt and adapt itself to the casting.

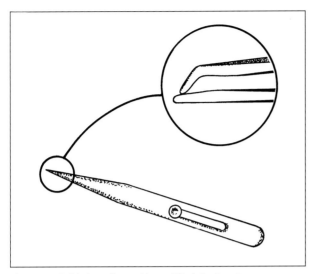

Fig 27-31 Soldering pliers with modified tip *(inset)*.

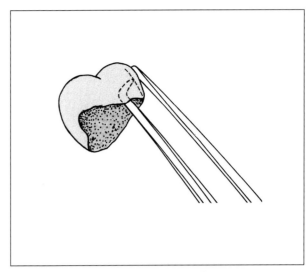

Fig 27-32 Holding crown with soldering pliers.

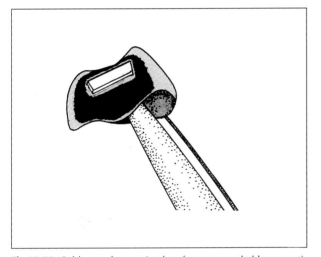

Fig 27-33 Solder on the proximal surface surrounded by an anti-flux (pencil mark).

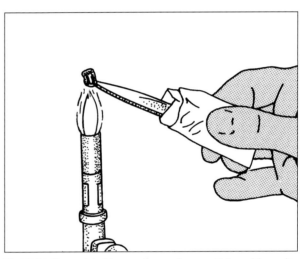

Fig 27-34 Crown is held over a burner flame until the solder melts.

Remove the casting from the flame. Allow a gold alloy casting to cool until the metal loses its glow and then quench it in water. Air abrade it with 50 μm aluminum oxide. If the casting is made of a base metal alloy, allow it to cool for at least 5 minutes before quenching it. Clean it with aluminum oxide abrasive. Then finish it to the proper contour and return it to the mouth for final adjustment of the contact area.

Repairing Casting Voids

There are some deficiencies in casting that can be repaired by soldering. "Blow holes" or voids extending all the way through a casting on an axial surface, or pits that do not extend all the way through, are candidates for solder repairs. Solder should not be used to repair:

1. *Deficient margins.* It is impossible to get an acceptably adapted margin by adding solder.
2. *Occlusal holes.* Holes in the occlusal surface cannot be successfully soldered because of the risk of solder running over the entire surface. Aside from the technique difficulties, the presence of a hole on the occlusal surface of a crown is usually symptomatic of inadequate occlusal reduction in the preparation.

Efforts to "patch" poor castings of this variety result in a compromise at best (and more often in a casting that is still poor). Inordinate amounts of time can be expended to salvage a restoration of questionable value when that same time could have been spent in remaking it properly. A remake is never a satisfying effort, but as Forrest Gump said, "It happens."

Armamentarium

1. Straight handpiece, no. 2 round bur
2. Bunsen burner, tripod, and screen
3. Matches
4. No. 2 pencil
5. Locking soldering pliers
6. Solder (650 fine), soldering flux
7. Platinum foil
8. PKT (Thomas) instrument (no. 1)
9. Sticky wax
10. Blowpipe, casting tongs

To repair a pit, outline the area around it with a no. 2 pencil. Grasp the crown with the modified locking soldering pliers, the handle of which is wrapped in a wet paper towel. Warm the casting slightly and put a dab of flux into the pit. Stick a corner of a triangular-shaped piece of solder, 1 × 2 mm, into the pit. Hold the casting over the Bunsen burner until the solder flows, remove it from the flame, let it cool, and then quench it. Air abrade it with 50 μm aluminum oxide, wash it, and finish down the newly soldered area.

To repair a hole that extends all the way through a crown, mark the die through the hole with a very fine lead. Remove the casting and place a small piece of platinum foil over the mark on the die. Reseat the crown over the foil and apply a bead of sticky wax to the hole with a PKT no. 1. When it has cooled, remove the casting from the die. The small piece of foil should be stuck to the inside of the casting. It will serve as a matrix over which the solder can flow. Fill the casting with investment and set it down in a small patty of investment.

When the investment has set, pick off the bead of sticky wax over the hole to be repaired. Antiflux the area around the hole with a no. 2 pencil. Place the casting on a tripod and warm it slightly. Apply a small amount of flux to the hole and the foil visible through the hole. Continue heating the casting and add a square of solder slightly larger than the hole. Heat the casting, not the solder. When the solder flows, remove the flame. Put the invested casting in a casting well or on a heat-safe benchtop. If it is a gold casting, wait 2 or 3 minutes to quench. Then air abrade it with 50 μm aluminum oxide. Wash the casting and finish the outward-facing surface of the axial wall. The platinum foil will be stuck to the inside of the casting. If it is left there, it will prevent the casting from seating completely. Use a no. 2 round bur to remove it.

Breaking Solder Joints

It is sometimes necessary to break a previously soldered fixed partial denture. The most common reason for this is the failure of the soldered fixed partial denture to fit the abutment teeth. The following technique will work on a soldered type III gold fixed partial denture. It cannot be used on prostheses with ceramic or resin veneers.

Armamentarium

1. Bunsen burner, matches
2. Locking soldering pliers
3. Paper towel
4. No. 7 wax spatula
5. Straight handpiece, carborundum disc on mandrel

Place a wadded-up wet paper towel on the bench next to the Bunsen burner. Grasp the fixed partial denture by the pontic with locking soldering pliers whose handle has been wrapped with a wet paper towel. Be careful not to contact the margins with the pliers. Contrary to the principles of soldering, in this situation the joint is heated directly. Hold the solder joint to be unsoldered directly at the tip of the blue cone of the Bunsen burner. When the solder starts to get glossy, quickly move the fixed partial denture over the wet paper towel. While holding the fixed partial denture about 0.5 inch above the table, tap the crown next to the melted joint. If the joint was heated sufficiently, the crown will fall off.

Clean the parts of a gold fixed partial denture by aluminum oxide air abrasion. Normally, some solder will remain on each of the parts. Grind off all of this solder with a carborundum disc and finish the surfaces with a Burlew disc before resoldering.

Soldering Metal-Ceramic Alloys

Although an effort is made to fabricate metal-ceramic fixed partial dentures as a single unit, it is sometimes necessary to solder the units together. This may occur if: *(1)* there is distortion in a single-piece fixed partial denture casting; *(2)* one retainer has inadequate margins and must be redone; *(3)* the fixed partial denture length is too great for an accurate single-piece casting; or *(4)* type III partial veneer retainers are used in an otherwise metal-ceramic fixed partial denture.

If all units of the fixed partial denture requiring soldering are of a metal-ceramic alloy, the fixed partial denture may be assembled in one of two ways. *Preveneer soldering* uses a high-fusing solder that is melted by torch before porcelain is added. Preceramic pontic soldering allows a diagonal joint through the middle of a pontic (Fig

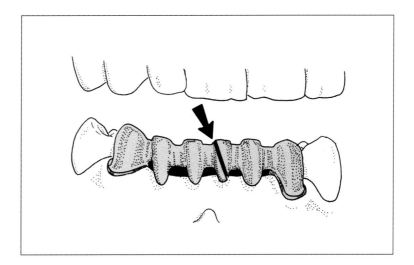

Fig 27-35 The diagonal cut across the left central incisor *(arrow)* provides more surface area for greater strength of the solder joint than would an interproximal joint.

27-35),[25] which produces stronger joints than soldering in the interproximal connector area,[28] and it is technically easier.[29] In *postveneer soldering,* a low-fusing solder is melted in the oven after porcelain has been baked on the fixed partial denture. Postceramic soldering compensates for any tooth movement in the mouth between final impression and restoration and it eliminates the significance of any distortion that might occur during porcelain firing.

If the fixed partial denture includes a type III gold alloy retainer, it can be assembled only by postveneer soldering. The high temperatures reached during the porcelain firing cycle would melt the type III gold alloy if it were soldered to the fixed partial denture before the porcelain had been added.

For many years, soldering was done with a gas-air blowpipe. With the development of metal-ceramic restorations, a need for oven soldering developed. Oven-soldered postveneer solder joints are at least as strong as torch-soldered preveneer solder joints,[30] and several investigators found the postveneer joints to be stronger.[13,31–33] Certainly, postveneer soldering does present special problems. Soldering investment, flux, and solder must be kept from contacting the porcelain to prevent discoloration or fracture of the porcelain.

In recent years a third method of soldering has been developed that utilizes an infrared soldering machine (JM Ney Co, Bloomfield, CT). The device focuses a concentrated beam of infrared energy from a tungsten iodine lamp that operates at 3,400°C in a closed chamber under a controlled atmosphere. No apparent differences in porosity and strength have been found between torch-soldered and infrared-soldered joints,[34,35] although infrared soldering has been found to require more time than torch soldering.[34]

Preveneer Metal-Ceramic Alloy Soldering

Although some investigators have found postveneer to be stronger than preveneer solder joints,[13,31–33] preveneer soldering remains more popular with ceramists. This is because postveneer soldering takes more time, skill, and attention to detail to keep the investment, flux, and solder from touching porcelain. When it does, there may be "greening" or crazing of the porcelain, which in turn can require the reapplication of porcelain and resoldering.

The apparent superiority of the postveneer solder joints also may be offset by the fact that unlike the standardized joint size in the laboratory studies, clinical postveneer joints frequently are smaller because of the ceramist's fear of causing damage to the ceramic by contacting it with solder.

The example demonstrated here is of a six-unit metal-ceramic fixed partial denture (FPD) with two retainers at one end, fabricated as a five-unit FPD (canine to lateral incisor) with the second retainer, a canine, made separately to facilitate margination of the proximal surfaces of the contiguous retainers (Fig 27-36). These restorations should be fabricated so that there will be parallel surfaces in the solder joint area, with adequate separation for a solder joint with optimum strength and minimum distortion (Fig 27-37).

To accurately transfer the segments to be joined to the laboratory bench, tack them together with an autopolymerizing acrylic resin (Duralay) index (Fig 27-38). Place monomer and polymer in separate Dappen dishes or medicine cups. Make sure that the segments of the FPD are completely seated and stable in the mouth. If one is not stable, hold it down with a finger. Dry the area with compressed air and isolate it with cotton rolls. Use a disposable brush to apply a few drops of monomer between the two retainers. Then dip the brush in polymer and

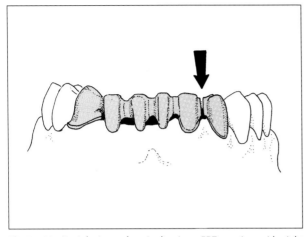

Fig 27-36 Facial view of a single-piece FPD casting with right canine and left lateral incisor retainers and an as yet unattached left canine retainer. Arrow marks area to be soldered.

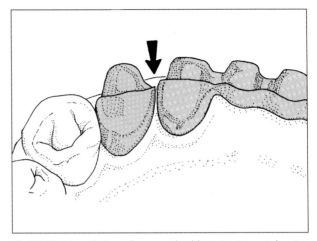

Fig 27-37 Lingual view of proposed solder joint *(arrow)* showing separation and alignment of surfaces to be joined.

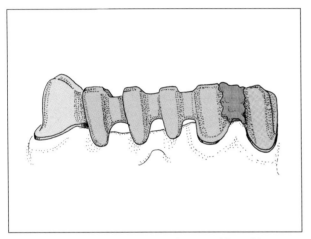

Fig 27-38 Facial view: Crowns to be joined by soldering are attached with autopolymerizing acrylic resin (Duralay).

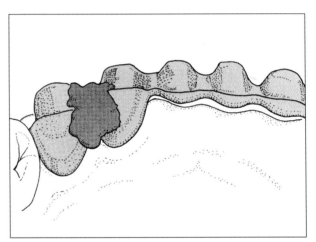

Fig 27-39 Lingual view of resin index between the canine and lateral incisor retainers.

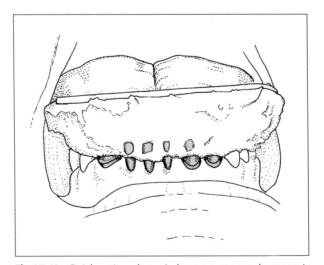

Fig 27-40 Quick-setting plaster index on a tongue depressor is shown in place in the mouth.

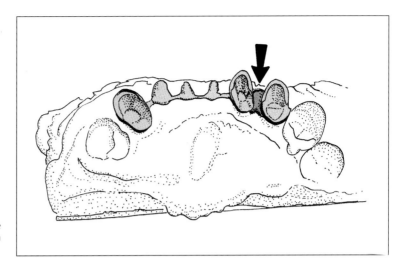

Fig 27-41 Inverted view of the FPD embedded in the plaster index after removal from the mouth. Resin index is indicated by arrow.

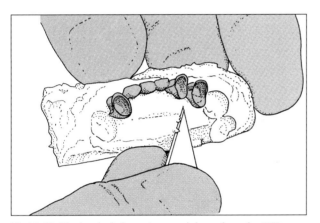

Fig 27-42 The level of plaster is carved down from the FPD.

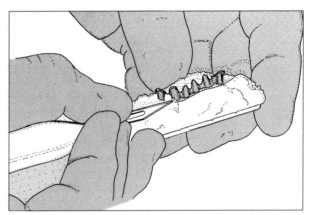

Fig 27-43 Each pontic and retainer is carefully cut around.

apply a small amount of powder to the joint. Continue alternating small quantities of liquid and powder, making sure that the material between the retainers is always wet. Build the index so that it extends onto adjacent surfaces of the two retainers (Fig 27-39).

Make a backup plaster index on a tongue depressor. Mix quick-setting plaster and place it on a wet depressor, creating a ridge of plaster that extends the length of the tongue depressor. Apply it to the teeth while the plaster is still fluid. If any cracks appear in the plaster, remove the material, wash the FPD thoroughly, and remake the index. Hold the index until the plaster is completely set (Fig 27-40). If left untended, it could shift or slip, necessitating a remake. Remove the index along the path of insertion of the abutment preparations. Examine it thoroughly to see if the components are securely embedded (Fig 27-41).

Carve the surface of the index surrounding the FPD, exposing the pontics and retainers (Fig 27-42). Very carefully expose each pontic and retainer (Fig 27-43).

Cut around, but do not disturb the resin. If the components are still firmly embedded in the plaster, they can be left there and invested from the plaster index using the technique previously described. The resin will serve as a filler in the solder joint.

Those who are more experienced at soldering may prefer to lift the components from the plaster. If the resin remains intact, mix some investment (Hi-Heat Soldering Investment, Whip Mix Corp) and gently vibrate it into the retainers (Fig 27-44). Use your fingers as a cushion between the vibrator and the FPD components. Place a quantity of investment large enough to contain the FPD on a ceramic or hard resin tile (Fig 27-45).

Invert the framework, whose retainers are filled with investment, and place it into the top of the soft mound of investment (Fig 27-46). With light finger pressure, partially submerge the luted-together castings into the investment. The incisal half of the castings (approximately) should protrude from the investment. Add a little investment over the units that will not be directly involved in sol-

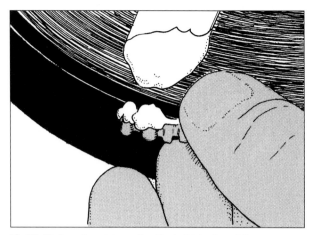

Fig 27-44 Investment is gently vibrated into the retainers.

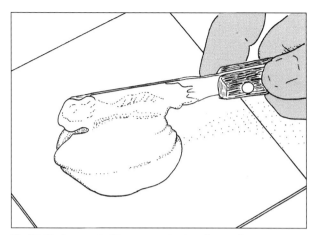

Fig 27-45 A mound of investment is placed on a tile.

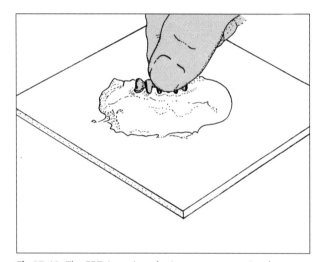

Fig 27-46 The FPD is set into the investment, margins down.

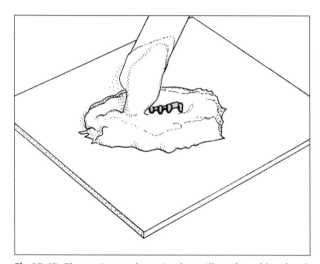

Fig 27-47 The retainer and pontics that will not be soldered with investment are covered.

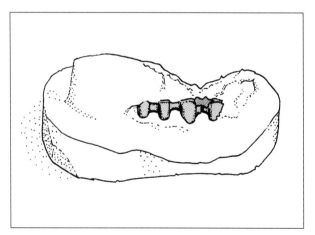

Fig 27-48 The edge of the block is trimmed to produce an even bulk of investment.

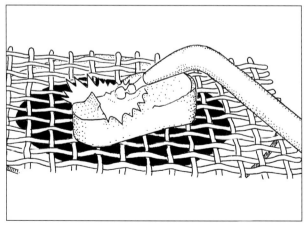

Fig 27-49 The flame is directed against the lingual surface of the block of investment.

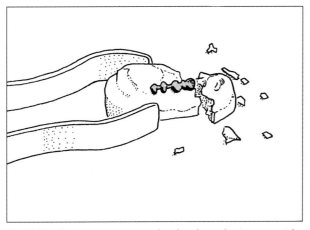

Fig 27-50 Casting tongs are used to break up the investment by tapping it on a benchtop.

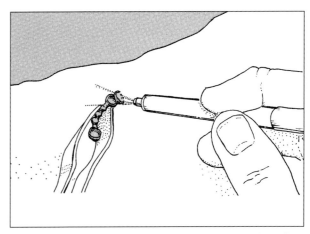

Fig 27-51 The casting is air abraded with aluminum oxide to clean the casting surface.

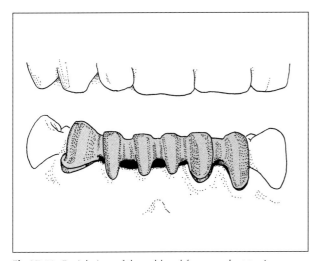

Fig 27-52 Facial view of the soldered framework at try-in.

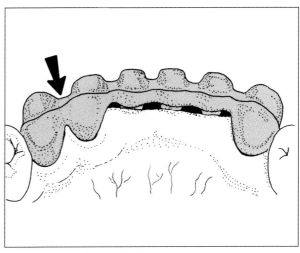

Fig 27-53 Lingual view of soldered area *(arrow)*.

dering (Fig 27-47). Allow the investment to set hard. When it does, trim the periphery to produce a near-even bulk of investment around the castings (Fig 27-48).

Preheat the invested castings in a burnout furnace at 650 to 815°C (1,200 to 1,500°F, depending on availability of furnaces). When the invested block has reached the desired temperature, use casting tongs to transfer it to the wire mesh or some other area that will not be damaged by flame. Several 2 × 3-mm pieces of solder can be laid in the lingual notch, or a strip of solder in a hemostat can be fed into the embrasure after it gets hot. The solder used is Olympic Pre-Solder (JF Jelenko, Armonk, NY), whose melting range is 1,050 to 1,150°C (1,922 to 2,100°F). Brush the investment with a gas-oxygen flame until the block glows if the flame is held in one spot for a few seconds. Hold the flame on the lingual surface of the block of investment (Fig 27-49). Then direct the torch into

the lingual notch as solder is fed into the facial notch. Heat will draw the solder through the joint area.

Remove the soldered FPD from the tripod and place it in a casting well or some other safe place where someone will not be able to touch it and be burned. When it has cooled to room temperature, break the investment by picking it up with casting tongs and tapping it on the bottom of a casting well or a heat-resistant benchtop (Fig 27-50). Retrieve the FPD from among the bits of soldering investment and clean it up. Air abrade the surface with 50 μm aluminum oxide (Fig 27-51).

When the restoration is tried in (Fig 27-52), all margins should be closed without any special force needing to be applied anywhere. Check for any encroachment on the interdental papilla on the facial or especially on the lingual aspect (Fig 27-53). If there is any, remove the restoration from the mouth and relieve the affected area.

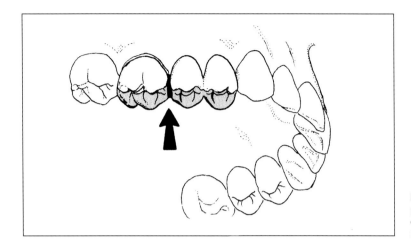

Fig 27-54 Three-unit maxillary metal-ceramic fixed partial denture. The arrow marks the area to be soldered between the premolar pontic and the molar retainer.

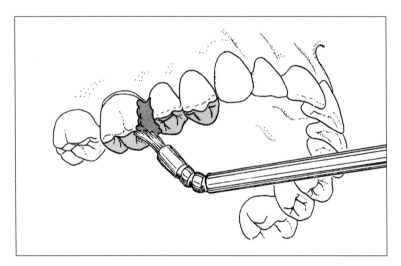

Fig 27-55 A disposable brush is used to apply monomer and polymer between the retainer and the pontic.

Postveneer Metal-Ceramic Alloy Soldering

The technique that follows is for the soldering of a gold-palladium alloy (Olympia, JF Jelenko). Both preveneer and postveneer soldering produce a stronger joint in Olympia than was possible previously in Jelenko "O."[36] All phases of the porcelain addition, including glazing, must be completed before the soldering process. The solder (Alboro LF [low fusing], JF Jelenko) has a melting range of 710 to 740°C (1,310 to 1,370°F), and it is used with M20-129 flux (Vident, Brea, CA).

Try the units in the mouth and make whatever adjustments are necessary. This technique is often employed without prior intent; ie, a fixed partial denture is carried to completion in expectation of cementing it without any type of try-in, only to find that it does not seat. The best joint esthetically, strengthwise, or both, is selected for separation, using a very thin (0.009 in or 0.23 mm) disk (Ultra-Thin Abrasive Disks, Dedeco, International).

Remove the FPD from the mouth. Cut the joint using the disk on a lathe. This allows the use of both hands to hold the FPD, and the disk remains steady, which definitely would not be the case if it were in a hand-held handpiece. These disks are very easily broken. After separation of the two parts of the prosthesis, try the retainers in the mouth to see if they fit individually. If they do, continue with the soldering procedure. A soldering index can be made of quick-setting impression plaster, resin, or zinc oxide–eugenol bite registration paste as previously described.

Finish those areas of the crown that are to be soldered with extra-fine sandpaper discs. Use no rouge or polishing compounds. Outline the area to be soldered with a no. 2 pencil, which will serve as an antiflux. Reseat the components of the fixed partial denture in the mouth (Fig 27-54). With the two parts of the FPD firmly seated, pour monomer and polymer into separate containers. Dry the

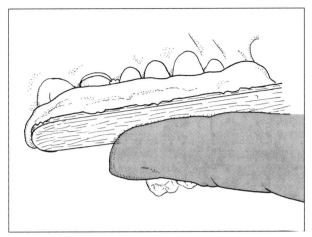

Fig 27-56 A tongue depressor is used to support a plaster index.

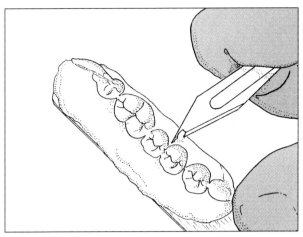

Fig 27-57 A flat surface with shallow imprints is carved on the index.

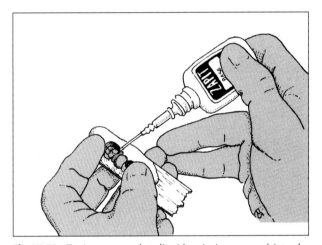

Fig 27-58 Zapit cyanoacrylate liquid resin is squeezed into the joint.

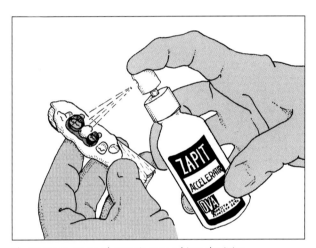

Fig 27-59 Zapit accelerator is sprayed into the joint.

area with compressed air and isolate it with cotton rolls. Use a disposable brush to apply monomer between the retainer and the pontic.

Next dip the brush in polymer and apply a small amount to the joint. Continue alternating small quantities of liquid and powder, making sure that the material between the retainer and the pontic is always wet. Build the index so that it extends onto adjacent surfaces of the two castings (Fig 27-55).

Fabricate a secondary plaster index on a tongue depressor. Arrange quick-setting plaster on a wet depressor, making a ridge of plaster that extends the length of the tongue depressor. Apply it to the teeth while the plaster is fluid. Stabilize the index until the plaster is completely set (Fig 27-56). Remove the index along the path of insertion of the abutment preparations.

Carve the surface of the index around the FPD components, creating a flat surface with shallow imprints (Fig 27-57). Rearrange the parts of the FPD on the plaster index. If the resin index has come loose, make sure that it is back in place between segments of the FPD, without any spaces. Squeeze a cyanoacrylate liquid resin (Zapit, Dental Ventures of America, Anaheim Hills, CA) in and around the joint while holding the parts securely (Fig 27-58). Then spray the Zapit accelerator over the joint (Fig 27-59). Zapit is the material of choice when indexing on a cast in the laboratory, but it should not be used in the oral cavity because its safety has not been proven.[22] Duralay is the material of choice for use in the mouth.[22]

To prevent investment from contaminating the ceramic veneer covering much of the fixed partial denture, place a 1.0-mm-thick layer of ivory wax over the gingival one-half to two-thirds of the facial surfaces of the retainers and pontic (Fig 27-60). The wax for this step and those following should overlap the metal by 1.0 mm. Turn the restoration over and apply a coat of wax to the gingival and lingual aspects of the pontic (Fig 27-61). Be sure to apply wax to any exposed ceramic that is part of a porce-

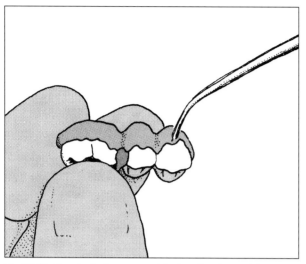

Fig 27-60 The gingival segment of the facial surfaces of the FPD is covered with 1.0-mm-thick wax.

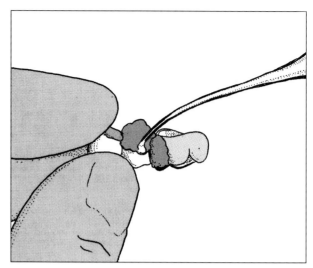

Fig 27-61 The gingival of the pontic is covered with wax.

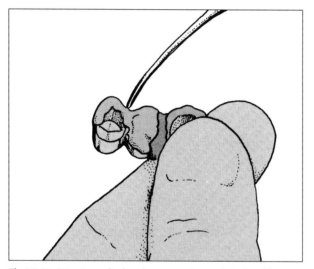

Fig 27-62 Wax is applied to the exposed porcelain shoulder.

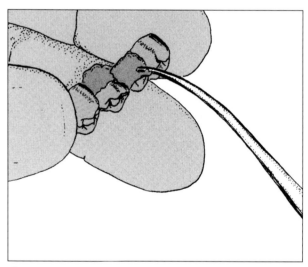

Fig 27-63 Wax is added to the joint area to increase access for solder.

lain shoulder (Fig 27-62). Add wax to the joint area to insure access for the solder after the restoration has been invested (Fig 27-63).

Mix a small amount of soldering investment and carefully vibrate it into the crowns (Fig 27-64). Be sure that the metal-ceramic crowns are filled completely with investment, since this is the major support for the crowns in the block. Avoid vibrating the castings directly to prevent the crowns from being loosened. Build a mound of investment on a flat surface (Fig 27-65) and set the inverted FPD, margins first, into the investment (Fig 27-66). Push up a ridge of investment with a spatula to cover most of the lingual surfaces of the retainers and pontic (Fig 27-67).

When the investment has set, trim it to within 3.0 mm of the castings. Create a wide bevel around the entire

periphery of the invested block with a laboratory knife equipped with a no. 25 blade (Fig 27-68). Then carve a V-shaped notch on the lingual aspect to insure adequate access to the solder joint (Fig 27-69). Flush out the wax with boiling water. When the FPD was embedded in investment, the wax prevented contact between investment and porcelain (Fig 27-70). After the wax has been removed, there is a space surrounding the porcelain, including any all-porcelain shoulders (Fig 27-71).

Place the invested castings in front of a porcelain oven to warm slowly for 10 minutes. Open the muffle of the oven (≈540°C or 1,000°F) and warm the castings for 5 more minutes.

Add a couple of 2 × 3-mm pieces of fluxed solder to the solder joint, making sure that they contact only the

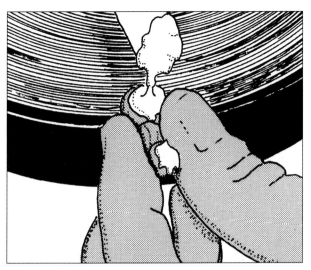

Fig 27-64 Crowns are filled with soldering investment.

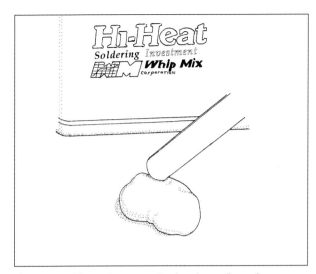

Fig 27-65 Soldering investment is placed on a flat surface.

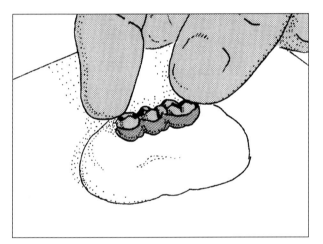

Fig 27-66 The FPD is put into the investment.

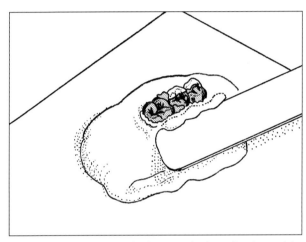

Fig 27-67 Investment is pushed up over the lingual surfaces of the FPD.

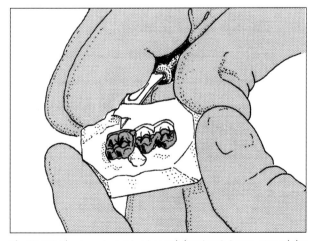

Fig 27-68 The investment is trimmed, leaving 3.0 mm around the castings. The entire block is beveled.

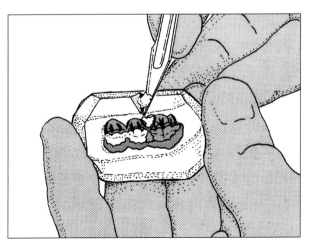

Fig 27-69 A V-shaped notch is carved on the lingual.

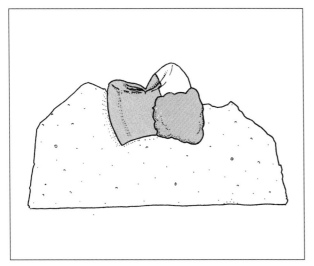

Fig 27-70 The wax layer separates the investment and porcelain.

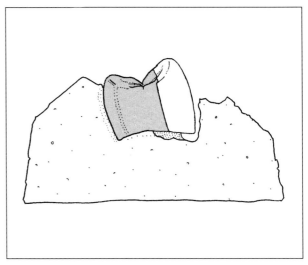

Fig 27-71 After wax removal, a space between porcelain and investment protects the porcelain.

metal framework of the fixed partial denture. Place the castings in the oven, turn on the vacuum, and raise the temperature to 815°C (1,500°F) at the rate of 42°C (75°F) per minute. Check the castings for completion of soldering. If the solder has not yet fused, continue raising the temperature in the oven until it reaches 870°C (1,600°F). The final temperature used will vary with different solders. Be sure to use the solder recommended by the manufacturer for the specific alloy being used.

Break the vacuum and remove the invested fixed partial denture from the oven. Allow the casting to cool to room temperature. The castings cannot be quenched, as the porcelain may fracture. When the fixed partial denture has cooled, remove the investment. Cover the porcelain with masking tape and air abrade the FPD.

Soldering can be done on base metal fixed partial dentures with gold solder in a manner similar to that used for gold-palladium metal-ceramic alloys.[37–39] While restorations of base metal alloys can be soldered, they tend to be quite technique sensitive,[39–42] with variable results.[43] Overheating of the metal substrate and excessive flux have been faulted,[40] while surface oxides have been blamed by others.[41] Closed vacuum furnaces were suggested as a solution for this problem,[41] and testing by Lima Verde and Stein confirmed that soldering under vacuum resulted in mean tensile strengths that were as much as 40% greater than those soldered in air.[42] High- and low-temperature solders are capable of producing joints with adequate tensile strength that will not lose that strength in a corrosive environment.[44] Gold solder used with high-resistance nickel-chromium alloy prevents corrosion, while silver solder used on the same alloy permits corrosion.[45] Silver solder joints become porous from corrosion along the interface between the solder and the nickel-chromium substrate. This does not occur with gold solder.[46]

Nonrigid Connectors

There are several situations in which the use of nonrigid connectors is indicated, either to relieve stress or to accommodate malaligned fixed partial denture abutments. Among those used are dovetails (key-keyways),[47] split pontics (connector inside the pontic),[48] or tapered pins.[49]

Dovetail

When a fixed partial denture is fabricated with a nonrigid connector, it is necessary to align the path of insertion of the keyway with that of the distal abutment. This technique is best suited for relieving stress at midspan on long pontics.

The wax pattern for the retainer on the pier abutment is fabricated on the working cast. When a plastic pattern is used for the key and keyway (PD, or plastic dovetail, pattern, APM-Sterngold, Attleboro, MA) (Fig 27-72), a deep box form is carved into the distal surface of the wax pattern to create space for the placement of the plastic keyway pattern. Adequate depth and a parallel path of insertion are essential when preparing the box form in the distal of this abutment.

Place the working cast, with the wax pattern seated, on the table of a surveyor. Assemble the key and keyway portions of the connector, and lock the mandrel that extends from the top of the key portion of the pattern into the vertical spindle of the surveying instrument. Manipulate the surveyor table until the mandrel and attachments are parallel with the path of insertion of the distal preparation. Then lower the plastic pattern to the middle retainer wax pattern and lute it in place with sticky wax (Fig 27-73). Remove the key portion and complete the middle retainer wax pattern by blending the distal surface with the keyway.

The pattern is then invested, burned out, and cast. After the casting has been cleaned and air abraded, carefully cut off any part of the keyway portion of the attachment that protrudes above the occlusal surface.

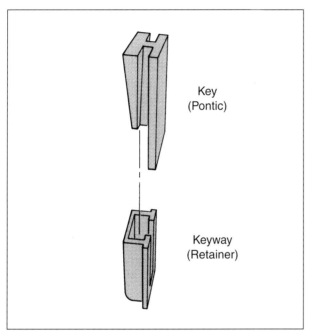

Fig 27-72 The nonrigid connector is composed of a key and keyway. The keyway is recessed into the proximal contour of the retainer, and the key extends from the pontic. (From Shillingburg and Fisher.[47])

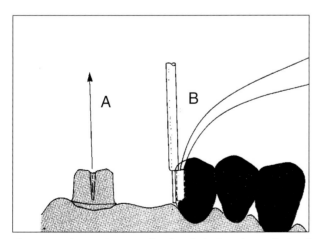

Fig 27-73 The cast is manipulated until the insertion path (A) of the distal abutment preparation parallels the mandrel (B) projecting from the key-keyway assembly. The keyway pattern is luted to the retainer wax pattern on the surveyor to maintain this relationship. (From Shillingburg and Fisher.[47])

Place the casting on the working cast, and place the prefabricated plastic pattern for the key into the keyway. At this point the pontic wax pattern is attached to the plastic key. The pontic pattern is completed, removed from the working cast, invested, burned out, and cast. After the casting is recovered from the investment, the mandrel and any excess on the top portion of the key are carefully reduced so the key and keyway are flush.

For a semiprecision attachment, the wax pattern for the middle retainer is first completed. Cut a keyway or T-shaped preparation in the distal surface of the wax pattern with a no. 170L bur. The path of insertion of the keyway can be checked against the path of insertion of the tooth preparation for the distal retainer by use of a surveyor or by visual examination. After the prepared wax pattern has been cast in gold, return it to the working cast. Refine and finish the tapered keyway preparation in the casting with a no. 169L or no. 170L bur. Lubricate the casting and form the key by placing acrylic resin in the keyway. After the acrylic key has polymerized, attach it to the wax pontic. The pontic wax pattern, incorporating the resin key, is then removed, invested, burned out, and cast. Because a precise fit is essential to prevent undue movement and stress in this long-span fixed partial denture, the rigid three-unit anterior segment is joined before try-in.

At the time of try-in, verify the fit of each individual unit. Then trial seat all of the units: the three-unit anterior combination with the distal pontic keyed into it, the pier abutment retainer, and the distal retainer. Make a soldering index of all the units with zinc oxide–eugenol bite registration paste or fast-setting impression plaster. Place the distal two units in their respective imprints and invest for soldering.

Try the finished soldering components in the mouth again at a subsequent appointment and make occlusal adjustments if necessary. When the restoration is cemented, place the mesial three-unit segment first (Fig 27-74) and seat the distal two-unit portion immediately afterward. No cement should be placed in the keyway (Fig 27-75).

Split Pontic

This is an attachment that is placed entirely within the pontic. It is particularly useful in tilted abutment cases, where the use of a conventional dovetail would necessitate the preparation of a very drastic box in the distal aspect of the pier abutment.[48] The wax pattern for the anterior three-unit segment (mesial retainer–pontic–pier retainer) is fabricated first, with a distal arm attached to the pier retainer. The underside of the arm is shaped like the tissue-contacting area of a pontic (which, in fact, it is). A surveyor is used to position either the key or the keyway segment of a PD pattern (see Fig 27-72), pointing occlusally. This segment must align (draw) with the distal abutment preparation.

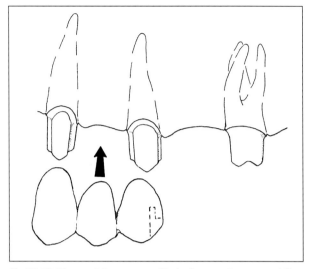

Fig 27-74 The mesial segment, with the keyway, is cemented first.

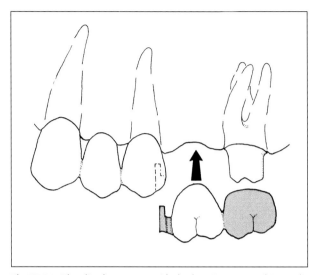

Fig 27-75 The distal segment, with the key, is cemented immediately after.

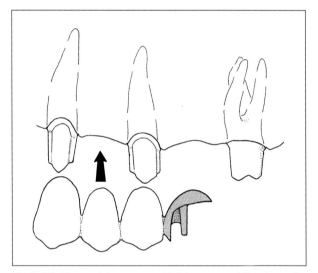

Fig 27-76 The mesial segment, which is cemented first, has a distal shoe that is the gingival portion of the pontic.

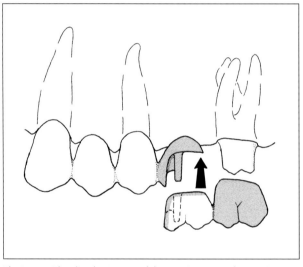

Fig 27-77 The distal segment of the pontic covers the mesiogingival part of the pontic when the distal retainer is cemented.

Invest, burn out, and cast the mesial three-and-a-half-unit segment. After preliminary finishing, seat the cast segment on the working cast. Place the plastic pattern down into it (if the keyway is in the casting), or down onto it (if the key was left facing upward on the pontic base). Wax the distal retainer and the disto-occlusal two-thirds of the pontic pattern. The pontic can be metal-ceramic, but there should be a thin collar of metal around the periphery of the ceramic section. Try it on the prepared teeth in the mouth, making adjustments as necessary. Cement the mesial segment first (Fig 27-76), followed immediately by the distal segment (Fig 27-77). No cement should be placed between the two segments of the pontic.

Cross-pin and Wing

The cross-pin and wing are the working elements of a two-piece pontic system that allows the two segments to be rigidly fixed after the retainers have been cemented on their respective abutment preparations.[49] The design will find use primarily in accommodating abutment teeth with disparate long axes. The path of insertion of each tooth preparation is made to parallel the long axis of that tooth.

Attach a vertical wing, cut out of a piece of baseplate wax, to the mesial surface of the distal retainer wax pattern. The wing should parallel the path of insertion of the mesial abutment preparation, extend out 3.0 mm mesially from the distal retainer, have a 1.0-mm thickness faciolingually, be 1.0 mm short of the occlusal surface, and

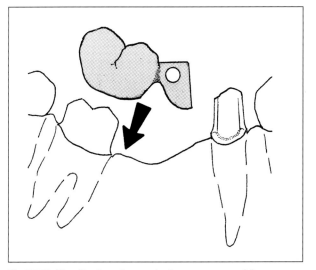

Fig 27-78 The distal retainer and wing are cemented first.

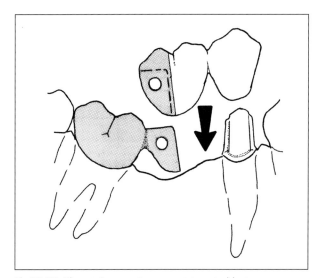

Fig 27-79 The retainer-pontic segment is seated last.

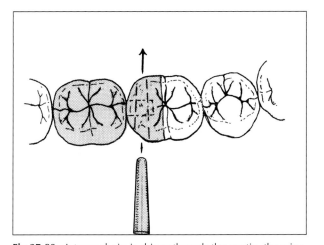

Fig 27-80 A tapered pin is driven through the pontic, the wing, and back out through the pontic.

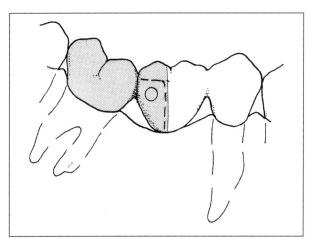

Fig 27-81 Completed cross-pin and wing fixed partial denture.

have an undersurface that follows the intended contour of the underside of the pontic.[49]

Invest, burn out, and cast the distal retainer, with wing. Seat the retainer on the cast, and drill a 0.7-mm hole through the wing with a twist drill in a handpiece. Place a 0.7-mm-diameter pencil lead through the hole and build the wax pattern around the lead and the wing. Remove the lead, withdraw the retainer-pontic wax pattern, and replace the 0.7-mm lead in the hole in the pontic pattern to maintain the patency of the hole during investing and casting.

Assemble the two parts of the fixed partial denture on the working cast. Use a tapered 8/0 machinist reamer to ream a smooth, tapered hole through the pontic and wing, following the pilot hole produced by the 0.7-mm pencil lead.

Fabricate a pin of the same alloy used for the fixed par-tial denture casting. A mold can be made by drilling a hole in a piece of aluminum with the machinist reamer and filling the hole with autopolymerizing resin (Duralay). An impression of the reamer can be made with polyvinyl siloxane impression material and filled with resin or molten wax. Invest, burn out, and cast it. It must be long enough to extend all the way through the pontic-wing assembly. Try the pin for fit in the components on the cast.

Cement the retainer with the wing first (Fig 27-78), followed by the retainer-pontic segment (Fig 27-79). Seat the pin in the hole with a punch and mallet (Fig 27-80). Remove excess length from the pin both facially and lingually. If it is ever necessary to remove part of this fixed partial denture, the pin can be tapped out and the parts dealt with separately. This technique requires no special patterns and does allow for a completely rigid prosthesis when completed (Fig 27-81).

References

1. Anusavice KJ: *Phillips' Science of Dental Materials,* ed 10. Philadelphia, WB Saunders Co, 1996, pp 619–630.

2. El-Ebrashi MK, Asgar K, Bigelow WC: Electron microscopy of gold soldered joints. *J Dent Res* 1968; 47:5–11.

3. Ryge G: Dental soldering procedures. *Dent Clin North Am* 1958; 2:747–757.

4. Phillips RW: *Skinner's Science of Dental Materials,* ed 8. Philadelphia, WB Saunders Co, 1982, pp 534–546.

5. Rasmussen EJ, Goodkind RJ, Gerberich WW: An investigation of tensile strength of dental solder joints. *J Prosthet Dent* 1979; 41:418–423.

6. Fusayama T, Wakumoto S, Hosoda H: Accuracy of fixed partial dentures made by various soldering techniques and one-piece casting. *J Prosthet Dent* 1964; 14:334–342.

7. Saas FA, Eames WB: Fit of unit-cast fixed partial dentures related to casting ring size and shape. *J Prosthet Dent* 1980; 43:163–167.

8. Hinman RW, Tesk JA, Parry EE, Eden GT: Improving the casting accuracy of fixed partial dentures. *J Prosthet Dent* 1985; 53:466–471.

9. Bruce RW: Evaluation of multiple unit castings for fixed partial dentures. *J Prosthet Dent* 1964; 14:939–943.

10. Bruce RW: Clinical applications of multiple unit castings for fixed prostheses. *J Prosthet Dent* 1967; 18:359–364.

11. Schiffleger BE, Ziebert GJ, Dhuru VB, Brantley WA, Sigaroudi K: Comparison of accuracy of multiunit one-piece castings. *J Prosthet Dent* 1985; 54:770–776.

12. Ziebert GJ, Hurtado A, Glapa C, Schiffleger BE: Accuracy of one-piece castings, preceramic and postceramic soldering. *J Prosthet Dent* 1986; 55:312–317.

13. Stade EH, Reisbick MH, Preston JD: Preceramic and postceramic solder joints. *J Prosthet Dent* 1975; 34:527–532.

14. Stackhouse JA: Assembly of dental units by soldering. *J Prosthet Dent* 1967; 18:131–139.

15. Johnston JF, Dykema RW, Mumford G, Phillips RW: Construction and assembly of porcelain veneer gold crowns and pontics. *J Prosthet Dent* 1962; 12:1125–1137.

16. Pruden WH: Solder connections with porcelain fused to gold. *J Prosthet Dent* 1969; 22:679–681.

17. Meyer FS: The elimination of distortion during soldering. *J Prosthet Dent* 1959; 9:441–447.

18. Patterson JC: A technique for accurate soldering. *J Prosthet Dent* 1972; 28:552–556.

19. Chang JC, Hutst TL, Johnson CD, Duong J: A soldering index made with 4-META adhesive resin. *J Prosthet Dent* 1994; 72:430–432.

20. Harper JC, Nicholls JI: Distortion in indexing methods and investing media for soldering and remounting procedures. *J Prosthet Dent* 1979; 42:172–179.

21. Moon PC, Eshleman JR, Douglas HB, Garrett SG: Comparison of accuracy of soldering indices for fixed prostheses. *J Prosthet Dent* 1978; 40:35–38.

22. Dixon DL, Breeding LC, Lindquist TJ: Linear dimensional variability and tensile strengths of three solder index materials. *J Prosthet Dent* 1992; 67:726–729.

23. Smyd ES: Wax, refractory investments and related subjects in dental technology. *J Prosthet Dent* 1955; 5:514–526.

24. Willis LM, Nicholls JI: Distortion in dental soldering as affected by gap distance. *J Prosthet Dent* 1980; 43:272–278.

25. Butson TJ, Nicholls JI, Ma T, Harper RJ: Fatigue life of preceramic soldered and postsoldered joints. *Int J Prosthodont* 1993; 6:468–474.

26. Steinman RR: Warpage produced by soldering with dental solders and gold alloys. *J Prosthet Dent* 1954; 4:384–395.

27. Kimondollo PM: A procedure for restoring proximal contact surfaces of cast gold restorations with solder. *J Prosthet Dent* 1991; 66:408–409.

28. Ferencz JL: Tensile strength analysis of midpontic soldering. *J Prosthet Dent* 1987; 57:696–703.

29. Foerster JG, Meyers RD, Butler GV, Brousseau JS: Midpontic soldering of the modified sanitary pontic. *J Prosthet Dent* 1994; 71:541.

30. Monday JJL, Asgar K: Tensile strength comparison of presoldered and postsoldered joints. *J Prosthet Dent* 1986; 55:23–27.

31. Staffanou RS, Radke RA, Jendersen MD: Strength properties of soldered joints from various ceramic-metal combinations. *J Prosthet Dent* 1980; 43:31–39.

32. Lorenzana RE, Staffanou RS, Marker VA, Okabe T: Strength properties of soldered joints for a gold-palladium alloy and a palladium alloy. *J Prosthet Dent* 1987; 57:450–454.

33. Rosen H: Ceramic/metal solder connectors. *J Prosthet Dent* 1986; 56:671–677.

34. Cattaneo G, Wagnild G, Marshall G, Watanabe L: Comparison of tensile strength of solder joints by infrared and conventional torch technique. *J Prosthet Dent* 1992; 68:33–37.

35. Tehini GE, Stein RS: Comparative analysis of two techniques for soldered connectors. *J Prosthet Dent* 1993; 69:16–19.

36. Nicholls JI, Lemm RW: Tensile strength of presoldered and postsoldered joints. *J Prosthet Dent* 1985; 53:476–482.

37. Blustein R, DePaul BM, Barnhart RC, Green KA: A reliable technique of post soldering of non–precious ceramic units. *J Prosthet Dent* 1976; 36:112–114.

38. Saxton PL: Post soldering of nonprecious alloys. *J Prosthet Dent* 1980; 43:592–595.

39. Sloan RM, Reisbick MH, Preston JD: Post–ceramic soldering of various alloys. *J Prosthet Dent* 1982; 48:686–689.

40. Anusavice KJ, Okabe T, Galloway SE, Hoyt DJ, Morse PK: Flexure test evaluation of presoldered base metal alloys. *J Prosthet Dent* 1985; 54:507–517.

41. Kaylakie WG, Brukl CE: Comparative tensile strengths of nonnoble dental alloy solders. *J Prosthet Dent* 1985; 53:455–462.

42. Lima Verde MAR, Stein RS: Evaluation of soldered connectors of two base metal ceramic alloys. *J Prosthet Dent* 1994; 71:339–344.

43. Townsend LWA, Vermilyea SG, Griswold WH: Soldering nonnoble alloys. *J Prosthet Dent* 1983; 50:51–53.

44. Hawbolt EB, MacFntee MI, Zahel JI: The tensile strength and appearance of solder joints in three base metal alloys made with high- and low-temperature solders. *J Prosthet Dent* 1983; 50:362–367.

45. Shigeto N, Yanagihara T, Hamada T, Budtz-Jørgensen E: Corrosion properties of soldered joints. Part I: Electrochemical action of dental solder and dental nickel-chromium alloy. *J Prosthet Dent* 1989; 62:512–515.

46. Shigeto N, Yanagihara T, Murakami S, Hamada T: Corrosion properties of soldered joints. Part II: Corrosion pattern of dental solder and dental nickel-chromium alloy. *J Prosthet Dent* 1991; 66:607–610.

47. Shillingburg HT, Fisher DW: Nonrigid connectors for fixed partial dentures. *J Am Dent Assoc* 1973; 87:1195–1199.

48. O'Connor RP, Caughman WF, Bemis C: Use of the split pontic connector with the tilted molar abutment. *J Prosthet Dent* 1986; 56:249–251.

49. Eichmiller FC, Parry EE: Tapered cross-pin attachments for fixed bridges. *Oper Dent* 1994; 19:7–10.

Chapter 28

Resin-Bonded Fixed Partial Dentures

Unquestionably one of the disadvantages of a conventional fixed partial denture with either full veneer or partial veneer crown retainers is the destruction of tooth structure required for the abutment preparations upon which the retainers will be placed. The prospect of the destruction of what is frequently sound tooth structure may well cause the patient to ask, "Is it really necessary to cut away all that good tooth?" This question has troubled conscientious dentists in prescribing the replacement of a missing tooth, as they have tried to balance the periodontal, occlusal, and esthetic benefits of the prosthesis against the damage to the abutment teeth.

Various solutions for this problem have been tried through the years. Inlay retainers have been used, in part to save tooth structure, but also to save time before the advent of air-turbine handpieces. Some dentists have tried to minimize the problem by eliminating one of the abutment teeth and fabricating a cantilever fixed partial denture. While this type of restoration does have its place in carefully selected situations, its indiscriminate use can result in failures that are costly both in money spent for subsequent replacement and in loss of periodontal support around previously sound teeth. Others have tried to use unilateral removable partial dentures to avoid undesirable destruction of tooth structure, but these restorations are usually wanting in both retention and stability. Additionally, they present the risk of aspiration if they become dislodged.

The development of acid etching of enamel to improve the retention of resin, first described by Buonocore in 1955,[1] has proven to be a means of attaching fixed partial dentures to teeth by less destructive means. Ibsen first described the attachment of an acrylic resin pontic to an unprepared tooth using a composite bonding resin.[2] Others since that time have utilized the technique,[3–7] but it is probably best suited for use as a long-term provisional restoration or intermediate replacement of a missing tooth.[8,9]

Metal Framework

The addition of a metal substructure and "wings," or retainers, extending onto the abutment teeth was a logical progression in the development of the restoration. The following classification of resin-bonded fixed partial dentures (Rochette bridge, Maryland bridge, cast mesh FPD, Virginia bridge) is a reflection of the metal surface finishing technique employed as much as anything else. The restoration has continued to evolve for nearly a quarter of a century.

Rochette Bridge

The first use of wing-like retainers, with funnel-shaped perforations through them to enhance resin retention (Fig 28-1), is attributed to Rochette in 1973,[10] who combined mechanical retention with a silane coupling agent to produce adhesion to the metal.[11] The perforated retainer became the standard design for several years, being used for both anterior[12–15] and posterior fixed partial dentures.[16]

Maryland Bridge

Livaditis and Thompson postulated that the retentive resin "rivets" extruding through the perforated framework were exposed to increased stresses as well as abrasion and leakage that diminished their longevity.[17] They adapted an electrochemical pit corroding technique that had been used by Dunn and Reisbick in a study of ceramic bonding to base metal alloys.[18] Tanaka et al had used a similar technique to produce pitting corrosion of metal for retaining acrylic resin facings on metal copings.[19]

Livaditis and Thompson used a 3.5% solution of nitric acid with a current of 250 mA/cm^2 for 5 minutes, followed

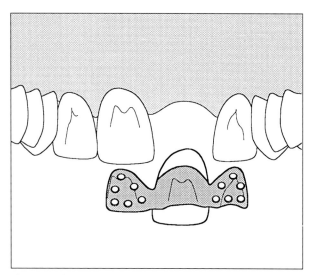

Fig 28-1 The metal retainers of the Rochette resin-bonded fixed partial denture used multiple perforations for retention.

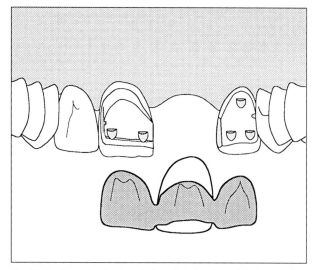

Fig 28-2 The Maryland resin-bonded fixed partial denture has solid metal retainers and relies on the etched inner surface of the retainers for its retention.

by immersion in an 18% hydrochloric acid solution in an ultrasonic cleaner for 10 minutes, to etch the internal surfaces of solid base metal retainers for resin-bonded fixed partial dentures[17] (Fig 28-2). This type of etched-metal prosthesis is frequently called the *Maryland bridge*. The authors measured a resin-alloy bond strength of 27.3 MPa (3,960 psi), compared with resin-enamel bonds of 8.5 to 9.9 MPa (1,200 to 1,400 psi). The acid solution and technique were specific to the nonberyllium nickel-chromium alloy that they tested.

Subsequently, Thompson et al reported that 10% sulfuric acid at 300 mA/cm^2, followed by the same cleaning procedures, would produce similar results with a beryllium-containing nickel-chromium alloy.[20] Dhillon et al found that an electrochemically etched surface was approximately 2.9 times as retentive as a perforated one.[21] A tendency toward greater retention in etched retainers was detected by Sloan et al, but they also found tremendous variability from one laboratory to another and from one retainer to another.[22] This was later confirmed by Hussey et al.[23]

McLaughlin proposed a much faster technique for etching retainers by immersing them in a beaker of a combined solution of sulfuric and hydrochloric acids placed in an activated ultrasonic cleaner for 99 seconds while electrical current is passed through the fixed partial denture and solution.[24] Subsequent in vitro testing of specimens treated by the one- and two-step techniques showed retainers treated by the one-step technique to be equally as retentive as those done by the two-step method.[25]

Electrochemical etching is technique-sensitive. Overetching produces an electro*polished* surface, and contamination of the surface reduces bond strength.[26] Because of the unpredictability of the etching technique and its dependence on the use of certain base metal

alloys, for the past several years there has been interest in alternative ways of creating metal surfaces capable of retaining resin bonding materials.

Other surface-treatment techniques have been developed. Livaditis reported acceptable results with a non-electrolytic technique that requires a nickel-chromium-beryllium alloy to be placed in an etching solution for 1 hour in a water bath at 70°C (158°F).[27] A form of chemical etching with a stable aqua regia gel was substituted for electrochemical etching by Doukoudakis.[28]

Some investigators reported slightly less[29] or slightly more retention[30] with acid gel chemical treatment than with electrochemical etching. Others found that metals etched electrochemically were still more retentive.[31,32] The use of an acid gel requires no special equipment, and the prosthesis can be fabricated and bonded in just two clinical sessions. It is easily accomplished in either the laboratory or the dental office. Unfortunately, it may not produce the results offered by other etchants with unfilled/filled composite resins.

Retainers coated with pyrolized silane (Silicoater, Kulzer, Irvine, CA) have been shown to be 47% to 104% more retentive than retainers treated by etching alone,[29] and 23% to 124% more retentive than retainers bonded by other composite-to-metal bonding systems.[33] Air abrading metal with 250 µm abrasive increases bonding strength remarkably when used in conjunction with silane.[34]

Cast Mesh Fixed Partial Denture

Techniques that produce roughness before the alloy is cast, or use a nonetching method after casting, have also been employed. A net-like nylon mesh (Klett-O-Bond,

Denerica, Northfield, IL) can be placed over the lingual surfaces of the abutment teeth on the working cast. It is then covered by and incorporated into the retainer wax pattern, with the undersurface of the retainer becoming a mesh-like surface when the retainer is cast. It eliminates the need for etching, and it permits the use of noble-metal alloys.[35–37] The material tends to be stiff, making it somewhat difficult to adapt to detail of the abutment tooth, and if wax runs too freely into the mesh, blocking out the undercuts, its retentive ability is compromised.

Virginia Bridge

Moon and Hudgins et al produced *particle-roughened* retainers by incorporating salt crystals into the retainer patterns to produce roughness on the inner surfaces.[38–40] In this method, also known as the *lost salt* technique for producing *Virginia bridges,* the framework is outlined on the die with a wax pencil, and the area to be bonded is coated first with model spray and then with lubricant. Sieved cubic salt crystals (NaCl), ranging in size from 149 to 250 μm (Virginia Technique Kit, Richmond, VA), are sprinkled over the outlined area.[41] The retainer patterns are fabricated from resin, leaving a 0.5- to 1.0-mm-wide, crystal-free margin around the outlined area.

When the resin has polymerized, the patterns are removed from the cast, cleaned with a solvent, and then placed in water in an ultrasonic cleaner to dissolve the salt crystals. This leaves cubic voids in the surface that are reproduced in the cast retainers, producing retention for the fixed partial denture. Subsequent investigation showed that retainers fabricated by this technique could be 30% to 150% more retentive than retainers prepared by the electrochemical technique, depending on the resin used.[42]

Air abrasion with aluminum oxide has been used as the sole means of surface treatment, as well as the precursor for other treatments. Tanaka et al used 50 μm aluminum oxide air abrasion to prepare cobalt-chromium castings for bonding with 4-META resin.[43] The difference here was not in the treatment of the metal surface as much as it was in the adhesive properties of the cement. Nickel-chromium alloys required oxidation with a dilute solution of sulfuric acid and potassium manganate as well.

Tanaka et al were also able to create a suitable surface for bonding with the same 4-META resin by inducing a heat-accumulated copper oxide deposit on noble-metal alloys in conjunction with 50 μm aluminum oxide air abrasion.[44] Wiltshire used air abrasion with 250 μm aluminum oxide and found that it was not significantly different from electrochemical etching in effectiveness,[45] while other investigators obtained better retention by air abrading with 250 μm aluminum oxide particles than with electrochemical etching.[42]

Resin Cements

The first resin-bonded restorations described by Rochette,[10] which were splints, were held in place by an unfilled resin, poly(methyl methacrylate) (Sevriton), attached to etched enamel, based on the work of Laswell et al.[46] While a whole generation of resin-bonded fixed partial dentures would bear the title of *Rochette bridges,* they made use only of the perforated retainers described by Rochette, ignoring the silane coupling with which he augmented resin attachment to the metal framework.[10]

Unfilled/filled composite resins (Adaptic/Adaptic Bonding Agent, J&J Dental Products Co, East Windsor, NJ,[12] and Concise Composite and Enamel Bond System, 3M Co, St Paul, MN[14,47]) were used with perforated retainers. Then a modified unfilled/filled composite resin with a thin film thickness specifically intended for luting resin-bonded fixed partial dentures was released, closely following the development of electrolytic etching.[16,17,48]

The next step was "chemically active"[11] (adhesive) resin cements: 4-META, or 4-<u>m</u>ethacryloxy<u>e</u>thyl <u>t</u>rimellitate <u>a</u>nhydride (C&B Metabond, Parkell Corp, Farmingdale, NY)[43] and MDP, or 10-<u>m</u>ethacryloyloxy<u>d</u>ecyl dihydrogen <u>p</u>hosphate (Panavia EX, Kuraray Co, Osaka, Japan).[49,50] These cements rely on adhesion to the metal and not on microretention in the surface of the metal for bond strength. Etching was no longer necessary.[51]

Air abrasion with small-particle aluminum oxide (50 μm or less) thus becomes part of the cleaning of the metal surface in preparation for chemical bonding and not a mechanism for roughening the surface to provide microscopic undercuts for the resin. Tin plating can make noble metals very good candidates for bonding.[52] Imbery et al[53] found the greatest bonding strength with a gold-palladium alloy (Olympia, JF Jelenko, Armonk, NY) that had been air abraded, tin plated, and bonded with a filled bis-GMA resin and phosphate ester monomer (Panavia EX), and a nickel-chromium-beryllium alloy (Rexillium III, Jeneric/Pentron, Wallingford, CT) that had been air abraded, silicoated, and cemented with a 4-META resin (C & B Metabond, Parkell). Breeding and Dixon[54] reported similar results: high noble (Olympia) and noble (Jelstar, Jeneric/Pentron) displayed shear bond strengths similar to that of a base metal alloy (Rexillium III).

Pros and Cons

There are situations in which resin-bonded fixed partial dentures should or should not be used, as well as features that should be considered in deciding that one is the treatment of choice for replacing a lost tooth.

Advantages

Reduced Cost. This is probably not as significant as was first thought when little or no preparation was involved with the technique. However, with the increased use of preparation features, more of the dentist's time and skill are required, and the cost differential between a conventional prosthesis and a resin-bonded fixed partial denture has become less.

No Anesthetic Needed. An anesthetic is not required because most of the preparation will be done in enamel.

Supragingival Margins. Although supragingival margins can be used with conventional retainers, they are mandatory for the resin-bonded fixed partial denture.

Minimal Tooth Preparation. Little tooth structure has to be removed for this technique, making it more conservative and less likely to create problems in unblemished abutment teeth.

Rebonding Possible. Resin-bonded fixed partial dentures can be rebonded if the "wings" or axial extensions are not sprung or bent when the restoration debonds. Commonly, one retainer does become loose before the other. If this goes undetected for any significant period of time, caries can develop on the abutment under the retainer and a new, conventional fixed partial denture may have to be constructed. However, if the debonding is detected early enough, the retainer that remained attached must be removed without damage to the tooth or to the restoration. This can be quite difficult if the tooth has been well-prepared. Removal of resin-bonded restorations by the use of specially designed ultrasonic scaler tips has been described.[55,56] The KJS, a straight chisel, is used to develop a fracture in resin along the incisal edge, and the KJC, a curved chisel, is used at the gingival margin.[56]

Disadvantages

Irreversible. The resin-bonded fixed partial denture, as it is frequently used today, requires the removal of enough tooth structure that it should be considered irreversible. Whether this is really a disadvantage or not is debatable, but the point is raised simply to remind the reader that it is necessary to do some preparation of the tooth.

Uncertain Longevity. The resin-bonded fixed partial denture is not new and totally untested, but there is still some concern about the longevity of this type of prosthesis. The results of 27 studies on resin-bonded FPD longevity are shown in Table 28-1.[13–15, 39,47,48,57–77] In a study by Marinello et al, the success rate dropped from 95% after 3 months to 91% at 6 months, 81.5% at 1 year, and 73% at 18 months.[65]

A review of about 60 publications on the clinical survival of resin-bonded FPDs put the 4-year survival rate at 74%.[78] By contrast, a similar study done on 552 three-unit conventional fixed partial dentures by Kerschbaum and Gaa showed that 96% of those prostheses were still in use after 4 years.[79] Another study of 487 metal-ceramic fixed partial denture retainers 18 to 23 years after their placement revealed a success rate of 95%.[80] While higher survival rates certainly would be more reassuring, it should be kept in mind that many of these studies have monitored the early development of the restoration. As an indication of what can be done with well-thought planning and attention to detail, Barrack reports a success rate of nearly 93% on 127 resin-bonded restorations placed in the mouths of his private patients over a span of 11 years.[75]

No Space Correction. Although some porcelain can be added to the metal retainer on the adjacent abutment teeth, there are definite limitations on what can be done if the edentulous space is significantly wider than the mesiodistal width of the tooth that would normally occupy the space.

No Alignment Correction. It is impossible to correct alignment problems with this restoration, inasmuch as nothing is done to the facial, proximal, and incisal areas of the abutment teeth.

Difficult Temporization. A provisional fixed partial denture cannot be fabricated with this type of restoration. If a missing tooth is to be replaced while the fixed partial denture is being made, it must be accomplished with a mucoadhesion temporary removable partial denture.

Indications

Caries-free Abutment Teeth. If the edentulous span is not too long, the resin-bonded fixed partial denture allows tooth replacement with minimal destruction of tooth structure on undamaged abutment teeth.

Mandibular Incisor Replacements. The acid-etched resin-bonded fixed partial denture is the restoration of choice for replacing one or two missing mandibular incisors when the abutment teeth are unblemished.

Maxillary Incisor Replacements. Maxillary incisors can be replaced if they are in an open-bite, end-to-end, or moderate overbite situation.

Periodontal Splints. The splinting of periodontally involved teeth comprised the first published report of the use of a resin-bonded prosthesis by Rochette,[10] and other authors described the use of resin-bonded, perforated[81] and etched-metal[82] splints for long-term usage. However, abutment mobility has been cited as one of the causes of failure by Barrack,[83] and the study by Marinello et al indicated that the failure rate for splints was 13% greater than that for fixed partial dentures.[66] If a resin-bonded prosthesis is to be used as a splint, careful attention must be paid to resistance features on the abutment preparations. In the previously cited study by Marinello et al, the use of grooves on abutments for splints improved the chances for success by nearly 15%.[66]

Single Posterior Tooth Replacements. While replacement of multiple teeth can be done with this type of prosthesis, it becomes a higher-risk procedure. Resin-bond-

Table 28–1   *Longevity of Resin-Bonded Fixed Partial Dentures*[13-15,39,47,48,57-77]

Author	Year	Type of Retention	Months in mouth	Number placed	Number retained	Percent successful
Barrack/Bretz[75]	1993	Etched	68	127	118	93
Bergendahl et al[58]	1983	Perforated	33	100	71	71
Chang et al[72]	1991	Etched	47	43	28	53
Clyde/Boyd[68]	1988	Etched	60	122	109	89
Creugers et al[63]	1986	Perforated	18	32	24	75
		Perforated (prox ext)	18	29	23	79
		Etched metal	18	40	38	95
Creugers et al[71]	1990	—	60	203	126	62
Denehy/Howe[14]	1979	Perforated	36	30	27	90
Ekstrand[61]	1984	—	36	120	98	82
Eshleman et al[15]	1979	Perforated	36	39	33	85
Ferrari et al[70]	1989	Etched	30	209	188	90
Hansson/Moberg[74]	1992	Etched	41	34	32	94
Hudgins[39]	1985	Particle roughened	18	27	26	96
Kuhlke/Drennon[13]	1977	Perforated	48	23	20	87
La Barre/Ward[60]	1984	Etched	12	45	41	91
Livaditis[48]	1981	Etched	12	66	64	96
Marinello et al[65]	1987	Etched metal FPD	18	153	127	83
		Cast metal FPD	18	127	112	88
		Perforated FPD	18	44	25	57
		Air-abraded FPD	18	54	48	89
Marinello et al[66]	1988	Etched metal splints	18	95	66	70
		Cast mesh splints	18	17	11	65
		Air-abraded splints	18	5	4	80
Olin et al[73]	1990	Etched	60	96	85	89
Priest/Donatelli[67]	1988	Perforated	51	3	1	33
		Cast mesh	42	2	2	100
		Electrochemical etch	26	38	30	79
		Chemical etch	7	15	15	100
Rammelsberg et al[76]	1993	Etched	84	141	117	83
Shaw/Tay[47]	1982	Perforated	44	46	37	80
Thayer et al[77]	1993	Perforated	87	44	27	61
		Etched metal	87	41	25	61
Thompson/Wood[62]	1986	—	41	180	140	78
van der Veen et al[64]	1987	Perforated	72	64	54	84
Williams et al[59]	1984	Perforated	72	63	53	84
Williams et al[69]	1989	Perforated and etched	120	90	100	83
Yankelson/Myers[57]	1980	Perforated	24	97	75	77

ed fixed partial dentures of more than three units have a 10% higher failure rate than those that are only three units in length.[66] Resin-bonded FPDs of greater than three-unit length should be used only if there is some mitigating treatment-planning consideration, such as opposing a removable partial denture, which would result in less occlusal stress. Fixed partial dentures with more than two retainers have a failure rate 2.5 times that of resin-bonded FPDs with only two retainers.[72]

Contraindications

Extensive Caries. Because the resin-bonded partial denture covers relatively little surface area and relies on bonding to enamel for its retention, the presence of caries of any size will require the use of a more conventional prosthesis.

Nickel Sensitivity. Since most resin-bonded partial dentures are etched nickel-chromium restorations, nickel sensitivity in a patient requires that another alloy be used or that another type of prosthesis be employed.

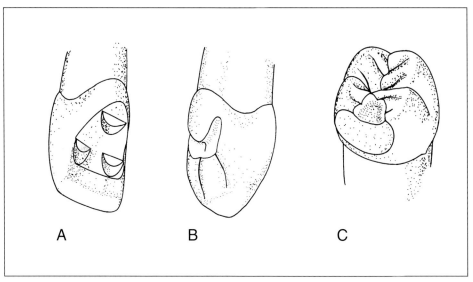

Fig 28-3 Vertical stops for a resin-bonded fixed partial denture can be a countersink (A), a V-shaped cingulum rest (B), or an occlusal rest seat (C).

Table 28–2 *Lingual Enamel Thickness of Maxillary Anterior Teeth (in millimeters)[94]*

Tooth	Millimeters from cementoenamel junction					
	1	2	3	4	5	6
Central incisor	0.3	0.5	0.6	0.7	0.7	0.7
Lateral incisor	0.4	0.5	0.5	0.6	0.7	0.7
Canine	0.2	0.4	0.6	0.7	0.9	0.9

Deep Vertical Overbite. So much enamel must be removed from the lingual surface of a maxillary incisor in this occlusal relationship that retention would be drastically reduced because of the poor bonding strength afforded by the exposed dentin.

Tooth Preparation

The early use of acid-etched resin-bonded fixed partial dentures was accomplished with no preparation of the abutment teeth.[10,12] Although some authors advocate little or no tooth preparation for this type of prosthesis, emphasizing its reversibility,[84,85] preparation features are used by many to enhance the resistance of resin-bonded fixed partial dentures.

The tooth preparation includes axial reduction and guide planes on the proximal surfaces with a slight extension onto the facial surface to achieve a faciolingual lock.[86–88] The preparation should encompass at least 180 degrees of the tooth to enhance the resistance of the retainer.[89] The preparation must be extended as far as possible to provide maximum bonding area. This has been a problem in the past. A number of the early restorations that failed covered too little surface area to give them the adequate strength needed to resist displacement.[90] There should be a finish line even though it will be nothing more than a very light chamfer, and it should be placed about 1.0 mm supragingivally.[47,83,89,91]

Occlusal clearance is needed on very few teeth that are prepared as abutments for acid-etched resin-bonded fixed partial dentures. Specifically, 0.5 mm is needed on maxillary incisors, where preparation is done on the lingual surface of the teeth.[59,92,93] The thicknesses of enamel on the lingual surfaces of maxillary anterior teeth are shown in Table 28-2.[94] Because of the limited thickness of enamel near the cementoenamel junction, this type of restoration cannot be used on patients with a severe Class II vertical overlap.[95]

Vertical stops are placed on all the preparations. This will consist of two or three flat countersinks on the lingual surface of an incisor,[83,90,96] a cingulum rest on a canine,[86] or an occlusal rest seat on a premolar or molar (Fig 28-3).[51,97] Wilkes found rests to be the dominant feature in a preparation, contributing to both resistance and rigidity.[98] The occlusal rest directs the applied force from the pontic to the abutments.[99] Barrack strongly recommends the use of two rests.[51,100]

The resistance features used in a tooth preparation for an acid-etched resin-bonded retainer will normally be grooves (Fig 28-4, A).[60,89,101,102] Grooves were found to increase resistance to displacement on anterior preparations 31% to 77% in one study[103] and 81% in another.[86] However, if there is an existing amalgam, all of the amalgam, or at least all of its surface, is removed so that the

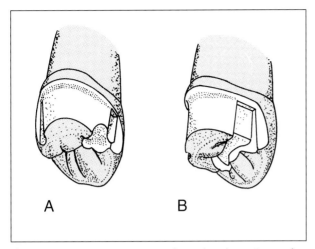

Fig 28-4 Grooves are most commonly employed as resistance features on resin-bonded fixed partial denture abutments (A), but the box form of an existing amalgam can also be converted for that purpose (B).

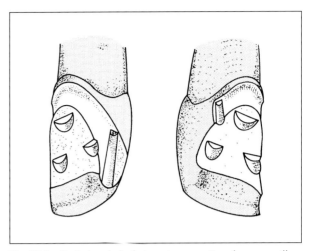

Fig 28-5 Resin-bonded abutment preparation for a maxillary incisor.

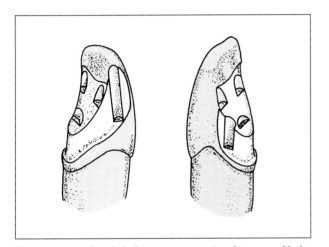

Fig 28-6 Resin-bonded abutment preparation for a mandibular incisor.

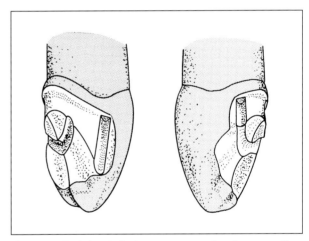

Fig 28-7 Resin-bonded abutment preparation for a maxillary canine.

box form can be utilized (Fig 28-4, B).[104] The entire occlusal outline of the existing amalgam restoration is included within the outline of the retainer's occlusal rest.[75] If the retainer margins cross over an amalgam-enamel margin, there is a high probability of leakage occurring around that margin.[104]

Examples of the preparations used on the different teeth include those made for a maxillary (Fig 28-5) or a mandibular incisor (Fig 28-6), a canine (Fig 28-7), maxillary premolars (Fig 28-8), and a mandibular second premolar (Fig 28-9), all of which have a proximal groove near the facioproximal line angle adjacent to the edentulous space. There is a second groove on the opposite side of the cingulum or lingual cusp of the tooth, which creates a wraparound effect in the retainer and produces resistance in the process. Both grooves should be placed in enamel.

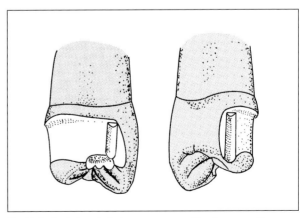

Fig 28-8 Resin-bonded abutment preparation for a maxillary premolar.

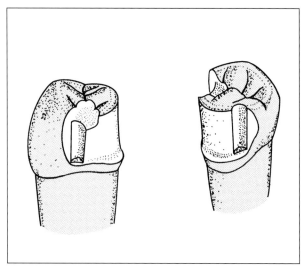

Fig 28-9 Resin-bonded abutment preparation for a mandibular second premolar.

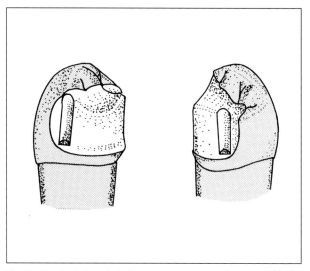

Fig 28-10 Resin-bonded abutment preparation for a mandibular first premolar.

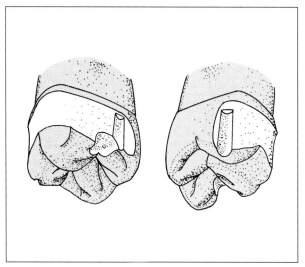

Fig 28-11 Resin-bonded abutment preparation for a maxillary molar.

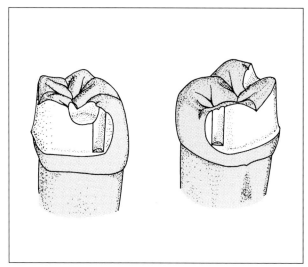

Fig 28-12 Resin-bonded abutment preparation for a mandibular molar.

Fig 28-13 Posterior resin-bonded fixed partial denture framework configurations include:

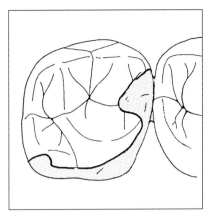 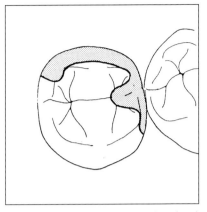 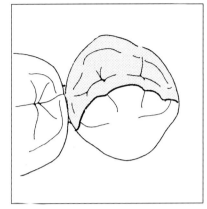

A. *Standard.* There are two grooves, one near the facioproximal angle adjacent to the edentulous space and one at the opposite linguoproximal corner, with 180+ degrees of axial wall coverage.

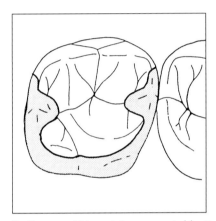 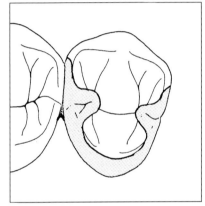

B. *Two rests.* This variation, suggested by Barrack,[51] has axial coverage on both proximal walls and two rest seats located near the central groove at the mesio-occlusal and disto-occlusal. They resist displacement by occlusal forces.

The preparation for a mandibular first premolar (Fig 28-10) is slightly different from that for other premolar preparations. Because the placement of a rest seat would leave very little solid tooth structure in the small lingual cusp of many first premolars, coverage of the entire small lingual cusp is substituted. Lingual cusp coverage, when it does not interfere with occlusion, is an excellent means of increasing surface area and reinforcing the retainer.[105] The last preparation to be considered is that for the molar. Its preparation in either the maxillary (Fig 28-11) or mandibular arch (Fig 28-12) is very similar to the preparation used on a premolar.

The framework can be bolstered by capping the lingual cusps as described for premolars (Fig 28-13), which produces rigidity. Occlusal inlays can be attached to anatomic grooves, such as lingual or distolingual grooves. Axial coverage can be extended through the proximal contact to connect with occlusal rests or inlays. Any extension of an occlusal groove can be used to good advantage in preventing the flexing of the ends of axial coverage, or a "wing."

Fig 28-13 *continued*

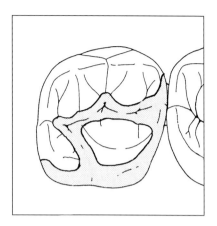

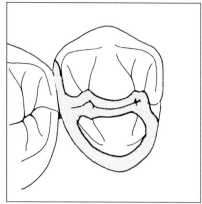

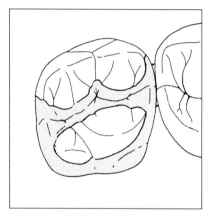

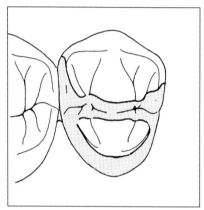

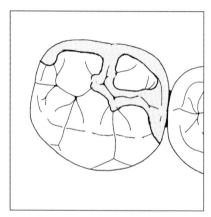

C. *Loops.* These features are formed by occlusal inlays being joined to a groove on a lingual or proximal surface. They brace the arms.

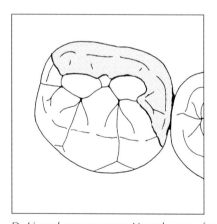

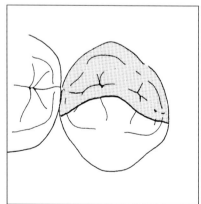

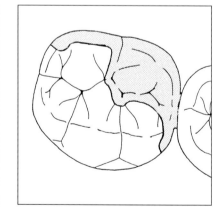

D. *Lingual cusp coverage.* Lingual cusps of mandibular molars and premolars can be covered to bolster the retainer against deformation.

E. *Tilted molars.* The mesial and particularly the mesiolingual cusps of mandibular molars that have tipped and are out of occlusion can be covered to improve occlusion and remove subocclusal food

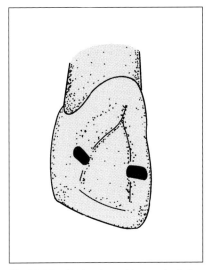

Fig 28-14 Occlusal marking: articulation paper.

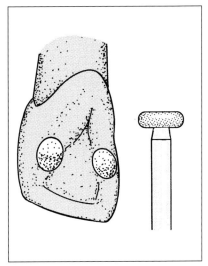

Fig 28-15 Occlusal clearance: small wheel diamond.

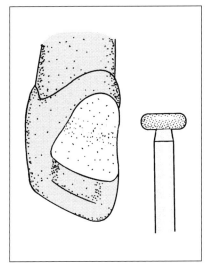

Fig 28-16 Lingual reduction: small wheel diamond.

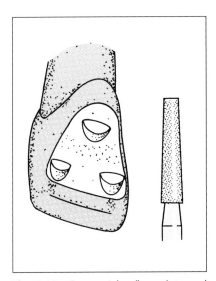

Fig 28-17 Countersinks: flat-end tapered diamond.

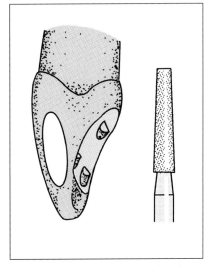

Fig 28-18 Proximal reduction (facial segment): flat-end tapered diamond.

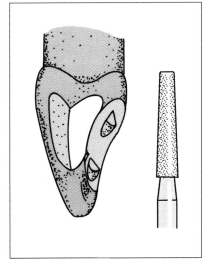

Fig 28-19 Proximal reduction (lingual segment): flat-end tapered diamond.

Preparation Armamentarium

1. High-speed handpiece
2. Articulating ribbon
3. Small wheel and short needle diamonds
4. Flat-end and round-end tapered diamonds

Preparation Sequence

The preparation sequence shown is for a maxillary incisor. First, the centric occlusal contacts are marked with articulating ribbon (Fig 28-14).[96] To insure adequate occlusal clearance in this area, use a small wheel diamond to remove 0.5 mm of tooth structure (Fig 28-15).

This particular step is necessary only on maxillary anterior teeth.

Use the same small wheel diamond to create a concave reduction on the entire cingulum surface of the incisor, producing 0.5 mm of lingual clearance (Fig 28-16). End this reduction 1.5 to 2.0 mm from the incisal edge, or just incisal to the incisalmost occlusal contact, whichever is closer to the incisal edge. Use a flat-end tapered diamond to prepare flat notches or countersinks on the lingual surface of the tooth to provide resistance to gingival displacement (Fig 28-17).

Proximal reduction on the surface adjacent to the edentulous space is done with a round-end tapered diamond, producing a small plane that extends slightly facial to the facioproximal line angle (Fig 28-18). This helps pro-

547

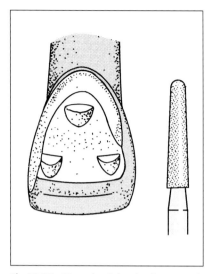

Fig 28-20 Lingual axial reduction: round-end tapered diamond.

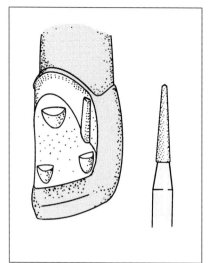

Fig 28-21 Cingulum groove: short needle diamond.

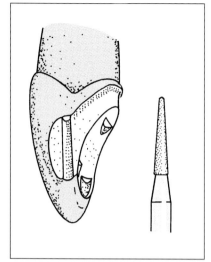

Fig 28-22 Proximal groove: short needle diamond.

duce facial wraparound to enhance resistance, a feature that will be less prominent on maxillary anterior teeth than on mandibular teeth. A second plane is produced lingual to the first with the same diamond (Fig 28-19).

Light upright lingual axial reduction is done from the biplanar proximal axial reduction around the cingulum to a point just short of the proximal contact on the opposite side of the cingulum from the edentulous space (Fig 28-20). The thickness of the axial walls of the retainer will be greater than the amount of axial tooth structure removed, leading to overcontouring of the axial walls of the cast retainer. To minimize any deleterious effect on the periodontium, the very light chamfer finish line should remain approximately 1.0 mm supragingival throughout its length.

A short groove is placed at the facialmost extension of the reduction on the opposite side of the cingulum with a short needle diamond (Fig 28-21). In addition to bolstering the rigidity of the retainer, the groove will serve to enhance its resistance. Use the same thin diamond to place a groove in the vicinity of the wraparound or break between the facial and lingual planes of proximal axial reduction adjacent to the edentulous space (Fig 28-22).

Framework Fabrication

Framework design for the resin-bonded fixed partial denture is important. It cannot be divorced from the preparation since the extensions for the retainers will be determined by the preparation. There must be an adequate thickness of the metal in the finished restoration so that it will be immune to distortion and/or dislodgment.

Caputo et al found through the use of photoelastic stress analysis that stresses could be lowered significantly by thickening the wraparound arms of the retainer to 0.6 mm and including proximal extensions.[99] Failure to reduce stress in the arms of the retainer will be translated into fatigue failure of the underlying resin bonding material.

Duplication Armamentarium

1. Full-arch master stone cast
2. Flat-surface metal sprue former block-out pin
3. PKT no. 1 waxing instrument, sticky wax, Bunsen burner
4. Duplicating flask, modeling clay, duplicating hydrocolloid
5. 500-cc Vac-U-Mixer, vacuum tubing
6. Vibrator
7. Water measure, spatula, brush, investment
8. Conical metal sprue former

Master Cast Duplication

The framework pattern is finished on a refractory cast, which is made by duplicating the full-arch master stone cast made from the first pour of the impression. The cast that is to be duplicated should be complete, with a smooth center (Fig 28-23). "Horseshoe" casts, or those with uneven, rough areas in the lingual space, are not acceptable. To avoid undercuts, the periphery of the cast is trimmed so that its sides are perpendicular to the base (Fig 28-24). If it is trimmed so that it slants in toward the

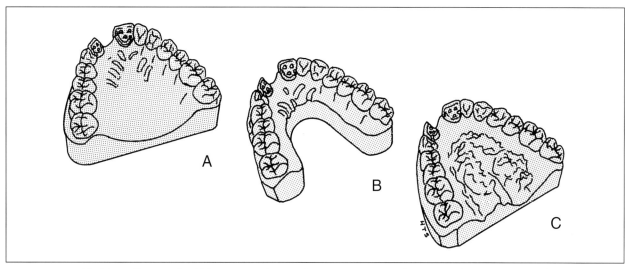

Fig 28-23 The cast should have a smooth, complete center (A). Horseshoe casts with no center (B) and casts with rough piles of stone in the center (C) are unacceptable.

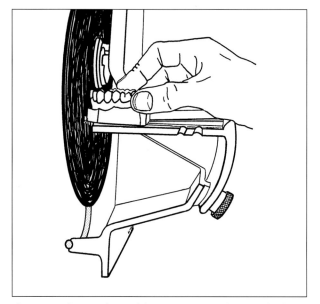

Fig 28-24 The periphery of the cast is trimmed perpendicular to the base for duplicating.

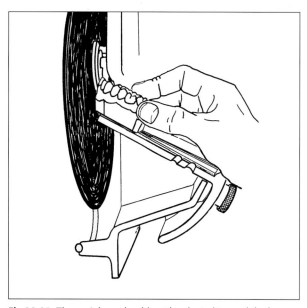

Fig 28-25 The periphery should not be slanted toward the base as shown here.

base (Fig 28-25), the resultant severe undercut will interfere with removal of the cast from the duplicating material. An extra step of "blocking out" will be required.

Fill in voids and any deep tissue undercuts in the vestibular area with modeling clay. Lute a flat-surface metal sprue former block-out pin in place (Fig 28-26). Soak the cast by placing the base in water for approximately 30 minutes. Immersing the entire cast may erode the surface of the cast in the area of the abutment preparations, whose accurate reproduction is essential.

Set the cast on the base of the duplicating flask and hold it in place with a small piece of modeling clay on either side of the cast (Fig 28-27). Fill in any undercuts around the periphery of the base. Place a thin strip of modeling clay around the periphery of the flask base so that it will form a seal when the flask is seated on the base. Position the top of the flask over the base and fill it with duplicating hydrocolloid (Ready-Mix Duplicating Material, Ticonium Co, Albany, NY) (Fig 28-28). Place the flask in a circulating water bath and allow it to cool for 45 minutes.

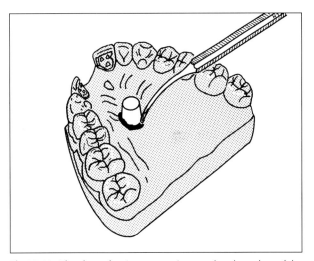

Fig 28-26 The short aluminum cone is waxed to the palate of the cast.

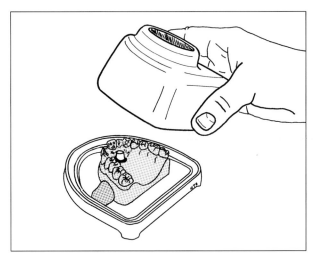

Fig 28-27 The cast is placed on the base of a duplicating flask and the top is put over it.

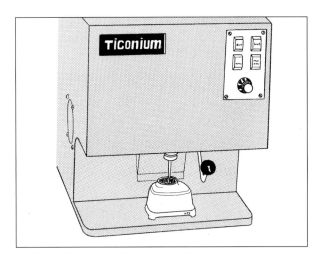

Fig 28-28 The flask is filled with duplicating material.

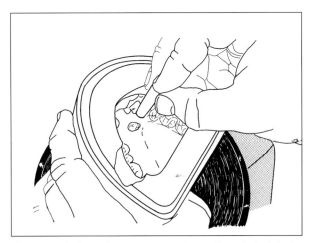

Fig 28-29 The long aluminum cone is inserted into the hole in the palate of the mold.

After the duplicating material has set, remove the base from the bottom of the flask and separate the cast from the hydrocolloid. Mix the investment (Investic, Ticonium Co) and place the conical metal sprue former into the conical depression created in the palatal area of the mold by the block-out pin (Fig 28-29). Pour the investment into the mold and allow it to set for 60 minutes (Fig 28-30).

After 1 hour, break away the duplicating material and remove the sprue former from the center of the cast (Fig 28-31). Trim the refractory cast on a model trimmer. Place it in a drying oven for 1 hour at 82 to 93°C (180 to 200°F). Put the refractory cast in the metal basket of a deep fryer, and immerse it in beeswax that has been preheated to 149°C (300°F) (Fig 28-32). When the wax bubbles, time it for 15 seconds. Remove the cast and allow it to cool. This will seal the cast and provide a smooth, dense surface for waxing (Fig 28-33). Set the refractory cast aside in a safe place where it will not be damaged and begin the pattern by fabricating resin copings.

Pattern Armamentarium

1. Stone die
2. Saw frame, jeweler's blade
3. Die lubricant, small brush
4. Monomer and polymer (Duralay)
5. Dappen dishes (2)
6. Straight handpiece, sandpaper disk on mandrel, large acrylic bur
7. Iwanson thickness gauge
8. Bunsen burner, PKT no. 2 waxing instrument, beaver-tail burnisher
9. Blue inlay wax
10. Hollenbeck carver, cleoid carver, spoon excavator
11. Cotton pliers

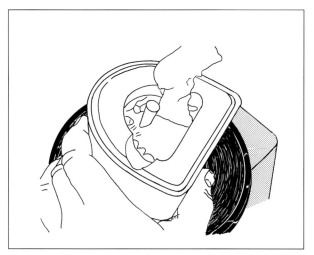

Fig 28-30 Investment is carefully poured into the mold from one side, vibrating the flask gently.

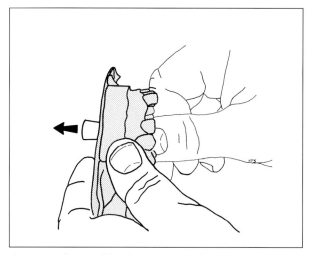

Fig 28-31 The top of the aluminum sprue former is pushed forcefully to remove it from the cast.

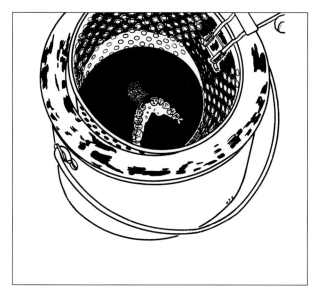

Fig 28-32 The cast is dipped in hot beeswax to seal it.

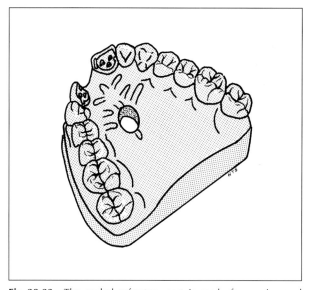

Fig 28-33 The sealed refractory cast is ready for waxing and investing.

Resin Coping Fabrication

Make a second pour, in densite stone, of just the prepared abutment teeth in the master impression. After the stone has set, remove the cast from the impression and trim away any excess stone from the preparations. Separate the prepared teeth with either a saw or a separating disk. Trim the dies thus formed, removing the stone apical to the gingival finish lines without producing any marked concavity in the area.

Apply an oily die lubricant to each of the dies and shake off the excess (Fig 28-34). Apply one or two drops of monomer (Duralay, Reliance Dental Manufacturing Co,

Worth, IL) to each die (Fig 28-35). Sprinkle on enough polymer to cover the entire surface of the preparation (Fig 28-36). Add another drop of monomer and repeat the process until the lingual surface of the die is covered with resin. Place each die in water to allow polymerization to occur without evaporation of the monomer (Fig 28-37). Tease the resin coping off the die. Remove the thin area of marginal flash by rubbing your fingertip across the margin. Any areas that are too thick to be removed in this fashion should be trimmed off with a sandpaper disk (Fig 28-38).

Cut the margins back 0.5 to 1.0 mm so they do not extend all the way to the finish lines. This will allow sealing of the margins in wax on the refractory cast later

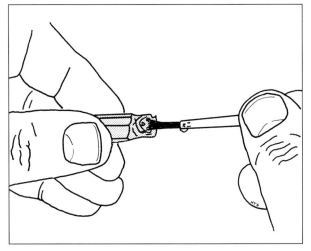

Fig 28-34 The die is painted with lubricant.

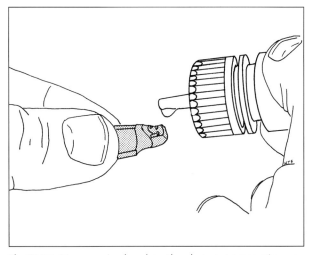

Fig 28-35 Monomer is placed on the abutment preparation portion of the die.

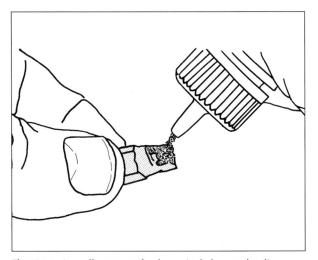

Fig 28-36 A small amount of polymer is shaken on the die.

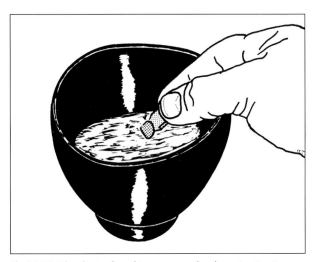

Fig 28-37 The die is placed in water until polymerization is complete.

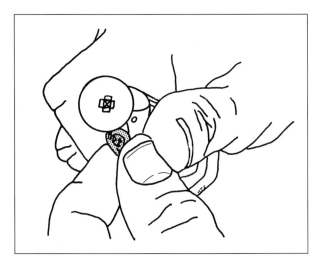

Fig 28-38 The coping margins are trimmed with a sandpaper disk.

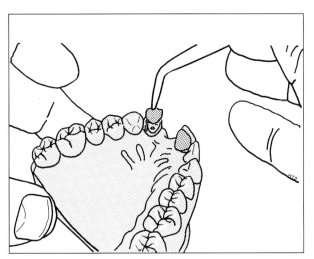

Fig 28-39 The resin coping is set on the abutment preparation on the master cast.

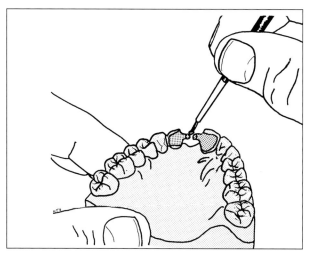

Fig 28-40 The resin projections are built across the edentulous space until they almost touch.

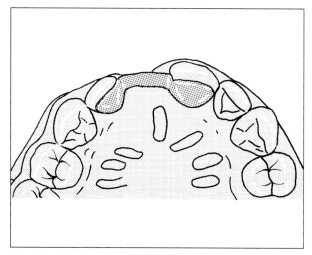

Fig 28-41 The resin bar should be thick enough faciolingually so that it will not break without extending too far facially or lingually.

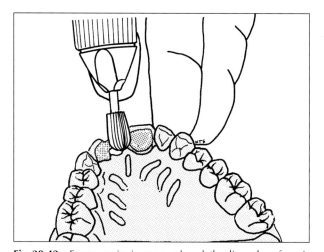

Fig 28-42 Excess resin is removed and the lingual surface is smoothed with an acrylic bur.

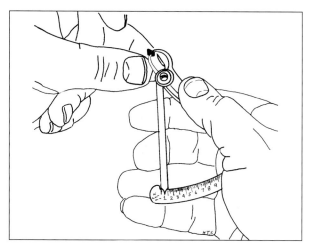

Fig 28-43 Thickness of the retainers is measured with an Iwanson gauge.

when the entire pattern has been completed. Place the copings back on their respective dies to insure that all of the margins have been sufficiently relieved.

Lubricate the stone master cast with the same oily die lubricant used on the dies. Transfer the copings to the stone master cast (Fig 28-39). Build a small projection into the edentulous space from the proximal surface of each coping, dipping a small brush first into monomer and then polymer (Fig 28-40). Do not build them into contact at this time. Set the cast aside for a while and allow the resin to polymerize. This allows much of the shrinkage distortion to occur before the retainers are joined together into one piece, where the shrinkage could warp the fixed partial denture framework.

Examine the lingual thickness of the resin copings and adjoining bar (Fig 28-41). Check them in occlusion against the opposing cast, and if they are too thick, remove the excess with a large acrylic bur (Fig 28-42).

Remove the pattern from the cast and check the thickness of the lingual surface of the retainer resin copings with an Iwanson thickness gauge (Fig 28-43). The thickness should be no less than 0.4 mm and preferably closer to 0.6 mm.

Wax Pattern

Add blue inlay wax to the bar of resin connecting the two retainers. Build up the wax to the full contour of the final pontic (Fig 28-44). Carve it flush on the lingual surface so that it blends with the milled lingual surface of the resin bar (Fig 28-45). If there are any voids in the resin, fill them in with wax and carve them flush. Use a spoon excavator or a discoid carver to cut 1.0-mm-deep grooves into the facial, lingual, and gingival surfaces of the pontic. The

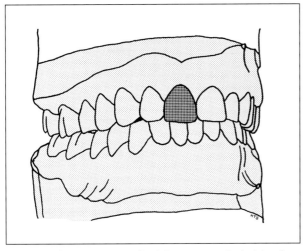

Fig 28-44 The pontic is waxed to full contour on the facial surface.

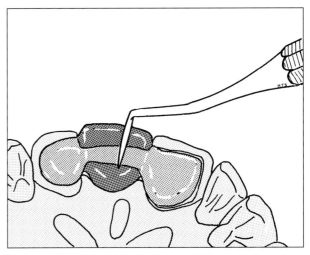

Fig 28-45 Wax is carved flush with the resin bar on the lingual surface.

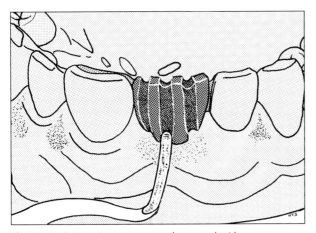

Fig 28-46 Orientation grooves can be carved with a spoon excavator.

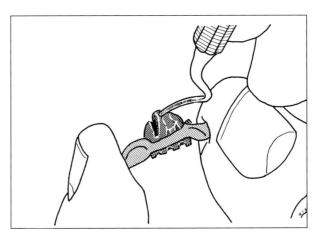

Fig 28-47 Wax between the grooves is removed to complete the cutback.

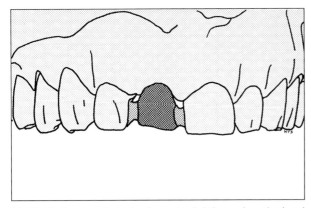

Fig 28-48 Because the cutback pontic slightly overlaps the facial aspect of the ridge, no space is visible.

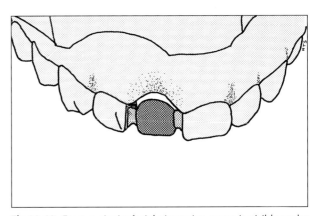

Fig 28-49 From a gingivofacial viewpoint, space is visible under the cutback pontic.

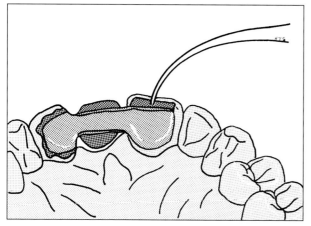

Fig 28-50 On the refractory cast, inlay wax is added in the marginal area around both retainers with a PKT no. 2.

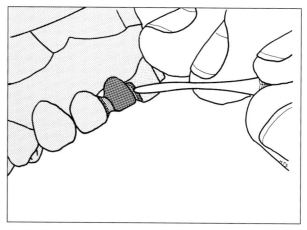

Fig 28-51 Facial margins are burnished and carved with a beavertail burnisher.

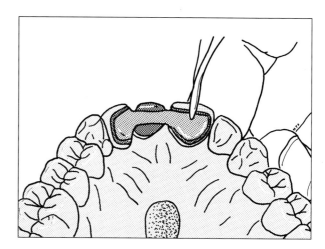

Fig 28-52 Margins on the lingual are finished with a beavertail burnisher.

grooves on the incisal edge should be 1.5 mm deep (Fig 28-46). These grooves will insure an adequate thickness of porcelain when it is added to the metal framework later. Carve away the wax to the depth of the grooves (Fig 28-47), duplicating the outer contours of the full-sized pontic in the cutback version.

To insure uniform space for porcelain under the pontic, and to prevent overshortening of the supportive metal framework in the gingival area, no space should be visible under the pontic when it is viewed from the facial surface (Fig 28-48). However, when the cast is tilted, there should be space under the pontic when it is viewed from a gingivofacial (Fig 28-49) or incisolingual direction.

Retrieve the refractory cast and, without painting any lubricant on the cast, transfer the pattern to it. Add blue inlay wax around the entire periphery of both retainer copings with a PKT no. 2 waxing instrument (Fig 28-50). The wax pattern will not be removed from this cast, and investing will take place directly on it. Carefully carve the margins with a heated, dull-edged beavertail burnisher on the facial (Fig 28-51) and lingual surfaces (Fig 28-52).

Investing and Casting Armamentarium

1. Bunsen burner
2. Cotton pliers, brush
3. Hollenbeck carver, PKT no. 2 waxing instrument
4. 8-gauge wax sprue, conical metal sprue former
5. 500-cc Vac-U-Mixer, vacuum tubing
6. Investment, split casting ring
7. Vibrator
8. Water measure, spatula
9. Modeling clay, 5-inch plastic square
10. Bench knife
11. 8.0 dwt of casting alloy

Investing and Casting

Attach an 8-gauge wax sprue to the lingual surface of the pontic. Cut it off over the hole in the palate that will accommodate the conical metal sprue former (Fig 28-

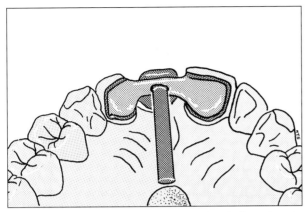

Fig 28-53 An 8-gauge wax sprue is attached to the lingual aspect of the pontic.

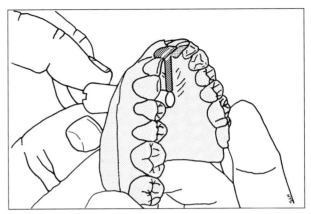

Fig 28-54 The conical sprue former is inserted through the tapered hole in the palate of the refractory cast.

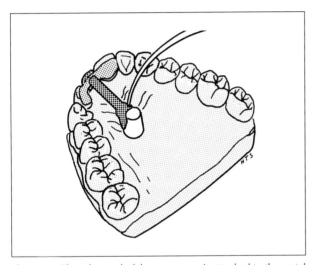

Fig 28-55 The other end of the wax sprue is attached to the metal sprue former.

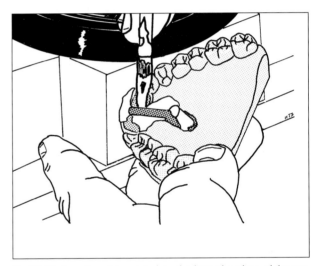

Fig 28-56 Investment is painted on the lingual surface of the pattern.

53). Then insert the sprue former through the hole until the cone is completely seated (Fig 28-54). It should contact the end of the wax sprue, or come close to it. Attach the wax sprue smoothly to the metal sprue former (Fig 28-55).

Vacuum mix the investment material, and with a large brush flow the material onto the lingual surface of the pattern, painting investment around all of the margins and under the wax sprue (Fig 28-56). Be sure to paint investment under the pontic so all of that space is completely filled with investment. The hand holding the brush is rested on the vibrator, but the cast itself is not vibrated. Turn the cast over and paint material on the facial surface of the anterior portion of the refractory cast. Take care to paint investment along all of the facial margins of the retainers.

With modeling clay, seal a split casting ring to a 5-inch ceramic tile or plastic square. Then fill the split ring with investment flush with the top. Grasping the cast by its

sides, place the molar end of the cast into the investment in the center of the ring. Wiggling the cast gently, immerse it completely in the investment, rotating it 90 degrees to an inverted position with the base of the cast parallel with the bottom of the ring. The teeth on the cast are toward the table, and the metal sprue former should protrude slightly from the investment.

When the investment has set completely, remove the investment-filled ring from its base. Use a bench knife to bevel into the base of the metal sprue former. When there is adequate access to grasp the sprue former, remove it from the investment. Burn out the invested pattern in a burnout furnace, going from room temperature to 732°C (1,350°F) in 45 minutes. Heat soak the ring at that temperature for 90 minutes. Transfer the ring to the cradle of an induction casting machine (Ticomatic 3001-C, Ticonium Co) and cast the fixed partial denture with a sufficient weight of suitable casting alloy. For the

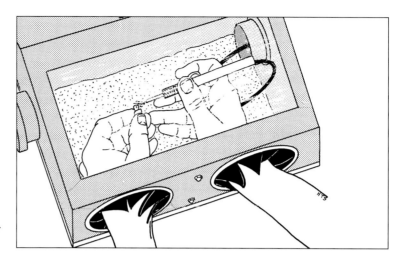

Fig 28-57 Cleaning of the casting is finished by air abrading it with aluminum oxide.

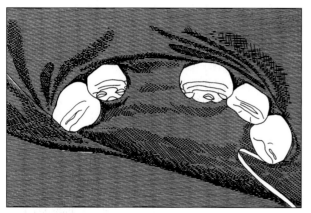

Fig 28-58 Abutment teeth are isolated with a well-inverted rubber dam.

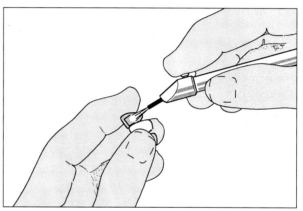

Fig 28-59 The fixed partial denture is air abraded after try-in at the beginning of the cementation appointment.

machine described here, the minimum amount of alloy is 8.0 dwt (Rexillium III, Jeneric/Pentron).

Allow the ring to cool to room temperature before breaking the casting out. After removing the large pieces of investment with sharp instruments, remove the final layer with aluminum oxide air abrasion (Fig 28-57). Using the technique described in Chapter 22, finish the portions of the framework on the lingual surface that will remain unveneered.

Porcelain can be added at this point, although the novice operator would be well-advised to try the casting in the mouth to insure its fit before proceeding. Even if the metal framework is tried in, there will be a try-in after porcelain has been added to insure the maximum esthetic result. Unless the particle-roughened or cast mesh technique has been employed in the fabrication of the fixed partial denture, it is now ready for air abrading.

Delivery Armamentarium

1. Rubber dam, clamp, and frame
2. Low-speed contra-angle handpiece, rubber prophy cup, pumice
3. Etchant, cotton pellets
4. Small brush, mixing well
5. Mixing pad, plastic spatula
6. Mylar strip, dental floss
7. Explorer, scaler
8. Complete adhesive resin kit

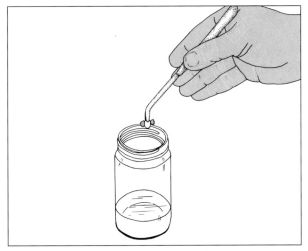

Fig 28-60 The abraded FPD is placed in dishwashing detergent in an ultrasonic unit.

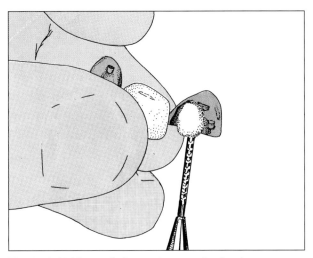

Fig 28-61 Noble-metal alloy retainers are tin plated.

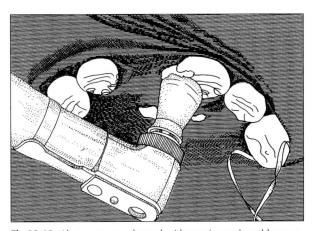

Fig 28-62 Abutments are cleaned with pumice and a rubber cup.

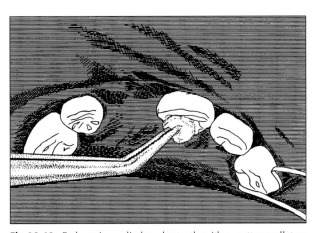

Fig 28-63 Etchant is applied to the teeth with a cotton pellet or small rubber sponge.

Delivery Sequence

The delivery sequence is an important procedure that must be accomplished efficiently because of the limited working time of bonding resins. It is also critically important to the longevity of the prosthesis. Contamination or improper seating of the fixed partial denture at this time will adversely affect the success of the restoration. The technique described here is for Panavia 21 (Kuraray Co).

The process begins with the isolation of the abutment teeth with a rubber dam (Fig 28-58).[89,97,106] Refresh the tooth-facing surfaces of the retainers by air abrading them again just before inserting the restoration. Use 30 to 50 μm aluminum oxide with a hand-held etcher (Micro-etcher, Danville Engineering). Two to three seconds per cm^2 at 4.2 to 7 kg/cm^2 (60 to 100 psi) pressure should be sufficient to restore the matte finish (Fig 28-59). Wash the casting in running water for 1 minute, place it in dish-

washing liquid in an ultrasonic unit for 2 minutes (Fig 28-60), and then rinse.

If the FPD is made of a high noble alloy, such as Olympia, the inner surfaces of the retainers should now be plated with a layer of tin approximately 0.5 μm thick. Ground the tin plating instrument (Micro-tin, Danville Engineering) to the pontic metal. Rub the active tip with a pellet soaked with plating solution over the inner surfaces of the retainers for 5 to 10 seconds each (Fig 28-61). The surface will become a slightly lighter shade of gray.[97] Rinse the restoration thoroughly in water and again for 2 minutes in detergent in an ultrasonic cleaner. Rinse, blow the FPD dry, and place it in an accessible but protected place.

The next step is to clean the tooth preparations with unflavored, nonfluoridated pumice and a rubber prophy cup (Fig 28-62). Wash off the pumice and apply a 40% to 50% phosphoric acid solution to the abutment prepara-

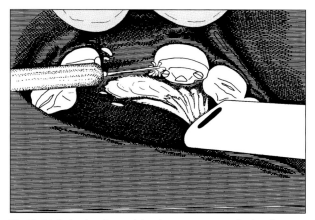

Fig 28-64 Etched surfaces of the abutments are washed with water.

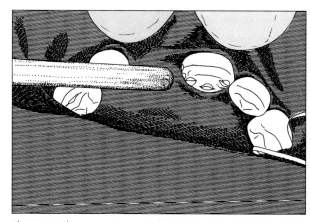

Fig 28-65 The preparations are dried with compressed air.

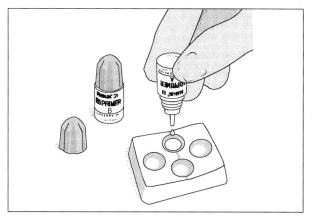

Fig 28-66 One drop each of A and B primer liquids is dispensed.

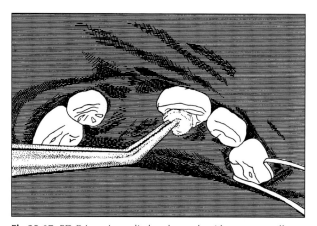

Fig 28-67 ED Primer is applied to the teeth with a cotton pellet or small pledget.

tions with a cotton pellet (Fig 28-63).[107] Leave the etchant on for 60 seconds, rinse, dry, and reapply for 15 seconds.[97] Wash the abutment preparations thoroughly with water for 20 seconds (Fig 28-64), followed by drying (Fig 28-65). Play a light stream of air over the preparation. Place a Mylar strip between each abutment and the neighboring tooth.

Now you are ready to mix the primer and the resin to bond the prosthesis in place. Dispense one drop each of ED Primer liquids A and B into a well in the mixing dish and mix for 4 seconds (Fig 28-66). Use a sponge pledget to apply the mixture to the preparations (Fig 28-67). Allow it to set for 60 seconds and then apply a gentle stream of air to evaporate the volatile substances, leaving a glossy surface. *Do not* apply primer to the metal; *do not* rinse.

Remove the cap from the dispenser and slowly rotate the rectangular "knob" clockwise one full turn, dispens-

ing the material onto the mixing pad (Fig 28-68). Stop when it clicks. If you think you have too small a quantity for the restoration you are placing, turn the handle another full turn until it clicks again. Mix the two stripes of paste for 20 to 30 seconds over a wide area (Fig 28-69). The material is anaerobic, so it will set only if oxygen is kept from it. Therefore, spreading it out will keep it from setting prematurely.

Apply a thin, bubble-free layer of paste to the retainers (Fig 28-70). Do *not* place any on the tooth, as the primer will accelerate it and the restoration will not seat completely. Seat the restoration with firm finger pressure (Fig 28-71) and hold it for 60 seconds. Use a small brush (Proxabrush, John O. Butler Co, Chicago, IL) to clean away excess resin.

Use a disposable brush to apply Oxyguard II to the margins of the retainers to keep oxygen away from the setting resin (Fig 28-72). The Mylar strips placed

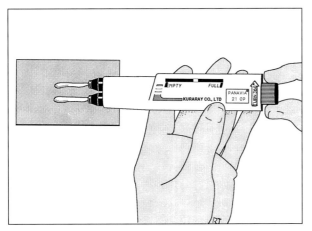

Fig 28-68 Resin pastes are dispensed by turning the knob one full turn.

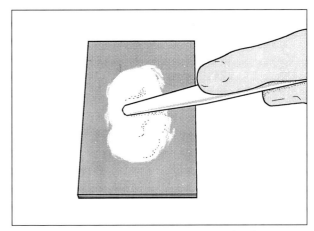

Fig 28-69 Resin paste is mixed over a wide area for about 25 seconds.

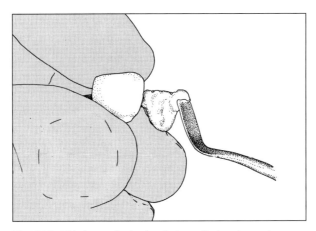

Fig 28-70 Thin layer of mixed resin is applied to the retainers.

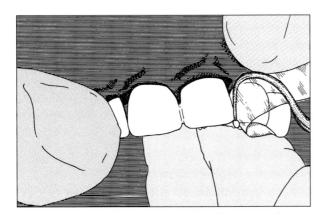

Fig 28-71 The FPD is held securely in place for 60 seconds.

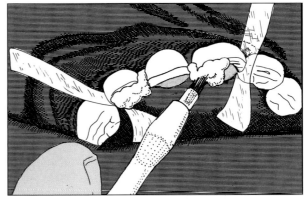

Fig 28-72 Oxyguard II is applied to protect the resin from exposure to oxygen.

between each abutment tooth and the tooth adjacent will insure that they do not bond together. A piece of floss can also be positioned between the abutment tooth and its neighbor when the fixed partial denture is placed. It is pulled out through the contacts before the resin has set completely. After 5 minutes remove the Oxyguard II with cotton rolls and a water spray.

Before the resin has become too hard, the excess must be removed because it will become irritating to the gingival tissue. An explorer or scaler can be used around the gingival margins and those exposed areas that can be reached. Floss should be run through the proximal contacts of the abutment teeth and of the adjacent teeth as well. The interproximal area between each retainer and its adjacent neighbor should be very carefully cleaned and examined.

References

1. Buonocore MG: A simplified method of increasing the adhesion of acrylic filling materials to enamel surfaces. *J Dent Res* 1955; 34:849–853.

2. Ibsen RL: One-appointment technique using an adhesive composite. *Dent Survey* 1973; 49:30–32.

3. Heymann HO: Resin-retained fixed partial dentures: The acrylic denture-tooth pontic. *Gen Dent* 1984; 32:113–117.

4. Scheer B, Silverstone LM: Replacement of missing anterior teeth by etch retained fixed partial dentures. *J Int Assoc Dent Child* 1975; 6:17–19.

5. Lambert PM, Moore DL, Elletson HH: In vitro retentive strength of fixed partial dentures constructed with acrylic pontics and an ultraviolet light polymerized resin. *J Am Dent Assoc* 1976; 92:740–743.

6. Stolpa JB: An adhesive technique for small anterior fixed partial dentures. *J Prosthet Dent* 1975; 34:513–519.

7. Sweeney EJ, Moore DC, Dooner JJ: Retentive strength of acid etched anterior fixed partial dentures. An in vitro comparison of attachment technique. *J Am Dent Assoc* 1980; 100:198–202.

8. Kochavi D, Stern N, Grajower R: A temporary space maintainer using acrylic resin teeth and a composite resin. *J Prosthet Dent* 1977; 37:522–526.

9. Jordan RE, Suzuki M, Sills PS, Gratton DR, Gwinnett JA: Temporary fixed partial dentures fabricated by means of the acid-etch resin technique: A report of 86 cases followed for up to three years. *J Am Dent Assoc* 1978; 96:994–1001.

10. Rochette AL: Attachment of a splint to enamel of lower anterior teeth. *J Prosthet Dent* 1973; 30:418–423.

11. Saunders WP: Resin bonded bridgework: A review. *J Dent* 1989; 17:255–265.

12. Howe DF, Denehy GE: Anterior fixed partial dentures utilizing the acid-etch technique and a cast metal framework. *J Prosthet Dent* 1977; 37:28–31.

13. Kuhlke KL, Drennon DC: An alternative to the anterior single tooth removable partial denture. *J Int Assoc Dent Child* 1977, 8:11–14.

14. Denehy GE, Howe DF: A conservative approach to the missing anterior tooth. *Quintessence Int* 1979; 7:23–29.

15. Eshleman JR, Douglas HB, Barnes D: The acid etch bonded porcelain fused to metal fixed partial denture. *Va Dent J* 1979, 56:16–19.

16. Livaditis GJ: Cast metal resin-bonded retainers for posterior teeth. *J Am Dent Assoc* 1980; 110:926–929.

17. Livaditis J, Thompson VP: Etched castings: An improved retentive mechanism for resin-bonded retainers. *J Prosthet Dent* 1982; 47:52–58.

18. Dunn B, Reisbick MH: Adherance of ceramic coatings on chromium cobalt structures. *J Dent Res* 1976; 55:328–332.

19. Tanaka T, Atsuta M, Uchiyama Y, Kawashima I: Pitting corrosion for retaining acrylic resin facings. *J Prosthet Dent* 1979; 42:282–291.

20. Thompson VP, Del Castillo E, Livaditis GJ: Resin-bonded retainers. Part I: Resin bond to electrolytically etched non-precious alloys. *J Prosthet Dent* 1983; 50:771–779.

21. Dhillon M, Fenton AH, Watson PA: Bond strengths of composite to perforated and etched metal surfaces [abstract 1219]. *J Dent Res* 1983; 62:304.

22. Sloan KM, Lory RE, Myers GE: Evaluation of laboratory etching of cast metal resin-bonded retainers [abstract 1220]. *J Dent Res* 1983; 62:305.

23. Hussey DL, Gratton DR, McConnell RJ, Sands TD: The quality of bonded retainers from commercial laboratories [abstract 424]. *J Dent Res* 1989; 68:919.

24. McLaughlin G: One hundred second etch technique for etched-metal fixed partial dentures. *J Mich Dent Assoc* 1982; 64:347–349.

25. McLaughlin G, Masek J: Comparison of bond strengths using one-step and two-step alloy etching techniques. *J Prosthet Dent* 1985; 53:516–520.

26. Wiltshire WA: A classification of resin-bonded fixed partial dentures based on the evolutionary changes of the different technique types. *Quintessence Dent Technol* 1987; 11:253–258.

27. Livaditis GJ: A chemical etching system for creating micromechanical retention in resin-bonded retainers. *J Prosthet Dent* 1986; 56:181–188.

28. Doukoudakis S, Cohen B, Tsoutsos A: A new chemical method for etching metal frameworks of the acid etched prosthesis. *J Prosthet Dent* 1987; 58:421–423.

29. Re GJ, Kaiser DA, Malone WFP, Garcia-Godoy F: Shear bond strength and scanning electron microscope evaluation of three different retentive methods for resin bonded retainers. *J Prosthet Dent* 1988; 59:568–573.

30. El-Sherif MH, Shillingburg HT, Duncanson MG: Comparison of the bond strength of resin-bonded retainers using two metal etching techniques. *Quintessence Int* 1989; 20:385–388.

31. Aquilino SA, Diaz-Arnold AM: Tensile bond strengths of electrolytically and chemically etched base metals [abstract]. *J Dent Res* 1989; 68:250.

32. Sedberry D, Burgess J, Schwartz R: Tensile bond strengths of three chemical and one electrolytic etching systems for a base metal alloy. *J Prosthet Dent* 1992; 68:606–610.

33. Naegeli DG, Duke ES, Schwartz R, Norling BK: Adhesive bonding of composites to a casting alloy. *J Prosthet Dent* 1988; 59:568–573.

34. Mukai M, Fukui H, Hasegawa J: Relationship between sandblasting and composite resin-alloy bond strength by a silica coating. *J Prosthet Dent* 1995; 74:151–155.

35. Heinenberg BJ: The formation of retention wings. *Quintessence Dent Technol* 1984; 8:573–576.

36. Taleghani M, Gerbo LR: Using a mesh framework for resin-bonded retainers. *Compend Contin Educ Dent* 1987; 8:166–170.

37. Taleghani M, Leinfelder KF, Taleghani AM: An alternative to cast etched retainers. *J Prosthet Dent* 1987; 58:424–428.

38. Moon PC: The Virginia resin bonded fixed partial denture: A restorative material report. *Va Dent J* 1984; 61:9–11.

39. Hudgins JL, Moon PC, Knap FJ: Particle-roughened resin-bonded retainers. *J Prosthet Dent* 1985; 53:471–476.

40. Moon PC: Bond strengths of the lost salt procedure: A new retention method for resin-bonded fixed prostheses. *J Prosthet Dent* 1987; 57:435–439.

41. Moon PC: The laboratory procedure for the Virginia resin bonded fixed partial denture. *Trends & Techniques* 1985; 1:22–28.

42. El-Sherif MH, El-Messery A, Halhoul MN: The effects of alloy surface treatments and resins on the retention of resin-bonded retainers. *J Prosthet Dent* 1991; 65:782–786.

43. Tanaka T, Fujiyama E, Shimizu H, Takaki A, Atsuta M: Surface treatment of nonprecious alloys for adhesion-fixed partial dentures. *J Prosthet Dent* 1986; 55:456–462.

44. Tanaka T, Atsuta M, Nakabayashi N, Masuhara E, Nagata K, Takeyama M: Surface treatment of gold alloys for adhesion. *J Prosthet Dent* 1988; 60:271–279.

45. Wiltshire WA: Tensile bond strengths of various alloy surface treatments for resin-bonded fixed partial dentures. *Quintessence Dent Technol* 1986; 10:227–233.

46. Laswell HR, Welk DA, Regenos JW: Attachment of resin restorations to acid pretreated enamel. *J Am Dent Assoc* 1971; 82:558–563.

47. Shaw MJ, Tay WM: Clinical performance of resin-bonded cast metal fixed partial dentures (Rochette fixed partial dentures). *Br Dent J* 1982; 152:378–380.

48. Livaditis GJ: Resin-bonded cast restorations: Clinical study. *Int J Periodont Rest Dent* 1981; 1(4):70–79.

49. Thompson VP, Grolman KM, Liao R: Bonding of adhesive resins to various nonprecious alloys [abstract 1258]. *J Dent Res* 1985; 64:314.

50. Jenkins CBG, Aboush YEY: The bond strength of a new adhesive recommended for resin bonded bridges [abstract 18]. *J Dent Res* 1985; 64:664.

51. Barrack G: The etched cast restoration—Clinical techniques and long-term results. *Quintessence Int* 1993; 24:701–713.

52. Eakle WS, Lacy AM: A clinical technique for bonding gold castings to teeth. *Quintessence Int* 1991; 22:491–494.

53. Imbery TA, Burgess JO, Naylor WP: Tensile strength of three resin cements following two alloy surface treatments. *Int J Prosthodont* 1992; 5:59–67.

54. Breeding LC, Dixon DL: The effect of metal surface treatment on the shear bond strengths of base and noble metals bonded to enamel. *J Prosthet Dent* 1996; 76:390–393.

55. Jordan RD, Krell KV, Aquilino SA, Denehy GE, Svare CW, Thayer KE, Williams VD: Removal of acid-etched fixed partial dentures with modified ultrasonic scaler tips. *J Am Dent Assoc* 1986; 112:505–507.

56. Krell KV, Jordan RD: Ultrasonic debonding of anterior etched-metal resin-bonded retainers. *Gen Dent* 1986; 34:379–380.

57. Yankelson M, Myers GE: Acid-etch bridges: Results of a 24 month clinical trial [abstract 917]. *J Dent Res* 1980; 59:496.

58. Bergendahl B, Hallonsten A-L, Koch G, et al: Composite retained onlay bridges. *Swed Dent J* 1983; 7:217–225.

59. Williams VD, Denehy GE, Thayer KE, Boyer DB: Acid-etched retained cast metal prostheses: A seven year retrospective study. *J Am Dent Assoc* 1984; 108:629–631.

60. LaBarre EE, Ward HE: An alternative resin-bonded restoration. *J Prosthet Dent* 1984; 52:247–249.

61. Ekstrand K: Erfarenheter av 120 kompositretinerade palaggsbroar. *Tandlakartidningen* 1984; 18:987–993.

62. Thompson VP, Wood M: Etched casting bonded retainer recalls: Results at 3–5 years [abstract 1282]. *J Dent Res* 1986; 65:311.

63. Creugers NHJ, van't Hof MA, Vrijhoef MMA: A clinical comparison of three types of resin-retained cast metal prostheses. *J Prosthet Dent* 1986; 56:297–300.

64. van der Veen H, Bronsdijk B, van de Poel F: Clinical evaluation of resin-bonded fixed partial dentures with perforated retainers—Six-year results. *Quintessence Dent Technol* 1987; 11:51–56.

65. Marinello CP, Kerschbaum T, Heinenberg B, Hinz R, Peters S, Pfeiffer P, Reppel PD, Schwickerath H: Experiences with resin-bonded bridges and splints—A retrospective study. *J Oral Rehabil* 1987; 14:251–260.

66. Marinello CP, Kerschbaum T, Heinenberg B, Hinz R, Peters S, Pfeiffer P, Reppel PD, Schwickerath H: Experiences with resin-bonded fixed partial dentures and splints—A cross-sectional retrospective study, part II. *J Oral Rehabil* 1988; 15:223–235.

67. Priest GF, Donatelli HA: A four-year clinical evaluation of resin-bonded fixed partial dentures. *J Prosthet Dent* 1988; 59:542–546.

68. Clyde JS, Boyd T: The etched cast metal resin-bonded (Maryland) bridge: A clinical review. *J Dent* 1988; 16:22–26.

69. Williams VD, Thayer KE, Denehy GE, Boyer DB: Cast metal, resin-bonded prostheses: A 10-year retrospective study. *J Prosthet Dent* 1989; 61:436–441.

70. Ferrari M, Mason PN, Cagidiaco D, Cagidiaco MC: Clinical evaluation of resin bonded retainers. *Int J Periodont Rest Dent* 1989; 9:207–219.

71. Creugers NHJ, Snoek PA, Van 'T Hof MA, Käyser AF: Clinical performance of resin-bonded bridges: A 5-year prospective study. Part III: failure characteristics and survival after rebonding. *J Oral Rehabil* 1990; 17:179–186.

72. Chang HK, Zidan O, Lee IK, Gomez-Marin O: Resin-bonded fixed partial dentures: A recall study. *J Prosthet Dent* 1991; 65:778–781.

73. Olin PS, Hill EME, Donahue JL. Clinical evaluation of resin-bonded bridges: A retrospective study. *Quintessence Int* 1991; 22:873–877.

74. Hansson O, Moberg LA: Clinical evaluation of resin-bonded prostheses. *Int J Prosthodont* 1992; 5:533–541.

75. Barrack G, Bretz WA: A long-term prospective study of the etched-cast restoration. *Int J Prosthodont* 1993; 6:428–434.

76. Rammelsberg P, Pospiech P, Gernet W: Clinical factors affecting adhesive fixed partial dentures: A 6-year study. *J Prosthet Dent* 1993; 70:300–307.

77. Thayer KE, Williams VD, Diaz-Arnold AM, Boyer DB: Acid-etched, resin-bonded cast metal prostheses: A retrospective study of 5- to 15-year-old restorations. *Int J Prosthodont* 1993; 6:264–269.

78. Creugers NHJ, Van 'T Hof MA: An analysis of clinical studies on resin-bonded bridges. *J Dent Res* 1991; 70:146–149.

79. Kerschbaum T, Gaa M: Longitudinale Analyse von festsitzendem Zahnersatz privatversicherter Patienten. *Dtsch Zahnärtzl Z* 1987; 42:345–351.

80. Palmqvist S, Swartz B: Artificial crowns and fixed partial dentures 18 to 23 years after placement. *Int J Prosthodont* 1993; 6:279–285.

81. Buchanan WT: Periodontal splinting: Two conservative procedures. *Gen Dent* 1984; 32:486–488.

82. Lyon HE: Etched-metal splint: A conservative approach to long-term splinting. *Gen Dent* 1984; 32:512–514.

83. Barrack G: Etched cast restorations. *Quintessence Int* 1985; 16:27–34.

84. Denehy GE: Cast anterior fixed partial dentures utilizing composite resin. *Pediatric Dent* 1982; 4:44–47.

85. Yanover L, Croft W, Pulver F: The acid-etched fixed prosthesis. *J Am Dent Assoc* 1982; 104:325–328.

86. Burgess JO, McCartney JG: Anterior retainer design for resin-bonded acid-etched fixed partial dentures. *J Prosthet Dent* 1989; 61:433–436.

87. Livaditis GJ: Etched metal resin-bonded restorations: Principles in retainer design. *Int J Periodont Rest Dent* 1983; 3(4):35–47.

88. Simon JF, Gartrell RG, Grogono A: Improved retention of acid-etched fixed partial dentures: A longitudinal study. *J Prosthet Dent* 1992; 68:611–615.

89. Barrack G: Recent advances in etched cast restorations. *J Prosthet Dent* 1984; 52:619–626.

90. Eshleman JR, Moon PC, Barnes RF: Clinical evaluation of cast metal resin-bonded anterior fixed partial dentures. *J Prosthet Dent* 1984; 51:761–764.

91. Thompson VP, Livaditis GJ: Etched casting acid etch composite bonded posterior bridges. *Pediatric Dent* 1982; 4:38–43.

92. Heymann HO: Resin-retained fixed partial dentures: The porcelain-fused-to-metal "winged" pontic. *Gen Dent* 1984; 32:203–208.

93. Wood M: Etched casting resin bonded retainers: an improved technique for periodontal splinting. *Int J Periodont Rest Dent* 1982; 2(4):9–25.

94. Shillingburg HT, Grace CS: Thickness of enamel and dentin. *J South Calif Dent Assoc* 1973; 41:33–52.

95. Synnott SA: Resin-bonded fixed partial dentures: An update. *Gen Dent* 1984; 32:211–215.

96. Simonsen R, Thompson VP, Barrack G: General considerations in framework design and anterior tooth modification. *Quintessence Dent Technol* 1983; 7:21–25.

97. Wood M, Thompson VP: Resin-bonded prosthodontics. An update. *Dent Clin North Am* 1993; 37:445–455.

98. Wilkes PW: *Effects of Resistance Form on Bonding Strength of Resin Retained Castings* [Master's thesis]. University of Oklahoma Health Sciences Center, Oklahoma City, 1992.

99. Caputo AA, Gonidis D, Matyas J: Analysis of stresses in resin bonded fixed partial dentures. *Quintessence Int* 1986; 17:89–93.

100. Pegoraro LF, Barrack G: A comparison of bond strengths of adhesive cast restorations using different designs, bonding agents, and luting resins. *J Prosthet Dent* 1987; 57:133–138.

101. Eshleman JR, Janus CE, Jones CR: Tooth preparation designs for resin-bonded fixed partial dentures related to enamel thickness. *J Prosthet Dent* 1988; 60:18–22.

102. Rubinstein S, Jekkals V: Preparations for anterior resin-bonded retainers. *Compend Contin Educ Dent* 1986; 7:631–634.

103. Saad AA, Claffey N, Byrne D, Hussey D: Effects of groove placement on retention/resistance of maxillary anterior resin-bonded retainers. *J Prosthet Dent* 1995; 74:133–139.

104. Hembree JH, Sneed WD, Looper S: In vitro marginal leakage of acid-etched composite resin bonded castings. *Quintessence Int* 1986; 17:479–482.

105. Murakami I, Barrack GM: Relationship of surface area and design to the bond strength of etched cast restorations: An in vitro study. *J Prosthet Dent* 1986; 56:539–545.

106. McLaughlin G: Composite bonding of etched metal anterior splints. *Compend Contin Educ Dent* 1981; 2:279–283.

107. McLaughlin G: Composite bonding for the clinician. *NY State Dent J* 1982; 48:232–235.

Index